D1557593

Handbook of
Urgent Care Medicine

Second Edition

Handbook of Urgent Care Medicine

Second Edition

Michelle H. Biros, MS, MD

Professor of Emergency Medicine
University of Minnesota Medical School
Research Director
Department of Emergency Medicine
Hennepin County Medical Center
Minneapolis, Minnesota

Steve Sterner, MD

Associate Professor of Clinical Emergency Medicine
University of Minnesota Medical School
Assistant Chief, Department of Emergency Medicine
Medical Director, Adult Emergency Department
Medical Director, Urgent Care
Hennepin County Medical Center
Minneapolis, Minnesota

E. Corradin Vogel, MD

Departments of Emergency and Critical Care Medicine
Aurora Baycare Medical Center
Green Bay, Wisconsin

HANLEY & BELFUS, INC. / Philadelphia

Publisher: HANLEY & BELFUS, INC.
              Medical Publishers
              210 South 13th Street
              Philadelphia, PA 19107
              (215) 546-7293; 800-962-1892
              FAX (215) 790-9330
              Web site: http://www.hanleyandbelfus.com

RC
86.8
·H36
2002

Note to the reader: Although the information in this book has been carefully reviewed for correctness of dosage and indications, neither the authors nor the editors nor the publisher can accept any legal responsibility for any errors or omissions that may be made. Neither the publisher nor the editors make any warranty, expressed or implied, with respect to the material contained herein. Before prescribing any drug, the reader must review the manufacturer's current product information (package inserts) for accepted indications, absolute dosage recommendations, and other information pertinent to the safe and effective use of the product described.

Handbook of urgent care medicine / edited by Michelle H. Biros, Steve Sterner, E. Corradin
Vogel.—2nd ed.
        p. ; cm.
    Includes bibliographical references and index.
    ISBN 1-56053-448-6 (alk. paper)
        1. Emergency medicine—Handbooks, manuals, etc. 2. Medical
emergencies—Handbooks, manuals, etc. I. Biros, Michelle H. II. Sterner, Steve. III.
Vogel, E. Corradin. IV. Series.
    [DNLM: 1. Emergencies—Handbooks. 2. Emergency Medicine—Handbooks. WB 39
H2368 2001]
    RC86.8.H36 2001
    616.02'5—dc21
                                                                2001039727

HANDBOOK OF URGENT CARE MEDICINE, 2nd edition   ISBN 1-56053-448-6

Last digit is the print number: 9 8 7 6 5 4 3 2 1

Contents

Contributors

Cheryl Adkinson, MD, FACEP
Associate Professor of Clinical Emergency Medicine, Department of Emergency Medicine, University of Minnesota Medical School; Hennepin County Medical Center, Minneapolis, Minnesota

Christopher L. Baker, MD
Assistant Professor, Department of Emergency Medicine, Eastern Virginia Medical School, Norfolk, Virginia

Jill L. Benson, MD
Department of Emergency Medicine, Hennepin County Medical Center, Minneapolis, Minnesota

Michelle H. Biros, MS, MD
Professor of Emergency Medicine, University of Minnesota Medical School; Research Director, Department of Emergency Medicine, Hennepin County Medical Center, Minneapolis, Minnesota

Cara Ellman Black, MD
Department of Emergency Medicine, Fairview-University Medical Center, Minneapolis, Minnesota

Jennifer Block, MD
Department of Emergency Medicine, Methodist Hospital, St. Louis Park, Minnesota

Douglas D. Brunette, MD
Director, Residency Program, Department of Emergency Medicine, Hennepin County Medical Center, Minneapolis, Minnesota

Joseph E. Clinton, MD
Professor, Department of Emergency Medicine, University of Minnesota Medical School; Chief of Emergency Medicine, Hennepin County Medical Center, Minneapolis, Minnesota

Joshua Cochrane, MD
Staff Physician, Frye Regional Medical Center, Hickory, North Carolina

Peter Craig, MD
Department of Emergency Medicine, Hennepin County Medical Center, Minneapolis, Minnesota

Mark Erlandson, MD
Emergency Medicine Physician, Methodist Hospital, St. Louis Park, Minnesota

Scott A. Freiwald, MD
Department of Emergency Medicine, Hennepin County Medical Center, Minneapolis, Minnesota

Scott R. Gunn, MD
Assistant Professor of Critical Care and Emergency Medicine, Department of Critical Care, University of Pittsburgh School of Medicine; Presbyterian-University Hospital, Pittsburgh, Pennsylvania

Howard J. Haines, MD, MS
Department of Emergency Medicine, Methodist Hospital, St. Louis Park, Minnesota

William G. Heegaard, MD, MPH
Associate Staff Physician, Department of Emergency Medicine, University of Minnesota Medical School; Hennepin County Medical Center, Minneapolis, Minnesota

Travis Heining, MD
Department of Emergency Medicine, Hennepin County Medical Center, Minneapolis, Minnesota

Brian A. Isaacson, MD
Department of Emergency Medicine, Ridgeview Medical Center, Waconia, Minnesota

Christine A. Kletti, MD
Faculty, Department of Emergency Medicine, Hennepin County Medical Center, Minneapolis, Minnesota

Susan L. Krieg, MD
Department of Emergency Medicine, Hennepin County Medical Center, Minneapolis, Minnesota

Karen Kuo, MD
Department of Emergency Medicine, Hennepin County Medical Center, Minneapolis, Minnesota

Louis J. Ling, MD, FACEP, FACMT
Professor of Clinical Emergency Medicine and Pharmacy, University of Minnesota Medical School; Medical Director, Hennepin Regional Poison Center; Associate Medical Director for Education, Hennepin County Medical Center, Minneapolis, Minnesota

Marc Martel, MD
Department of Emergency Medicine, Hennepin County Medical Center, Minneapolis, Minnesota

James R. Miner, MD
Assistant Professor of Clinical Emergency Medicine, Department of Emergency Medicine, University of Minnesota Medical School; Hennepin County Medical Center, Minneapolis, Minnesota

Terrence D. Morton, Jr., MD, FACEP
Department of Emergency Medicine, University Hospital, Charlotte, North Carolina; Iredell Memorial Hospital, Statesville, North Carolina; Lincoln Medical Center, Lincolnton, North Carolina; Piedmont Emergency Medicine Associates, Charlotte, North Carolina

Daniel T. O'Laughlin, MD
Assistant Professor of Clinical Emergency Medicine, University of Minnesota Medical School, Minneapolis, Minnesota; Assistant Medical Director of Emergency Medicine, Fairview Southdale Hospital, Edina, Minnesota

Mitchell N. Palmer, MD
Emergency Physician, Fairview Southdale Hospital, Edina, Minnesota

David Plummer, MD
Director, Performance Improvement, Ultrasound Education, Department of Emergency Medicine, Hennepin County Medical Center, Minneapolis, Minnesota

Catherine A. Ripkey, MD
Medical Staff, Department of Emergency Medicine, Ravenswood Hospital, Chicago, Illinois

Ernest Ruiz, MD
Professor Emeritus of Emergency Medicine, Department of Emergency Medicine, University of Minnesota Medical School, Minneapolis, Minnesota

Robert Rusnak, MD
Associate Physician and Director, Medical Student Education, Department of Emergency Medicine, Hennepin County Medical Center, Minneapolis, Minnesota

Laura Schrag, MD
North Memorial Medical Center, Robbinsdale, Minnesota

Steve Sterner, MD
Associate Professor of Clinical Emergency Medicine, University of Minnesota Medical School; Assistant Chief, Department of Emergency Medicine; Medical Director, Adult Emergency Department; Medical Director, Urgent Care, Hennepin County Medical Center, Minneapolis, Minnesota

Rodney L. Thompson, MD
Department of Emergency Medicine, Providence Portland Medical Center, Portland, Oregon

Carrie D. Tibbles, MD
Assistant Residency Director, Department of Emergency Medicine, Harvard Affiliated Emergency Medicine Residency; Beth Israel Deaconess Medical Center, Boston, Massachusetts

E. Corradin Vogel, MD
Departments of Emergency and Critical Care Medicine, Aurora Baycare Medical Center, Green Bay, Wisconsin

James P. Winter, MD, FACEP
Emergency Associates and Consulting, Coeur d'Alene, Idaho

Erich Zeitz, MD, JD
Assistant Professor, Department of Family Practice, University of Minnesota Medical School, Minneapolis, Minnesota; Chief of Emergency Medicine, Methodist Hospital, St. Louis Park, Minnesota

Preface to the Second Edition

Since the publication of the first edition of this handbook in 1990, the challenges of the practice of medicine have drastically changed. Because of shifting social and economic needs and pressures, urgent care centers and emergency departments have become primary resources for patients who may otherwise find it difficult or impossible to obtain urgent medical assessment and treatment. With this in mind, and at the request of primary care providers who read our first edition, we have updated and revised this book. Our goal remains the same as it was in 1990—to provide a rapid reference in the diagnosis and treatment of patients with medical and surgical urgencies.

Patients presenting to urgent care centers have a broad scope of minor medical illnesses and injuries, and the urgent care clinicians who treat them have a diverse range of clinical training and expertise. No textbook can provide a comprehensive, all-inclusive guide to the management of all medical and traumatic problems that may present urgently, and no textbook can remain truly current. No specialty training or curriculum exists for urgent care physicians, who may have backgrounds in primary care, emergency medicine, or perhaps even no specialty training. Therefore, this book is designed for health care providers at all levels and targets pathologies most likely to be seen in the urgent care setting.

Our clinical approach is tempered by our personal experiences as emergency practitioners as well as by what we find recommended in the clinical literature. Our book reflects a conservative approach in most circumstances because we, as emergency physicians, tend to err on the side of sickness rather than of health. Therefore, in addition to describing the pathology, the differential diagnosis, and management of the various urgencies, we also describe pitfalls we believe clinicians should be aware of as they evaluate urgent care patients.

It is our hope that this handbook serves its intended purpose and provides a basis for thoughtful evaluation of the urgent care patient. We thank our loved ones, residents, patients, and colleagues for their support as we completed this book and for their critical useful evaluation of the work itself.

Michelle H. Biros, MS, MD
Steve Sterner, MD
E. Corradin Vogel, MD

Preface to the First Edition

This book is designed for use by clinicians as a rapid reference in the diagnosis and treatment of patients who are likely to present to an urgent care center with a broad spectrum of minor illnesses and injuries. The urgent care physician is targeted as the audience because the background and training of these physicians tends to be diverse, strong in some areas yet weak in others. Other physicians, medical students, nurses, and allied health professionals working in a similar medical setting may also find this book useful.

The format of the book facilitates this purpose. The organization is based on presenting symptoms and body systems. The information is presented in a brief and concise manner, with frequent use of tables and figures. The scope is broad, with attention given to many minor problems that may be difficult to research in other texts. Serious illnesses that should be included in the differential diagnosis of presenting complaints as well as complications of minor problems are also described.

This book is not an all-inclusive, authoritative text. It is a reference that can be used quickly and easily to assist the clinician as patient care is being delivered. References are cited in the event that further reading in more detail is desired. The authors are members of the Department of Emergency Medicine of Hennepin County Medical Center. In addition to their Emergency Department experience, they have worked in an urgent care center and have assisted in the development of an urgent care training program.

The editors would like to thank Dr. Ronald B. Goodspeed, MSCH, FACP, for his thoughtful review of this book. His comments were helpful in our final evaluation of the scope and intent of our work.

Michelle H. Biros, MD
Steve Sterner, MD

Chapter 1

Fielding True Emergencies in an Urgent Care Center

Ernest Ruiz, MD
E. Corradin Vogel, MD

Expectations

The public expects medical facilities and personnel to be prepared for emergencies. It is not difficult for an urgent care center (UCC) to attain a satisfactory degree of readiness with some planning and thoughtful preparation.

Depending on its location relative to other medical facilities and its ease of access to and from population or industrial centers, the UCC can expect certain types of emergency patients to appear occasionally at its door. Some UCCs can count on seeing an occasional severely ill infant or child, whereas others, depending on their location, are more likely to encounter a severely injured industrial worker. A UCC that appears to be a free-standing, quasi-emergency medical facility probably has a greater obligation, from the public's viewpoint, to be prepared to provide at least basic care for true emergencies than a physician's office or clinic. Adequate preparation for all types of emergencies is not difficult to achieve and should be the goal.

Preparations

The first step in preparing for true emergencies is to assess the availability, capabilities, and equipment carried by first and second responders of the local emergency medical services (EMS) system. As a general rule, the UCC should be supplied at least with the equipment that the first responders carry: oxygen cylinders with masks and nasal prongs, a bag-valve-mask apparatus, nasal and oral airways, esophageal obturator airways, cervical collars, and trauma dressings. Some first responder teams are equipped with automated external defibrillator (AED) units. Medications, monitors and defibrillators, intravenous (IV) equipment and fluids, and intubating equipment are generally carried by the second responders (paramedics).

In addition to being familiar with the equipment offered by the EMS system, UCC personnel should be knowledgeable about the rules of operation of the system. In some systems the radio control physician at the base station gives any and all orders to paramedics. Some systems allow physicians at the scene to give orders, and other systems mandate that any physician who gives orders in the field must accompany the patient to the hospital. It behooves the urgent care physician to become familiar with the standing orders that paramedics are allowed to follow without physician input as well as the procedures and medications that they are allowed to administer on a physician's order. The paramedics are operating under the medical license of their medical director, who has given them specific orders as to what they can and cannot do. A visit to the local medical director of the ambulance service helps familiarize the urgent care physician with the rules governing a particular system. Another important aspect of the local EMS system that may affect the UCC is its rules about acceptable "Do Not Resuscitate" orders and other care-limiting orders. EMS systems may require specific forms and procedures to be followed before honoring such directives.

It is obviously important for the UCC physicians and nurses to be familiar with the local EMS system. The best way to activate the system should be thoroughly understood, and the number, usually 911, should be posted for ready reference. In some systems, activation means that fire fighters with full gear will enter the UCC, alarming patients and personnel. Observers must understand that this is the best way to get immediate response and that the rescue personnel need to be prepared to leave for a fire at any time.

In most situations, at least when the UCC is free-standing, the standard medications and procedures included in the American Heart Association's Advanced Cardiac Life Support course should be available in the UCC.[1] A monitor or defibrillator is required in the UCC unless the response time of the EMS system is exceptionally short and consistent. Airway management, IV access, dysrhythmia recognition and management, and life support of arrest states in adults and children are included in this course.

Recognition and Immediate Management of Emergencies

Most true emergencies are obvious and should result in the immediate activation of the EMS system. Chapter 18 describes emergency conditions in children. True emergencies in adults are listed in Appendix A, along with steps that should be taken immediately while preparing for the arrival of EMS personnel and transportation of the patient to a full-service emergency department.

Transport to an Emergency Hospital

Protocols should be established in each UCC about the destination of patients being transferred for emergency care. Generally, patients should go to the nearest hospital that has sufficient facilities and expertise for definitive management of their problem.[2] The emergency physician at the receiving hospital should be called and informed of the patient's condition and estimated time of arrival. The emergency physician may suggest or request further intervention before transfer. Personnel at the receiving hospital can then be fully prepared to manage the patient on arrival.

Conclusion

Patients with true life- and limb-threatening emergencies occasionally present to the UCC. Planning and preparation can ensure that such patients receive appropriate initial care, enter the local EMS system quickly and efficiently, and are transported to the facility best able to care for them.

References

1. American Heart Association: Guidelines 2000 for cardiopulmonary resuscitation and emergency cardiovascular care. Circulation 102:I22–I357, 2000.
2. Lilja GP, Swor RA: Emergency Medical Services. In Tintinalli JE, Kelen GB, Stapczynski JS (eds): Emergency Medicine: A Comprehensive Study Guide, 5th ed. New York, McGraw-Hill, 2000, pp 1–6.

Appendix A

Ernest Ruiz, MD
E. Corradin Vogel, MD

Condition	Immediate Action
Cardiac emergencies	
General	1. Administer oxygen. If no history of chronic obstructive pulmonary disease (COPD), mask at 10 L/min, or if the patient cannot tolerate the mask, nasal cannula at 4–6 L/min. If history of COPD, use cannula at 2–3 L/min. 2. Obtain vital signs and estimate patient's weight. 3. Perform appropriate physical examination while obtaining pertinent history, including history of allergies. 4. Start IV of normal saline and run to keep open. 5. Attach electrocardiograph (ECG) leads and monitor rhythm.
Suspected myocardial infarction • Chest pain/pressure in any patient >30 y/o • Syncopal episode in any patient over age 50 (without suspicion of stroke) • Atypical chest pain, i.e., shoulder, arm, or jaw pain in absence of chest pain; patients with cardiac risk factors • Acute onset of fatigue, shortness of breath, or diaphoresis in patients with cardiac risk factors • Unexplained respiratory distress	1. Consider nitroglycerin (0.4 mg sublingual tablet and/or spray) for chest pain if patient not hypotensive (SBP >110 mmHg). May repeat every 5 min x 2. Monitor blood pressure before and after administration. 2. Morphine sulfate (4–10 mg IV slowly) for chest pain. Monitor respirations. 3. Administer adult aspirin tablet. Have patient chew aspirin to decrease absorption time.
Suspected pulmonary edema • Characterized by tachypnea, labored respirations, anxiety and agitation, fatigue, rales, jugular venous distension, peripheral edema, frothy sputum, and/or cyanosis	1. Allow patient to remain semiupright. 2. Administer high-flow oxygen. Consider positive-pressure ventilatory assistance. 3. Follow immediate action for "suspected myocardial infarction," and monitor ECG. 4. Administer furosemide (40 mg IV). 5. Consider morphine sulfate (4–10 mg IV slowly). 6. Consider nitroglycerin (0.3–0.4 mg sublingually). 7. Consider nebulized albuterol (2.5 mg).
Dysrhythmias associated with myocardial ischemia • Premature ventricular contractions (PVCs)	1. Administer high-flow oxygen. 2. Monitor blood pressure and ECG closely.
• Bradyarrhythmias	1. If any of the following signs or symptoms are present, administer atropine 0.5 mg IV and place transcutaneous pacemaker if available. • Systolic blood pressure less than 90 mmHg or symptoms of shock • Altered level of consciousness • Chest pain • PVCs or ventricular escape beats • Dyspnea

(Cont'd on next page)

Condition	Immediate Action
• Bradyarrhythmias (*cont'd*)	2. Repeat atropine as necessary up to total of 2 mg.
Narrow complex tachycardia • Paroxysmal supraventricular tachycardia (PSVT) • Atrial flutter • Atrial fibrillation	1. If patient without serious signs or symptoms (e.g., chest pain, dyspnea, hypotension [< 90 SBP], hypoxia), monitor blood pressure and ECG and transport. 2. For PSVT only: • Attempt Valsalva maneuver. • If Valsalva unsuccessful, administer adenosine 6 mg IV rapid push. May repeat adenosine dose at 12 mg IV, if necessary. For significantly symptomatic atrial flutter, fibrillation, and unsuccessful intervention of PVST, consider synchronized monophasic cardioversion at 50, 100, 200, 300, 360 J.
• Ventricular tachycardia with palpable pulse and with serious signs or symptoms	If patient is deteriorating, consider synchronized cardioversion at 100, 200, 300, 360 J with sedation if conscious.
Cardiac arrest states • Ventricular fibrillation and pulseless ventricular tachycardia	1. Precordial thump if witnessed, initiate CPR. 2. Immediately defibrillate up to 3 times at 200, 300, 360 J. 3. If defibrillation is unsuccessful after three attempts, start cardiopulmonary resuscitation (CPR) and manage airway. Start IV (normal saline) and give 1 mg epinephrine (10 ml of 1:10,000 solution IV) or vasopressin 40 U IV single dose, then defibrillate again at 360 J. Treat resulting rhythm per ACLS guidelines.
• Asystole	1. Consider precordial thump if witnessed. 2. If fine ventricular fibrillation is a possibility, follow ACLS protocol for ventricular fibrillation. 3. Manage airway and start IV. 4. Give 1 mg epinephrine (10 ml of 1:10,000 solution IV). 5. Continue considering atropine IV treatment per current ACLS protocol.
• All other nonperfusing rhythms	1. Start CPR, manage airway, and start IV. 2. Look for underlying cause (hypovolemia, cardiac tamponade, tension pneumothorax, hypoxia). 3. Consider fluid challenge if pulseless electrical activity is present. 4. Consider drug therapy with epinephrine, atropine, calcium chloride, bicarbonate per current ACLS protocol.
Nontraumatic shock Suspected hemorrhagic (gastrointestinal bleeding, ruptured abdominal aortic aneurysm, ectopic pregnancy) or nonhemorrhagic (septic, cardiogenic, overdose, unknown) shock	1. Monitor blood pressure, administer oxygen. 2. Start IV of normal saline. Consider bolus administration for hypertension.
Anaphylactic shock	1. Administer oxygen as needed. 2. If patient is in respiratory distress or hypotensive, administer epinephrine (0.3 mg of 1:1,000 solution subcutaneously). 3. Start IV of normal saline. Consider bolus administration for hypotension. 4. Consider placing venous tourniquet proximal to sting or injection site, and/or ice pack at sting or injection site. 5. May administer diphenhydramine HCl 25 mg IV/50 mg IM.
Asthma/COPD	A. For patients in respiratory distress: airway. 1. Insert oral airway and begin positive pressure ventilation. Attempt orotracheal intubation if properly trained or consider other artificial airway device if available (e.g., laryngeal mask airway, combitube, EOA). Avoid hyperinflation by bagging patient at rate of 8–10 breath/min, allowing for prolonged expiratory pulse.

(Cont'd on next page)

Condition	Immediate Action

Asthma/COPD *(cont'd)*	2. Insert IV.
	3. Refer to medical interventions listed below.
	B. For patients in respiratory distress: medications.
	  1. Begin oxygen by nasal cannula at 2 to 3 L/min. or by facemask for higher oxygen requirements.
	  2. Administer nebulized albuterol 2.5 mg with or without atrovent 0.5 mg.
	  3. Consider epinephrine (0.3 mg of 1:1,000 solution subcutaneously) or terbutaline (0.25 mg subcutaneously) for increasing respiratory distress. Use with caution in elders and patients with coronary artery disease. Place ECG monitoring on these patients.

Obstructed airway	1. Heimlich maneuver, back blows, abdominal thrusts, and chest compressions per BCLS protocols. 2. Finger sweeps and direct laryngoscopy for removal of foreign body. 3. Administer oxygen and manage airway.
Status epilepticus seizures	1. Clear and maintain airway. 2. Administer oxygen and be ready to turn patient on side if patient vomits. 3. Start IV and administer benzodiazepine to halt seizure. If unable to obtain IV, consider IM, PR administration. 4. Consider causes of seizure (hypoglycemia, meningitis, space-occupying lesion, trauma, etc.).
Coma of unknown etiology	1. Administer oxygen. Manage airway. 2. Start IV and get blood sample for measurement of glucose level. 3. Give 50 ml of 50% dextrose IV if blood glucose < 60. If unable to place IV, may give glucagon 1 mg IM. 4. If suspected narcotics overdose, consider 2 mg Narcan IV. 5. Monitor blood pressure and ECG.
Insulin reaction/hypoglycemia	1. If patient is conscious, give sugar or 50 ml of 50% dextrose to drink. 2. If unable to drink, start IV with dextrose (5% in water) and give 50 ml of 50% dextrose IV. If possible, obtain blood to test for glucose level before giving 50% dextrose. 3. May give glucagon, 1 mg IM, if unable to place IV.
Suspected cerebrovascular accident	1. Manage airway. Administer oxygen. Monitor blood pressure and ECG. 2. Start IV with normal saline at "to keep open" rate. 3. Expedite transfer to hospital for further management. (CT scan, thrombolytics)
Severe hyperthermia (temperature 105° F or higher)	1. If patient is alert, administer antipyretics. 2. Undress, apply tepid (not cold) water/mist and use fan to improve cooling.
Traumatic emergencies Suspected cervical spine injury	1. Apply hard cervical collar. 2. Transport on spine board if any paresthesia or weakness.
Bleeding wounds	1. Apply direct pressure to control bleeding. 2. Start IV or normal saline with large-bore needle.

Chapter 2

Common Lower Respiratory Problems

Peter Craig, MD
Carrie Tibbles, MD
Jennifer Block, MD

Although the urgent care physician occasionally encounters the critically ill patient requiring immediate referral and transport to an emergency department, the vast majority of patients presenting with respiratory complaints can be managed in the urgent care setting. The following sections outline the common lower respiratory problems, their evaluation, and management.

Lower respiratory infections (i.e., pneumonia and acute bronchitis) are the most common infectious diseases in patients with respiratory complaints. Although it is often difficult to determine conclusively the nature of a lower respiratory tract infection, the physician must (1) distinguish bronchitis from pneumonia, (2) determine the most likely etiologic agents, and (3) determine the overall health of the patient. Patients with impairment of any aspect of normal host defenses are predisposed to lower respiratory infections and at increased risk for infection by atypical pathogens. These considerations allow appropriate therapy and disposition even when the infecting organism is unidentified.

All patients presenting with respiratory complaints require immediate assessment for evidence of life-threatening respiratory failure. The two main principles in this initial evaluation are (1) assurance of a patent airway for ventilation and removal of secretions and (2) assurance of adequate oxygenation. Immediate threats to these processes must be sought while evaluating patients for the less emergent pathologies discussed in this chapter. Table 1 lists several common emergent conditions that can present as acute respiratory distress.

Table 1. Emergent Conditions Causing Acute Respiratory Distress

Foreign body in the airway	Pulmonary edema
Epiglottis	Pneumothorax
Anaphylaxis	Pulmonary emboli
Status asthmaticus	Acute myocardial ischemia and infarction
Aspiration	

Pulse oximetry offers a valuable, immediate, noninvasive indicator of arterial oxygenation and may contribute diagnostically if measured before supplemental oxygen is given. Supplemental oxygen should not be delayed or withheld, however, from the patient with probable hypoxia.

Signs of significant hypoxia include tachypnea, labored breathing, mental status changes, lethargy, agitation, diaphoresis, and cyanosis. Stridor or sonorous respirations indicate airway obstruction. Patients with these signs require immediate intervention, possibly including mechanical airway assistance to improve ventilation.

Dyspnea

Differential Diagnosis. Dyspnea may be defined as the uncomfortable perception of breathing or labored breathing. Patients may describe "air hunger," tightness in the chest, or shortness of breath. The differential diagnosis of this complaint is broad and best approached by first classifying the dyspnea as acute or chronic and its etiologies as pulmonary or nonpulmonary.

Chronic dyspnea most often results from either pulmonary disorders, such as asthma or chronic obstructive pulmonary disease (COPD), or cardiac conditions, such as cardiomyopathy or valvular heart disease. More often in the urgent care setting, patients present with the acute onset of dyspnea, or an increase in the level of dyspnea. Both require prompt and thorough evaluation, because a number of serious or life-threatening conditions can present in either manner. The differential diagnosis of acute or acute-on-chronic dyspnea includes pulmonary conditions (pneumonia, pneumothorax, pulmonary embolism, asthma exacerbation, chest wall or pleuritic pain, aspirations, noncardiogenic pulmonary edema), cardiac conditions (cardiogenic pulmonary edema, congestive heart failure, myocardial ischemia/infarction, pericarditis), and other conditions (thyroid disease, gastrointestinal reflux, anemia, sepsis, acidosis, and neuromuscular diseases).

History and Physical Examination. The history should focus on the onset of symptoms as well as duration and exacerbating or alleviating factors. Are symptoms present only with exertion, or do they persist at rest? Associated symptoms such as chest pain, fever, or cough, as well as any history of recent trauma, should be elicited. In addition, risk factors for cardiac disease (smoking, hypertension, diabetes, hypercholesterolism, family history) and pulmonary embolism (recent surgery or immobilization, neoplastic disease, personal or family history of deep venous thrombosis or pulmonary embolism) should be sought. Use of tobacco or illicit drugs is also important.

A focused physical exam includes evaluation of vital signs, such as pulse oximetry and, as indicated, peak flow measurement. In patients with suspected bronchospasm, peak flow measurement also provides a useful means of determining response to treatment. High fever points to an infectious etiology, but low-grade fever can be seen with pulmonary embolus (PE) and other causes of dyspnea.[1]

The patient's general appearance and work of breathing should be noted. The head, ear, eye, nose, and throat (HEENT) exam may reveal pallor suggestive of anemia or exopthalmus suggestive of hyperthyroidism. Neck exam may reveal a goiter or increased jugular venous pressure related to pulmonary edema. Auscultation of the heart should focus on the presence of a murmur or rub. Ausculation of the lungs may reveal wheezing and a prolonged expiratory phase, pointing more toward obstructive disease. Localized rhonchi or rales may suggest pneumonia, whereas bilateral rales suggest pulmonary edema. Decreased breath sounds may be due to COPD, effusion, or pneumothorax. Finally, the presence of peripheral edema should be noted.

Diagnostic Aids. The history and physical exam determine the need for ancillary tests. A chest x-ray may be obtained to rule out pneumothorax, pulmonary edema, effusion, or pneumonia. An electrocardiogram should be considered in patients with chest pain or those at risk for silent myocardial ischemia, such as diabetics and the elderly. Ventilation-perfusion (VQ) scan or computed tomography (CT) using the PE protocol (i.e., spiral chest CT) may be performed if this diagnosis is suspected. Hemoglobin level is helpful if anemia is suspected. The white blood cell count is nonspecific but, if markedly elevated, suggests an infectious etiology. Further lab work may be obtained if such conditions as acidosis or thyroid disease are in the differential. Arterial blood gas also may be considered, particularly if ventilatory status is in question.

Management. Specific management of dyspnea is directed at treatment of the underlying cause. General measures, such as placement of supplementary oxygen and perhaps a trial of a beta agonist, may be undertaken while the work-up is in progress. Obviously, any patient with apparent respiratory distress requires definitive management of airway and respiratory status before the initiation of ancillary testing.

Disposition. Whether the patient can be discharged home depends on both the underlying cause and how acutely ill he or she is. Patients with reversible airway disease such as asthma, which responds to treatment, can usually be safely discharged. In general, those with significant hypoxia or ventilatory compromise should not be sent home, regardless of the cause of their symptoms.

Pitfalls in Practice. Attributing the feeling of shortness of breath or air hunger to psychological causes runs the risk of missing serious, possibly life-threatening pathology. All patients with unexplained dyspnea should be referred immediately for additional diagnostic evaluation and management.

Pneumonia

Differential Diagnosis. Pneumonia refers to an inflammation of the lung parenchyma. Although both acute and chronic forms of pneumonia exist, this chapter reviews only acute infectious pneumonia.

Clinical differentiation of bronchitis from pneumonia relies on history, general appearance of the patient, chest examination, and chest x-ray (Table 2). The physician should also distinguish pneumonia from exacerbation of COPD, pulmonary edema, pulmonary

Table 2. Clinical Distinction of Pneumonia from Bronchitis

Distinguishing Feature	Bronchitis	Pneumonia
General appearance	Not toxic	Toxic, patient is dyspneic
Vital signs		
Respiratory rate	Usually normal	Elevated
Temperature	Usually normal	Usually elevated
Sputum	Small volumes	Large volumes; hemoptysis likely
Chest examination	Usually normal, or occasional coarse rhonchi	Rales, consolidation; decreased breath sounds, dullness to percussion
Chest x-ray	Usually normal or peribronchial infiltrate	Acute infiltrate (alveolar, interstitial, patchy)

infarction, atelectasis, tumors, toxic peneumonitis, and pulmonary hemorrhage. Once the diagnosis of acute infectious pneumonia is made, management depends on (1) characterization of the patient and (2) determination of likely infecting organisms.

History and Physical Examination. The general symptoms of bronchitis, COPD exacerbation, and pneumonia overlap and thus contribute little to specific diagnosis. However, some symptoms may be indicative of certain pathogens (e.g. "currant jelly" sputum in *Klebsiella* infection, subacute clinical course in mycoplasmal infection). Although general symptoms may contribute less to determination of etiologies, other history may be invaluable. Recent exposures or travel history, hospitalizations, and suspicions of an immunocompromised host may significantly alter diagnostic choices and management. Risks of aspiration are sometimes overlooked, even though aspiration is a common cause of pneumonia (as many as 70% of patients with altered mental status aspirate oropharyngeal contents and up to 45% of otherwise normal people have significant aspiration during sleep).[2]

Physical examination typically reveals an acutely ill, toxic-appearing patient with abnormal vital signs (commonly tachypnea, fever, and tachycardia). Patients have varying degrees of dyspnea, cough, and sputum production. Chest auscultation often reveals crackles, rhonchi, or evidence of consolidation, such as tubular or bronchial breath sounds, egophony, or dullness to percussion. Chest pain may be musculoskeletal or truly pleuritic, and chest wall expansion may be asymmetric.

Diagnostic Aids. A chest radiograph is not necessary in all patients with lower respiratory tract infections, and fairly good data support its omission when pneumonia is not clinically evident.[3] In addition, radiographic features in community-acquired pneumonia do not differentiate common etiologies (*Streptococcus pneumoniae*, *Mycoplasma*, *Legionella* species, *Staphylococcus aureus*) and are not exclusive of nonbacterial processes.[4] However, in suspected pneumonia, indicators of severity (i.e., effusion, multilobar involvement) or nonbacterial pathology (i.e., carcinoma) may be found on chest x-ray. Thus, in healthy persons with community acquired pneumonia, it may be reasonable to omit radiographs; if disposition is equivocal or there are other pulmonary concerns, chest x-ray is indicated.

The measurement of pulse oximetry is easy and noninvasive, and often contributes to the overall clinical picture in determining the severity of illness. Pulse oximetry should be routinely measured for patients with respiratory complaints.

Blood cultures, pleural fluid cultures, serologic testing, sputum Gram stains, and cultures are generally helpful only for patients who fit hospitalization criteria. The results are not available quickly; thus, such studies are not useful for decision making in the urgent care setting. However, obtaining such studies before hospital admission and administration of antibiotics is often helpful in determining the final diagnosis and etiologic agent.

Arterial blood gases should be considered in patients who have other confounding illness, are > 60 years old, or are being considered for hospital admission.

Disposition. The first disposition decision is whether the patient can be managed safely in the outpatient setting. If inpatient management is indicated, it is necessary to determine whether the patient requires placement in an intensive care unit. The decision depends on the clinical picture. Vital signs may help. Increased mortality rates have been shown with temperature > 40° C or < 35° C; pulse > 125; respiratory rate > 30; or systolic blood pressure < 90 mmHg.[5]

Management. Nonspecific treatment includes adequate hydration, administration of expectorants, and avoidance of cough suppression. Chest physiotherapy is also helpful but is difficult to provide for outpatients. Avoidance of cough suppression is important, particularly in bacterial pneumonia, unless the patient demonstrates intercostal strain, barotraumas, or significant sleep disturbance.

It is important, from a therapeutic standpoint, to distinguish bacterial from nonbacterial causes of pneumonia. Table 3 compares characteristics of bacterial and nonbacterial pneumonia and highlights the differences between their clinical presentations.

Table 3. Bacterial Compared to Nonbacterial Pneumonia

Distinguishing Feature	Bacterial	Nonbacterial
Age of patient	Any age	Children and young adults
Toxicity	Toxic	Less toxic
Sputum	Large volume; purulent	Scant; no bacteria
Chest examination	Rales; consolidation	Rales
Chest x-ray	Infiltrate (patchy, lobar, segmental); pleural effusion	Interstitial infiltrate
White blood cell count	High	Usually normal or low

Accurate identification of the infecting organism requires cultures of properly obtained sputum. As previously noted, this process is of limited value in guiding initial therapy and frequently requires up to 2 days for results. Nevertheless, consideration of the clinical setting and possibly chest x-ray usually guide initial therapy and disposition. Table 4 summarizes characteristics of infectious pneumonia caused by the common etiologic agents.

Table 4. Characteristics of Common Pneumonia

Etiologic Agent	Presentation	Chest Roentgenography
Viral	Usually seen in children and young adults; fine rales	Nonlobar, nonsegmental, interstitial infiltrate
Streptococcal		
Nongroup A	Abrupt onset	Lobar or segmental; consolidation is common
Group A	Not common; abrupt onset, high fever, pleuritic pain	Pleural effusion
Mycoplasmal	Seen in young adults; not toxic	Interstitial infiltrate, nonlobar, nonsegmental; occasional pleural effusion
Staphylococcal	Toxic, hectic fever pattern	Multiple infiltrate; cavitation
Legionnaires' disease	Toxic; high fever, encephalopathy, abdominal pain, diarrhea	Early: patchy infiltrate Late: consolidation, cavitation
Haemophilus influenzae	Seen in young children and immunosuppressed patients	Patchy infiltrate, multilobar

Streptococcal pneumonia (nongroup A) is the most common acute pneumonia. It accounts for up to 60% of community-acquired pneumonias.[3] Presentation may be atypical in immunosuppressed patients. Uncomplicated cases usually respond well to outpatient treatment with oral macrolides. Table 5 presents common antibiotic regimens suggested for the outpatient treatment of community acquired pneumonia.

Table 5. Common Regimens for Outpatient Treatment of Community-acquired Pneumonia

Pediatric (1 month–18 years)
• Erythromycin, 10 mg/kg/dose orally 4 times/day × 10–14 days
• Clarithromycin, 7.5 mg/kg/dose orally twice daily × 10–14 days
• Consider initiating treatment with a single dose of parenteral antibiotics: erythromycin, 10 mg/kg IV (maximum of 1 gm) + cefuroxime, 50 mg/kg IV (maximum of 1 gm)
Common etiologies: *S. pneumoniae, H. influenzae* (1–24 months), *Chlamydia pneumoniae, Mycoplasma* sp., respiratory syncytial virus (1–24 months), often viral.

Adults ≤ 60 years old, no comorbidity
• Azithromycin, 500 mg orally × 1; then 250 mg/day orally × 4 days
• Erythromycin, 500 mg orally 4 times/day × 14 days (not in areas with resistant *S. pneumoniae*; also variably effective against *H. influenzae*)
• Doxycycline 100 mg twice daily for 10–14 days
Common etiologies: *S. pneumoniae, Mycoplasma* sp., *Chlamydia pneumoniae, Legionella* sp., *H. influenzae.*

Adults < 60 years old, smoker, chronic illness, alcohol
• Azithromycin, 500 mg orally × 1; then 250 mg/day orally × 4 days
• If any suspicion of resistant *S. pneumoniae*: levofloxacin, 500 mg/day orally × 10–14 days
• If any suspicion of aspiration: amoxicillin/clavulanate, 500 mg orally 3 times/day × 10–14 days
Common etiologies: *S. pneumoniae, H. influenzae, M. catarrhalis, Legionella* sp., *Chlamydia pneumoniae*, coliforms.

Adults > 60 years old with no significant comorbidity
• Azithromycin
• Levofloxacin (CDC recommendations state that levofloxacin should be withheld in cases of macrolide failure or allergy)

Influenzal pneumonia typifies viral pneumonias. It most often occurs in children, elderly patients, or debilitated patients. Onset is usually nonspecific with myalgia, coryza, and malaise. Pneumonia appears within 2 days of onset when it is purely viral. Bacterial superinfection is common and begins later in the course. Such patients usually present with a high fever and a dry, nonproductive cough. Chest x-rays reveal a patchy interstitial infiltrate. Amantadine may shorten the duration of symptoms if a treatment regimen is started within 2 days of the onset of the symptom complex.

Pitfalls in Practice. In general, patients respond well to outpatient treatment if (1) the offending organism is not highly virulent, (2) the patient does not appear toxic, and (3) the patient is otherwise healthy. Patients at risk for rapid progression require parenteral antibiotic treatment as inpatients. Examples include immunosuppressed patients, patients with chronic cardiac or pulmonary disease, debilitated patients, and patients with poor judgment or insight about their disease.

Patients normally do well with close follow-up as long as significant comorbidities or risk factors are not overlooked. Thorough history is the key to avoiding these pitfalls.

Acute Bronchitis

Differential Diagnosis. Acute tracheobronchitis is defined as inflammation of the trachea and bronchi. It is caused chiefly by infection, but noninfectious causes include allergy and irritants (e.g., smoke, pollution). Clinical differentiation of bronchitis from pneumonia relies on history, general appearance of the patient, and chest examination (see Table 2). Chest x-ray may be helpful.

Acute bronchitis is usually associated with respiratory viruses, most commonly the common cold viruses (i.e., rhinovirus and coronavirus). However, influenza also should be considered, particularly in epidemics. *Mycoplasma pneumoniae*, *Chlamydia pneumoniae*, and *Bordetella pertussis* are the most common bacterial causes of acute bronchitis. Table 6 offers a differential diagnosis of acute bronchitis.

Table 6. Differential Diagnosis of Acute Bronchitis

Disease Process	Signs and Symptoms
Reactive airway diseases	
Asthma	Evidence of airway obstruction even when not infected
Allergic aspergillosis	Transient pulmonary infiltrates; eosinophilia in sputum and peripheral blood smear
Occupational exposures	Symptoms worse during work week, improve on weekends, holidays, and vacations
Chronic bronchitis	Chronic cough with sputum production on a daily basis for a minimum of 3 months; seen in smokers
Respiratory infection	
Sinusitis	Tenderness over sinuses; postnasal drainage
Common cold	Upper airway inflammation and no evidence of bronchial wheezing
Pneumonia	Infiltrate on x-ray, usually febrile
Other causes	
Congestive heart failure	Basilar rales, S_3 gallop, orthopnea, cardiomegaly, increased interstitial or alveolar fluid on chest x-ray
Bronchogenic tumor	Constitutional signs often present; cough chronic, sometimes with hemoptysis
Other aspiration syndromes	Usually related to a precipitating event, such as smoke inhalation; vomiting, decreased level of consciousness

Adapted from Hueston W, Mainous A: Acute bronchitis. Am Fam Physician 57:1270–1276, 1281–1282, 1998, with permission.

Bronchitis must be differentiated from other causes of similar symptoms, such as reactive airway diseases (e.g., asthma, occupational exposures), other respiratory infections (e.g., sinusitis, pneumonia, common cold), or other causes (e.g., congestive heart failure, reflux esophagitis, aspiration syndromes).

History and Physical Examination. Patients with bronchitis typically present with cough, with or without fever, and sputum production. The patient may have musculoskeletal chest pain. The chest examination is usually normal, although coarse rhonchi are common. Diffuse wheezing indicative of small airway obstruction from reactive bronchospasm or mucous secretions also may be present. The history and physical exam should rule out other causes of cough, particularly parenchymal lung disease or cardiovascular disease.

Diagnostic Aids. In general, a Gram stain of sputum is not necessary in the diagnosis or treatment of acute bronchitis. A chest x-ray is usually not required but may be helpful in considering other pulmonary disease. Influenza A nasal washing also can be done if this infectious etiology is suspected.

Management. Appropriate treatment varies, depending on (1) the overall health of the patient and (2) the most likely cause of the bronchitis. Patients with good pulmonary function usually respond well to outpatient treatment aimed at the most likely etiologic agents.

The course of the illness may help determine its cause. If the time between exposure and development of the illness is known to be less than 1 week, it is most likely viral.

During a known influenza outbreak or if the influenza A test is positive, consider a course of amantadine (100 mg twice daily × 5 days), which, if given in the first 48 hours, may shorten the duration of the illness. Several recent studies have demonstrated relief of symptoms with bronchodilators such as albuterol in acute bronchitis, since pulmonary function testing is similar in acute bronchitis and asthma.[6,7] Antitussive therapy at night and expectorants also may provide symptomatic relief.

Recent studies have consistently failed to show a significant clinical benefit of antibiotic therapy in acute bronchitis.[8,9] In general, antibiotics are no longer recommended in patients with acute bronchitis. Exceptions to this general guideline include patients with COPD, who have minimal functional lung reserve[10]; adults and children with suspected pertussis[11]; and children with cystic fibrosis.[12]

Patients with poor pulmonary reserve, including patients with COPD or other chronic pulmonary disease, cardiac diseases, or immunosuppression, may require hospital admission for oxygen therapy and observation. Patients with acute bronchitis superimposed on chronic bronchitis may require treatment with broad-spectrum antibiotics. This approach is discussed further in the section on COPD (see below).

Pitfalls in Practice. Consider potentially serious causes of cough, such as pulmonary emboli or cardiac asthma, before making the diagnosis of acute bronchitis, particularly if the cough has been persistent. Most cases of acute bronchitis do not require antibiotics, and overprescribing practices contribute to antimicrobial resistance. Studies demonstrate that satisfaction with the physician encounter is the same whether or not the patient with acute bronchitis is prescribed an antibiotic, as long as the physician's rationale for withholding antibiotics is explained adequately.[13]

Respiratory Infections in Immunocompromised Patients

Immunocompromised patients are susceptible to respiratory infections, both with common and unusual pathogens. Those at risk for immune compromise include people with acquired immunodeficiency syndrome, organ transplant recipients, and patients with congenital immune deficiencies or on chemotherapy or steroids. Table 7 lists the common pathogens seen in the various types of immunocompromised patients.

Table 7. Characteristics of Respiratory Infections Common in Immunocompromised Patients

Infection	Characteristics
Pneumocystis carinii pneumonia (PCP)	Most common opportunistic infection in HIV; seen when CD4 count < 200 cells/mm^3 Subacute course: mortality up to 10% with first episode
Tuberculosis (TB)	Common in HIV; spread by inhalation droplets; presents as fever, cough, hemoptysis, night sweats, weight loss
Mycobacterium avium infection	In HIV, CD4 count < 50 cells/mm^3; spectrum of disease from asymptomatic to disseminated disease
Histoplasmosis	Endemic to Mississippi and Ohio River valleys
Blastomyces	Mississippi and Ohio River valleys, Wisconsin, Michigan, Minnesota
Coccidioides	Southwestern United States, Mexico
Cryptococcus	Isolated pulmonary disease uncommon; presents as meningitis or disseminated disease
Aspergillus	Common in transplant patients

In evaluating respiratory infections in immunocompromised patients it is important to consider the acuity of the infection, because many of the opportunistic infections have a subacute clinical course. The appearance of the chest x-ray also may be helpful. It is also important to consider geographic factors, patient's travel history and local patterns of disease.[14]

Pneumocystis carinii Pneumonia

Differential Diagnosis. *Pneumocystis carinii* pneumonia (PCP) has become the most common opportunistic infection in HIV, typically seen when the CD4 count is below 200 cells/mm.[14] It is usually insidious in onset, and patients may have symptoms, most often a dry, nonproductive cough, for weeks prior to diagnosis. Physical exam should include evaluation for other signs of immunocompromise, such as candidiasis, Kaposi's sarcoma, or lymphadenopathy. Ausculatory exam may reveal rales.

Diagnostic Aids. Pulse oximetry and possibly arterial blood gases may be helpful to assess the degree of hypoxia. A decline in oxygen saturation may be induced by a brief period of exercise. Serum lactate dehydrogenase is often elevated. The white blood cell count is usually normal. The most common chest x-ray finding is diffuse bilateral perihilar interstitial infiltrates (i.e., the "batwing appearance"). However, up to 20% of patients have normal chest x-rays at presentation.[15] The diagnostic procedure of choice is sputum induction with direct fluorescent antibody; if this test is negative, bronchoscopy with bronchial alveolar lavage is recommended.

Management. A patient with a new diagnosis of suspected PCP should be admitted to the hospital. Trimethoprim-sulfamethoxazole (TMP-SMX) (20 mg/kg/day based on TMP given orally 3 times/day × 21 days) is the first-line treatment. Patients with a $PO_2 < 70$ are usually started on a 21-day course of steroids. Oxygen supplementation should be provided to hypoxic patients. Mildly ill patients with HIV and undifferentiated pneumonia may have a trial of outpatient therapy if the patient is compliant and has adequate home support systems. The TMP-SMX used for PCP prophylaxis (TMP, 5 mg/kg/day in 2 doses) is often effective for suppressing PCP as well as pneumonia from other bacterial causes.[16] If no improvement is seen in 2 days, hospitalization is warranted.

Pitfalls in Practice. PCP often presents subacutely and may be the first opportunistic infection in a patient with AIDS not receiving PCP prophylaxis. Pulse oximetry or arterial blood gas analysis after exercise may be necessary to assess accurately the degree of hypoxia.

Asthma

Asthma is a chronic inflammatory disease of the airways that affects 14–15 million people in the United States and accounts for 5000 deaths annually. The NIH expert panel on asthma has formulated a useful definition of asthma based on current research and understanding:

Asthma is a chronic inflammatory disorder of the airways in which many cells and cellular elements play a role, in particular, mast cells, eosinophils, T-lymphocytes, macrophages, neutrophils, and epithelial cells. In susceptible individuals, this inflammation causes recurrent episodes of wheezing, breathlessness, and chest tightness and coughing, particularly at night or in the early morning. These episodes are usually associated with widespread but variable airflow obstruction that is often reversible either spontaneously or with treatment. The inflammation also causes an associated increase in the existing bronchial hyper responsiveness to a variety of stimuli.[17]

The differential diagnosis of asthma in adults includes COPD, acute bronchitis, congestive heart failure, pulmonary embolus, upper airway obstruction or laryngeal dysfunction, anaphylaxis, pneumonia, or cough secondary to medications. The clinician must be aware of these alternative diagnoses and pursue them if warranted. In particular, the clinician should be wary of attributing wheezing to asthma in patients who do not carry a previous diagnosis of asthma, especially in the elderly population. Further work-up may be indicated in such cases.

History and Physical Examination. The triad of wheezing, dyspnea, and cough is the most common presentation. Patients with an acute asthma exacerbation require immediate assessment with a directed history and physical exam, progressing quickly to treatment. A brief history includes time of onset of symptoms, the likely cause of the episode (i.e., the trigger), significant prior cardiopulmonary disease, and current medications. Questions about previous hospitalizations, including intensive care admissions and intubations, frequency of ED/UC visits, and steroid use can help determine the severity of the underlying disease. The objectives of the physical exam are to assess the severity of the exacerbation and the current status of the patient, to rule out upper airway obstruction, and to identify complications (e.g., pneumothorax).

Diagnostic Aids. Spirometry or peak flow assessment helps determine the degree of obstruction and improvement with therapy. It is particularly useful if the patient knows his or her baseline values. Pulse oximetry is invaluable to assess the degree of hypoxia. Arterial blood gases are not usually necessary in typical asthma exacerbations. Chest x-ray, electrocardiography, sputum analysis, and complete blood count are not routinely needed unless the clinician suspects more severe underlying cardiopulmonary disease such as pneumonia.

Management. The aims of therapy in acute asthma exacerbation are to reverse bronchoconstriction and to decrease airway inflammation. Patients also should receive supplemental oxygen by nasal cannula or facemask, as needed, to maintain adequate oxygen saturations.

Short-acting inhaled beta$_2$ agonists are the mainstay of treatment for the relief of acute bronchoconstriction. Terbutaline also can be given subcutaneously for severe exacerbations, when the respiratory distress or the bronchospasm is so severe that inhaled medications are not adequately delivered. The addition of inhaled ipratropium (an anticholinergic) can provide added benefit. Patients with moderate-to-severe exacerbations should be given a short course of oral steroids to speed resolution of the inflammation and prevent recurrent exacerbations. Table 8 describes suggested medications and doses for the management of acute asthma exacerbations.

The decision whether to admit a patient with an acute asthma attack must be individualized for each patient and based on the severity and duration of the exacerbation and the response to treatment received in the urgent care setting. The comorbidities, such as cardiopulmonary disease or psychiatric illness, and social support system, including access to medical care, are also important considerations in deciding the appropriate disposition for the asthmatic patient.

Table 8. Dosages of Drugs for Asthma Exacerbations

Albuterol	
Nebulizer solution 5 mg/ml	2.5–5 mg every 20 minutes for 3 doses, then 2.5–10 mg every 1–4 hours as needed or continuously
Metered-dose inhaler (90 µg/puff)	4–8 puffs every 20 minutes up to 4 hours, then every 1–4 hours as needed
Ipratropium bromide	
Nebulizer solution (0.25 mg/ml)	0.5 mg every 20 minutes for 3 doses, then every 2–4 hours as needed
Metered-dose inhaler (18 µg/puff)	4–8 puffs as needed
Terbutaline (1 mg/ml)	0.25 mg every 20 minutes for 3 doses subcutaneously
Epinephrine 1:1000 (1 mg/ml)	0.3–0.5 mg every 20 minutes for 3 doses subcutaneously
Prednisone	40–60 mg/day orally for 5 days

Pitfalls in Practice. Omission of steroid treatment on discharge is probably the most common cause of early relapse. Both physician and patients often underestimate the severity and rapid progression of an acute asthma attack. Therefore, patients should be evaluated immediately and treated promptly.

Chronic Obstructive Pulmonary Disease

COPD comprises a group of distinct disorders that demonstrate irreversible changes in airway architecture that result in small airway obstruction. Although many diseases ultimately progress to COPD, the most common are emphysema and chronic bronchitis. Table 9 summarizes the clinical aspects of these two syndromes.

Table 9. Chronic Obstructive Pulmonary Diseases

Distinguishing Feature	Emphysema	Bronchitis
Patient's appearance	"Pink puffer"	"Blue bloater"
Symptoms	Dyspnea	Cough
Chest x-rays	Hyperinflated, small heart	Normal volumes until late; cardiomegaly
Cor pulmonale	Late	Early
Habitus	Cachexia; pursed lips	Overweight; barrel chest

Differential Diagnosis. Patients with COPD have little pulmonary reserve. Frequently, other primary pulmonary problems, such as pneumothorax, pnuemopericardium, pneumomediastinum, pulmonary embolus, pneumonia, atelectasis, or acute bronchitis, can present as an exacerbation of COPD. Asthma, anaphylaxis, upper airway obstruction, or endobronchial lesions also present as exacerbations of COPD. Evaluation of the chest x-ray, hematocrit, and arterial blood gases is important in distinguishing these entities.

History and Physical Examination. Patients with an exacerbation of COPD invariably present with acute shortness of breath. They have variable degrees of cough and sputum production. They almost always have a significant smoking history and a long history of dyspnea. On physical examination, patients have evidence of hyperlucency, increased intercostal spaces, and flattened diaphragms. Although many patients initially have some reversible component (asthma), almost all eventually have poor reversibility with bronchodilators. Patients with COPD frequently present with pulmonary infections, cor pulmonale, or respiratory failure.

The severity of the disease is based on the patient's initial presentation and response to treatment. Patients presenting with imminent respiratory failure, marked agitation, or decreased level of consciousness require immediate endotracheal intubation and further evaluation. Vital signs are important and accurate indicators of severity. Elevated pulse, respiratory rate, or pulsus paradoxus indicates severe exacerbation. Accessory respiratory muscle use is evident in severe exacerbation.

Diagnostic Aids. Pulse oximetry should be measured in all patients. The degree of hypoxia demonstrated on pulse oximetry is an important indicator of the patient's respiratory status and helps follow response to acute therapy.

If obtained, arterial blood gases commonly show baseline hypoxia in advanced COPD. The degree of compromise in forced expiratory volume in 1 second (FEV_1) is often poorly correlated with degree of hypoxia. Hypercapnia is seen in exacerbations or advanced cases of COPD with primarily bronchitic etiology, whereas emphysema usually causes only mild hypoxia with little or no hypercapnia, except in advanced cases. Often the FEV_1 is the only available method of measurement of current respiratory status in an urgent care setting, but spirometry is perhaps the most important of the diagnostic aids. Patients usually become symptomatic when the FEV_1 drops to 1–1.5 L. In the setting of airway obstruction, FEV_1 indicates severity without the need for FVC measurement of forced vital capacity (FVC). If FEV_1 can be measured, the predicted % FEV can be compared to the actual FEV to indicate the severity of airflow limitation. Severe COPD will present with an FEV of < 50% predicted; moderate disease will present with FEV < 70%.[18]

Radiographic findings on chest x-ray often correlate poorly with the severity of symptoms in acute COPD, but are useful if the diagnosis is unclear. The chest x-ray may reveal other pathologies, or complications of COPD (such as pneumothorax).

An electrocardiogram may help identify occult myocardial ischemia but also may reveal multifocal arterial tachycardia, arterial fibrillation or flutter, or p-pulmonale, which can present in acute respiratory distress.

Management. Oxygen. Improving airflow and relieving hypoxia are the goals of treatment. All patients with COPD require supplemental oxygen. Small increases in the fraction of inspired oxygen (FiO_2) provided by a rebreather mask (24–28%) reduce the risk of carbon dioxide retention.

Pharmacologic Therapy. The mainstay of pharmacologic treatment in COPD is cholinergic blockade. Ipratropium bromide is the usual first-line anticholinergic agent, but tiotropium bromide, if available, is superior because of increased receptor specificity. Beta agonists should be added to therapy because often there is some reversible component of airway narrowing in COPD. The long-acting agents (salmeterol, formoterol) are the best choices for management. Oral prednisone also should be routinely given in any significant COPD exacerbation.

Smoking Cessation. Smoking cessation is the only way to reduce the rate of decline in lung function in patients with COPD and can significantly prolong and improve the quality of life. Bupropion (Zyban) appears to be effective in aiding smoking cessation and may be superior to nicotine patches.[19]

Antibiotics. In acute exacerbation of COPD with a bronchitic component, antibiotics are often indicated. Primary targeted organisms are *Haemophilus influenzae, Mycobacterium catarrhalis, Streptococcus pneumoniae, Klebiella* sp., and anaerobes. If cost is a factor, SMX-TMP (2 times/day orally × 10 days) should be prescribed. Otherwise macrolides (Table 10) or fluoroquinolones are effective.

Immunization. Once the acute exacerbation has been relieved, influenza and pneumococcal vaccines should be considered when the patient is at baseline. Many patients with an acute COPD exacerbation require hospitalization, but others may be managed in the outpatient setting. Table 10 presents an example of a reasonable treatment regimen.

Table 10. Suggested Treatment Program for Acute COPD Exacerbations

1. Oxygen (with consideration for home oxygen by Ventori mask).
2. Ipratropium (Atrovent) MDI, 2–4 puffs 4 times/day.
3. Salmeterol (Serevent), 2 puffs twice daily.
4. Prednisone, 40 mg orally 4 times/day × 2 weeks with subsequent tapering under care of primary care provider.
5. Consider antibiotics (TMP-SMX, macrolides, or fluoroquinolones).
6. Bupropion (Zyban), 150 mg orally each morning × 3 days, then 150 mg orally twice daily × 7–12 weeks. Target quit date after at least 1 week of therapy; write "dispense behavioral modification kit" on first prescription.

Pitfalls in Practice. The major pitfalls in management of patients with acute exacerbations of COPD involve delay or withholding of oxygen therapy. All patients with COPD exacerbations are hypoxic. This hypoxia represents an immediate threat to life. There should be no delay in providing supplemental oxygen therapy while waiting for test results or for fear of carbon dioxide retention.

The physician must actively evaluate the patient for several conditions associated with severe and refractory COPD exacerbations, including acute bronchitis, pneumonia, and pneumothorax. Such conditions require prompt treatment when identified. Avoidance of precipitating factors, particularly smoking, is critical to address before discharge.

Patients with severe exacerbations of COPD should be transported by ambulance to an ED for evaluation and further treatment. Oxygen should be provided en route, and inhaled therapies should be initiated in the urgent care setting while awaiting ACLS transport.

References

1. Shah SM, Searles L: The febrile adult. Part II: Differential diagnosis and management of infectious and noninfectious syndromes. E,erg Med Reports 19(8):183–190, 1998.
2. Huxley EJ, Viroslav J, Gray WR, et al: Pharyngeal aspiration in normal adults with depressed levels of consciousness. Am J Med 64:564–568, 1978.
3. Woodhead M: Management of pneumonia in the outpatient setting. Semin Respir Infect 13(1):8–16, 1998.
4. DeBlieux PM, Slaven EM: Community acquired pneumonia: Deciding whom to admit and which antibiotics to use. Emerg Med Proc 1(4):1–24, 1999.
5. Fine MJ, et al: A pPrediction rule to identify low-reach patients with community acquired pneumonia. N Engl J Med 336:243–250, 1997.
6. Hueston WJ: A comparison of albuterol and erythromycin for the treatment of acute bronchitis. J Fam Pract 39(5):437–440, 1994.

7. Hueston WJ: Albuterol delivered by metered dose inhaler to treat acute bronchitis. J Fam Pract 39(5):437–440, 1994.
8. Orr PH, Schere K, MacDonald A, Moffatt ME: Randomized placebo-controlled trials of antibiotics for acute bronchitis: A critical review of the literature. J Fam Pract 36(5):507–512, 1993.
9. Bent S, Saint S, Vittinghoff E, Grady D: Antibiotics in acute bronchitis: A meta-analysis. Am J Med 107:62–67, 1999.
10. Saint S, Bent S, Vittinghoff E, Grady D: Antibiotics in chronic obstructive pulmonary disease exacerbations. JAMA 273:957–960, 1995.
11. Gonzales R, Bartlett J, Besser RE, et al: Principles of appropriate antibiotic use for treatment of uncomplicated acute bronchitis: Background. Ann Int Med 134(6):521–529, 2001.
12. O'Brien K, Dowell SF, Schwartz B, et al: Cough illness/bronchitis: Principles of judicious use of antimicrobial agents. Pediatrics 101:178–181, 1998.
13. Hamm RM, Hicks RJ, Bemben DA: Antibiotics and respiratory infections: Are patients more satisfied when expectations are met? J Fam Pract 43:56–62, 1996.
14. Zwanger M: Pneumonia in immunocompromised patients. In Tintinalli J, Ruiz E, Krome R (eds): Emergency Medicine: A Comprehensive Study Guide, 4th ed. New York, McGraw-Hill, 1996, pp 413–418.
15. Goodman J, Tashkin D: PCP with normal CXRs and arterial oxygen tension. Arch Int Med 143:1981–1982, 1983.
16. Emerman C: CAP Update Year 2000: Current antibiotic guidelines and outcome effective management. Part 1. Emerg Med Rep 20(24):237–248, 1999.
17. National Asthma Education and Prevention Program: Expert Panel Report 2: Guidelines for the Diagnosis and Management of Asthma. National Institutes of Health Pub No 97-4051A. Bethesda, MD, 1997.
18. American Thoracic Society: Lung function testing: Selection of reference values and interpretive strategies. Am Rev Resp Dis 144:1202–1218, 1991.
19. Barns PJ: New therapies for chronic obstructive pulmonary disease. Thorax 53(2):137–147, 1998.
20. Bosker G: CAP in the geriatric patient: Evaluation, risk stratification, and antimicrobial treatment guidelines for inpatient and outpatient management. Emerg Med Rep 21:217–234, 2000.

Chapter 3

Diagnosis and Management of Chest Pain in the Urgent Care Setting

Scott R. Gunn, MD
Mark Erlandson, MD

Chest pain is a common complaint and a diagnostic challenge. Even with current liberal admission standards for chest pain, physicians erroneously discharge approximately 5% of patients with acute myocardial infarctions.[1] Causes of chest pain range from benign to life-threatening (Table 1, next page). Ischemic heart disease should always be considered in patients presenting with the chief complaint of chest pain. The history is the most useful tool in guiding further evaluation. Physical exam findings and ancillary test results are neither sensitive nor specific enough to make the definitive diagnosis in many clinical situations.[6,9] Management goals of chest pain in an urgent care setting include recognizing life-threatening causes, anticipating potential problems, and protecting the patient with appropriate therapy and disposition. Selected causes of life-threatening and non-threatening chest pain are described in Tables 2 and 3 (pages 23–25).

History

A careful history is essential in establishing the most probable cause of chest pain. Allow the patient a few minutes to tell his or her own story with as little interruption as possible. One common mistake is to provide descriptions of chest pain to the patient who does not immediately give a cogent account. Unable to describe their own symptoms adequately, the patient may agree to your suggestions, leading to an inaccurate representation.[2] After the first few minutes, it may be necessary to focus the history by asking specific questions. An adequate history should include a clear description of the chest pain, associated symptoms, previous episodes of chest pain, and past medical and social history.

The important historical variables of chest pain include precipitating and alleviating factors, location and radiation, quality, severity, and duration.[3] The timing of pain in relation to precipitating and alleviating factors is most significant.[4] Chest pain that is provoked by activity or stress and relieved by rest or nitroglycerin is most specific for cardiac ischemia. Nevertheless, up to 25% of patients with ischemic chest pain present with atypical signs and symptoms.[5] Location and radiation are rarely helpful in assessing the significance of chest pain. Many types of chest pain start in the left chest and radiate to

Table 1. Differential Diagnoses of Chest Pain by Type and Cause

Chest pain (nonpleuritic)	Chest pain (pleuritic)

1. Cardiovascular
    Myocardial ischemia/infarction
    Myocarditis
    Chest pain associated with mitral valve
       prolapse
    Dissecting aortic aneurysm
	1. Cardiac
	    Pericarditis
	    Postpericardiotomy/Dressler syndrome

2. Pulmonary and mediastinal
    Neoplasm
    Pneumonia
    Pulmonary embolism/infarction
    Mediastinal tumors: lymphoma,
       thymoma
	2. Pulmonary
	    Pneumothorax
	    Hemothorax
	    Pulmonary embolism/infarction
	    Pneumonia
	    Empyema
	    Neoplasm
	    Bronchiectasis
	    Tuberculosis
	    Carcinomatous effusion

3. Gastrointestinal
    Esophageal: spasm, rupture, esophagitis,
       ulceration, neoplasm, achalasia,
       diverticula, foreign body
    Gastric and duodenal: hiatal hernia,
       neoplasm, peptic ulcer disease
    Gallbladder and biliary: cholecystitis,
       cholelithiasis, impacted stone,
       neoplasm
    Pancreatic: pancreatitis, neoplasm
    Referred pain from subdiaphragmatic
       gastrointestinal structures
	3. Gastrointestinal
	    Liver abscess
	    Pancreatitis
	    Whipple's disease with associated pericarditis or pleuritis
	    Subdiaphragmatic abscess

4. Soft tissue
    Herpes zoster
    Mastitis
    Cervical spondylosis
	4. Soft tissue
	    Costochondritis
	    Chest wall trauma
	    Fractured rib
	    Interstitial fibrositis
	    Myositis
	    Strain of pectoralis muscle
	    Herpes zoster
	    Soft tissue and bone tumors
	    Collagen-vascular diseases with pleuritis

5. Other
    Psychoneurosis
	5. Other
	    Familial Mediterranean fever
	    Psychoneurosis

the left arm. Pain quality is either visceral or somatic. Somatic pain is sharp and easy to localize. Generally, benign pleural and chest wall pains have a somatic quality. Visceral pain is deep, dull, and difficult to localize. Ischemic myocardial pain can present with either visceral or somatic qualities. Pain perception and the reaction to pain can vary. Assessment of pain severity can be difficult in the stoic or hysterical patient. Onset and duration of pain can be helpful in narrowing the differential diagnosis. Pain that lasts for only seconds is generally not life-threatening. Likewise, pain that has been constant for days is rarely ischemic.[5]

Symptoms associated with ischemic chest pain include nausea, vomiting, diaphoresis, palpitations, syncope, and dyspnea. Some investigators consider diaphoresis associated with chest pain as a significant predictor of ischemic cardiac pain.[6] The clinician should also inquire about previous episodes of chest pain and compare and contrast this episode to prior episodes.

Past medical history, such as coronary, esophageal, peptic ulcer, hepatobiliary, or pulmonary disease leads to a more focused differential diagnosis. By obtaining a complete

Table 2. Selected Life-Threatening Causes of Chest Pain

Cause	History	Examination	Diagnostic Aids	Treatment	Disposition
Unstable angina	Substernal chest pain (oppressive, dull, heavy), recent onset, changing character of pain; may occur at rest	Usually normal; tachycardia, bradycardia	Electrocardiogram (ECG), graded exercise tolerance test, coronary angiogram	Oxygen, IV, cardiac monitor, pain control with nitroglycerin or morphine sulfate (MS)	Ambulance transfer; admit patient to monitored bed; high risk of infarction and death if untreated
Acute myocardial infarction	Substernal chest pain (severe, crushing), duration longer than 15 min Associated symptoms: diaphoresis, nausea, vomiting, dyspnea, syncope, fatigue	Usually normal; possible signs of congestive heart failure, hypotension; tachycardia, bradycardia	ECG, echocardiogram, cardiac enzymes	Oxygen, IV cardiac monitor, pain control with nitroglycerin or MS, early thrombolytic therapy	Ambulance transfer; admit patient to intensive care unit
Aortic dissection	Severe chest or interscapular pain, sudden onset Predisposing factors: hypertension, pregnancy, coarctation, Marfan's syndrome	Difference in bilateral upper extremity pulses and blood pressures; murmur of aortic insufficiency; possible signs of congestive heart failure; possible focal neurologic signs (present in 30% of cases)	Chest films (may show wide mediastinum, left hemothorax, intimal calcification separated from outer aortic margin) Aortogram Chest CT	Oxygen, IV, cardiac monitor, nitroprusside and beta blockers as needed, surgery	Same
Pulmonary embolus	Pleuritic chest pains, dyspnea, apprehension, cough, hemoptysis, syncope Risk factors: immobilization, prior trauma, cancer, deep venous thrombosis, use of oral contraceptives	Tachypnea, tachycardia, increased loudness of second pulmonic heart sound (S_2P), hypotension, fever, possible phlebitis	Room air (alveolar-arterial) gradient (may be elevated), ECG (may show $S_1Q_3T_3$, or non-specific ST-T changes), chest films (may be normal, show volume loss, pleural effusion, infiltrate, rounded pleural-based density, decreased distal vascular markings), ventilation-perfusion scan, pulmonary angiogram, chest CT	Oxygen, IV, cardiac monitor, heparin or thrombolytic agents	Same
Pneumothorax	Sharp chest pain, sudden onset, dyspnea, cough	Tachypnea, tachycardia, decreased breath sounds, hyperresonance: possible jugular venous distention, signs of tension pneumothorax (i.e., tracheal deviation, hypotension)	Chest films	Oxygen, IV, cardiac monitor, early tube thoracostomy	Ambulance transfer; admit patient to hospital

Table 3. Selected Non–Life-Threatening Causes of Chest Pain

Cause	History	Examination	Diagnostic Aids	Treatment	Disposition
Angina pectoris	Substernal chest that may radiate. Pain is dull, heavy, usually not sharp. Pain is exertional, relieved with rest and nitroglycerin. Duration is 3–10 min; similar to previous episodes of chest pain.	Usually normal	ECG (normal in 50% of cases; should be unchanged from baseline ECG)	Oxygen and nitroglycerin	Home if angina is stable Admission if unstable or increasing in duration or frequency
Pericarditis	Retrosternal chest pain that may radiate. Pain is sharp or dull, has long duration. Dyspnea, recent viral illness.	Fever, improvement of pain by sitting or leaning forward, pericardial rub, possible signs of cardiac tamponade	Complete blood count, blood urea nitrogen, ECG (may show diffuse ST elevation and PR depression), echocardiogram (for pericardial effusion)	Pericardiocentesis for tamponade, aspirin, indomethacin	Ambulance transfer; admit patient to hospital
Esophageal spasm	Chest pain may be similar to that of angina, may be relieved with nitroglycerin; brought on or made worse by alcohol or cold liquids Dysphagia	Usually normal	Esophagoscopy	May need to treat as angina or myocardial infarction if diagnosis is not certain IV glucagon	Ambulance transfer; admit patient to hospital if ischemic heart disease cannot be ruled out
Chest wall syndrome	Sharp chest pain that is generally short-lived and worsens with activity, position changes, respiratory effort	Local tenderness to palpation	Nonspecific	Heat, aspirin, nonsteroidal anti-inflammatory drugs (NSAIDs), steroids	Home
Rib fractures	History of chest wall trauma, pleuritic chest pain, dyspnea	Point tenderness of chest wall, anteroposterior and lateral-lateral chest compression painful, tachypnea, tachycardia; possible organ damage	Chest films (50% of single rib fractures are missed) Suspect neurovascular injuries with fractures of ribs 1–3 and visceral damage with fractures of ribs 9–12	Treat complications, (i.e., pneumothorax, hemothorax, pulmonary contusion, cardiac contusion)	Admit patient to hospital for complications; otherwise, home with pain control
Palpitations	Pounding, skipping sensation Emotional stress Use of tobacco, coffee, cocaine, bronchodilators, decongestants	Fever, anemia, thyrotoxicosis, murmur (i.e., aortic insufficiency, mitral regurgitation), anxiety	ECG and rhythm strip, complete blood count, glucose level, urine toxin screen, thyroid function tests	Education Eliminate cause if possible	Home if hemodynamics and ECG are benign

(Cont'd on next page)

Table 3. Selected Non–Life-Threatening Causes of Chest Pain *(Continued)*

Cause	History	Examination	Diagnostic Aids	Treatment	Disposition
Endocarditis	Nonspecific complaints of long duration (i.e., fatigue, malaise, weight loss, fevers, sweats) History of valvular disease, IV drug use	Possible signs of heart failure, fever, microvascular or petechial lesions, new murmur or change in existing murmur, splenomegaly	Complete blood count, sedimentation rate, uric acid measurements, blood cultures	Antibiotics Surgery if needed	Ambulance transfer for hospital admission

list of medications, you are often able to decipher a significant portion of the patient's medical history. The social history should specifically contain information about tobacco and cocaine use. Identify risk factors for coronary artery disease, such as cigarette smoking, hypertension, diabetes, hypercholesterolemia, or a family history of ischemic heart disease.

Physical Examination

Next to the history, more information is gleaned from a careful physical exam than any other diagnostic aid. Information gained in the history steers the physical examination. Specific areas on which to focus include an assessment of the patient's airway, breathing, and circulation (ABCs), as described in the American Heart Association's Advanced Cardiac Life Support (ACLS) course. Problems with the ABCs should be corrected as they arise. In addition to a quick but thorough assessment of the ABCs, a detailed examination of the patient's general appearance, cardiovascular system, lungs, abdomen, and extremities should be performed.

The patient's **general appearance and vital signs** are important to note. Sweating, pallor, cyanosis, or decreases in mental status are worrisome signs. Peripheral pulses and blood pressure in both arms as well as with the patient supine and standing may yield valuable data about vascular pathology and intravascular volume. An elevated temperature generally indicates an infectious cause of chest pain. However, myocardial infarction and pulmonary embolus can also cause fever.

Examination of the **heart and cardiovascular system** should start with palpation of the heart. A displaced point of maximum impulse indicates cardiomegaly or hypertrophy. The presence of cardiac thrills point to valvular dysfunction. Auscultation of the heart over each of the respective valves may reveal murmurs. S_3 or S_4 gallops may indicate congestive heart failure or decreased ventricular compliance, respectively. Loss of physiologic splitting of the S_2 heart sound is a sign of ischemic dysfunction. Rubs point to pericardial disease. In addition to the examination of the heart, inspection of the neck for jugulovenous distention and carotid pulse is important.

Examination of the **chest and lungs** must include inspection, palpation, percussion, and auscultation. The patient must be disrobed for thorough inspection and examination. Intercostal muscle retraction and use of accessory respiratory muscles indicate respiratory compromise. Focal chest wall tenderness and crepitation point to chest wall syndromes and pneumothorax, respectively. Dullness to percussion leads to consideration of an effusion or infiltrate. Focal hyperresonance is evident only with a large pneumothorax. If rales are present on auscultation, coupled with jugulovenous distention and peripheral edema, congestive heart failure is likely. Focal rales point to consolidation and collapse of lung tissue, as in pneumonia. Other signs of consolidation include egophony and tactile fremitus. Expiratory rhonchi indicate an airflow obstruction, as in asthma or emphysema.

Examination of the **abdomen and extremities** may suggest further diagnostic possibilities. Peptic ulcer disease, cholelithiasis, pancreatitis, and gastritis can cause upper epigastric or chest pain. In addition, examination of the lower extremities is important. Congestive heart failure can result in bilateral edema. Unilateral edema, cords, and pain with palpation of the calf (Homan's sign) suggest deep venous thrombosis; in patients with chest pain, these signs suggest pulmonary embolus as an etiology.

Diagnostic Aids

Ancillary studies can aid the clinician in the work-up of chest pain when used appropriately. Their central use should be to confirm or rule out a limited number of differential diagnoses. Tools for the diagnosis of chest pain in the urgent care physician's armamentarium include the resting electrocardiogram, chest radiograph, and basic laboratory studies.

Obtaining an **electrocardiogram** (ECG) should be routine in the evaluation of all patients with acute chest pain unless the cause is clearly of a noncardiac nature.[1] The ECG can be normal in up to half of patients with coronary artery disease; it is therefore important to use the ECG as an ancillary test only and not to rule out ischemic chest pain solely on the basis of a normal ECG.[7] A detailed review of ECG interpretation is beyond the scope of this chapter. However, ECG interpretation should start with an assessment of rate, rhythm, and axis. Next, examine the QRS morphology. It may show signs of intraventricular conduction delay or bundle-branch block. ST-segment elevation and T-wave inversion are difficult to evaluate in the presence of left bundle-branch block. Finally, review the ST-segments and T-waves for signs of ischemia or injury. The definitive sign of ischemia is ST-segment elevation greater than 1 mm in contiguous leads. Concordant ST-segment elevation in the face of left bundle-branch block is also worrisome. Other non-specific signs of injury include hyperacute T-waves, ST-segment depression, inverted T-waves, or Q-waves. If past ECGs are available, comparison with present ECGs is useful. Any changes should be concerning.

The **chest radiograph** is most helpful in diagnosing pulmonary, pleural, or bony causes of chest pain. It is diagnostic of pneumothorax, rib fractures, infiltrates, and effusions. Increased heart size and pulmonary-vasculature cephalization aid in the diagnosis of congestive heart failure.

Laboratory studies are of little use in the urgent care setting. Elevation of the alveolar-arterial (A-a) oxygen gradient from an arterial-blood gas sample may suggest pulmonary embolism. Unfortunately, the A-a gradient is not sensitive or specific enough to confirm or rule out a suspected diagnosis of pulmonary embolism. Complete blood counts can point toward infectious causes of chest pain. Cardiac markers are rarely available in the urgent care center. If they are available, a single low level should not be used to rule out myocardial ischemia.

Management

Obviously, a complete description of all management options for the many causes of chest pain is beyond the scope of this chapter. Approach each patient with acute chest pain as having a life-threatening condition. Such patients need to take priority over other, less urgent patients. If there are problems with the ABCs, resuscitation should begin immediately, following standard ACLS guidelines.[8] If the initial presentation is judged to be significant or if vital signs are abnormal, oxygen therapy, intravenous access, and cardiac monitoring should be initiated as soon as possible. Interventions may need to take place before the history and physical examination are completed.

Time is of the essence in cardiac ischemia. Unless it is contraindicated by allergy, administer an aspirin to all patients suspected of having ischemia as a cause of chest pain. Treat ischemic pain with sublingual nitroglycerin and morphine sulfate within blood pressure constraints. Arrange transfer to a hospital via ambulance for further diagnosis and treatment.

Disposition

Disposition is intimately related to diagnosis. In essence, only two possibilities exist. Either the diagnosis is apparent or it is not. In some cases, there is no doubt that the patient requires admission to a hospital because of life-threatening chest pain. Likewise, if the diagnosis is clearly not life-threatening, implement appropriate treatment and arrange for discharge. All patients need referral for follow-up care after discharge.

The greatest challenge arises when the diagnosis is not immediately clear. No single diagnostic criterion is uniformly effective at predicting low-risk patients. Telephone consultation with the patient's primary care physician and local emergency medicine physicians may be helpful. If exclusion of potentially life-threatening causes of chest pain is impossible, transfer the patient to an emergency department for further evaluation. Transfer should be by ambulance personnel, not by private car.

Pitfalls in Practice

Errors can occur in the diagnosis, management and disposition of patients with chest pain. **Errors in diagnosis** typically result from overreliance on negative results from ancillary studies to identify low-risk patients. As stated earlier, ancillary studies are neither sensitive nor specific enough to diagnose many causes of chest pain. The rate of false-negative errors can be unacceptably high. The clinician may fail to recognize chest pain emergencies. **Errors in treatment** stem from misdiagnosis or failure to manage problems appropriately as they arise. Delay of appropriate therapy results in increased risks of preventable disease progression and complications of therapy. The most serious **error of disposition** is typically inappropriate discharge.

References

1. American College of Emergency Physicians: Clinical policy for the initial approach to adults presenting with a chief compliant of chest pain, with no history of trauma. Ann Emerg Med 25:274–299, 1995.
2. Burnum M: Evaluation of chest pain. In Goroll AH, May LA, Mulley AG (eds): Primary Care Medicine, 3rd ed. Philadelphia, Lippincott-Raven, 1995, pp 94–101.
3. Ferri F: Differential diagnosis of chest pain. In Ferri FF (ed): Practical Guide to the Care of the Medical Patient, 3rd ed. St. Louis, Mosby, 1995, pp 51–52.
4. Plotnick GD, Fisher ML: Risk stratification: A cost-effective approach to the treatment of patients with chest pain. Arch Intern Med 145:41–42, 1985.
5. Aufderhiede TP, Gibler WB: Acute ischemic coronary syndrome. In Rosen P, Barkin RM, et al (eds): Emergency Medicine: Concepts and Clinical Practice, 4th ed. St. Louis, Mosby, 1998, pp 1655–1716.
6. Goldman L, Weinberg M, Weisberg M, et al: A computer-derived protocol to aid in the diagnosis of emergency room patients with acute chest pain. N Engl J Med 307:588, 1982.
7. Lee TH, Cook E, Weisberg M, et al: Acute chest pain in the emergency room—Identification and examination of low-risk patients. Arch Intern Med 145:65–69, 1985.
8. American Heart Association: Advanced Cardiac Life Support. Dallas, AHA, 2000.

Chapter 4

Evaluation of Abdominal Complaints

Joseph E. Clinton, MD
Daniel T. O'Laughlin, MD

The urgent care patient commonly presents with vague, perplexing complaints referable to the abdomen or anorectal area. Pain, gastrointestinal dysfunction, fever, and bleeding may be present in varying combinations. Numerous conditions and agents are possible causes of the presenting complaints. The physician must work from the general to the specific in a rapidly narrowing search for the correct diagnosis. Tools applied to the search are patient history, physical examination, and, if necessary, laboratory and radiologic studies. Once a confident diagnosis has been reached, rational therapy can be administered.

The goals of urgent care evaluation of patients with abdominal and anorectal complaints are threefold: (1) to determine whether the patient has an abdominal problem requiring emergent surgery or medical stabilization, (2) to begin diagnostic evaluation of patients with nonsurgical abdominal problems, and (3) to provide supportive and definitive treatment to patients with established diagnoses.

Abdominal Pain

The potential causes of abdominal pain are numerous. Sources for abdominal pain are not limited to the intra-abdominal organs. Extra-abdominal organ systems such as the cardiovascular and pulmonary systems, frequently have abdominal pain as the presenting complaint. The history and physical findings usually narrow the search quickly to a few possibilities. Further laboratory or radiologic examination may lead to a definitive diagnosis. If not, at least a confident classification of disease severity and the need for surgical intervention should result from such examination.

Differential Diagnosis. History and Physical Examination. The cause of abdominal pain is often strongly suggested by the historical findings. Gathering certain important differential information is essential for every patient with abdominal pain (Table 1, next page). Although the usual approach to history taking is to use open-ended questions, it is more efficient to ask direct questions about these items in the urgent care setting. For example, a thorough menstrual and pregnancy history is seldom elicited without direct questioning.

The initial task of the physical examination is to differentiate patients with an acute problem requiring immediate surgery or major medical intervention from those with less

Table 1. Historical Information in Abdominal Pain

Women	All patients *(cont.)*
Last menstrual period, including time and character	Duration of pain
Parity	Previous episodes
Contraceptive use and type	Appetite
All patients	Last bowel movement
Fever, chills, sweats	Melena or hematochezia
Onset of pain	Urinary complaints
Character	Medication history
Is the pain constant or intermittent?	Any medical history that includes HIV, inflammatory bowel
Radiation of pain	disease, cancer, cholelithiasis, pancreatitis, or renal disease
Severity	Surgical history, specifically abdominal surgery
Aggravating factors	Acquaintances or family members with similar problem
Alleviating factors	

serious disease. Important signs and symptoms of acute abdominal problems requiring emergent surgery are listed in Table 2. Physical examination may be all that is necessary to be sure of the diagnosis. Physical findings must be interpreted in the context of any underlying disease states.

Table 2. Symptoms and Signs of an Acute Surgical Abdomen

History and Symptoms	Signs
Pain	Localized pain
Rebound	Percussive tenderness
Characteristic progression	Absent bowel sounds
Duration < 48 hours	Persistent findings
Followed by vomiting	Progressive findings
Anorexia	
Emesis	Free air on abdominal x-ray
Persistent, progressive	
Absence of diarrhea	
Advanced age	
Prior surgical procedure	
Decreased bowel movement	

Examination should begin with a review of the patient's vital signs. Evidence of fever, hypotension, tachycardia, and/or tachypnea requires further evaluation and, when significant, necessitates transfer of the patient to an emergency department (ED). Observation of the patient's posture at rest gives an indication of the degree of abdominal distress. The abdomen should be observed to assess the degree of distention. Bowel sound presence and activity are important clues to the diagnosis. Palpation and percussion of the abdomen indicate the likelihood of peritonitis and its location. An examination attempting to identify peritonitis is best performed by gentle percussion of the abdomen rather than by attempting to elicit "rebound pain" by deep palpation and sudden release.[1] Rectal examination with testing of the stool for blood must be routine. Likewise, pelvic examination should be performed on nearly all women who present with abdominal pain. Exceptions occur only when the diagnosis is certain. Tables 3 and 4 list many causes of abdominal pain that present with localizing or diffuse signs and symptoms.

Table 3. Common Causes of Localized Abdominal Pain

Quadrant	Right	Left	Either or Both
Upper	Hepatitis	Gastritis	Lower lobe pneumonia
	Liver congestion	Gastric ulcer	Pulmonary emboli
	Hepatic abscess	Splenic infarction	Pancreatitis
	Leaking duodenal ulcer	Splenic rupture (delayed)	Myocardial ischemia
	Gallbladder disease	Leaking splenic artery aneurysm	Myocardial infarction
	Retrocecal appendicitis	Mononucleosis	Renal stones
		Diverticulitis	Subphrenic abscess
Lower	Gallbladder disease	Diverticulitis	Ureteral stones
	Mesenteric adenitis	Volvulus	Aortic aneurysm
	Regional enteritis		Testicular torsion
	Meckel's diverticulum		Epididymitis
	Appendicitis		Prostatitis
	Leaking duodenal ulcer		Cystitis
			Pelvic inflammatory disease
			Tubo-ovarian abscess
			Ectopic pregnancy
			Dysmenorrhea
			Mittelschmerz
			Ovarian cyst

Table 4. Causes of Non-localizing Abdominal Pain

Mesenteric ischemia	Hematoma	Carcinomatosis	Gastroenteritis
Diffuse peritonitis	Retroperitoneal	Colitis	Intestinal obstruction
Hemoperitoneum	Mesenteric	Conversion reaction	Inflammatory bowel disease

Diagnostic Aids. Diagnostic studies alone rarely identify the source of abdominal pain. When diagnostic testing is performed, results should be considered in conjunction with the history and physical exam. A urine pregnancy test should be performed for every woman of child-bearing age who presents with abdominal pain. The only exception to this rule is a woman who has had a total abdominal hysterectomy. Urinalysis should be obtained in any patient with urinary tract complaints or lower abdominal or flank pain. Consider obtaining the urinalysis by catheter if potential contamination is a concern. In general, the complete blood count (CBC) is notoriously misleading in the context of abdominal pain and should not be obtained unless the results will alter the course of management. However, a CBC with differential can be useful in some subgroups such as elderly or immunocompromised patients. Leukocytosis in such patients with abdominal pain is worrisome. Serum lipase or pancreatic amylase can be useful in distinguishing pancreatitis from other sources of abdominal pain. However, the decision to discharge or transfer a patient to the hospital for pancreatitis should be based on clinical grounds, not on laboratory values. Hepatic function testing can help to distinguish cholecystitis, obstructive cholelithiasis, and hepatitis. Evaluation of serum electrolytes, blood urea nitrogen, and serum creatinine should be reserved for patients who appear ill, have underlying medical problems or have any change in mental status, or have been ill for longer than 24 hours. An electrocardiogram should be obtained in patients with upper abdominal pain without a clear cause.

Although abdominal films are infrequently diagnostic in the entire patient group, they should be obtained when the possibility of obstruction or ruptured viscus is entertained.

Patients may need to be referred if further diagnostic testing is indicated. Abdominal ultrasonography can be helpful in the diagnosis of pelvic pain in young women of childbearing age to demonstrate an intrauterine pregnancy or to evaluate for adnexal pathology. Abdominal pain due to cholecystitis also may be diagnosed by ultrasonography of the gallbladder. The abdominal computed tomographic (CT) scan gives excellent visualization of the retroperitoneal structures, liver, and spleen. The CT scan also is frequently used to assist in the assessment of abdominal pain that may be caused by appendicitis, but is not clinically clear.

Management. Patients with a problem requiring emergent surgery must be stabilized and transported by ambulance to a facility capable of the necessary surgery. Local circumstances dictate the best site for surgical evaluation. In most cases, evaluation occurs after transfer. Prompt surgical attention should be sought in all cases in which the urgent care evaluation suggests a surgical diagnosis.

Management of patients with nonsurgical conditions is highly dependent on the presumed diagnosis. Supportive care with close follow-up is often practiced when the cause is uncertain. The urgent care physician must arrange careful follow-up to avoid missed diagnoses of serious conditions. If timely follow-up with a primary physician cannot be arranged, the patient should be re-evaluated in an ED in 8–12 hours—sooner if the pain worsens. Dietary manipulation and antacid therapy are often of value when peptic disease or gastroenteritis is suspected. Analgesics may be useful in gynecologic or urinary conditions but should be avoided when a gastrointestinal diagnosis is suspected. The analgesics appropriate for outpatient management of abdominal pain are the nonnarcotic anti-inflammatory agents and antipyretics. Use of these agents is limited, however, by their tendency to aggravate gastrointestinal complaints. Severe pain believed to require narcotic therapy may imply the need for surgical evaluation.

Pitfalls in Practice. Appropriate disposition and follow-up are sometimes more important than the final diagnosis. A diagnosis of abdominal pain of unclear etiology is better than an inappropriate more benign diagnosis (i.e., gastroenteritis, constipation, urinary tract infection), which may bias subsequent work-up and management. Patients in higher risk groups, such as the elderly and the immunocompromised, require a more detailed evaluation and close follow-up if a firm diagnosis cannot be made. Diagnoses that may represent a need for emergent surgical intervention or a potential threat to life need to be ruled out by history, physical exam, and available ancillary studies before the patient is discharged. If these cannot be ruled out, the patient should be transferred to an appropriate facility where further evaluation can be obtained. Patients in whom a diagnosis of early appendicitis, cholecystitis, or other surgical complaint is suspected should be re-examined in 12–24 hours if symptoms do not resolve.

VOMITING

Differential Diagnosis. Noxious stimuli to the gastrointestinal tract often result in nonspecific manifestations of vomiting, diarrhea, or both. The presentation is so common that the urgent care physician must start with a broad differential diagnosis (Table 5). Vomiting may result from direct gastric irritation with increased peristalsis or from gastric atony due to ileus or bowel obstruction.

Table 5. Emesis Syndromes

Condition	Presentation	Examination	Etiology	Diagnosis	Treatment	Follow-Up
Appendicitis	Anorexia, peri-umbilical to right lower quadrant pain, no stools.	Right lower quadrant tenderness, decreased bowel sounds.	Infected appendix; appendo-lithiasis.	Clinical suspicion with compatible history and examination. Leukocytosis often present.	Appendectomy; observe if not sure.	Monitor for return of appetite; monitor for recurrent post-op fever.
Gastro-enteritis	Malaise, myalgia; diarrhea often present as well. Epidemic occurrence.	Nontender abdomen, hyperactive bowel sounds, low-grade fever. Condition usually not toxic.	Self-limited viral infection; rotavirus; enterovirus; adenovirus; Norwalk agent.	Compatible history and examination.	Supportive. Avoid dairy products. Liquid diet until symp-toms abate, then pro-gressive diet.	Reevaluate vomiting lasting more than 24 hours.
Gastric outlet obstruction	Vomiting shortly after eating, little nausea, crampy abdominal pain; history of peptic disease or surgery in adults. Bile in vomitus excludes diagnosis.	Peritoneal findings sug-gest pene-trating ulcer. Abdomen often nontender. Succussion splash may be present.	Infants: congenital pyloric stenosis. Adults: scarring due to peptic ulcer disease; tumor.	Compatible history and examination. Abdominal film showing distention, endoscopy.	Nasogastric suction, intravenous hydration, surgery.	Hospitalize for acute treatment.
Small bowel obstruction	Spasmodic epigastric or periumbilical pain; early, severe bilious vomiting. Distension late. Feculent vomitus if low small intestine obstruction.	Distention, tympanitic to percussion, pain variable, rushes and tinkles on auscultation; bowel sounds decreased late in course.	Adhesions; hernia; tumor; intussus-ception.	Flat and upright abdominal films, ladder-like pattern on abdominal films, distended loops in small bowel, minimal gas in colon.	Nasogastric suction, barium enema in intussus-ception, surgery.	Hospitalize for acute treatment.
Large bowel obstruction	Vomiting late, feculent: abdominal distention.	Similar to small bowel obstruction.	Strangulated hernia; intus-susception; carcinoma; volvulus; abscess.	Abdominal films, barium enema. Colonoscopy	As above.	Hospitalize for acute treatment.
Vascular catastrophe	Varied pain response; patient usually in distress.	Ischemia, dif-fuse findings; hemorrhage, expanding mass.	Mesenteric thrombosis; ruptured abdominal aortic aneu-rysm; splenic artery aneurysm.	Laparotomy, plain abdom-inal film, abdominal ultrasonog-raphy.	Emergency surgery.	Hospitalize for acute treatment.

(Cont'd on next page)

Table 5. Emesis Syndromes

Condition	Presentation	Examination	Etiology	Diagnosis	Treatment	Follow-Up
Drug-induced	Often other effects apparent (e.g., vision changes); dysrhythmia with digitalis, theophylline.	History of drug use or ingestion, related effects.	Ingested agent.	History, serum levels.	Specific for drug.	Psychiatric evaluation if ingestion was intentional.
Ileus	Abdominal distention, vomiting Patient may have dull pain.	Abdominal distention, bowel sounds absent, abdomen tympanitic.	Electrolyte imbalance; reflex ileus (e.g., vertebral fracture with ileus).	Differentiate from infarction.	Nasogastric suction, fluid replacement, correction of electrolyte imbalance when present.	Prevention; monitor hydration. Probable hospitalization.
Hepatitis	Right upper quadrant tenderness, possible dermatitis; icterus often present.	Right upper quadrant tenderness, palpable liver.	Hepatitis virus	Hepatic enzyme elevation, jaundice.	Supportive, usually outpatient management; high caloric diet best tolerated in morning. Hospitalize for dehydration, toxicity. Restrict activity.	Monitor laboratory enzymes, antigen and antibody status.
Peptic ulcer disease	Burning epigastric pain. Pain is frequently relieved by vomiting. Vomiting may occur during or soon after food ingestion.	Generally epigastric discomfort with palpation. Peritoneal findings suggest perforation of ulcer.	Multifactorial	Clinical suspicion with compatible history and examination.	Initial treatment of uncomplicated episodes includes liquid antacids and H_2 receptor antagonist.	Hospitalization for any complicated episodes (hemorrhage, perforation, pyloric stenosis).
Pancreatitis	Moderate to severe epigastric pain, hypotension in severe cases.	Epigastric pain	Chronic alcohol abuse, biliary tract disease; mumps; toxins.	Serum lipase	Nasogastric suction; maintain hydration, treat underlying cause.	Monitor for pseudocyst formation, treat alcoholism.
Cholecystitis	Fatty food intolerance, right upper quadrant pain to scapula; episodic.	Right upper quadrant pain, Murphy's sign; gallbladder palpable in 30–70% of cases; possible icterus.	Cholelithiasis; bacterial invasion.	Ultrasonography, CT scan for stones, technetium scan of biliary tree.	Meperidine for pain, antibiotics if suppuration suspected.	Hospitalization and monitor for infectious complications.
Reye's syndrome	Emesis, lethargy after viral illness, influenza.	Lethargy, dehydration, signs of increased intracranial pressure. Hepatomegaly may be present.	Infection (influenza virus, varicella); salicylate use associated.	Serum ammonia level, serum glucose level, intracranial pressure measurement, liver biopsy.	Aggressive intracranial pressure control, serum glucose maintenance, intensive care.	Hospitalize for acute treatment.

(Cont'd on next page)

Table 5. Emesis Syndromes *(Continued)*

Condition	Presentation	Examination	Etiology	Diagnosis	Treatment	Follow-Up
Intracranial processes	Vomiting may be without nausea, associated neurologic deficits, vertigo.	Dysarthria, ataxia, mixed cranial nerve findings.	Hemorrhage into or ischemia of posterior fossa and brainstem, elevated intracranial pressure, hydrocephalus, intracranial lesions and meningitis.	CT scan of head Consider lumbar puncture as indicated after CT scan obtained.	Neurosurgical intensive care may be needed. Patient may require emergency decompression of hemorrhages if mass effect.	
Migraine headache	History of migraines; improved after sleep.	No neurologic deficit or signs of intracranial pressure increase, normal examination.	Vascular	Diagnosis of exclusion of more serious etiologies.	Ergotamine, 1 mg orally; repeat to maximum of 5 mg per attack, 20 mg/wk. Droperidol 2.5 mg with diphenhydramine 25 mg both intramuscularly.	Neurologic follow-up mandatory.
Meniere's syndrome, labyrinthitis	Whirling vertigo, nausea, vomiting, tinnitus, sensorineuronal hearing loss.	Nystagmus; hearing loss may be present.	Unknown; distention of membranous labyrinth.	Exclude vertigo basilar etiology, posterior fossa mass; differentiate postural vertigo, labyrinthitis.	Salt restriction, diuretics, antihistamine.	Neurologic and otolaryngologic evaluation mandatory.
Ischemic heart disease	Nausea, vomiting, gastrointestinal upset usually associated with low chest or upper abdominal discomfort.	Diaphoresis may be present; abdominal examination normal; S4 gallop may be heard.	Myocardial infarction; angina due to atherosclerotic heart disease.	Index of suspicion, electrocardiogram.	Oxygen, nitroglycerin, and morphine sulfate. In addition, give ASA 325 mg orally if able.	Admission to cardiac care unit.
Diabetes mellitus, gastroparesis	Vomiting several hours after meals.	Examination unremarkable; gastric distention may be present.	Delayed gastric emptying due to autonomic neuropathy.	Typical history; differentiate from early outlet obstruction.	Nasogastric suction; assess diabetic control.	Close diabetic control.
Addison's disease	Weakness, hyperpigmentation, hypotension; diarrhea associated.	Hyperpigmentation, postural hypotension.	Adrenal insufficiency	Physical/laboratory findings: hypotension, hypoglycemia, hyponatremia, hyperkalemia, hypercalcemia, serum cortisol, adrenocorticotropic hormone levels	Crystalloid volume replacement; correct hypoglycemia, electrolyte disturbance; glucocorticoid administration.	Maintenance steroids Admission may be required

History and Physical Examination. Historical inquiry should seek to characterize the emesis. Bilious emesis may indicate an obstruction distal to the ampulla of Vater. Bilious emesis is often present with pyloric obstruction, however, because the obstruction is usually incomplete. Bloody emesis, whether red or coffee-ground in appearance, indicates bleeding proximal to the ligament of Treitz.[2] Feculent emesis indicates a colonic obstruction that has been present for some time. The frequency of emesis gives the physician an idea of the severity of the gastrointestinal disturbance. A history of isolated early-morning vomiting may suggest the diagnosis of pregnancy or uremia. Intermittent projectile vomiting without nausea may suggest the diagnosis of increased intracranial pressure with hydrocephalus. Other pertinent historical data that should be obtained are listed in Table 6.

Table 6. Historical Information for the Differentiation of Vomiting

Age	Any changes in stool habits?
When does the vomiting occur?	Any fevers?
How often and for how long?	Any weight loss?
Is there any abdominal pain?	What does the emesis look like?
Central nervous system findings (i.e., head-	Any chest discomfort or shortness of breath?
ache, unsteady gait, focal weakness)?	Any dysuria?
How does eating affect the vomiting?	Last menstrual period (if female)?

Associated symptoms may indicate the cause of the emesis. Headache or other neurologic symptoms occurring with emesis suggest a central nervous system etiology, such as migraine headache or increased intracranial pressure. Vertigo followed by vomiting suggests a middle ear disorder, such as infection, Ménière's syndrome, or a posterior fossa mass. Associated neurologic deficit, ataxia, dysarthria, or diplopia should prompt consideration of posterior fossa cerebrovascular accident or mass lesion. If vomiting is thought to be secondary to intracranial pathology, a detailed neurologic examination is required and a CT scan of the head must be obtained.

Vomiting that occurs immediately after a meal may be related to peptic ulcer disease or psychogenic causes. Vomiting that is delayed more than 1 hour after meals may be related to gastric outlet obstruction or motility disorders.

A medical history of similar problems may provide an established diagnosis and give important clues about the expected course of the presumed recurrence. A family history of similar complaints may be helpful in establishing a diagnosis in patients with a first-time presentation.

Age is an important factor affecting the differential diagnosis. Malrotation, Meckel's diverticulum, and pyloric stenosis must be considered in the very young. Ischemic bowel disease, diverticulitis, and adenocarcinoma are etiologic considerations only in older patients. The diagnosis of appendicitis is frequently overlooked in elders, apparently because other possibilities receive greater attention[3] and presentation is often atypical.[4]

Protracted vomiting after a minor illness should raise suspicion of Reye's syndrome, especially during influenza season. Associated somnolence and history of aspirin use during the preceding illness should heighten the suspicion of Reye's syndrome.[5]

Associated disease may produce abdominal pain and secondary vomiting. Atherosclerosis may produce ischemia and infarction of the bowel. Hematologic disease may affect spleen size and fragility. Anticoagulants or coagulopathy may lead to occult hemorrhage and abdominal complaints. Adverse drug reaction is a common cause of abdominal complaints. Associated disease and drug history are important historical data.

Many legitimate drugs may produce abdominal complaints. Gastric irritants such as alcohol, aspirin, and nonsteroidal anti-inflammatory agents are common offenders. Theophylline preparations or digoxin may be responsible. Accidental ingestion by children or dependent adults should be considered. Street drugs and their adulterants may be the direct cause of gastrointestinal dysfunction, or it may be produced indirectly through improper administration.

The association of nausea, emesis, and abdominal pain places appendicitis high in the differential diagnosis. Right upper quadrant pain after consumption of fatty foods should prompt a search for cholecystitis. Conversely, the association of malaise, myalgia, and diarrhea may signify a relatively benign case of viral gastroenteritis, especially if experience indicates that an epidemic of the disease is current in the community.

Prior surgery should prompt consideration of bowel obstruction due to adhesion formation. Simple abdominal radiography may confirm such a suspicion. Feculent vomiting with abdominal distention suggests an obstruction in the large bowel. History may help in the diagnosis of emesis of endocrine origin. The diabetic patient may develop gastroparesis as a complication of diabetes. When this occurs, hospitalization may be necessary.[6] A patient who appears to be hyperpigmented, complains of weakness, and has orthostatic hypotension may have Addison's disease.

Physical examination of the patient with vomiting or diarrhea includes assessment of the degree of distention of the abdomen, bowel and vascular sounds, and location and quality of the pain. Distention of the abdomen indicates dilated intestines or an extraluminal collection of air or fluid (ascitic, exudative, or blood).

Auscultation can reveal important information. Hyperactive bowel sounds indicate some form of enteritis. High-pitched tinkles and rushes suggest obstruction. The presence of a bruit may indicate aortic disease compromising blood supply to the gut.

Initial light palpation of the abdomen localizes the pain and allows the examiner to get an idea of the location of voluntary guarding. Tenderness to gentle percussion may identify peritoneal irritation. Murphy's sign in cholecystitis (right upper quadrant tenderness on inspiration) and Rovsing's sign in appendicitis (pain in the right lower quadrant while the examiner is palpating the left lower quadrant) are examples of peritoneal irritation.

Bloody emesis should prompt a search for the site and amount of bleeding. Gastric intubation should be performed to confirm the complaint. Endoscopy eventually determines whether the esophagus, stomach, or duodenum is the source.

Diagnostic Aids. History and physical examination are often not sufficient to characterize the patient presenting with emesis. Laboratory considerations are similar to those discussed with abdominal pain. Blood count and urinalysis are important screening tools. Gastrointestinal fluid losses and electrolyte losses may be significant in the patient with emesis. Accordingly, serum electrolytes should be evaluated. Likewise, arterial blood gas determination may be necessary to detect metabolic alkalosis. Serum ammonia levels should be obtained if Reye's syndrome is a possibility.

The middle-aged person at risk for cardiovascular disease should receive an electrocardiogram when the cause of vomiting is obscure. The urgent care physician must always remain sensitive to nausea and vomiting as presenting symptoms of cardiac disease.[7] An awareness that cardiac disease can occur in younger patients also needs to be maintained.

Radiologic studies are subject to the same considerations described above for abdominal pain. Patients with gastroenteritis frequently display the troublesome radiologic findings of air in the small bowel. When air in the bowel is seen in this context, clinical correlation is necessary. Air-fluid levels in the small bowel demand evaluation of the possibility of peritonitis or bowel obstruction. The amount of air seen in gastroenteritis is small, without dilation of bowel loops or significant air fluid levels. Air and fluid located in the distal ileum and cecum suggest appendicitis. Dilation of the cecum and ileum associated with right lower quadrant haze is called appendiceal ileus because of its association with the disease.[8] Sentinel loops in the left upper quadrant in the area of the proximal jejunum suggest pancreatitis, but the findings are present in only a minority of cases. The sign is nonspecific but, if present, contributes to the total clinical picture.[9]

Abdominal radiographs must be scrutinized for presence or loss of psoas shadows as an indication of peritonitis. Flank stripes and "dog ears" signs indicate intraperitoneal fluid accumulation. Flank stripes are seen as separations of the colon gas from the peritoneal fat stripe by a gap that represents fluid. The normal situation is for the colon to abut the peritoneal fat. Collection of fluid around the bladder gives the appearance of a dog's head with two ears protruding superiorly. The "ears" are the fluid collections, and the "head" is the bladder.

Free air on abdominal radiographs is best demonstrated by placing the patient in the left lateral decubitus position for 10–20 minutes before taking the film. A second film is taken with the patient in the upright position to reveal any collection of air between the liver and diaphragm. This technique has been shown to demonstrate as little as one milliliter of intra-abdominal air.[10] If the patient is ambulatory, an upright chest film is the optimal choice to demonstrate free intra-abdominal air because of its collection under the diaphragm. The patient with free intra-abdominal air who has had no penetrating wounds of the abdomen has a ruptured viscus until proved otherwise. Barring history or physical findings suggesting a source of the free air remote from the abdomen, laparotomy is indicated to repair the ruptured viscus.

Management. The degree of medical intervention is determined by the severity of the disease. Differentiation of surgical emergencies from cases that can be managed medically is the paramount consideration. Most patients can be readily categorized into a surgical or nonsurgical grouping on the basis of the initial evaluation. Nevertheless, the status of certain patients may be indeterminate. Such patients often require observation to determine the severity of the illness. Hospitalization for observation or close outpatient follow-up may be elected, depending on the degree of suspicion and the nature of the disease suspected.

Management always includes supportive therapy. Rehydration therapy and correction of any electrolyte disturbances are the initial steps in treatment. Diagnosis of the specific condition often allows the choice of additional therapy that will cure or curtail the disease. Nonsurgical reasons for hospitalization include metabolic complications of vomiting (e.g., profound dehydration), central nervous system or cardiac effects of electrolyte imbalance, acid-base disturbance, and lack of appropriate care facilities in the home. Specific pharmacologic therapy may be indicated in selected patients. For example, the patient with vertigo may be helped by meclizine (25 mg 3 times/day), which inhibits vestibular system afferent innervation. Phenothiazines inhibit the chemoreceptor trigger zone and decrease afferent impulses from the gastrointestinal tract. Patients should be cautioned about the sedative effect that phenothiazines can cause. Outpatient management requires patient instruction in oral hydration with a clear liquid diet or electrolyte solutions. Whenever outpatient management is elected, close follow-up is mandatory.

Pitfalls in Practice. Failure to perform a rectal and pelvic examination in any patient with abdominal complaints may delay diagnosis and result in significant morbidity. Failure to examine the rest of the patient is a surprisingly frequent mistake made in the evaluation of abdominal complaints. The head and neck, nervous system, lungs, heart, and genitalia may be involved in the disease process and hold important clues to the etiology of vomiting. Diagnosis of neurogenic and metabolic causes of vomiting demands a thorough examination. For example, a strangulated hernia can cause intestinal obstruction, but failure to examine the patient completely may result in missing the diagnosis.

Diarrhea

Differential Diagnosis. Diarrhea is generally defined as abnormally frequent episodes of stooling that contain more water than normal. Most cases of diarrhea seen by the urgent care physician are infectious and occur in epidemic fashion. The approach to patients with diarrheal illness must separate those with benign, self-limited disease from those with an etiology demanding specific therapeutic intervention. Diarrhea of acute onset may be initially evaluated in the urgent care environment but may require further investigation if it does not resolve in a timely fashion. Generally, patients who give a history of chronic diarrhea require an evaluation beyond the capabilities of most urgent care facilities. This section focuses on acute diarrheal syndromes of infectious etiology. Table 7 (next page) describes the most common infectious diarrhea syndromes.

Infectious diarrhea can result from a toxin that diminishes the absorptive capacities of the gut or from direct invasion of the mucosa by the offending agent. The first type of diarrhea is exemplified by staphylococcal food poisoning and enterotoxic *Escherichia coli*. Parasitic disease and bacteria such as *Shigella* species produce diarrhea by direct invasion of the bowel wall.

History and Physical Examination. The most common cause of diarrhea is viral gastroenteritis. The onset is acute and often associated with myalgia and fever. The tendency of the condition to occur in outbreaks simplifies the diagnosis after the first few cases have been seen. The duration of the illness is typically 1–2 days, but it may last as long as 2 weeks.

The presence of mucoid or bloody stools suggests a diagnosis other than viral gastroenteritis. Invasion of the mucosa of the gastrointestinal tract by bacteria or parasites produces this type of exudative diarrhea. The patient appears ill, and sepsis is a possibility. Symptoms typically are longer-lasting and more severe than in viral diarrhea, and the degree of dehydration may be greater.

Outbreaks of diarrhea associated with food intake are common. Staphylococcal food poisoning characteristically occurs 1–8 hours after ingestion of contaminated products. Many people are commonly affected from a common food source. Infections with *Salmonella* and *Campylobacter* species are more commonly associated with poultry products. *Campylobacter* infections may also be seen from ingestion of milk or contaminated

Table 7. Infectious Diarrhea Syndromes

Condition	Presentation	Examination	Etiology	Diagnosis	Treatment	Follow-Up
Viral gastro-enteritis	Acute onset associated fever, malaise, myalgia, nausea, vomiting, diarrhea, cramps, headache.	Low-grade fever, hyperactive bowel sounds, benign abdomen, liquid stool, low white blood cell count in stool, varying degree of dehydration.	Rotavirus, Norwalk agent, enteric adenovirus, astrovirus, calcivirus. Fecal-oral transmission. Common causes of day care diarrhea.	Clinical characteristics, occurring in outbreak, short duration.	ORT Consider 1–2 L IV crystalloid if patient has signs of significant dehydration. Antispasmodic antinauseant (prochlorperazine or promethazine hydrochloride) may help decrease abdominal cramps. Antibiotics and antidiarrheals are not indicated.	Re-examine if diarrhea persists more than 48 hours; obtain stool for examination in such cases. Duration is generally 2–7 days.
Shigellosis	Intense fever, colicky pain, mucoid stools (may be bloody), true dysentary may develop. Within 48–72 hours of exposure, symptoms develop. Peripheral neuropathy in adults and seizures in children have also been seen.	Patient may have high fever, normal to hyperactive bowel sounds, mucoid stools.	*Shigella sonnei* (75%) *S. flexneri; S. dysenteriae.* Fecal-oral transmission. Usually penetrates enterocytes and produces shiga toxin, resulting in cell death and causes sloughing of large intestine. If no penetration occurs, then only a transient diarrhea may occur.	Polymorpho-nucleocytes (PMNs) in stool, shallow mucosal ulcerations. Culture positive in 90% of cases.	Self-limited course, usually does not require antibiotics, but adults with severe symptoms may benefit from ciprofloxacin 500 mg or norfloxacin 400 mg po every 12 hours times three doses.	Symptom resolution, hydration status, infection contacts.
Escherichia coli	Low-grade fever, abdominal cramping, nausea, and gradual or abrupt onset of diarrhea. Pain may be severe with certain types.	May have low-grade fever; normal to hyperactive bowel sounds.	Depending on type of bacteria, bacteria may cause diarrhea by toxin production or direct invasion of intestinal wall. Transmission is via contaminated food and water.	Stool culture, fecal leukocytes may be seen. Specific serotyping can be done it needed.	Frequently a self-limited disease. Treat with ORT. Ciprofloxacin may decrease the duration of disease in adults; however, antibiotics are considered a possible risk factor for developing hemolytic-uremic syndrome in VTEC. Antimotility agents are not indicated.	Usually resolves spontaneously in 2–3 days. Hospitalization in severe cases may be required.

(Cont'd on next page)

Table 7. Infectious Diarrhea Syndromes *(Continued)*

Condition	Presentation	Examination	Etiology	Diagnosis	Treatment	Follow-Up
Salmonel-losis	Nausea, vomiting, fever, cramping abdominal pain; mucoid, watery stools (may be bloody). Incubation, 8–48 hours. Typhoid: fever with relative brady-cardia, head-ache, malaise, abdominal pain, leukopenia, "rose" spots. Incubation is 10–14 days.	Diffuse abdominal tenderness, hyperactive bowel sounds. May affect several members of a family.	*Salmonella* bacteria (e.g., *S. typhi*) most commonly spread by infected food handlers and contaminated eggs and cheese.	PMNs in stool, characteristic outbreak, stool culture.	Antidiarrheal agents (prolong disease) and antibiotics (promote carrier state) are generally contraindicated. Exception is septic condition or serious underlying medical problem. If toxic, hospitalize patient for IV antibiotics. Typhoid: supportive care and ciprofloxa-cin 500 mg po twice a day or ceftriaxone 2 gm IV every day for 5 days. If shock or any change in mental status then add dexamethasone 3 mg/kg initial dose and then 1 mg/kg every 6 hours times eight doses.	Patient may shed organ-isms for weeks. Food handlers and health care workers should not return to work until stool cultures are negative.
Staphylo-coccal food poisoning	Onset 1–8 hours after ingestion; vomiting, abdominal cramping; diarrhea variable.	Diffuse abdominal tenderness (variable).	Enterotoxin; fever; food handler-related infection. Most cases are caused by *S. aureus.* Toxin is pro-duced within a few hours of food left out at room temperature (commonly mayon-naise, ham, potato and egg salad).	Characteristic outbreak, short incubation period, no PMNs in stool.	Supportive care, antiemetics, fluids; antidiarrheal agents not useful because of short course.	Investigate food handler source. Symptoms generally resolve within 6–10 hours.
Campylo-bacter species	Fever, cramping abdominal pain, diarrhea, anorexia, malaise, myalgia, head-ache, watery diarrhea (may be bloody); mimics inflammatory bowel disease. Onset is usually within 3–5 days of exposure.	Diffuse abdominal pain, hyper-active bowel sounds, fever.	*Campylobacter fetus* sub-species *jejuni* and *C. coli;* ingestion of contaminated poultry, milk or water; con-tamination from chickens or wild birds.	PMNs in stool, direct phase contrast microscopy (S-shaped bacteria seen), rule out in new cases of ulcerative colitis.	Most cases resolve spontaneously. Usually symptoms resolve within 2 weeks, but > 25% will relapse within a few weeks. Antibiotics are not commonly needed. May use ciprofloxa-cin 500 mg or norfloxacin 400 mg	Symptomatic follow-up; reculture only if symptoms persist.

(Cont'd on next page)

Table 7. Infectious Diarrhea Syndromes *(Continued)*

Condition	Presentation	Examination	Etiology	Diagnosis	Treatment	Follow-Up
Campylo-bacter species *(cont.)*					every 12 hours for 5 days. May also consider azithromycin 500 mg every day for 3 days or erythromycin stearate 500 mg every day for 5 days.	
Clostridium perfringens	Cramping, diarrhea, myalgia 6–24 hours after food ingestion.	Hyperactive bowel sounds, fever.	Heat stable toxin produced in contaminated food by *C. perfringens;* usually in pre-cooked or poorly reheated meats, poultry and gravies.	Typical history	Supportive; disease is self-limited; usually resolves within 24 hours.	Symptomatic follow-up.
Clostridium difficile	Pseudomem-branous colitis usually within 10 days of anti-biotic therapy or initiation of therapy, but can be longer. Resembles shigellosis.	Resembles shigellosis.	Overgrowth of bacteria after antibiotic use. Frequently seen in children on antibiotics.	Endoscopy, stool toxin assay. History of exposure to antibiotics.	Metronidazole 500 mg 3 times a day for 7–14 days. Vancomycin po 125 mg 4 times a day for 7–14 days as an alternative. Avoid antimotility agents. Discontinue responsible antibiotics if possible.	Symptomatic follow-up.
Yersinia species	Diarrheal illness similar to sal-monellosis; vomiting, colicky pain, fever; stools may be bloody. May cause mesen-teric adenitis mimicking appendicitis, regional enteritis.	Colicky pain, hyperactive bowel sounds.	*Yersinia enterocolitica;* mucosal invasion. Foodborne	Stool culture (requires special techniques).	Avoid antimotility agents. Self-limited diarrhea. Benefit of anti-biotics uncertain, not recommended.	Symptomatic follow-up; watch for abdominal pain.
Vibrio para-haemolyticus	Symptoms vary in severity; low-grade fever, chills, headache, vomiting, diar-rhea, cramping after seafood ingestion; 2–24 hour incubation.	Hyperactive bowel sounds, watery diarrhea.	Transmitted by raw or under-cooked oysters clams, crabs, or other seafood; unknown mechanism.	Typical presentation.	Supportive, liquids. Antibiotic therapy does not shorten course. Usually a self-limited course lasting < 72 hours	Symptomatic follow-up.

(Cont'd on next page)

Table 7. Infectious Diarrhea Syndromes *(Continued)*

Condition	Presentation	Examination	Etiology	Diagnosis	Treatment	Follow-Up
Vibrio cholera	Painless, explosive watery diarrhea. Often described as "rice water" diarrhea. Rapidly progressive to severe dehydration.	Intense watery diarrhea, signs of dehydration.	Food/water transmission. Bacteria produces enterotoxin which results in osmotic diarrhea.	Stool culture	Fluid losses can be 1 L/hour. Aggressive fluid management required with IV lactated Ringer's solution. Use glucose-containing oral solution, ~ 5% strength to stimulate and maintain sodium absorption. Antibiotics will reduce symptoms and speed clearance of organism. Use ciprofloxacin 1 gm as a single dose or norfloxacin 40 mg twice a day for 3 days.	Hospitalization in severe cases may be required.
Entamoeba histolytica	Asymptomatic state or fever, cramps, bloody diarrhea. Symptoms usually develop within 3 days to 2 weeks of contamination. Foul-smelling dysentery (syndrome of tenesmus with bloodstreaked copious watery diarrhea and abdominal pain).	Hyperactive bowel sounds, blood-streaked mucus in stools.	Fecal-oral spread by cysts; trophozoite invades colonic mucosa, producing ulceration. Waterborne. Can invade systemically causing abscess formation usually in the liver, but also brain and elsewhere.	Sigmoidoscopy; stool ova and parasite examination reveals trophozoites. Usually history of travel to an underdeveloped area.	For asymptomatic cases: Paromomycin 500 mg 3 times a day for 7 days or Iodoquinol 650 mg 3 times a day for 20 days. If diarrhea or dysentery: metronidazole 750 mg 3 times a day for 10 days, followed by Paromomycin or Iodoquinol as above.	Follow for relapse.
Giardia lamblia	Most common parasitic infection. Bloating, urge to defecate, cramping. Watery diarrhea, flatulence, anorexia, and nausea. Symptoms develop 1–3 weeks after exposure. Occasionally cholecystitis will develop.	Foul-smelling, frothy diarrhea; cysts passed in stool.	Fecal-oral spread; infected stream water; protozoa invades mucosa.	Demonstrate cysts in stool by ova or parasite examination. May need up to three specimens because cyst shedding is intermittent. Giardial antigen in the stool.	Metronidazole, 15 mg/kg in three divided doses, maximum dose of 250 mg 3 times a day for 5 days or albendazole 400 mg every day for 5 days.	Symptomatic follow-up; re-examine stools only if symptoms persist. Chronic infections are not uncommon.

(Cont'd on next page)

Table 7. Infectious Diarrhea Syndromes *(Continued)*

Condition	Presentation	Examination	Etiology	Diagnosis	Treatment	Follow-Up
Crypto-sporidium species	Profuse, watery diarrhea; common animal diarrhea agent. Three settings: people working with animals, children in day care, immuno-suppressed patients.	Nonbloody diarrhea; evidence of depressed immunity often but not always present.	Acquired by ingestion of oocysts; noninvasive; toxin. Fecal-oral transmission.	Acid-fast stain of stool for oocysts. Suspect in children in late summer, early fall.	Supportive care; remove immuno-suppressing drugs if possible. In healthy host it is self-limited. Major cause of chronic diarrhea in immuno-compromised patient.	Consider cause of immuno-deficiency.
Cyclospora cayetan-ensis	Watery, non-bloody diarrhea that begins days or weeks after foreign travel. Onset abrupt or gradual. Nausea, vomiting, anorexia, bloating, abdom-inal cramping, fatigue, and malaise also are frequently present.	Fecal leukocytes not usually seen.	Coccidian parasite present in fecally contaminated food and water.	Acid-fast stain of stool.	TMP-SMX DS, 1 tablet po 2 times a day for 7 days in immunocom-petent patients, for 10 days and then 1 po 3 times a week in immuno-compromised.	Consider cause of immuno-deficiency. Duration is 1–7 weeks with periods of remission.
Bacillus cereus	Abdominal pain, watery diarrhea, tenesmus, usually within 1–36 hours of consuming contaminated food.		Classically found in fried rice left on steam tables but can be obtained from gravies and meats.			
Listeria monocyto-genes			Food poisoning	Not detected in standard stool cultures.	Ampicillin 200 mg/kg IV every 6 hours.	

ORT = oral rehydration therapy, TMP-SMX = trimethoprim-sulfamethoxazole.

water. Chickens and wild birds are the primary reservoir. Shellfish may be the source of infection with *Vibrio parahaemoliticus*. Salads are notorious for transmission of *Shigella* species and fried rice for the transmission of *Bacillus cereus*. *Shigella*-related infections in the United States are often related to poor hygiene and crowded living conditions.[11]

Certain areas are endemic for parasitic diarrhea. Infection with *Giardia lamblia* may be contracted by drinking water containing oocysts deposited by animals. Beaver and deer have been blamed in endemic areas.

Infection with *Cryptosporidium* organisms also may present with diarrhea. The diarrhea is typically profuse and watery. The infection is most commonly seen in immunosuppressed patients. Its frequency is increasing in patients with acquired immunodeficiency syndrome (AIDS), in whom it may be life-threatening. Other populations in which this agent may be seen are people who work with animals and children in day-care centers.

A history of antibiotic use should be sought in patients who have been ill. Pseudomembranous colitis caused by the overgrowth of *Clostridium difficile* needs to be considered in such patients.[12]

The most urgent physical findings to evaluate in the patient with diarrhea relate to complications. The degree of dehydration must be assessed. Orthostatic blood pressure and pulse changes should be determined. The moisture of mucous membranes and the presence or absence of tearing in children should be noted. Prolonged dry diapers may indicate decreased urine output. A sunken fontanelle in an infant represents significant dehydration.[13]

Abdominal findings are nonspecific in patients with diarrhea. Hyperactive bowel sounds are usually present. Peritoneal findings are unusual. The patient may experience some discomfort during abdominal palpation but rarely demonstrates peritonitis or involuntary guarding.

Sigmoidoscopic examination is indicated in cases of diarrhea that persist longer than 14 days and are unresponsive to antibiotics and in any homosexual male with moderate-to-severe diarrhea.[14] Visualization of the bowel mucosa hastens the diagnosis of invasive diarrhea. Likewise, the patient suspected of *C. difficile* infection with pseudomembranous colitis requires sigmoidoscopic examination.

Diagnostic Aids. A rectal examination and an evaluation for occult blood should be done at the same time. Several studies have demonstrated that the presence of occult blood in the setting of acute diarrhea has the same clinical significance as large numbers of fecal leukocytes.[15] Stool cultures should be obtained when the diarrhea is severe, a specific diarrheal agent is suspected, occult blood or fecal leukocytes are present, fever is present, or the patient has persistent diarrhea after an unsuccessful course of antibiotics.

For the patient suspected of having a specific infectious diarrhea, stool specimens should be obtained for culture and ova and parasite examination, when appropriate. Negative cultures and parasite examinations should not be relied on if the patient's symptoms continue. Up to three specimens may be necessary to identify the parasite in some cases because the cysts or parasite may be shed only intermittently.

The blood count and electrolyte measurements are important determinations in ill patients with diarrhea. An elevated white blood cell count may indicate a more serious infection than previously suspected. A large number of bands with a relatively low total white blood cell count should prompt consideration of *Salmonella typhi* infection.[16] Loss of fluid and electrolytes in the stool may create a life-threatening electrolyte imbalance.

An abdominal film should be taken if inflammatory bowel disease is suspected. The flat plate of the abdomen may be diagnostic of toxic megacolon in such cases. Normally, however, the abdominal film is of little help in patients with diarrhea.

Management. Acute diarrheal disease is a self-limited process in most cases, even when it is bacterial. The patient with viral gastroenteritis who displays signs of mild dehydration usually needs only instruction in oral fluid maintenance. Intravenous rehydration in the urgent care setting may be considered occasionally. Patients who receive 1–2 L of crystalloid solution usually feel subjectively better and orthostatic abnormalities resolve.

The patient with severe persistent diarrhea may require hospitalization for diagnosis and treatment. Systemic antibiotics should be considered in shigellosis and salmonellosis in septic patients. Patients who are treated as outpatients should not be given antibiotics for the diagnosis of salmonellosis because antibiotics do not appear to change the duration or severity of the diarrhea and may induce a carrier state.[15] Antibiotic therapy is indicated in all cases of shigellosis because it shortens the duration of illness and reduces the health risk to contacts of the infected patient.[16] Normally, antidiarrheal agents such as loperamide are not given to patients with febrile dysentery. The decreased motility created by such agents is believed to prolong the disease by prolonging the contact time between the pathologic agent and the mucosa. It is more effective to treat the infection with an antibiotic and to maintain hydration as the bowel recovers.

Pitfalls in Practice. A common mistake in the management of diarrhea is to underestimate the seriousness of the disease. The physician must not ignore any disease that is prolonged, produces systemic toxicity, or causes bloody diarrhea. Such patients need further diagnostic studies. The degree of illness may require intravenous hydration and antibiotics for safe management. Contacts of patients with infectious diarrhea need to be instructed in hand-washing techniques to avoid spreading the infection.

Anorectal Pain and Bleeding

Differential Diagnosis. The patient with anorectal complaints is often in significant physical and emotional distress. It is not unusual to see patients who have delayed their visit in the hope that the symptoms would abate so that they could avoid an anorectal examination. Pain, bleeding, burning, and pruritus are the most common complaints suggesting anorectal disease. Change in bowel movement and character may be associated as well. Traumatic, anatomic, and infectious causes are responsible for anorectal disease (Table 8, next page).

History and Physical Examination. The correct etiology of anorectal disease can usually be surmised from the history and confirmed by physical examination. Confirmatory laboratory tests are rarely needed. Sudden anorectal pain during defecation or Valsalva maneuver is indicative of one of two conditions: an anal fissure during the passage of firm stool or an external anal hematoma, more commonly called a thrombosed external hemorrhoid. The patient with hematoma usually supplies the differentiating history of a painful lump near the anus. Such histories are highly characteristic and reproducible. Other anorectal conditions presenting with pain as a component of the condition do not have a sudden onset. The pain of abscess and other conditions is more gradual in onset and usually not severe, at least initially. The patient with an abscess may be in excruciating pain on arrival to the urgent care setting, but a history of a gradual increase in the pain over time can be elicited.

In contrast to external anal thromboses, internal hemorrhoids do not present with pain as a prominent part of the history. Painless bleeding is the initial symptom of internal hemorrhoidal disease. The varicosities of the anal hemorrhoidal veins may produce bloody streaking on the surface of stools, or the patient may notice blood in the toilet bowl or on tissue paper. Later, when the hemorrhoids enlarge, itching and burning develop. These symptoms result from engorgement, edema, and increased moisture in the perianal area due to prolapse of the hemorrhoids. Patients with severe hemorrhoids complain of a sensation of prolapse during defecation. As the disease progresses, the hemorrhoids may require digital reduction after a bowel movement. They may become irreducible.

Table 8. Anorectal Syndromes

Condition	Presentation	Examination	Etiology	Diagnosis	Treatment	Follow-Up
Anal fissure	Acute pain on Valsalva maneuver and defecation. May have rectal bleeding. May also have spasm of the anal sphincter.	Visual inspection with manual traction of anal skin. Avoid digital examination when intense pain or sphincter spasm present. 2% lidocaine gel applied to area may assist with the exam.	Tear due to passage of firm stool. Sphincter spasm retards healing, leads to chronic fissure with triad. Consider syphilis, gonorrhea, tuberculosis, inflammatory bowel disease, leukemic ulcer when history or examination is atypical.	Typical location at 12 or 6 o'clock. Triad of chronic fissures: fissure, "sentinel" skin tag, hypertrophied anal papilla. "Kissing" fissures suggest syphilis. VDRL or RPR should be considered in all cases. Investigate symptoms of inflammatory bowel disease.	Sitz bath twice a day, stool softener, and bulk laxative. Surgery may also be required. Topical agents such as Anusol may provide some relief.	Follow up any laboratory studies. Refer to a colorectal surgeon if not healing.
Thrombosed external hemorrhoid	Acute pain on Valsalva maneuver and defecation. May have rectal bleeding. History of a painful lump.	Visual inspection with manual traction of anal skin, digital examination, anoscopy.	Anal hematoma; extravasation of clot from perianal vein; straining at stool.	Inspection, subcutaneous hematoma below pectinate line. Distinguish from internal hemorrhoid extending above line (is not as painful). Internoexternal hemorrhoid is an an internal hemorrhoid that has extended beneath pectinate line, mimicking external hemorrhoid.	Local infiltration at base; incise, remove clot, excise redundant skin; warm sitz bath twice a day stool softener.	At 2 weeks. Discuss stool softener.
Internal hemorrhoids	Blood on tissue paper or stools, itching, burning, sensation of prolapse. May manually replace. Not painful unless incarcerated.	External examination, anoscopy with Valsalva maneuver. Grade according to degree of prolapse.	Digital hemorrhoidal veins, chronic straining during defecation. 50% of adults older than age 50 have some degree of hemorrhoids.	Distinguish from other causes of rectal bleeding; anoscopy. OK acutely if hemorrhoids found bleeding with typical history; schedule sigmoidoscopy.	Sitz bath twice a day, stool softeners, bulk laxatives, Anusol. Banding of hemorrhoids is treatment of choice when incarcerated.	At 2 weeks. Discuss stool softener.

(Cont'd on next page)

Table 8. Anorectal Syndromes *(Continued)*

Condition	Presentation	Examination	Etiology	Diagnosis	Treatment	Follow-Up
Abscess	Gradually increasing pain, fever.	External examination, digital examination, anoscopy, sigmoidoscopy when diagnosis unclear. Indurated perianal mass, seldom flucuant because of tense cavity, thick tissue.	Anal glands are likely source. *E. coli, Proteus* organisms; enterococci; *Bacteroides* organism; anaerobes.	Distinguish location (low anal submucosal, ischiorectal, supralevator), fullness, induration (external or on rectum). Fever with ischiorectal supralevator abscess.	Incise and drain all abscesses. Low anal: outpatient therapy. Others require hospitalization. Abscess must be unroofed to minimize recurrence, fistula formation. Antibiotics unnecessary as outpatient.	Re-examine after 24 hours; remove any wick at 24 hours; follow up with colorectal surgeon within 1 week.
Pruritus ani	Perianal itching (sensation of variable duration). Patient may have history of other perianal disease.	Perianal irritation, lichenification. Search for perianal disease; examine stool for ova, parasites; do tape test for pinworm.	Perianal disease; increasing moisture or poor hygiene; skin tab, warts; hemorrhoids; enterobius vermicularis, fissures, rectal prolapse.	Visual examination, anoscopy, sigmoidoscopy. Examine stool for ova, parasites; perianal tape examination for pinworm ova.	Treat underlying disease. Sitz baths. Improve perianal hygiene with nonvigorous cleaning of the region.	Rapid resolution if etiology defined. Intractable pruritus without detectable etiology is difficult to treat. If pinworm is identified, other household contacts need evaluation and possible treatment.
Foreign body	Low abdominal, rectal pain; history usually available; autoeroticism, self-treatment.	May be visually apparent or palpable on rectal examination. Radiography always recommended.	Autoeroticism; self-treatment; accident; trauma.	Examination, radiography	Sphincter block helpful: local infiltration in quadrants external to anal sphincter. Removal manually with forceps and balloon catheter usually possible; surgical removal occasionally necessary. Avoid cathartics and enemas.	Sigmoidoscopy after removal mandatory to diagnose potential injury; psychiatric evaluation may be indicated.
Rectal prolapse	Mass protruding from rectum.	Mucosal mass with radial or circumferential folds in mucosa.	Absent mesentery; lax anal sphincter; redundant sigmoid colon.	Visual examination. Consider intussusception in young children.	Manual reduction usually possible. Placement of sugar on rectal mucosa may aid in reduction. Discuss stool softeners, bowel habits. Consider surgery for redundant colon in adults.	Colorectal surgery referral in all cases; postreduction examination.

(Cont'd on next page)

Table 8. Anorectal Syndrome *(Continued)*

Condition	Presentation	Examination	Etiology	Diagnosis	Treatment	Follow-Up
Condyloma acuminata (anal warts)	Verrucous perianal tags.	Visual examination, anoscopy, sigmoidoscopy.	Papilloma virus; venereal spread.	Visual diagnosis. Extent of involvement of anal canal requires anoscopy and sigmoidoscopy before definitive treatment.	Isolated warts may be treated with topical podophyllin resin; multiple warts usually require fulguration in stages.	Colorectal surgery referral; explain etiology; encourage treatment of sexual partners.

The patient with a perianal abscess complains of anal pain and tenderness. Low-grade fever may be present as well. In all such patients, a thorough history should be taken for diabetes or conditions that increase susceptibility to infection.

Patients with perianal fistulas have a chronic disease of which they are usually aware. The cyclical symptoms include periodic pain followed by spontaneous drainage of the fistula with a decrease in the pain. Constant drainage of the fistulas can be annoying. The incidence of inflammatory bowel disease in this group of patients is high.

Perianal condyloma acuminata may be a mystery to the patient on initial presentation. Painless, warty growths surround the anus. They may become irritated and painful from trauma or as a result of poor hygiene exacerbated by their presence. Proctitis of obscure cause presents as vague discomfort with or without a history of loose stools. Anal discharge with staining of the underwear may be present. Condyloma and proctitis are more likely to be present and transmitted in the male homosexual population.

Proper interpretation of physical findings in anorectal disease requires an understanding of the anatomy of the anorectal region. Figure 1 (next page) is a cutaway view of the anus illustrating several structures that are important to an understanding of pathologic processes affecting the area.

The pectinate or dentate line marks an important anatomic demarcation point. Below the line innervation is by the pudendal nerve, and the skin of the area is richly supplied with pain fibers. Above the line the innervation is largely autonomic, with minimal pain sensation. Lymphatic drainage below the line goes to the inguinal nodes. The periaortic nodes receive drainage above the line. Venous drainage is also demarcated at that point. The hemorrhoidal veins responsible for internal hemorrhoids are situated above the line. Anal hematomas result from rupture of veins below the pectinate line. The columns of Morgagni are mucosal folds above the line that terminate at the anal papillae of the pectinate line. Between the papillae are the anal crypts, which are the site of origin of most low anal abscesses and fistulae. There are two layers of anal sphincter: the external and the internal.

Anal fissures usually occur in the posterior midline of the anus. The mucosal tear extends from the anal margin along the internal anal sphincter in an internal-to-external direction. The tear may be difficult to see on superficial examination. The intense sphincter spasm associated with the fissure causes the mucosa to be drawn into the anal canal. The examiner's fingers should be used to place gentle traction on the perianal skin to draw the tissue into view. Digital examination and anoscopy are painful to a patient with acute

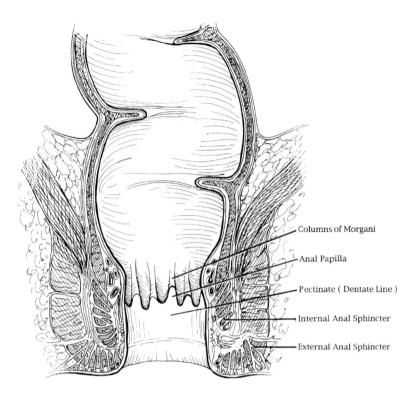

Anal Papilla

Columns of Morgani

Pectinate (Dentate Line)

Internal Anal Sphincter

External Anal Sphincter

Figure 1. Anorectal anatomy.

anal fissure. If a typical history is present and the fissure is visualized, there is no need to subject the patient to further instrumentation on the first visit. Conservative therapy should be tried and a more complete examination performed later when the acute pain has subsided. Care must be exercised not to mistake an anal ulcer, chancre, or squamous cell carcinoma for a fissure.

The patient with an anal hematoma presents with a painful superficial lump on the anal verge. It may have some purple coloration due to the contained clot. Such patients must have a digital and anoscopic examination to confirm that the lump is contained externally below the pectinate line. It should not be confused with a prolapsed internal hemorrhoid or an internal hemorrhoid varicosity that has dissected below the pectinate line. This differentiation is important to make before incising what is thought to be an external hemorrhoid. Anoscopy reveals a normal-appearing pectinate line and anal mucosa above.

The patient with internal hemorrhoids often has a normal external examination. Anoscopy reveals varicosities of the mucosa above the pectinate line. The mucosa is often friable and easily bleeds. The hemorrhoids swell and may prolapse when the patient is asked to perform a voluntary Valsalva maneuver. The degree of prolapse allows classification of the hemorrhoids. Swelling without prolapse is grade 1. Lesions that prolapse externally on Valsalva maneuver but reduce spontaneously are grade 2. Those requiring manual reduction are grade 3. Grade 4 hemorrhoids are chronically prolapsed and irreducible.[17]

Low perianal abscesses present as tense, painful swellings about the anus. They rarely are fluctuant, although they are virtually always full of pus. Ischiorectal abscesses are much larger and more angry-looking than low perianal abscesses. They may extend on both sides of the anus to form a "horseshoe" abscess. Pelvirectal abscesses are larger still and present in patients who are seriously ill.

High submucous rectal abscesses can be insidious. They may present as rectal pain and fever without obvious external swelling or abscess formation. Pilonidal abscesses are similar to low anal abscesses in appearance but occur in a typical location at the superior portion of the gluteal cleft over the sacrum.

Perianal condyloma presents as verrucous, warty growths on the external anal mucosa. Anoscopic examination often reveals that the lesions extend into the canal to and above the pectinate line.

The patient with proctitis has friable, easily bleeding mucosa on sigmoidoscopic examination. The appearance of the mucosa varies according to the agent producing the disease. Ulceration occurs with shigellosis and *Entamoeba histolytica*. Chlamydial infection and gonorrhea demonstrate uniformly inflamed mucosa.

The patient with an anal foreign body usually presents no diagnostic dilemma. The dilemma occurs at the time of removal of the agent. Injury to the anus must be avoided. Once the object has been removed, a thorough examination for injury must be carried out.

Rectal prolapse of differing types occurs in very young and elderly populations. Partial bowel wall prolapse may occur in infants and toddlers who strain at defecation. The prolapse is often easily reduced with relief of symptoms. When profound edema has complicated the prolapse, application of table sugar to the exposed tissue may reduce the swelling and allow reduction to be performed.[18] Careful examination must be done to ensure that the lesion does not represent an intussusception presenting at the rectum. Complete rectal prolapse occurs in patients with a lax anal sphincter and redundant sigmoid colon. The appearance of this prolapse is significantly different from that of partial prolapse. The mucosa of the complete prolapse has circumferential folds rather than the radial spokelike folds seen in partial prolapse.

Diagnostic Aids. Rectal cultures for gonorrhea and chlamydial infection and stool cultures for proctitis are common laboratory examinations in patients with anorectal disease. Any tissue excised from the anorectal area needs to be sent to pathology for microscopic examination to rule out squamous cell carcinoma. Patients with large perirectal abscesses need routine admission laboratory work before drainage of the abscesses in the operating suite. In patients with rectal pain and fever, a pelvic x-ray should be taken to investigate the possibility of a gas-forming infection with air in the soft tissues.

Management. The conservative management of many anorectal conditions involves the use of sitz baths and stool softeners. A sitz bath 2 or 3 times/day brings significant relief to patients after anorectal surgery as well as to patients who have conditions increasing perianal moisture. The stool softener renders defecation less stressful and may remove an aggravating factor from the patient's convalescence. The patient with an anal fissure is treated conservatively, with sitz baths initially to allow the fissure a chance to heal. A significant percentage of fissures become chronic because the fissure traps debris so that epithelial bridging cannot occur. A chronic fissure is recognized by the "sentinel" skin tag. The tag is actually hypertrophic scar tissue from the body's attempt to heal the fissure. Surgical treatment consists of division of the internal anal sphincter and excision of any redundant skin. The decrease in sphincter spasm allows the sphincter to heal.

The skin overlying an external anal hematoma may be excised and the clot removed with significant relief of symptoms. Good anesthesia for the procedure is obtained by injecting the distal sides of the hematoma base with lidocaine. This procedure is by no means mandatory. The natural history of the disease is spontaneous resolution. Again, the excised skin should be sent to pathology.

Internal hemorrhoids shrink with stool softeners and improved bowel habits. Sitz baths help with the burning and itching. Over-the-counter hemorrhoidal suppositories do not add any benefit to regular sitz baths. Banding of the hemorrhoids causes them to slough. The procedure is carried out by the proctologist over two or three office visits. Severe hemorrhoids require hemorrhoidectomy.

Perianal and pilonidal abscesses must be thoroughly unroofed to prevent fistula formation. The objective is to create a shallow-based ulcer configuration without overlying skin edges. The edges have a tendency to adhere to the wound, leading to recurrence or fistula formation. A cruciate incision with excision of the margins is recommended. Larger abscesses should be treated in the hospital. Patients with large abscesses tend to be chronically ill.

The patient with anal pruritus should undergo a search for an instigating cause. Most often the cause is a condition that increases perianal moisture (hemorrhoids, condyloma, or proctitis). Treatment is to remove the primary causes. Pruritus ani without another cause is a diagnosis of exclusion. Management of such patients can be difficult, requiring a long-term approach by the primary physician or proctologist.

Rectal prolapse often can be replaced manually. Surgical consultation is necessary for irreducible prolapse. Surgical procedures are available to prevent recurrence and can be offered to adult patients with prolapse.

Removing rectal foreign bodies requires an imaginative approach. A sphincter block should be used in all such patients. Removal of the object often can be accomplished with the hands alone when the sphincter block is in place. Sliding a catheter up the side of the foreign body to vent the colon above it breaks any vacuum holding the foreign body in the rectum. Delivery forceps have been used for fragile objects such as light bulbs. Occasionally, abdominal surgery is necessary to remove the object. Condyloma acuminata are removed in stages by means of electrocautery or laser excision. Papilloma virus has been demonstrated in the laser vapor; this finding emphasizes the need for care when using the instrument to remove warty growths.[19]

Pitfalls in Practice. Problems in anorectal disease management occur in both diagnostic and therapeutic areas. Anatomic examination should reduce the number of misdiagnoses (e.g., internal rather than external hemorrhoids). A syphilis test should be performed on every patient with anal fissure. An anal abscess must be drained; the patient should not be sent home to wait for the abscess to become fluctuant. Such a maneuver is always a mistake. If doubt exists about the presence of pus, needle aspiration is recommended. Failure to send excised tissue to pathology can lead to a missed diagnosis of serious disease. The patient with rectal pain and fever should be hospitalized until the source is found.

Conclusion

Abdominal complaints are common problems for the urgent care physician. The challenges of efficient, cost-effective, accurate diagnosis and treatment can be met with an organized approach. Skillful historical and physical examination provides the foundation for judicious use of laboratory and radiologic assistance. If a definitive diagnosis cannot be reached on the initial presentation, at least disease severity can be defined. Once the disease is characterized, the physician can make appropriate, safe management decisions.

References

1. Silen W: Cope's Early Diagnosis of the Acute Abdomen. 19th ed. New York, Oxford University Press, 1996, pp 34–35.
2. Laine L: Acute and chronic gastrointestinal bleeding. In Feldman M (ed): Sleisenger & Fordtran's Gastrointestinal and Liver Disease Pathophysiology, Diagnosis, Management. 6th ed. Philadelphia, W.B. Saunders, 1998, p 200.
3. McCallion J, Canning GP, Knight PV: Acute appendicitis in the elderly: A 5-year retrospective study. Age Ageing l6:256–260, 1987.
4. Sanson TG, O'Keefe KP: Evaluation of abdominal pain in the elderly. Emerg Med Clin North Am 14:615–627, 1996.
5. Hurwitz ES, Barrett MJ, Bregman D, et al: Public Health Service study of Reye's syndrome and medications: Report of the main study. JAMA 257:1905–1911, 1987 [erratum appears in JAMA 257:3366, 1987].
6. Camilleri M: Gastrointestinal problems in diabetes. Endocrinol Metabol Clin 25:361–378, 1996.
7. Hurst JW, Morris DC, Crawley IS, et al: The history: Past events and symptoms related to cardiovascular disease. In Hurst JW (ed): The Heart. New York, McGraw-Hill, 1986, pp 109–122.
8. Ominsky SH, Margulis AR: Appendicitis. In Replick JG, Haskin ME (eds): Surgical Radiology. Philadelphia, W.B. Saunders, 1981, pp 577–580.
9. Clements JL, Gonzalez AC, Weens HS: The pancreas. In Replick JG, Haskin ME (eds): Surgical Radiology. Philadelphia, W.B. Saunders; 1981, pp 1003–1012.
10. Miller RE, Nelson SW: The roentgenologic demonstration of tiny amounts of free intraperitoneal gas: Experimental and clinical studies. Am J Roentgenol 112:574–585, 1971.
11. American Academy of Pediatrics: Summaries of infectious diseases. In Pickering LK (ed): 2000 Red Book: Report of the Committee on Infectious Diseases, 25th ed. Elk Grove Village, IL, American Academy of Pediatrics; 2000, p 510.
12. Bitterman RA: Acute gastroenteritis and constipation. In Rosen P, Barkin RM (eds): Emergency Medicine Concepts and Clinical Practice, 4th ed. St. Louis, Mosby, l998, 1917–1958.
13. Shaw KN: Dehydration. In Fleisher GR (ed): Textbook of Pediatric Emergency Medicine, 4th ed. Philadelphia, Lippincott Williams & Wilkins, 2000, pp 198–199.
14. DuPont HL: Guidelines on acute infectious diarrhea in adults. Am J Gastroenterol 92:1962–1975, 1997.
15. Hargrett-Bean NT, Pavia AT, Tauxe RV: *Salmonella* isolates from humans in the United States 1984–1986. MMWR 37(SS-2):25–31, 1988.
16. Sensakovic JW, Smith LG: Oral antibiotic treatment of infectious diseases. Med Clin North Am 85:115–123, 2001.
17. Nelson H, Dozois RR: Disorders of the anal canal. In Townsend CM Jr (ed): Sabiston Textbook of Surgery, 16th ed. Philadelphia, W.B. Saunders , 2001, p 979.
18. Coburn WM III, Russell MA, Hofstetter WL: Sucrose as an aid to manual reduction of incarcerated rectal prolapse: A case report. Ann Emerg Med 30:347–349, 1997.
19. Garden SM, O'Banion MK. Shelnitz LS, et al: Papillomavirus in the vapor of carbon dioxide laser-treated verrucae. JAMA 259:1199–1202, 1988.

Chapter 5

Urgencies of the Genitourinary System

Catherine A. Ripkey, MD

Urinalysis Abnormalities

Hematuria

Differential Diagnosis. The differential diagnosis of he hematuria is extensive. Even the mildest blunt trauma of the abdomen or back may produce bleeding from anywhere within the urinary tract, often unmasking an asymptomatic abnormality. Nontraumatic hematuria must be considered an indication of serious urologic disease. The degree of hematuria is in no way indicative of the seriousness of its cause; the presence of more than five red blood cells per high-power field[1] is a significant finding in need of eventual evaluation. Table 1 lists common causes of nontraumatic hematuria.

Table 1. Common Causes of Nontraumatic Hematuria

Urinary tract infections	Glomerulonephritis
Cystitis	Drugs
Nephrolithiasis	Coagulopathies
Urinary tract neoplasms	Sickle cell disease
Congenital renal anomalies	Diabetic nephropathy

Infection is the leading cause of nontraumatic hematuria, followed by tumor, obstruction, and renal calculus. In infancy and childhood, hematuria often results from infection behind a congenital obstruction. In young adults, infection is much more common than calculus, and tumors are relatively rare. In adults older than 50 years, infection is still the most common cause, but tumors, benign prostatic hypertrophy (BPH), and nephrolithiasis also become common.

History and Physical Examination. The physical examination of the patient with hematuria includes assessment of the abdomen, flank, prostate, pelvis, and external genitalia. Many causes of hematuria are painless. If pain is present with hematuria, its source is frequently not well localized. Therefore, a careful examination is essential to ensure that bleeding is indeed from the urinary tract and not from surrounding structures. Frequently the physical examination is normal, and diagnosis depends on the history and laboratory studies.

Important clues to the cause of hematuria may be obtained from the history. The timing of the hematuria in relation to the urinary stream (initial, terminal, or total) is helpful.

Initial hematuria (as urination begins) implicates the urethra as the source of bleeding. Terminal hematuria usually originates in the prostate, bladder neck, or trigone. Total hematuria (throughout micturition) may originate from any site but usually signifies a source somewhere above the prostate.

Painful hematuria indicates an inflammatory (infectious) disorder or calculi, whereas painless hematuria most often results from tumors, BPH, or blood dyscrasia. Painless hematuria in children is attributable to glomerular disease until shown otherwise. Other considerations in childhood include polycystic kidney disease, sickle cell disease, porphyria, scurvy, bleeding dyscrasia, and Wilms' tumor. A history of the passage of blood clots is another helpful clue. Large, fresh clots typically originate in the bladder, whereas long, wormlike clots are casts of the collecting system and may signify renal neoplasm.

Diagnostic Aids. Careful interpretation of the urinalysis results may reveal the cause of hematuria. Red blood cell casts are characteristic of glomerular disease, crystals are frequently present with stones, and bacteria and pyuria are usually found with infection.

Management. Urgent care management of patients with hematuria involves determination of the need for immediate or routine diagnostic imaging, antibiotics, or referral (emergent or routine). All patients with gross hematuria must undergo diagnostic imaging as soon as possible unless they have an obvious genitourinary infection or a history of recent transurethral surgery. Routine blood studies, including complete blood count, prothrombin time, partial thromboplastin time, platelet count, blood urea nitrogen, and creatinine, are essential. If bleeding is continuous and severe (i.e., if evidence of hemodynamic compromise is seen) or if clots are passed, immediate urologic consultation is mandatory. Such patients should be stabilized with intravenous fluids and transferred by ambulance to a center equipped for further diagnostic imaging.

Management of microscopic hematuria consists of forcing fluids, encouraging frequent voiding, and administering antibiotics as indicated. In any patient older than 40 years who has microhematuria, a urine sample should be sent for cytologic studies. Malignant cells are difficult to detect in the presence of gross hematuria, and cytologic examination may be deferred in this setting. With the exception of patients with uncomplicated infection (who may be followed by their primary care physician), patients with microhematuria should be referred to a urologist for further investigation.

Pitfalls in Practice. Failure to appreciate the significance of hematuria after any type of trauma may result in delay in the diagnosis of serious urologic or other injury. All patients with hematuria require prearranged follow-up before discharge from the urgent care center. Many causes of nontraumatic hematuria (e.g., nephrolithiasis, cancer) can cause significant morbidity and mortality if final diagnosis and management are delayed.

Proteinuria

Differential Diagnosis. The finding of new-onset hypertension, edema, arthritis, or diabetes should prompt an investigation of the patient's urine for protein. Proteinuria also is commonly found on routine screening urinalysis. Table 2 lists the more common causes of proteinuria. In the healthy kidney, protein is present in the glomerular filtrate but is reabsorbed by tubular cells. Normal adults may excrete up to 150 mg of protein daily, only 10–15 mg of which is albumin. When glomerular damage is present, as in glomerulonephritis, albumin excretion may be excessive because normal filtration is lost.

When a disease process damages the tubules, as in amyloidosis, tubular reabsorption of low-molecular-weight protein is decreased, resulting in proteinuria. "Overflow" protein-uria occurs when a disease such as multiple myeloma causes an increase in plasma pro-tein concentration, thus exceeding the tubular reabsorptive capacity.

Table 2. Causes of Proteinuria

Glomerulonephritis (all types)	Chronic congestive heart failure
Connective tissue diseases	Renal vein thrombosis
Diabetes mellitus	Infections (hepatitis B, sepsis, herpes)
Multiple myeloma	Tumors (Hodgkin's, bone metastasis, chronic lymphocytic leukemia)
Amyloidosis	Interstitial nephritis
Allergic reactions (bee stings, drug reactions)	Hypertensive nephrosclerosis
Pericarditis	Obstructive uropathy
Nephrotic syndrome	Nephrocalcinosis
Preeclampsia	Exercise-induced proteinuria

History and Physical Examination. Once proteinuria is found on urinalysis, patients should be questioned about presence of systemic disease that can affect the kidneys. Bone pain (from multiple myeloma or bone metastasis), polyuria, fatigue and excessive thirst (from diabetes), congestive heart failure, and exposure to toxins are significant and may suggest the cause of proteinuria. Physical examination should include evaluation for hy-pertension, arthritis, edema, and retinal changes. The concomitant development of hyper-tension and proteinuria suggests primary renal disease. The combination of proteinuria, hypoproteinemia, and edema is consistent with the diagnosis of nephrotic syndrome. Arthritis, rashes, and proteinuria suggest a connective tissue disease. Funduscopic exami-nation may reveal changes consistent with systemic hypertension, diabetes, or vasculitis.

Management. The significance of proteinuria cannot be determined on a single urine dipstick test. If urinalysis by dipstick shows proteinuria of the 1+ level (about 300 mg/L) or more, close follow-up with a primary care physician is mandatory. Patients should re-ceive careful instructions in the proper technique of 24-hour urine collection for protein and creatinine. The results of such a collection aid the primary care physician in choosing further diagnostic tests. If 24-hour urine protein is > 150 mg, electrophoresis is done to determine the proportions of albumin and other proteins.[2] Excretion mainly of albumin signifies a glomerular lesion. By definition, when total daily protein excretion exceeds 3.5 gm, nephrotic syndrome is present. The presence of a large amount of Bence Jones protein suggests that multiple myeloma or another neoplastic process may be present.

Pitfalls in Practice. The patient with persistent, nonepisodic, asymptomatic, but signif-icant proteinuria has a definite risk of renal pathology and merits an intensive evaluation, possibly including a renal biopsy. Intravenous pyelography (IVP) should not be done in pa-tients suspected of having multiple myeloma because the dye may precipitate in the renal tubules when Bence Jones protein is present. The importance of continued evaluation of patients with new-onset hypertension for renal pathology cannot be overemphasized.

Urinary Tract Infections

Differential Diagnosis. Urinary tract infections (UTIs) affect all age groups, and dy-suria is a frequent complaint of urgent care patients. During the preschool years and into adulthood, UTI is more common in women than men. When infection occurs in boys and young men, serious congenital abnormalities or urinary tract disease are frequently present. Uncomplicated UTIs in adult men are infrequent until later years, when they are probably due to the onset of BPH with consequent urinary stasis.

History and Physical Examination. As with hematuria, the physical examination of patients with complaints of UTI can be nonspecific. Nonetheless, a careful examination, as described above, is essential. Historical points of significance include previous UTIs, underlying medical and urologic diseases, presenting signs and symptoms, systemic symptoms, and the patient's ability to comply with advised medical management.

Risk factors for the development of UTI are listed in Table 3. Urinary stasis increases the risk of UTI in various circumstances. Pregnancy results in decreased ureteral peristalsis, which contributes to urinary stasis. BPH with its resultant obstruction to urinary flow also leads to stasis. Urinary stasis explains the increased infection rate when mechanical or neurogenic malfunction is present as well as in infrequent voiders.

Table 3. Factors Predisposing to Urinary Tract Infection

Female sex	Incomplete bladder emptying
Advancing age	Infrequent voiding
Pregnancy	Diabetes
Prostatic hypertrophy	Sickle cell disease
Urinary calculi	Instrumentation, indwelling catheters
Vesicoureteral reflux	Obstruction
Congenital abnormalities	

Diagnosis of UTI requires collection of an acceptable urine specimen for urinalysis and potentially for culture. The midstream voiding specimen is appropriate for most adults. Females should be instructed to spread the labia and to sponge the periurethral area from front to back with povidone-iodine or liquid soap, to pass a small amount of urine into the toilet, and then to urinate into a sterile cup. Males should carefully cleanse the urethral meatus (retracting the foreskin if uncircumcised) and obtain a midstream specimen. Catheterization is indicated if the patient cannot void spontaneously, is menstruating, or is extremely obese. In small children, the collection of urine into a sterile collection bag can be attempted. Urethral catheterization is a more accurate technique for obtaining a specimen in young children.

Diagnostic Aids. Pyuria, bacteriuria, positive nitrite test, and the presence of leukocyte esterase in the urine are diagnostic aids obtainable from a urine specimen. Pyuria has been defined in women as more than 10 white blood cells per high-power field. However, some symptomatic women with low-grade pyuria (< 10 white blood cells per high-power field) have significant infections that will respond to antimicrobial therapy. This subgroup of women has what is termed the dysuria-pyuria syndrome, and frequently infection is caused by organisms other than typical coliform organisms (e.g., *Chlamydia* sp.).[3] In men, more than 1–2 white blood cells per high-power field can be significant in the presence of bacteria. Urethritis and prostatitis are far more common causes of pyuria in young men than UTI.

Bacteriuria is a sensitive indicator of UTI and, in a clean specimen (suggested by the absence of squamous epithelial cells), correlates to a high degree with culture results. A positive nitrate urine test has a high degree of specificity; because its sensitivity is low, however, it is a poor screening tool. The presence of leukocyte esterase in the urine is a sensitive indicator of the presence of pyuria and therefore is a good screening test. Although its specificity is somewhat low for predicting significant bacteriuria, it may be quite useful when microscopic examination is not available. The combination of a positive nitrite screen and leukocyte esterase achieves sensitivity of 65–98%.[4,5]

The classic definition of UTI has been a colony count of more than 10/ml on culture. This definition is changing, however, and more attention is directed toward the urinalysis as new knowledge of UTI is acquired. For example, cultures of urine from women with the dysuria-pyuria syndrome are frequently negative for UTI because colony counts are less than 10/ml, yet such women improve symptomatically with antibiotics.[3]

Most uncomplicated UTIs (i.e., those occurring in patients without underlying renal or neurologic disease) are caused by gram-negative aerobic bacilli from the gut; the vast majority of these are *Escherichia coli* (90% of first episodes), staphylococci followed by saphophytici (5–15%), and species of *Klebsiella*, *Proteus*, *Enterobacter*, and *Pseudomonas*.[3]

Management. When faced with a patient who has a UTI in the urgent care setting, the physician must decide whether hospital admission is indicated. If outpatient management is chosen, the physician must determine what antibiotic is needed and what type of follow-up is appropriate.

In patients with high fever (102–104°F), hypotension, or shaking chills, gram-negative bacteremia should be suspected, and hospital admission is mandatory. Similarly, patients with severe flank pain, nausea, and vomiting and patients whose condition appears to be toxic probably have pyelonephritis and usually require inpatient treatment. Physicians should readily admit patients who are pregnant, diabetic, elderly, or immunocompromised for any reason. The probability of patient compliance is another consideration in the decision of who should be admitted.

For patients who can be managed outside the hospital, there is at present no clear drug of choice or duration of therapy. Table 4 (next page) lists appropriate agents and dosages in outpatient management of UTI. A reasonable therapeutic approach is to guide antibiotic therapy according to the clinical setting and urinalysis results. In symptomatic, nonpregnant women, options include short-course therapy (3–5 days) and the traditional 7- to 10-day course of therapy. Single-dose therapy (with ampicillin 3.5 gm, amoxicillin 3.0 gm, cephalexin 2 gm, trimethoprim-sulfamethoxazole 2 tablets) has been advocated by some authorities, but short-course therapy is more effective than single-dose therapy.[3] Short-course therapy has improved compliance, lower cost, and fewer side effects than the traditional 7- to 10-day regimen, making it an attractive treatment option.[3] Short-course therapy also may be an option for uncomplicated UTI in children, particularly adolescent girls. Pregnant women with UTIs and men with UTIs should not be treated with single-dose or short-course therapies, because UTIs in these populations are considered complicated. Regardless of treatment regimen, patients should be reevaluated in 3–5 days, and, if pyuria or bacteriuria is still present, culture and sensitivity tests should be done.

Pitfalls in Practice. Treatment of UTIs with single-dose or short-course therapy warrants follow-up within 5 days because evidence of treatment failure may indicate subclinical

Table 4. Oral Antibiotic Therapy for Uncomplicated Urinary Tract Infections and Pyelonephritis in Adults

Agent	Conventional Treatment	Short-Course Treatment
Uncomplicated UTIs/cystitis		
Ciproflaxacin	250 mg PO × 7–10 days	250 mg PO bid × 3 days
Trimethoprim-sulfamethoxazole (TMP-SMX-DS)	160/800 mg PO bid 7–10 days	160/800 mg PO bid × 3 days
Nitrofurantoin	50–100 mg tid or qid × 7–10 days	
Doxycycline	100 mg PO bid × 7–10 days	
Amoxicillin-clavulanic acid	500 mg PO tid × 7–10 days	
Cephalexin	250–500 mg qid × 7–10 days	
Cephradine	250–500 mg qid × 7–10 days	
Cefadroxil	500 mg PO bid × 7–10 days	
Uncomplicated pyelonephritis (outpatient treatment)		
Ciprofloxacin	500 mg PO bid × 7–10 days	Not recommended in pyelonephritis
Levofloxacin	500 mg PO qd × 7–10 days	
Ofloxacin	400 mg PO bid × 7–10 days	
Amoxicillin-clavulanic acid	500 mg PO tid × 14 days	
Cephalosporins	500 mg PO tid × 14 days	
TMP-SMX-DS	2 tabs qd × 14 days	

bid = twice daily, tid = 3 times/day, qd = each day, PO = orally.

pyelonephritis, bacterial resistance, atypical pathogens, or underlying renal abnormalities ("staghorn" calculi, congenital anomalies, obstruction, or diabetes). In sexually active women with dysuria and low-grade pyuria with no bacteria seen on urinalysis, *Chlamydia* sp. should be considered as a possible cause of symptoms. A 10-day course of sulfonamides or doxycycline is standard treatment, although single-dose azithromycin has been advocated for greater compliance. Concurrent treatment for gonorrhea also must be considered.

UTIs in children deserve special consideration because they frequently signify underlying urinary tract defects. In addition, UTIs in young children typically present with nonspecific signs and symptoms. Neonatal UTIs present with feeding difficulties, irritability, and sluggishness. Children 1 month to 3 years of age typically present with fever, vomiting, abdominal pain, and irritability. To complicate matters further, the ability of urinalysis screening tests to detect UTI appears to be less reliable in young children than in older patients.[6] Urine cultures, therefore, are recommended by most authors for this age group. Children should be thoroughly evaluated with the first UTI for correctable urinary tract abnormalities. Of children with first infections, 80% have another within 18 months.[6] Waiting until a second infection is documented does not increase the diagnosis of correctable abnormalities, and deferring investigation appears to be unjustified.

UTIs during pregnancy require special consideration. Bacteriuria or pyuria, even if asymptomatic, warrant aggressive therapy. Several antibiotics are contraindicated in pregnancy; before prescribing treatment, the clinician should verify its safety for the patient at specific gestational stages.

Scrotal Pain

When a patient presents to the urgent care center with acute scrotal pain, the physician must evaluate and diagnose the problem rapidly. Torsion of the spermatic cord, which is a primary consideration, must be reversed within hours if testicular function is to be preserved. The goals of urgent care assessment are to determine the likelihood of this diagnosis compared with other causes of acute scrotal pain and the need for emergent or urgent evaluation.

Differential Diagnosis. The most common causes for scrotal pain are listed in Table 5. Often the diagnosis can be made on the basis of history and physical examination alone, provided that scrotal anatomy, the natural history of the problem, and predisposing factors of acute scrotal pain are known. Figure 1 depicts the basic anatomy of the scrotum, which must be understood to interpret properly the findings of the scrotal examination. The head of the epididymis is normally located above the testis, with the body and tail behind it.

Table 5. Diagnostic Considerations of Acute Scrotal Pain

Testicular torsion	Acute orchitis
Acute epididymitis	Torsion of the testicular appendage
Incarcerated hernia	Testicular malignancy with acute hemorrhage
Trauma	

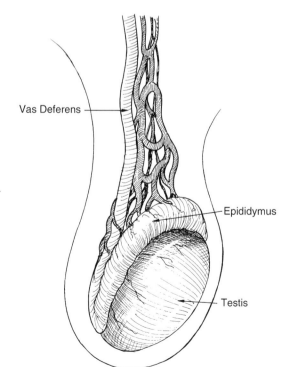

Figure 1. Anatomy of testis.

Vas Deferens

Epididymus

Testis

Table 6 lists the characteristics of testicular torsion and epididymitis that aid in differentiation. It can be extremely difficult, if not impossible, for even the most experienced clinician to distinguish torsion from epididymitis. Color Doppler ultrasonography is currently the method of choice to establish the diagnosis when clinical diagnosis cannot be made with absolute certainty.

Table 6. Characteristics of Testicular Torsion and Acute Epididymitis

Parameter	Torsion	Epididymitis
Age of patient	< 25 yr	> 25 yr
Onset	Sudden	Gradual (days)
Response to scrotal elevation	Increased pain	Decreased pain
Pyuria	Absent	Frequently present
Findings on Doppler ultrasonography	Flow decreased or absent	Flow normal

Doppler ultrasonography is helpful in distinguishing torsion from other entities. The finding of decreasing or absent flow is considered diagnostic of torsion. Nevertheless, false-negative examinations do occur (e.g., the detection of pulses in the presence of torsion). The use of Doppler ultrasonography or any imaging modality cannot be recommended if it delays necessary urologic consultation and management in patients suspected of having testicular torsion.

A history of trauma, prostatitis, or exposure to mumps may suggest the cause of scrotal pain. A history of severe, intermittent testicular pain with spontaneous remission should alert the physician to the possibility of torsion. The pain of testicular torsion is severe and often associated with nausea and vomiting. Diagnosis is made difficult by the extreme pain, which may permit only a superficial examination at best. The onset of pain in torsion is sudden, whereas in epididymitis the pain is usually more gradual in onset, reaching a peak over a period of days. The average age for epididymitis is 25 years, and the condition is extremely rare in patients younger than 20 years. There are two periods during which torsion is likely to occur: the first year of life (torsion outside the tunica vaginalis) and at puberty (torsion inside the tunica vaginalis). Torsion in men older than 30 years is rare but does occur.[8] Because the testicle can rotate 360°, the torsed epididymis can lie in its normal position posterior to the testes, making difficult the differentiation of torsion from epididymitis.

The appendix testes and other vestigial appendages may undergo torsion, causing sudden onset of point tenderness. A localized ecchymosis or blue-block dot may be noted on the scrotal sac. Orchitis usually follows a systemic viral infection. Scrotal discomfort and swelling (usually unilateral) typically start 7–10 days after the onset of mumps parotitis. The pain of orchitis is rarely as severe as that of epididymitis.

Testicular cancers are the second most frequent malignancy. Acute scrotal pain may be due to an incarcerated indirect inguinal hernia and occasionally can be mistaken for an abnormal testis or epididymis. The patient with an incarcerated scrotal hernia may present with signs and symptoms of intestinal obstruction or simply with a painful scrotum. A mass that extends from the external ring is palpable and distinct from the testis, which is normal. Bowel sounds may be heard on auscultation of the scrotum.

Management. The laboratory evaluation of patients with outer scrotal pain rarely helps in determining its cause.[7] Urinalysis, urine culture, and urethral swab for chlamydial infection and gonorrhea may assist in the eventual diagnosis. If testicular torsion is likely, immediate urologic consultation is mandatory. Torsion is a true surgical emergency because testicular infarction with subsequent loss of spermatogenesis ensues within 4–6 hours after strangulation.

The management of epididymitis consists of bed rest, scrotal elevation, ice packs, generous analgesia, and antimicrobial therapy. Patients with evidence of systemic infection (such as chills and temperature > 101°F) or abscess formation with a tender, fluctuant mass should be admitted and treated with intravenous antibiotics (aminoglycosides or ampicillin). Most patients with epididymitis can be treated on an outpatient basis. Most cases of epididymitis in heterosexual young men (under age 40) are caused by *Neisseria gonorrhoeae* or *Chlamydia* sp.[9] The phenomenon of asymptomatic gonorrhea or chlamydial infection has been well documented in this population: the same antibiotics are therefore suitable, even in the absence of penile discharge and organisms on Gram stain. Ceftriaxone is effective against both penicillin-resistant and tetracycline-resistant strains of *N. gonorrhoeae*; tetracycline covers the possibility of concomitant chlamydial infection. In the absence of a urethral discharge, boys, young teenagers, homosexuals, and older men (over age 40) should be presumed to have coliform infection and started on a broad-spectrum antimicrobial. Table 7 lists antibiotics recommended for outpatient therapy of epididymitis. For acute orchitis, treatment is symptomatic and consists of bed rest, local support, and analgesia. Neither corticosteroids nor antibiotics have been useful. Infiltration of a local anesthetic into the spermatic cord above the testis may relieve swelling and pain. As with torsion, the seminiferous elements may be destroyed; sterility may result from orchitis in patients with bilateral involvement.

Table 7. Outpatient Antibiotic Therapy for Epididymitis

Patients	Drug/Dose/Route
Young (< 35 years old)	1. Ceftriaxone 250 mg IM × 1 plus doxycycline 100 mg PO bid × 10 days or 2. Ofloxacin 300 mg PO bid × 10 days
Age > 35 years or homosexual males	1. Ciprofloxacin 500 mg PO bid × 10–14 days 2. Ofloxacin 200 mg PO bid × 10–14 days 3. Trimethoprim-sulfamethoxazole 1 tab bid × 10 days

IM = intramuscularly, PO = orally, bid = twice daily.

If a scrotal hernia is diagnosed as the cause of pain, immediate surgical consultation is warranted. Even if the painful hernia is reduced, the patient may need admission for observation to rule out infarcted bowel. Truly incarcerated scrotal hernias necessitate prompt surgical exploration.

Pitfalls in Practice. Testicular torsion and incarcerated scrotal hernias are surgical emergencies and require prompt recognition and referral to prevent significant morbidity. It cannot be overemphasized that emergent urologic evaluation is required for all patients in whom these diagnoses are suspected. In addition, suspicion of a testicular tumor as the cause of acute scrotal pain requires prompt surgical exploration and biopsy.

Nephrolithiasis

Differential Diagnosis. In the United States, approximately 12% of the population will experience nephrolithiasis at some point in their lifetime. The overwhelming majority of patients with kidney stones are Caucasians aged 30 to 50 years, with a ratio of men to women of 4:1. On the average, 80% of patients with documented ureteral calculi are treated as outpatients.

There are four basic types of urinary stones: calcium, struvite, uric acid, and cystine. Calcium stones are the most common. The next most common stone is the struvite (magnesium-ammonium phosphate complex) stone, which is nearly always associated with urea-splitting bacteria in the urine. Both uric acid and cystine stones are distinctly uncommon. Factors contributing to stone formation are listed in Table 8.

Table 8. Factors Contributing to Kidney Stone Formation

Dietary
Calcium-rich foods
Oxalate-rich foods (spinach, beets, greens, fruits, coffee, tea)
High-purine diets (meats, vegetables, beer, wine)

Metabolic

Dehydration	Primary hyperparathyroidism
Medications (antacids, chemotherapeutic agents)	Renal tubular acidosis
Gout	Hereditary cystinuria

Mechanical
Anatomic abnormalities causing urinary stasis
Phosphate precipitation in alkaline urine (produced by urea-splitting bacteria)

History and Physical Examination. Patients with nephrolithiasis usually present with sudden onset of severe, colicky pain. The patient is frequently writhing on the bed, and nausea and vomiting are common. The pain usually begins in the flank when the stone is high along the course of the ureter and then radiates into the low abdomen and groin as the stone progresses down the ureter. Men may describe testicular pain, and women may have pain in their labia. Hypertension and tachycardia, due primarily to severe pain, are common. Abdominal palpation may reveal moderate nonspecific tenderness, but the findings are usually unremarkable. Indeed, the patient's pain is markedly out of proportion to the physical findings.

On occasion the pain resolves or lessens before the physician sees the patient; in such cases, an accurate history is crucial for the diagnosis. Patients should be questioned about family history and prior episodes of renal colic. A history of low fluid intake or excessive intake of foods containing calcium, oxalate, or purine supports the diagnosis. Occasionally, patients with renal calculi present in a less dramatic way and may complain only of a dull flank pain. Patients with struvite stones may be pain-free and present with recurring UTIs.

Diagnostic Aids. A rapid urine dipstick test for heme should be immediately obtained to expedite treatment of this painful condition. A formal urinalysis is also imperative and usually reveals hematuria. However, if the stone has completely obstructed the ureter, hematuria may be absent. Patients presenting with a new diagnosis of renal colic should undergo diagnostic imaging to establish the diagnosis and evaluate the status of the urinary tract. Blood should be obtained for complete blood count and measurement of electrolytes, blood urea nitrogen, creatinine, and calcium.

The usefulness of the kidney-ureter-bladder flatplate film is questionable in the diagnosis of stones. It is usually a suboptimal film because of patient movement and overlying feces and bowel gas. Radiolucent stones cannot be seen, small stones are easily obscured, and various calcific densities can be mistaken for stones. A negative abdominal film does not exclude the presence of a stone.[10]

Imaging modalities used for the diagnosis of acute nephrolithiasis include helical CT and intravenous pyelography. Helical CT has been shown to have a high sensitivity (95–98%) and specificity (96–100%) for the diagnosis of nephrolithiasis.[11] This rapid, noninvasive test permits not only a rapid diagnosis but also excellent localization of the stone and determination of stone size. It also may provide alternative diagnosis.

Ultrasonography can assist in the diagnosis of nephrolithiasis if symptoms are classic and hydronephrosis or the stone itself is detected.[12] However, the presence of hydronephrosis depends on the degree and duration of ureteral obstruction; early in the clinical course, ultrasound may not provide the diagnosis. The main difficulty with ultrasound in establishing the diagnosis of nephrolithiasis is the presence of bowel gas that interferes with the image. In addition, ultrasound does not assess kidney function; creatinine concentration should be measured if the diagnosis of nephrolithiasis is being made by ultrasound alone.

Intravenous pyelography (IVP) can establish the diagnosis in 96% of cases,[10] but its use is being replaced by helical CT. Some patients have true allergies to IVP dye, and IVPs are contraindicated in children, pregnant women, and patients with renal insufficiency (creatinine > 2).[10] The most common sites for stones to lodge are the narrowest points in the urinary tract (at the ureterovesicular junction, the crossing of the iliac vessels at the pelvic brim, and the ureteropelvic junction). The size of the stone and its location are somewhat predictive of the clinical course.

Management. Indications for outpatient and inpatient management of nephrolithiasis are outlined in Table 9. Initial treatment of renal stones consists of adequate hydration and analgesia. Restoring normal fluid status is frequently all that is necessary to pass the stone from the ureter and to resolve the renal colic. It should be noted, however, that pushing IV fluids to "flush" the stone is no longer believed to be effective or indicated.

Table 9. Management of Patients with Renal Stones

Outpatient Criteria	Admission Criteria
Normal intravenous pyelogram	Stone diameter > 6 mm
Pain relief with oral analgesics	Single kidney
Tolerating oral fluids	Kidney transplant
	Suspicion of infection
	Dehydration
	Unrelenting pain
	Nausea, vomiting

After initial clinical assessment and a rapid urine dipstick test to confirm hematuria, adequate analgesia should be administered before further testing or the return of urinalysis results. Large doses of titrated narcotics are frequently required and may be accompanied by nonsteroidal anti-inflammatory drugs (NSAIDs, typically IV ketorolac). In addition to analgesic effects, NSAIDs decrease ureterospasm and renal capsular pressure.[13] Outpatient treatment is indicated for nephrolithiasis if imaging confirms the absence of complete obstruction, adequate pain relief can be achieved, and the patient can tolerate oral fluids and medications.

When the patient is sent home, a urine strainer should be given with instructions for use. The patient should be informed that the most important time to strain the urine is after the pain has ceased (signifying passage of a stone) and that the urine should be strained for 72 hours to ensure stone retrieval. Retrieved stones are analyzed by crystallography to determine their content and to guide the urologist in preventive therapy.

Most stones ≤ 4 mm in diameter are passed spontaneously. The chances of spontaneous passage drop dramatically to < 10% with stones > 8 mm. Some investigators recommend hospital admission for patients with stones > 6 mm in diameter.[14] If persistent nausea and vomiting are present or if oral narcotics do not relieve the pain, hospital admission is probably necessary.

Pitfalls in Practice. Patients with a classic history for nephrolithiasis but no hematuria may have complete ureteral obstruction. Diagnostic imaging should be considered to establish or refute the diagnosis. A heme-negative urine dipstick also should prompt the physician to reconsider the diagnosis to ensure that a catastrophe mimicking renal colic is not missed, particularly an abdominal aortic aneurysm (AAA). This process can be difficult, because properly communicating with and examining a patient with severe pain are extremely challenging. Findings suspicious for AAA are hypotension, abdominal mass, focal tenderness, abnormal pulsations or bruits, and distal extremity pulse deficits or age > 60 years. Other diagnoses to be considered include ectopic pregnancy, appendicitis, cholecystitis, renal infarction, and papillary necrosis. However, these disorders generally may be ruled out with proper history and analysis of urine and IVP results.

Acute Urinary Retention

Differential Diagnosis. Acute urinary retention (AUR) is the sudden inability to urinate. Although usually not life-threatening, AUR is very painful and may indicate serious underlying pathology. Common causes of AUR can be found in Table 10.

Table 10. Causes of Acute Urinary Retention

Cause	Examples
Obstructive (by location)	
Penis	Phimosis, paraphimosis, meatal stenosis, foreign body
Urethra	Tumor, calculus, foreign body, stricture, meatal stenosis (in women), urethritis, trauma, hematoma
Prostate	Benign prostatic hypertrophy, cancer, prostatitis, prostatic infarction, bladder neck contracture
Neurologic	
Motor paralytic	Spinal shock, spinal cord syndromes
Sensory paralytic	Diabetes, tabes dorsalis, multiple sclerosis, spinal cord syndromes, herpes zoster
Pharmacologic	
α-adrenergic stimulators	Ephedrine, "cold tablets," amphetamines
Other drugs	Antihistamines, anticholinergics, antispasmodics, tricyclic antidepressants

Obstructive retention is the most common cause of AUR. Benign prostatic hypertrophy (BPH) is responsible for most cases of AUR and typically is seen in men older than 50 years. The patient with BPH gives a history of progressively increasing symptoms of hesitancy, nocturia, diminished urinary stream, dribbling, and a sensation of incomplete bladder emptying. Increased fluid loads or medications may precipitate the AUR episode. Obstructive symptoms are a late complication of prostatic carcinoma but may be the presenting complaint.

Neurogenic retention arises from lesions directly or indirectly affecting the spinal cord or the bladder's motor or sensory nerves. Examples of cord lesions include trauma, herniated disc, tumor, epidural abscess, and multiple sclerosis. Bladder nerve damage most often results from either diseases such as diabetes mellitus, herpes, and syphilis or iatrogenic causes such as pelvic surgery. Herpes simplex-mediated transient vesical motor paralysis is also seen.

Pharmacologic retention results from disruption of intravesical neurotransmission. The bladder neck and sphincter have α-adrenergic receptors, which, when stimulated, promote urinary retention. The detrusor muscle of the bladder is parasympathetically innervated, and, when stimulated, promotes bladder emptying and micturition. Consequently, anticholinergic drugs inhibit bladder emptying and contribute to retention. In addition, central nervous system-depressant drugs, such as alcohol, may depress the brainstem center for micturition and contribute to urinary retention.

In children, AUR usually results from congenital obstructive lesions such as meatal stenosis, hypospadias, or posterior urethral valve.

History and Physical Examination. The patient with AUR is usually in acute distress, with lower abdominal pain and severe urgency. On physical examination, the bladder is palpated above the symphysis pubis and sometimes above the umbilicus. Palpation of the urethra may reveal induration suggestive of a stricture or stone. A careful neurologic examination may reveal decreased rectal tone (suggestive of neurologic disease), a pelvic mass, enlarged prostate, or prostatic nodules.

Management. Establishment of bladder drainage is the immediate goal. The insertion of a catheter is both diagnostic and therapeutic. A small 16-French catheter is usually adequate except in cases caused by clot retention, in which a large-caliber catheter is preferred to allow bladder irrigation. If difficulty is encountered in catheterizing patients with BPH, a large-caliber catheter, which is stiffer than a small one, should be used to overcome the resistance imposed by prostatic tissue. If this approach fails, an 18–French coudé catheter usually will pass. Lubrication with an anesthetic jelly (e.g., 1% lidocaine) eases catheter placement and reduces patient discomfort. In the presence of a urethral stricture, care should be taken not to injure the urethral mucosa. In this instance, passage of filiform and follower tubes is a gentler procedure than catheterization and prevents creation of a false passage. If catheterization fails, urologic consultation should be obtained.

If sent home, patients must be instructed to seek medical attention immediately for any symptoms of infection or recurrence of AUR. Follow-up within 2–3 days is advised. Patients sent home with an indwelling catheter should be seen by a urologist within 24–36 hours.

Pitfalls in Practice. Passage of a urinary catheter should never be forceful. If resistance is met, the attempt should be discontinued to avoid urethral injury or the creation of a false lumen. Relief of AUR in the urgent care setting is a temporizing measure. Because AUR can be due to serious underlying disease, failure to ensure follow-up can delay definitive diagnosis and management.

Hernias

Differential Diagnosis. A hernia is the protrusion of any viscus that is enclosed in a peritoneal sac from its normal position through an aperture in the surrounding structures. A reducible hernia can be returned to its normal anatomic position simply by manipulation. An incarcerated hernia is an irreducible hernia, which requires surgical intervention to restore normal anatomy. Incarceration may be acute or chronic. The risk of incarceration is greatest when the hernia occurs in the presence of a condition that causes increased intra-abdominal pressure (e.g., asthma, chronic obstructive pulmonary disease, BPH, constipation). Incarceration is also most likely to occur when the defect is small and the herniated contents large. Once incarceration occurs, edema develops. As it progresses, the hernia becomes increasingly difficult to reduce. Impingement on the vascular supply may occur, resulting in a strangulated hernia. If this vascular compromise is not relieved, gangrene ensues.

History and Physical Examination. Most inguinal hernias are asymptomatic and are detected either inadvertently by the patient or on routine physical examination. The most common complaint is a tender swelling in the groin. When incarceration occurs acutely, pain may develop suddenly, and the patient is unable to return the lump to its normal position. Acute incarcerations may be accompanied by nausea and vomiting if intestinal obstruction (partial or complete) has occurred. Strangulation may occur without signs and symptoms of intestinal obstruction if only a portion of the bowel wall is caught in the defect (Richter's hernia).[15]

Physical examination of the patient with an incarcerated inguinal hernia reveals a tender, abnormal groin swelling. The consistency of the mass depends on the contents of the sac. Mild fever and tachycardia are often present, and signs of intestinal obstruction may be present as well. If strangulation has occurred, perforation, abscess formation, peritonitis, and septic shock may ensue.

Management. Abnormal laboratory studies seen in acute incarceration may include a slightly elevated white blood cell count with a left shift and an elevated blood urea nitrogen level secondary to dehydration. In elderly patients, however, laboratory studies are not reliable indicators of the patient's physical state. Flat and upright abdominal films should be obtained to look for loops of bowel within the hernia sac as well as for air fluid levels and free air under the diaphragm.

If the incarceration is of recent onset, an attempt should be made to reduce the hernia. Immediate surgical consultation is necessary. Before any attempt at reduction is made, the patient should be placed in the Trendelenburg position and given mild sedation. Warm compresses placed over the area may ease reduction by decreasing swelling and relaxing abdominal musculature. Only gentle compression should be attempted, and nothing should be forced back into the abdomen. If there is any question about the duration of incarceration, no attempt should be made so that dead bowel is not reintroduced into the abdomen. If the incarceration cannot be reduced or if any signs of strangulation are present, the patient should be transferred for hospital admission. The patient should be given nothing by mouth, intravenous hydration should be started, and broad-spectrum antibiotics should be administered.

If the incarceration is reduced, the patient may be discharged to home with instructions to seek immediate medical care for any fevers, chills, nausea, vomiting, or abdominal pain. Any patient discharged from an urgent care center after reduction of an incarcerated hernia requires follow-up evaluation by a general surgeon for elective herniorrhaphy.

Pitfalls in Practice. Failure to recognize an incarcerated or strangulated hernia can result in significant morbidity and possible mortality. If any question exists about the diagnosis, the patient should be immediately evaluated by a surgeon. Groin hernias must not be mistaken for tender lymph nodes or hydrocele. Lymph nodes are generally firm, mobile, and multiple. Incarcerated hernias do not transilluminate and are tender, whereas hydroceles usually transilluminate and are not tender. If bowel is present in the hernia sac, bowel sounds may be heard and peristalsis may be seen.

Genital Infections in Men

Infectious Genital Lesions

Differential Diagnosis. Table 11 describes several infectious diseases that can cause genital lesions in men. Cutaneous lesions quickly gain the attention of the patient because of the concern over the possibility of a venereal disease or malignancy.

Table 11. Infectious Causes of Genital Lesions

Disease	Etiology	Characteristics	Presentation
Balanitis	Inflammation of glans penis	Usually uncircumcised patients; may be first symptom of diabetes.	Lesions due to excoriation; purulence, foul odor, tenderness of glans and of foreskin.
Syphilis	*Treponema pallidum*	Incubation: 3–4 weeks.	Solitary painless ulcer with clean base sharp borders.
Chancroid	*Hemophilus ducreyi*	Incubation: 3–14 days.	Multiple painful necrotic lesions, tender inguinal adenopathy.
Herpes progenitalis	Herpes simplex type 2	Primary illness lasts up to 3 weeks; recurrent illness. Virus can be dormant for years and then reactivate.	Multiple shallow ulcerations, painful erythematous papules and vesicles, bilateral tender inguinal adenopathy; occasionally fever, malaise, dysuria.
Genital warts (condyloma acuminatum)	Viral origin	Weeks to 1 year; resistant to therapy.	Cauliflower-shaped, painless lesions; intraurethral lesions may develop.
Granuloma inguinale	*Calymmatobacterium granulomatis*	Incubation: up to 3 months; rare in U.S.	Small, painless, papular, nodular, or vesicular lesions of mucous membranes and skin that develop into extensive granulomatous or ulcerative lesions.
Lymphogranuloma venereum	*Chlamydia trachomatis* immunotypes	Incubation: 3 days to 3 weeks.	Initially, small, transient, nonindurated painless vesicle that ulcerates and heals quickly; followed by tender, enlarged inguinal lymph nodes (pseudobuboes).

(Cont'd on next page)

Table 11. Infectious Causes of Genital Lesions *(Continued)*

Disease	Diagnosis	Management
Balanitis	Clinical	Cleanse with mild soap. Antifungals (nystatin or clotrimazole), or antibacterial agents as appropriate. Referral for circumcision.
Syphilis	Dark field microscopy, fluorescent treponemal antibody, Venereal Disease Research Laboratory test VDRL), rapid plasma reagin (RPR)	Benzathine penicillin G (2.4 µg IM × 1) or doxycycline (100 mg PO bid × 14 days) or tetracycline (500 mg PO qid × 14 days) Follow-up in 4 weeks with primary care physician.
Chancroid	Positive culture for Gram stain	Ceftriaxone (250 mg IM × 1 dose) or erythromycin (500 mg PO qid × 7 days) or azithromycin (1 gm PO × 1 dose) or amoxicillin clavulanate (500 mg PO tid × 7 days) or ciprofloxacin (500 mg PO bid × 3 days). Follow-up at 2 weeks with primary care physician.
Herpes progenitalis	Positive culture for multinucleated giant cells and acidophilic inclusion bodies from ulcer scrapings, positive viral cultures, rising serum antibody titers	Primary: acyclovir 400 mg PO tid or 200 mg 5 times/day × 10 days or famciclovir 250 mg PO tid × 5–10 days or valacyclovir 1000 mg PO bid × 10 days. Recurrent: acyclovir 400 mg PO tid × 5 days or famciclovir 125 mg PO bid × 5 days or valacyclovir 500 mg PO bid × 5 days. Follow-up at 2 weeks with primary care physician.
Genital warts (condyloma acuminatum)	Clinical	Podofilox (Condylox) 2× daily applied with cotton swab for 3 days followed by 4 days without rx; repeat cycle 4–6× as necessary, or 25% podophyllin in tincture of benzoin (Podocon-25) 1× weekly for up to 6 weeks; wash after 1–4 hr, or imiquimod (5% cream) applied 3×/week prior to sleep; remove 6–10 hr later when awake; continue until clear; max of 16 weeks, or obtain VDRL/RPR. Cryotherapy/electrosurgery. Referral to urologist or dermatologist for long-term care.
Granuloma inguinale	Histologic staining of granulo-matous lesions	Doxycycline 100 mg PO bid × 3–4 weeks, or trimethoprim-sulfamethoxazole bid × 3 weeks,or erythromycin 500 mg qid × 3 weeks or ciprofloxacin 750 mg PO qd × 3 weeks. Erythromycin 500 mg PO qid × 14 days. Referral to urologist for long-term care.
Lymphogranuloma	LGV complement fixation test (serum titer test); Frei skin test; culture of pseudobulbar aspirate for *Chlamydia*.	Doxycycline 100 mg PO bid × 21 days or erythromycin 500 mg PO qid × 21 days. Follow-up in 2–3 weeks with primary care physician.

IM = intramuscularly, qid = 4 times/day, PO = orally, tid = 3 times/day, bid = twice daily.

History and Physical Examination. Historical points that aid in the differentiation of in-fectious genital lesions include time since probable exposure, changes in the appearance of the lesion, previous similar episodes, and whether the lesion is painful. On physical examination, the number of lesions, their appearance, and additional local or systemic signs may suggest a particular disease entity. Specific differentiating points about the dis-ease processes can assist in the diagnosis.

Diagnostic Aids. Many of the laboratory studies used to diagnose infectious genital dis-eases (see Table 11) are not routinely available in the urgent care setting or require sev-eral hours to days until results are available. In general, diagnosis of such entities can be made by historical and clinical examination and confirmed when the results of the labo-ratory studies are ready.

Management. Specific management protocols for infectious genital diseases are listed in Table 11. The acute phase of some of these diseases (balanitis, syphilis, and chancroid) usually responds to therapy that can be initiated in the urgent care setting. On the other hand, effective therapy for genital warts and granuloma inguinale may require several months, and the urgent care patient should be referred to a specialist for long-range treatment.

Most of these diseases are effectively managed on an outpatient basis. The treatment of herpes progenitalis, however, is determined by the extent and severity of symptoms. Patients with severe symptoms may require topical and systemic analgesics, hospitalization, catheterization, and intravenous acyclovir.

Pitfalls in Practice. Unless the diagnosis of a benign disease is readily apparent, referral and possible biopsy of cutaneous genital lesions are indicated. Patients who present with painful genital lesions should be given analgesia in addition to the specifically indicated medical management. The possibility of sexual transmission of most genital infections should be discussed with the patient who requires specific treatment.

Penile Discharge

Differential Diagnosis. The complaint of dysuria and penile discharge suggests the presence of urethritis. Male infectious urethritis is either gonococcal or nongonococcal. Most patients with gonococcal urethritis have a copious purulent discharge. Nongonococcal urethritis can be asymptomatic. The penile discharge associated with symptomatic nongonococcal urethritis is often watery or mucoid.

Differentiation of the two types of urethritis by clinical examination is difficult. Gram stain of the penile discharge is a quick, helpful, sensitive and specific diagnostic tool that aids in the effort.[16] Patients with nongonococcal urethritis usually have leukocytes present on Gram stain of the discharge but no intracellular organisms. Because of the strong correlation between a Gram stain and positive culture for gonococci, most authorities agree that Gram stain alone is sufficient to make the diagnosis of gonococcal urethritis. Cultures of the discharge are important, however, to track the epidemiology of the disease and to document the emergence of strains of *N. gonorrhoeae*.

Nongonococcal infectious urethritis occurs alone or together with gonococcal urethritis. *Chlamydia trachomatis* has been implicated in this disease; other organisms, such as *Ureaplasma urealyticum*, also may be important.

Noninfectious causes of urethral syndrome in men include penile foreign bodies, urethral neoplasms, meatal ulcerations, or Reiter's syndrome. Periurethral abscesses and herpes virus can cause urethral irritation, dysuria, and inflammatory penile discharge. A careful physical examination should rule out these possible causes of urethral irritation.

Management. The management of infectious urethritis is outlined in Table 12 (next page). Patients with gonococcal urethritis are treated for presumed concurrent chlamydial infection. Patients with urethritis should be reevaluated 2 weeks after completion of therapy. Repeat cultures should be performed if symptoms persist at that time.

Pitfalls in Practice. Urethritis that persists in men despite adequate antimicrobial therapy suggests infection by a resistant organism. Urethritis is occasionally caused by herpes virus, *Trichomonas* organisms, and *Candida* organisms, which are not adequately treated by the standard recommended therapy. Recurrence of urethritis shortly after adequate

Table 12. Treatment of Gonorrhea/Chlamydial Urethritis

Gonorrhea	1. Ceftriaxone 125 mg IM × 1	Chlamydia	1. Azithromycin 1 gm PO × 1
	2. Cefixime 400 mg PO × 1		2. Doxycycline 100 mg PO bid × 7
	3. Ciprofloxacin 500 mg PO × 1		3. Ofloxacin 300 mg PO bid × 7
	4. Ofloxacin 400 mg PO × 1		

IM = intramuscularly, PO = orally, bid = twice daily.

therapy may be due to postgonococcal urethritis. This syndrome occurs if the initial infectious episode was due to an infection with both gonococci and chlamydial organisms, but treatment was given for only gonococcal urethritis. Treatment for chlamydial infection should be initiated.

Female sexual partners of patients with gonococcal urethritis or chlamydial infection are often asymptomatic at the early stages of infection. Failure to treat sexual partners of patients with these diseases can result in severe infection, such as pelvic inflammatory disease. Treated patients can become reinfected if partners are not treated simultaneously.

Prostatitis

Prostatitis (inflammation of the prostate) can be divided into two categories: acute bacterial prostatitis and chronic prostatitis. Acute prostatitis is the entity most commonly seen in the urgent care setting.

Acute Bacterial Prostatitis

Differential Diagnosis. Acute prostatitis usually occurs in men between the ages of 20 and 40 years and is typically dramatic in its presentation to the urgent care setting, making the diagnosis relatively easy. The patient frequently appears toxic, with fever, chills, and pain that may be suprapubic, perineal, low back, or rectal in location. The infection often begins with malaise, fever, arthralgia, and myalgia several days before the onset of prostatic inflammation, which produces the symptoms of dysuria, frequency, urgency, and even urinary retention.

General physical examination typically reveals findings of toxicity (i.e., fever, tachycardia). Examination of the prostate is often inadequate because of the exquisite pain caused by the examiner's finger but typically reveals a swollen, tender prostate that is firm and warm to the touch. Massage of the prostate may cause hematogenous spread and subsequent bacteremia.

If urethral discharge is present, a Gram stain should be done to exclude gonococcal infection. The bacteria most commonly implicated in acute prostatitis are *Escherichia coli*, *Pseudomonas* sp., enterococci, and *Klebsiella* sp. Rarely, *Salmonella* sp., *Clostridium* sp., tuberculosis, or fungus may cause an acute prostatitis.

Management. Any patient who appears to be toxic or who is febrile, has urinary retention, a prostatic abscess, or altered immune response requires hospital admission. For patients with AUR due to prostatitis, urethral catheterization should be avoided. Suprapubic needle aspiration is much safer and more comfortable for the patient.

Patients not requiring hospitalization require oral antibiotic therapy. Because of the anatomic location of the prostate (completely surrounding the urethra), the urine generally contains the infecting organism. Acute bacterial prostatitis is responsive to antibiotics that under normal circumstances diffuse poorly from plasma into prostatic fluid. Men younger than 35 years should be treated for gonorrhea and chlamydial infections, which are the most common organisms causing prostatitis in young men. Older patients (> 35 years) or those with a history of anal intercourse require coverage for *E. coli*, *Enterobacter*, *Klebsiella*, and *Proteus* spp. Appropriate antibiotics and their dosages are listed in Table 13. All patients treated for acute prostatitis require follow-up with their primary care physician for reexamination after completion of the antibiotic course.

Table 13. Outpatient Treatment of Acute Prostatitis

Men < 35 years old
  1. Ofloxacin 400 mg PO × 1, then 300 mg PO bid × 10 days
  2. Ceftriaxone 250 mg IM × 1, then doxycycline 100 mg PO bid × 10 days

Men > 35 years old or with a history of anal intercourse
  1. Ciprofloxacin 500 mg PO bid × 14–28 days
  2. Trimethoprim-sulfamethoxazole 1 tab PO bid × 14–28 days
  3. Ofloxacin 200 mg PO bid × 14–28 days

PO = orally, IM = intramuscularly, bid = twice daily.

Antipyretics, narcotic analgesics, and stool softeners also are indicated. NSAIDs and spasmolytics may be used for mild pain. Bed rest and sitz baths also make the patient more comfortable.

Pitfalls in Practice. Some experts maintain that if acute prostatitis is suspected, rectal examination should not be performed because of the potential for sepsis from bacterial seeding. This philosophy seems to ignore the differential diagnosis and the potential hazards of an incomplete physical examination. Missing a perirectal abscess or a rectal neoplasm can have tragic consequences. A reasonable compromise is to have only one examiner perform a gentle, brief rectal examination.

Failure to recognize the need for a prolonged course of antibiotics in treating acute prostatitis is another pitfall. Because of the relatively poor penetration of antibiotics into prostatic tissue as well as the risk of developing chronic bacterial prostatitis, most cases must be treated for at least 14–28 days.

Chronic Prostatitis

Differential Diagnosis. Chronic prostatitis is a relapsing, indolent disease, and the urgent care physician most often deals with an acute exacerbation. Clinical manifestations vary widely, but most patients complain of urinary symptoms (frequency, urgency, and dysuria), low back pain, and perineal pain. Low-grade fever, hematospermia, and suprapubic or testicular pain also may be present.

Physical examination of the patient is often noncontributory. The prostate examination is frequently normal, but the prostate is sometimes tender, boggy, or somewhat firm to the touch. Urine collected at the end of the patient's urinary stream after prostatic massage contains expressed prostatic secretions; urine collection, therefore, increases the chances of isolating the responsible organism. If no bacterial pathogen is identified, the term chronic nonbacterial prostatitis is used; it is postulated that this entity may be caused by organisms such as *Chlamydia* sp., *Ureaplasma urealyticum*, *Trichomonas vaginalis*, or *Mycoplasma hominis*.

Management. Whereas treatment of acute prostatitis is relatively easy and has a high success rate, the treatment of chronic prostatitis is difficult and frustrating to both patient and physician. Cure is difficult because most antimicrobial agents that are useful against the causative organisms diffuse poorly into the prostatic fluids. In addition, no organism is identified in the nonbacterial variant of chronic prostatitis.

On the basis of tissue levels and penetration, drugs that may be appropriate for use in chronic prostatitis include trimethoprim-sulfamethoxazole, doxycycline, erythromycin, and carbenicillin. Ciprofloxacin also is recommended. As in acute prostatitis, adequate analgesia, stool softeners, sitz baths, and avoidance of ejaculation are indicated. All patients with chronic prostatitis should be referred to a urologist for appropriate management.

Pitfalls in Practice. The relapsing nature of chronic prostatitis, as well as the need for a specialist, needs to be explained and emphasized to the patient to encourage compliance with both antibiotic therapy and follow-up care.

References

1. Fracchia JA, Mottoa J, Miller LS, et al: Evaluation of asymptomatic microhematuria. Urology 46:484–489, 1995.
2. Ahmed Z, Lee J: Asymptomatic urinary abnormalities: Hematuria, proteinuria. Med Clin North Am 81:641–652, 1997.
3. Hooton TM, Stamm WE: Diagnosis and treatment of uncomplicated UTIs. Infect Dis Clin North Am 11:551–581, 1997.
4. Shaw KN, McGowan KL, Gorelick MH, Schwartz JS: Screening for UTIs in infants in the ED: Which test is best? Pediatrics 101(6):E1, 1998.
5. Winberg J: Commentary: Progressive renal damage from infection with or without reflux. J Urol 148:1733–1734, 1992.
6. Gallagher S: Diagnosis and management of UTIs: A disease stratification model. Part I: Epidemiology, detection, and evaluation. Emerg Med Rep 20(4):33–40, 1999.
7. Burgher SW: Acute scrotal pain. Emerg Med Clin North Am 16:781–809, 1998.
8. Edelsburg JS, Surh YS: The acute scrotum. Emerg Med Clin North Am 6:521–546, 1988.
9. Stewart C, Bosker G: Common sexually transmitted diseases: Diagnosis and treatment of uncomplicated gonococcal and chlamydial infection. Emerg Med Rep 20:173–182, 1999.
10. Steward C: Nephrolithiasis. Emerg Med Clin North Am 6:617–630, 1988.
11. Boulay I, Holtz P, Foley WD, et al: Ureteral calculi: Diagnostic efficiency of helical CT and implications for treatment of patients. Am J Radiol 15:877–893, 1999.
12. Brown DF, Rosen CL, Wolfe RE: Renal ultrasonography. Emerg Med Clin North Am 15:877–893, 1997.
13. Larson RE, Shapiro MA: Sexually transmitted urogenital diseases. Emerg Med Clin North Am 6:487–508, 1988.
14. Drach GW: Urinary lithiasis: Etiology, diagnosis, medical management. In Walsh PC, Retik AB, Stanley TA, Vaughi ED (eds): Campbell's Urology, 6th ed, vol. 3. Philadelphia, W.B. Saunders, 1992.
15. Kadirov S, Sayan J, Friedman S, et al: Richter's hernia: A surgical pitfall. J Am Coll Surg 182:60, 1996.
16. Morris DL: Sexually transmitted diseases. In Tintinalli JE, Kelen GD, Stapczynski JS (eds): Emergency Medicine: A Comprehensive Study Guide, 5th ed. New York, McGraw-Hill, 2000, pp 943–946.

Chapter 6

Infectious Disease

Joshua Cochrane, MD
Terrence D. Morton, Jr., MD
Michelle H. Biros, MS, MD

Problems related to infectious diseases are commonly seen in the urgent care setting and also account for much of the medical advice given to patients or their caretakers over the telephone. Many diseases of infectious etiology are covered in other chapters that deal with the organ systems affected; this chapter presents additional problems and concepts of infectious disease.

Immunizations

Immunizations enhance the immune system to prevent or treat an infectious disease. Passive immunization occurs after the administration of immunologically active substances (i.e., immunoglobulins) derived from an outside source (human or animal) and given to the patient for immediate immunity against the infection. Active immunization occurs when the patient is administered a killed or attenuated live infectious agent, which stimulates the patient's natural defenses to develop immunity against the infectious organism. Active immunity develops 7–21 days after exposure to the antigen.

Passive immunization can be done for immediate protection when the time between exposure and possible infection is shorter than the time needed for development of active immunity. Passive immunization is also used when no antigen for active immunization is available or when active immunization is contraindicated (i.e., during pregnancy or in immunosuppressed patients). In general, passive immunity is of short duration, and frequent repeat dosing may be needed to offer continued protection. The immunogens given in passive immunization can serve as antigens, especially if animal serum is the source of the vaccine, and thus can cause serum sickness.

Although an urgent care center is not the ideal setting for patients to receive immunizations, patients may ask about recommendations for immunizations, side effects, timing of administration, and safety. Public policy about immunizations for infectious disease is constantly evolving; therefore, information in this handbook invariably will be revised as newer and more effective vaccines are developed.

Who Should Be Immunized?

This question initially sounds rhetorical and intuitive, but in certain situations the answer may not be so clear. Recommendations for childhood immunization have been made by a variety of authoritative groups. These recommendations cover immunizations against several infectious diseases from birth to the timing of boosters in the early teens. Table 1 provides a basic childhood immunization schedule; there may be state-specific modifications, depending on the patient population. Adherence to the recommendations is mandatory to attend public schools, but many children treated in an urgent care setting are of preschool age. Screening questions to determine compliance with recommended immunizations should be asked in the history.

Table 1. Routine Immunizations in Childhood

Vaccine	Age							
	Birth	*2 Mo*	*4 Mo*	*6 Mo*	*12 Mo*	*15 Mo*	*4–6 Yr*	*11–12 Yr*
Hepatitis B	HB-1	HB-2		HB-3				
Diphtheria, tetanus, pertussis		DTP	DTP	DTP	DTP or DTaP @ 15+ mo		DTP or DTaP	dT
Hemophilus influenzae type b		Hib	Hib	Hib	Hib			
Polio		OPV	OPV	OPV			OPV	
Measles, mumps, rubella					MMR		MMR	MMR

Some recommendations for immunizations extend beyond childhood. Pneumococcal disease is associated with thousands of deaths each year, affecting mostly elders and debilitated patients. Pneumococccal vaccinations are therefore frequently recommended for these subgroups.[1] Influenza epidemics are also associated with many thousands of deaths each year. Current recommendations for elders, health care workers, and chronically ill patients are yearly influenza vaccinations. Patients with asplenia, chronically ill patients, and elders should be immunized against pneumococci. Boosters for pneumococci are not recommended, except for patients with asplenia, renal failure, or transplant, because of increased occurrence of side effects with repeat vaccination.[1]

Who Should Not Be Immunized?

There are four broad categories of contraindications to immunizations: (1) a live virus should not be given to patients who cannot mount an immune response (i.e., patients with HIV/AIDS, cancer, leukemia, chemotherapy, radiation therapy, or high-dose steroids); (2) immunization should be avoided in a patient with a known severe reaction to one of the components of a vaccine; (3) live virus immunizations should be avoided in pregnant women; and (4) live immunization should be avoided in patients with active moderate-to-severe illness. Table 2 contains a list of common immunizations, possible side effects, and contraindications.

Who Should Be Given Passive Immunizations?

Passive immunization, the administration of preformed antibodies in anticipation of exposure or after exposure to a potentially infectious disease, may be necessary in treatment

Table 2. Common Immunizations

Vaccine or Immune Globulin	Type of Preparation	Population to Be Immunized	Common Adverse Reactions	Contraindications
Diphtheria toxoid	Toxoid	All	Local pain and swelling	
Tetanus toxoid	Toxoid	All	Local pain and swelling	
Tetanus immune globulin	High titer HIG	Unimmunized patient with wound	No significant reactions	Anaphylaxis to previous gammaglobulins or thimerosal.
Whole cell pertussis	Killed bacteria	All children	Fever, pain, local swelling, reported severe neurologic reactions and/or febrile seizure	Encephalopathy within 7 days of administration; neurologic disorder with progressive mental delay or neurologic change; age over 6 yr; fever > 105°F within 48 hr.
Acellular pertussis vaccine	Fractionated killed bacteria and toxoid	All	See above, but the reactions are more mild	See above.
Measles vaccine	Live attenuated virus	All children	Fever, rash	Anaphylaxis to eggs or neomycin; pregnancy: moderate to severe illness; immunodeficiency, although HIV positive alone not a contraindication.
Rubella	Live attenuated virus	All children and unimmunized women	Arthralgias, fever	Anaphylaxis to eggs or neomycin; pregnancy: moderate to severe illness; immunodeficiency, although HIV positive alone not a contraindication.
Mumps	Live attenuated virus	All children and young adults without history of mumps	Not significant	Anaphylaxis to eggs or neomycin; pregnancy: moderate to severe illness; immunodeficiency, although HIV positive alone not a contraindication.
Polio vaccine, oral	Live attenuated virus	All	Rare paralytic disease	HIV infection; immunodeficiency; household contacts with HIV or known immunodeficiency; moderate to severe systemic illness.
Polio vaccine parenteral	Killed virus	All	Not significant	Anaphylaxis to neomycin, polymyxin B, or streptomycin
Hemophilus influenzae, type B	Conjugated purified polysaccharide	All children and high-risk adults (asplenia)	Not significant	
Hepatitis B immune globulin	High-titered human gammaglobulin	Nonimmunized patients exposed to hepatitis B	Not significant	Anaphylaxis to previous gammaglobulins

(Cont'd on next page)

Table 2. Common Immunizations *(Continued)*

Vaccine or Immune Globulin	Type of Preparation	Population to Be Immunized	Common Adverse Reactions	Contraindications
Influenza vaccine	Killed virus; preparations change yearly	Persons at high risk (elders, chronically ill, health care employees)	Fever, local tenderness	Past history of anaphylaxis to eggs, flu vaccination, or aminoglycosides; Guillain-Barré disease; acute febrile illness
Meningococcal vaccine	Purified poly-saccharide	Only during disease epidemics or patients at high risk	Erythema at the site of injection	Moderate illness with or without fever
Rabies vaccine	Killed virus	Person bitten by possibly rabid animal or at high risk of exposure	Pain, urticaria, rare neurologic reactions	Anaphylaxis; acute illness
Rabies immune globulin	High-titered human gamma-globulin	Unimmunized persons with suspicious animal bite	Not significant	Anaphylaxis to previous gammaglobulins
Pneumococcal vaccine	Polyvalent purified polysaccharide	Persons with asplenia, chronic illness or elders	Erythema at the site of injection	Anaphylaxis; acute illness

of a previously unimmunized patient. Examples of passive immunization include tetanus immune globulin (TIG) and rabies prophylaxis.

Tetanus is a progressively debilitating disease, characterized by progressive muscle tetani from the central nervous system effects of *Clostridium tetani* toxin. It affects approximately 50 Americans a year.[2] Since tetanus immunization is part of the routine vaccinations of childhood, most cases occur in elders who have not had boosters or recent immigrants. Symptoms of the disease—increased muscle tone and generalized muscle spasms—typically occur within 4–21 days. Treatment is largely supportive. The prognosis is worse for neonates, chronically ill patients and elders. The sequelae of tetanus infection are entirely preventable with up-to-date immunizations or early immune globulin therapy. The Centers for Disease Control (CDC) has published recommendations for tetanus prophylaxis for routine wound management[3] (Table 3).

Table 3. Recommendations for Tetanus Prophylaxis

History of Absorbed Tetanus Toxoid	Clean, Minor Wounds		All Other Wounds	
	Td	TIG	Td	TIG
Uncertain or < 3 doses	Yes	No	Yes	Yes
≥ 3 doses*	No	No	No	No

* Last dose within 10 years for a clean wound and 5 years for a contaminated wound.
Td = 0.5 ml IM; TIG = 250 U IM

Rabies acquired within the United States is rare and preventable. The virus is spread by direct inoculation of tissue with infected secretions (i.e., bite) or, rarely, by inhaled aerosolized virus, ingestion, or organ or tissue transplant. In many parts of the world domestic animals are major carriers of the rabies virus, but in the U.S. this scenario is rare. Wild-life carnivores account for more than 90% of the suspected cases in the U.S.; wild skunks, bats, foxes, coyotes, raccoons, and bobcats are notorious carriers.[4] After exposure, the virus has a variable and often prolonged incubation period, ranging from 10 days to over 1 year. The virus initially replicates in the peripheral muscle tissues and then develops a specific affinity for nervous tissue, spreading centripetally up the nerve toward the central nervous system. Clinical manifestations are represented in the following four stages: (1) nonspecific prodrome (e.g., headache, fever, malaise, myalgia); (2) acute encephalitis (e.g., seizures, posturing, hallucinations); (3) profound brainstem dysfunction (bulbar palsies/neuritis, hydrophobia, suppressed respiratory drive); and (4) recovery (rare).

Animals bite approximately one million Americans yearly. Pre-exposure prophylaxis for rabies should be given to veterinarians, cave explorers, laboratory workers who handle rabies virus, and tourists traveling to highly endemic regions with significant exposure risk. The vaccine (human diploid cell vaccine, [HDCV]), rabies vaccine absorbed [RVA], or purified chick embryo cell culture [PCEC]), is given in three doses over 21–28 days. Receiving the pre-exposure vaccine does not eliminate the need for postexposure prophylaxis; it eliminates only the need to receive human rabies immune globulin (HRIG) and decreases the number of required vaccine doses to two.

Prophylaxis for rabies should be given as soon as possible after the exposure, preferably within 24 hours. The recommended treatment for postexposure prophylaxis includes administration of HRIG (20 IU/kg, as much as possible near the wound and the rest at an intramuscular site away from the intramuscular site of the vaccine) and initiation of the 5-dose vaccination series. Previously unimmunized patients should receive vaccine doses on days 0, 3, 7, 14, and 28.[5] For previously immunized patients, vaccine should be given on days 0 and 3.

Before initiating the postexposure protocol, the physician should consider the following questions: (1) Was there exposure to saliva? (2) Was the animal a known or suspected virus carrier? (3) Was the animal captured? If questions arise about whether a patient should be given postexposure rabies prophylaxis, the local state department of health should be contacted. A proposed set of clinical guidelines is presented in Figure 1 (next page).

Reportable Diseases

A reportable disease has been defined by a state's department of health as constituting a public health hazard because of its potential to spread to epidemic proportions or otherwise endanger the health of a specific population. Statistics about the number of cases of such diseases are kept by state health departments to help trace epidemiologic trends. Each state has a separate list of reportable diseases.

Every state's department of health requires the reporting of certain communicable diseases. The list commonly comprises diseases of epidemiologic concern: venereal diseases, diseases with high attack rates, and diseases of public health concern. It is the responsibility of the treating physician to report the diagnosis of a reportable disease to the local health authorities. Reporting may be done on an immediate (i.e., hepatitis A outbreak among food handlers) or delayed basis (i.e., giardiasis). Exact requirements are county- and state-dependent. Table 4 provides a list of selected reportable diseases.

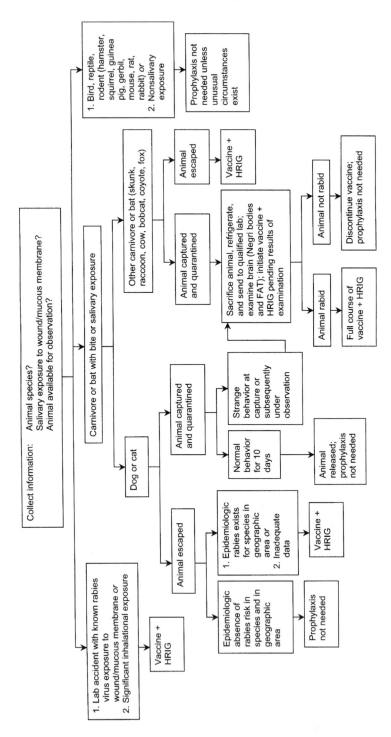

Figure 1. Clinical guidelines for administration of rabies postexposure prophylaxis. FAT = fluorescent antibody test; HRIG = human rabies immune globulin. (Adapted from Mann JR: Rabies risk: Systemic evaluation and management of animal bites. Compr Ther 7:53, 1981.)

Table 4. Selected Reportable Diseases

Acquired immunodeficiency syndrome (AIDS)	Herpes simplex (neonatal)	Psittacosis
	Kawasaki syndrome	Rabies
Amebiasis	Influenza, viral (laboratory confirmed)	Reye's syndrome
Animal bites	Lead poisoning	Rheumatic fever (Jones criteria only)
Anthrax	Legionellosis	Rocky Mountain spotted fever
Aseptic meningitis	Leprosy	Rubella and congenital rubella syndrome
Botulism	Leptospirosis	Salmonellosis
Brucellosis	Lyme disease	Septicemia in newborns
Chancroid	Lymphogranuloma venereum	Shigellosis
Chlamydia trachomatis infection	Malaria	Staphylococcus aureus (outbreaks only)
Cholera	Measles	Syphilis
Diphtheria	Meningitis	Tetanus
Encephalitis	Meningococcemia	Toxic shock syndrome
Giardiasis	Mumps	Trichinosis
Gonorrhea	Murine typhus fever	Tuberculosis
Granuloma inguinal	Pertussis	Tularemia
Hemophilus influenzae type b (invasive)	Plague	Typhoid fever
Hepatitis A, B, C	Poliomyelitis	Varicella

Physicians are also responsible for reporting outbreak of disease of known or unknown etiology, an incidence case of potential danger to public health, and an unusual manifestation of a communicable disease.

Communicable Diseases

Communicable disease is defined as illness that can be spread from human host to human host. The list of such diseases is obviously extensive, and the majority are covered in other chapters. This section highlights common viral communicable diseases capable of outbreaks into community epidemics.

Differential Diagnosis. The differential diagnosis of community-acquired illness is broad. Table 5 provides a truncated list of common viral communicable diseases, their epidemiology, presentation, diagnosis, treatment, and follow-up issues. History-taking clues that may help in making a diagnosis include information about immunization status, ill contacts, presence of a prodromal syndrome, location or progression of rash, and associated symptoms. Travel history and community outbreak trends also may be helpful in eliciting a diagnosis.

Management. Management of the most common communicable diseases is largely supportive, although evidence indicates that early treatment (i.e., within 48 hours of symptoms) with amantadine or rimantadine may foreshorten the symptoms of influenza A.[6] Details of management and treatment of some viral diseases are included in Table 5. Of note are the potential morbidity and mortality associated with exposure of high-risk populations to certain highly contagious viruses (i.e., influenza in elders, varicella in pregnant women). Precautions should be taken to avoid contact between the newly diagnosed patient and at-risk groups.

Pitfalls in Practice. Many communicable viral diseases pose serious morbidity and mortality risks to certain high-risk populations. It is important to stress the need for isolation, if the patient may be in contact with the immunocompromised, pregnant, or elderly people.

Table 5. Communicable Viral Illnesses

Disease	Epidemiology	Presentation	Diagnosis	Treatment	Follow-up Issues
Measles	Incubation: 7–14 days Incidence greatest: 5–7 yr Route of spread: nasopharyngeal secretions Communicability: high before prodrome to 4 days after rash Immunity: lifelong after infection Epidemic: every 2–3 yr Prevention: MMR immunization	Prodrome: fever, cough, coryza, conjunctivitis, pharyngitis, Koplik's spots, rash (starts on face).	Clinical, exposure history	Symptomatic	Patient may return to work or school 5 days after rash disappears.
Mumps	Incubation: 2–3 wk Incidence greatest: ages 5–14 yr Route of spread: res- piratory secretions Communicability: from 6 days before to 9 days after parotitis Immunity: lifelong after infection Prevention: MMR vaccine	Prodrome: fever, headache, swollen, tender single or multiple salivary glands. Unilateral orchitis, oophoritis, aseptic meningitis.	Clinical, usual exposure history	Symptomatic	Patient may return to school or work when swollen glands subside. Potential complications: staphylococcal parotitis or sterility (very rare).
Varicella (chicken pox)	Incubation: 14–18 days Incidence greatest: 2–8 yr Route of spread: res- piratory secretions Communicability: highly contagious when lesions open and weeping Immunity: lifelong	Mild (no prodrome) Characteristic vesicular rash starting on trunk with crops of lesions of varying ages.	Clinical, exposure history, Tzank smear	Symptomatic: varicella zoster IG within 72 hr of exposure for high-risk con- tacts (immuno- compromised and neonates), acyclovir, foscarnet	Congenitally acquired in- fection associated with significant mortality and morbidity. Reye's syndrome asso- ciated with chicken pox and aspirin. Potential complications: secondary pneumonia. Patients may return to school or work after last of lesions have crusted.
Mononucleo- sis (Epstein- Barr virus)	Incubation: 2–4 wk Incidence greatest: all ages Route of spread: saliva Communicability: uncertain Immunity: lifelong	Fever, cervical lymphadenop- athy, spleno- megaly, pharyn- gitis; occasional hepatitis, rash, pneumonitis, myopericarditis, CNS involvement.	Clinical, atypical lymphocytes on smear, positive serum heterophil antibody test	Supportive	Complete recovery in 2–4 wk Potential complications: fatigue and malaise that may persist for months Splenic rupture No contact sports for at least 4 wk; longer if spleen is still palpable or tender at follow-up.

(Cont'd on next page)

Table 5. Communicable Viral Illnesses *(Continued)*

Disease	Epidemiology	Presentation	Diagnosis	Treatment	Follow-up Issues
Roseola infantum	Incubation: 10 days Incidence greatest: 6 mo to 3 yr, most common in the fall and spring Route of spread: uncertain Communicability: mildly contagious Immunity: lifelong	Begins with acute onset of fever lasting 3–5 days. Temperatures up to 41° C with child active and alert. Fine, rose-colored maculopapular rash on trunk after breaking fever; may spread to face and hands.	Clinical; leukopenia on day 3 to 4 is suggestive, though nonspecific	Supportive; acetaminophen for fever	Most common exanthem in patients < 2 years of age, self limited. High fevers may result in febrile seizures.
Erythema infectiosum	Incubation: 4–14 days Incidence: usually between 2 and 12 yr Route of spread: respiratory secretions Communicability: mildly contagious	Few constitutional symptoms Three staged rash: 1. "Slapped cheeks" with circumoral palor 2. Erythematous maculopapular rash spreading to trunk and extremities, fades in approximately 1 wk 3. Recurrence of rash precipitated by minor trauma, sunlight, cold	Clinical	Supportive	Adults with more serious course: fever, adenopathy, malaise and arthritis. Rarely associated aplastic crisis in patients with chronic hemolytic anemia; may require blood transfusion.
Influenza	Incubation: 18–72 hr Incidence: all ages, capable of epidemics Route of spread: respiratory secretions Communicability: highly contagious Immunity: annual change in serotypes prevents significant immunity	Syndrome: abrupt onset of fever (up to 106° F) lasting 3–7 days, chills, myalgias, headache and malaise Cough, nasal discharge, sore throat appear when systemic symptoms wane Cough and weakness last 2 weeks or longer.	Clinical; nasopharyngeal swab	Treatment: amantadine or rimantadine taken within 2 days of the onset of symptoms may reduce the duration of fever and systemic symptoms by 1–2 days. Otherwise supportive	Complications: pulmonary—range from mild airway hyperactivity to ARDS. Secondary pneumonia. Rare: myositis, Guillain-Barré disease, Reye's syndrome.

ARDS = acute respiratory distress syndrome, CNS = central nervous system.

Parasitic Diseases

Although endemic parasitic disease is not prevalent in much of the metropolitan United States, primary care physicians need to be familiar with recognizing, diagnosing, and treating parasitic illness because (1) U.S. citizens are traveling more often to endemic international destinations; (2) an increasing number of people from southeast Asia, Africa,

Central, and South America are immigrating to metropolitan U.S.; (3) patients with acquired immunodeficiency syndrome are at risk for enteric parasites; and (4) many rural areas in the U.S. are endemic for certain parasitic diseases.

Differential Diagnosis. The signs and symptoms of parasitic illness are often protean and nonspecific. The urgent care physician must keep a high index of suspicion and should direct the history toward possible exposure to a parasitic agent. Gastrointestinal symptoms, including diarrhea, abdominal discomfort, and visualization of the passage of parasites, are common, but parasitic illness can affect any organ system.

Management. Table 6 divides the more common parasitic infections into affected organ system, morphology, epidemiology, presentation, diagnosis, and treatment.

Table 6. Common Parasitic Infections

System	Parasite	Morphology	Epidemiology
Gastrointestinal disorders	*Giardia lamblia*	Extracellular protozoan	Found worldwide. Ingestion of food or water contaminated by cysts. Beavers may be an animal reservoir. Transmission from person-to-person contact, venereal disease in male homosexual population.
	Ascaris lumbricoides	6–14 inch long, tan to pink worm with curved posterior end	Greatest incidence in tropical areas and southeastern U.S. Transmission: food and water contaminated with eggs.
	Strongyloides stercoralis	Filariform and rhaditiform larvae	Greatest incidence in warm, moist areas, including southeastern U.S. Transmission: larvae from stool contaminated soil penetrate lower extremity integument.
	Ancylostoma duodenale, Necator americanus (hookworm)	½ inch long, cylindrical worm with flexed end	Greatest incidence in warm, moist areas, including southeastern U.S. Transmission: larvae from sewage-contaminated soil penetrate lower extremity integument.
	Taenia saginata (beef tapeworm)	10–30 inch long worm with flat segmented body	Endemic wherever undercooked beef is eaten, common in the U.S.
	Trichuris trichiura (whipworm)	2 inch long, threadlike worm with "whip" end and thick "handle" end	Greatest incidence in tropical areas and the southeastern U.S., especially in institutionalized patients. Transmission: food and water contaminated by eggs.
	Enterobius vermicularis (pinworm)	¼–½ inch long, round white worm with cephalic swelling	Greatest incidence in children, group spread is common. Spread via anus to mouth secondary to scratching.
	Hymenolepsis nana (dwarf tapeworm)	1–2 inch long worm	Endemic: most common tapeworm in the U.S., mostly children. Transmission: fecal-oral.
Cardiovascular	*Trypanosoma cruzi* (Chagas disease)	C-shaped flagellated protozoa	Endemic to South America. Transmission: fecal-oral.
	Trichinella spiralis (trichinosis)	Usually not visualized	Endemic where pork is eaten

(Columns cont'd on next page)

Pitfalls in Practice. The signs and symptoms of parasitic illness often may be insidious. The history may provide the only clues to a diagnosis. Travel history, country of origin and time in the U.S., and possible exposure to undercooked meat or suspect water should be included in the physician's standard history questions. In addition, toxoplasmosis titers probably should be checked in cat owners before pregnancy.

Immunocompromised Patients

Differential Diagnosis. Immunocompromise may result from one of several etiologies: (1) inborn errors of the immune system (i.e., antibody, cell-mediated, phagocytic, or complement deficiencies); (2) iatrogenic causes (i.e., steroids or chemotherapeutic

Table 6. *(Columns continued)*

Presentation	Diagnosis	Treatment
Abdominal distention, malodorous diarrhea or soft stool, crampy midepigastric abdominal pain.	Cysts or trophozoites in stool, duodenal "fuzzy string test," endoscopy with biopsy.	Metronidazole 250 mg PO tid × 5 days In pregnancy paromomycin 500 mg PO tid × 7 days
Vague abdominal pain, may initiate biliary colic during migration. Larval stage in the lungs causes fever, chills, dyspnea, cough, malaise, pneumonia.	Diagnosis by clinical suspicion; eosinophilia, passage of eggs or adult worms in the stool	Mebendazole 100 mg PO bid × 3 days or pyrantel pamoate 11 mg/kg × 1 dose
"Creeping eruption" migrating linear urticarial eruption, pneumonia, midepigastric or RUQ pain. Major concern for the immunodeficient— violation of bowel integrity, CNS infection.	Papanicolaou-stained gastric aspirate, indirect hemaggluti- nation or ELISA test.	Thiabendazole 50 mg/kg/day bid × 2–5 days
Cramping epigastric pain, nausea, diarrhea or constipation, anemia with large worm burden.	Eggs or larvae in stool.	Mebendazole 100 mg PO bid for 3 days. Treat anemia if necessary.
Asymptomatic to vague midepigastric discomfort, diarrhea and hunger pains.	Passage of eggs or body segments.	Niclosamide (2 gm PO × 1 or, for children, < 34 kg, 1 gm PO × 1)
Usually asymptomatic. Severe infestations: anorexia, vomiting, abdominal pain. May cause iron deficiency anemia.	Eggs found in stool, eosinophilia.	Mild infections require no treatment. Severe infections: children and adults—mebendazole 100 mg bid × 4 days
Perianal pruritus, cystitis, enuresis, vaginitis; may be asymptomatic.	Clinical, clear tape test for eggs.	Mebendazole 100 mg PO or pyrantel pamoate 11 mg/kg; repeat in 2 wk. Treat entire family or exposed group
Usually asymptomatic. If severe: abdominal pain, diarrhea, dizziness, headache, toxemia.	Eggs in stool.	Niclosamide (2 gm PO for 5 days, or for children < 34 kg, 1 gm PO for 5 days). Recheck stool after treatment.
Myocarditis, conduction system damage (RBBB), ventricular aneurysms, CHF; lymphedema; may have CNS involvement—seizures, cerebral edema.	Peripheral smear complement-fixation tests, indirect hemagglutination.	Nifurtimox 1.25 mg/kg qid increasing by 2 mg/kg/day every 2 weeks until 15–17 mg/kg/day.
Usually asymptomatic, but larvae may invade cardiac muscle tissue resulting in inflammatory response—myocarditis, CHF. May also produce facial edema, CNS symptoms.	Biopsy or skin test: after 2–5 weeks.	Prevention—cooking or freezing pork. For severe infections: steroids and mebendazole 200–400 mg PO tid × 10 days.

(Cont'd on next page)

Table 6. Common Parasitic Infections *(Continued)*

System	Parasite	Morphology	Epidemiology
Pulmonary	*Ascaris lumbricoides, Ancyclostoma duodenale, Ncctor americanus*	See above.	See above.
	Paragonimus westermani (lung fluke)	Flat worm	Ingestion of tainted, undercooked fresh water crab or crayfish.
	Taenia solium (pork tapeworm; cysticercosis)	Tapeworm	Ingestion of contaminated pork containing larval cysts. Most common in tropical climates, but often seen in U.S.
	Echinococcus granulosus	Tapeworm	Ingestion of food or water contaminated by ova from sheep or cattle infected by an adult worm. Seen commonly in U.S.
	Toxoplasma gondii (toxoplasmosis)	Intracytoplasmic protozoan	Greatest incidence in warm climates, but endemic in U.S. Cats are the primary hosts. Transmission: soil or litter boxes soiled with infected cat stool.

RUQ = right upper quadrant, CNS = central nervous system, RBBB = right bundle-branch block, CHF = congestive heart failure, GI = gastrointestinal, PO = orally, bid = 2 times/day, tid = 3 times/day.

agents); (3) acquired deficiency (AIDS); (4) chronic disease (renal or hepatic failure); or (5) chronic alcohol or drug abuse. Because such patients have an impaired ability to fight infection, they are much more likely to contract, harbor, and develop severe infectious disease than immuncompetent people. Therefore early and thorough assessment, diagnosis, and treatment of patients who present with immunocompromise and suggestions of an infectious illness are critical to avoid significant morbidity and mortality.

Most patients who present to an urgent care or emergency department with immunocompromise have been previously diagnosed. Multiple bacterial pneumonias or the presence of opportunistic infections may lead to a new diagnosis of immunodeficiency. Table 7 (next page) lists common causes of immunocompromise and typical associated pathogens.

Management. Physical exam must be extraordinarily thorough in evaluating a patient with immunocompromise and a fever. Increased temperature may be the only overt sign of infection because the patient's baseline immune response is impaired. The urgent care physician must examine carefully the skin, oral pharynx, lungs, heart, perineum, and vascular access sites for possible sources of infection.

If the history and physical exam suggest systemic illness, a complete laboratory workup should be initiated before hospital admission. Evaluation includes complete blood count with differential; urine, sputum, and blood for culture; urinanalysis; chest x-ray; and, possibly, stool for white blood cells, ova, and parasites as well as cerebral spinal fluid. An initial course of broad-spectrum antibiotics should be started as soon as possible.

Table 6. *(Columns continued)*

Presentation	Diagnosis	Treatment
In addition to GI symptoms, the migratory life-cycle of these parasites can cause a pneumonitis as larvae burrow through alveolar wall.	See above.	See above.
Pneumonia with persistent cough, hemoptysis, chest pain, symptoms similar to tuberculosis (TB).	Eggs in sputum or stool, also have complement-fixation, indirect hemagglutination tests. Patients often are TB skin test positive.	Praziquantel 25 mg/kg PO tid.
Migration of larvae into CNS and subsequent cyst formation causes an inflammatory reaction: inflammation fibrosis, and calcification. Enlargement causes brain compression and may be manifested by seizures.	Clinical: first-time seizure coupled with risk of exposure and CT scan with ring enhancing lesion. Biopsy.	Praziquantel 50 mg/kg/day divided tid × 15 days.
Migration and encystment of larvae: liver most common, but also CNS. Seizures are a common presentation.	CT scan, serum or CNS complement fixation testing.	Careful surgical excision.
Usually asymptomatic but severe infections may occur in immunocompromise: i.e., seizures. High risk for birth defects if acquired during pregnancy.	Serologic testing.	Adults: pyrimethamine (7 mg/kg/day × 3 days, then 0.3 mg/kg/day) Children: sulfadiazine (100 mg/kg/day) Pregnancy: clindamycin (need obstetric consult).

RUQ = right upper quadrant, CNS = central nervous system, RBBB = right bundle-branch block, CHF = congestive heart failure, GI = gastrointestinal, PO = orally, bid = 2 times/day, tid = 3 times/day.

Table 7. Causes of Immunocompromise

Cause of Immunocompromise	Typical Infectious Pathogens
Neutropenia (maligancy, treatment with cytotoxic chemotherapy)	Gram-negative bacilli: *Escherichia coli, Klebsiella, Pseudomonas, Enterobacter, Proteus* spp. Gram-positive cocci: *Staphylococcus epidermidis, S. aureus,* alpha hemolytic streptococci). Fungi: *Candida* and *Aspergillus* spp.
Cell-mediated immunity (CMI) deficiency (i.e., chemotherapy, high dose steroids, leukemia, lymphoma, AIDS)	Bacteria (intracellular): *Listeria, Salmonella, Mycobacterium tuberculosis* and *avium intracellulare, Legionella, Nocardia* spp. Fungi: cryptococci, histoplasmosis, *Coccidioides, Candida, Aspergillus* spp. Viruses: Herpes simplex, varicella zoster, cytomegalovirus, Epstein-Barr virus. Parasites: *Pneumocystis, Toxoplasma, Cryptosporidium, Strongyloides* spp.
Renal failure (impairment of CMI, granulocyte dysfunction and mucocutaneous barriers)	Gram-positive bacteria: Staphylococcus aureus (many patients on hemodialysis are chronic carriers), coagulase-negative staphylococci, streptococci. Gram-negative rods: *Escherichia coli.* Atypicals: mycobacteria, *Nocardia* sp. Fungi: *Coccidioides* sp., histoplasmosis.
Asplenia (true and functional)	Encapsulated organisms: *Streptococcus pneumoniae, Hemophilus influenzae, Neisseria meningitidis.*
Alcoholism	Polymicrobial infections: aspiration pneumonias, spontaneous bacterial peritonitis.
Miscellaneous	Malnourishment, burns, vascular insufficiency, chronic individual catheters.

Pitfalls in Practice. There are several scenarios in which a physician may put an immunocompromised patient at risk. Vaccination with live attenuated viruses is absolutely contraindicated in immunocompromised patients, who may be unable to mount a response to even a genetically weakened virus. The morbidity and mortality associated with immunocompromise and infection after active immunization places such patients at extreme risk.

Any immunocompromised patient who presents with symptoms of an acute infection requires very careful follow-up, if admission is not necessary. If compliance with follow-up is a question, the threshold for hospitalization should be lowered, and the patient should be admitted.

Infectious Disease and Travel

Approximately 25–40 million Americans travel to a foreign destination annually. Ten percent visit third-world countries, with a significant exposure to infectious diseases uncommonly encountered in the U.S. Many travelers seek medical attention before departure to obtain advice and vaccinations. In deciding what immunizations a patient should receive, it may be helpful to stratify risk into three categories: (1) low (the business traveler staying at a world-class hotel in a metropolitan area); (2) high (the low-budget traveler, exploring the rural third world with significant exposure risk); or (3) medium (most travelers, who fit somewhere between). This information may help determine the immunizations and education that the traveler needs.

Immunization requirements vary from country to country; each country has its own requirements and endemic risks. Legal entry may be denied in some countries that require specific immunizations if the vaccinations have not been obtained before arrival. Currently the only two legally required vaccines for countries in endemic zones are yellow fever and cholera.[7] *Health Information for International Travel* (Centers for Disease Control and Prevention, Atlanta, GA 30333) and *Vaccination Certificate Requirements for International Travel and Health Advice to Travelers* (World Health Organization Publication Center, 49 Sheridan Ave., Albany, NY 12210) are helpful guides that provide updated information about vaccines and health tips for international travelers. Table 8 (next page) provides lists common vaccines along with general recommendations.

Traveler's Diarrhea

Differential Diagnosis. Diarrhea is a common symptom, affecting 20–50% of international travelers. The differential diagnosis includes toxin-mediated, bacterial, viral, and parasitic diseases. Fortunately, most cases of traveler's diarrhea are self-limited and require only adequate hydration to replace fluid losses. Table 9 provides a brief list of causes of traveler's diarrhea and proper management. Parasitic causes of diarrhea (see Table 6) are usually insidious in onset and may be present for months. Typical description of traveler's diarrhea includes abrupt onset of several watery or loose stools, which may or may not be accompanied by abdominal pain. Clinically the patient may appear dehydrated; orthostatics should be obtained. Hemoccult of the stool should be tested; a positive result suggests invasive organisms, which should be treated with antibiotics.

Table 8. Common Vaccines for Travelers

Vaccine	Route of Administration	Recommendations/Comments
Yellow fever (live attenuated virus)	Subcutaneous (SC) injection Effective immunity: 10 yr	Highly effective, may be a requirement to enter endemic countries (central Africa and South America). Not recommended for age < 9 mo. Contraindicated in pregnancy or egg hypersensitivity.
Cholera (killed virus)	SC or intramuscular (IM) injection Immunity for 6 mo	Poorly effective vaccine, but may be required for entrance into some African countries. Attack rate for cholera in tourist is very low and the vaccine is of limited efficacy; therefore, if not required, recommend consumption of only cooked foods and bottled/boiled water over vaccination.
Typhoid fever (inactivated or live attenuated)	SC parenteral vaccine Effective for 3 yr or Oral vaccine Effective for 5 yr	Effective vaccine; advised for travelers to rural areas of developing countries (greatest risk in South America and Indian subcontinent). Parenteral: local pain, swelling, fever, malaise for 1–3 days. Oral: 4 doses over 7 days; must not take antibiotics during week of administration.
Poliomyelitis (killed or live attenuated)	SC or oral	Recommend for travel to developing countries. Inactivated virus is preferable in unimmunized adults (risk of paralysis is less). Observe precautions for live oral vaccine.
Tetanus and diphtheria (toxoid)	IM injection Booster every 10 yr	All travelers should be up to date.
Hepatitis A (immune globulin (IG) or killed virus)	IM injection of pooled IG Efficacy: 6 mo	Endemic in many parts of the world. Spread through contamination of food or water. IG very effective in prevention.
Hepatitis B (recombinant proteins)	Series of IM injections	Spread through sexual contact. High endemic rate in Africa and Southeast Asia. Vaccine very effective.
Meningococcal disease (quadravalent vaccine)	SC injection Efficacy: 3–5 yr	Advised to travelers of endemic areas (India, sub-Saharan Africa, Saudi Arabia, Nepal, Tanzania, Burundi). Contact the CDC for information about destination country's risk.
Japanese encephalitis (inactivated virus)	SC injection Series: weekly injection × 3 Boosters every 1–4 yr	Mosquito-borne encephalitis, endemic in China and Southeast Asia. Increased risk in rural regions with high mosquito exposure. Vaccine with low to moderate rate of side effects: malaise, fever, headaches, myalgias.

Diagnostic Aids. Prolonged illness after traveling should be investigated with a stool culture for fecal leukocytes, erthrocytes, ova, and parasites. Stool culture may be useful in patients with a fever and fecal leukocytes, especially for assessing a possible organism for antibiotic resistance. A complete blood count with eosinophilia may suggest a parasitic pathogen.

Management. The first line of treatment for prolonged travelers diarrhea is adequate hydration. Severe dehydration may result from continual gastrointestinal fluid loss, and patients may require intravenous rehydration and electrolyte replacement. The use of antimotility agents should be avoided because they increase stool transit time, therefore increasing exposure of the intestinal mucosa to bacterial colonization, invasion, and toxin. Antibiotics may be used for severe infection (see Table 8). Because of the growing resistance to trimethoprim-sulfamethoxazole, fluoroquinolones are becoming a first-line treatment.[7]

Table 9. Causes and Suggested Management of Traveler's Diarrhea

Organism	Source	Characteristics	Management
Enterotoxigenic *Escherichia coli*	Contaminated food or water	Onset: abrupt, within 24–72 hr of ingestion. Duration: seldom more than 3 days. Stool examination: no fecal leukocytes.	IV fluid rehydration. Antibiotics only for severe cases.
Shigella sp.	Contaminated food or water (fecal-oral spread)	Onset: Abrupt, within 24–48 hr. of ingestion. Abdominal pain and fever precedes diarrhea. Duration: usually brief, but may last up to 2 wk. Stool examination: may see red blood cells.	Ciprofloxacin or norfloxacin PO every 12 hr × 3 days. or Trimethoprim-sulfamethoxazole (TMP-SMX) DS every 12 hr × 3 days (resistance is high).
Salmonella sp.	Contaminated food or water	Onset: abrupt, within 8–24 hr of ingestion. Duration: 3–10 days. Stool examination: fecal leukocytes	If mild, no treatment. If severe or immunocompromised, ciprofloxacin or norfloxacin bid × 3–7 days. Second line: TMP-SMX DS (resistance is high)
Vibrio sp.	Raw or under-cooked fish	Onset: within hours to days after ingestion. Duration: usually 48 hr. Stool examination: leukocytes, occasionally erythrocytes. *V. vulnificus* can cause septicemia in immunocompromised patients.	Ciprofloxacin or doxycycline PO
Campylobacter sp.	Usually infected poultry or milk	Onset: abrupt, within 2–5 days of ingestion; diarrhea lags 1–2 days behind fever, abdominal pain. Duration: more than 7 days. Stool examination: fecal leukocytes, erythrocytes	Ciprofloxacin or norfloxacin × 5 days or Azithromycin × 3 days or Erythromycin × 5 days

IV = intravenous, PO = orally, bid = 2 times/day.

Many travelers visit physicians before traveling abroad to seek antibiotics for prevention of diarrheal illness. Most authorities recommend against antibiotic prophylaxis for travelers diarrhea, because the risks often outweigh the benefits.[7] Some indications in which the benefits of prophylaxis may exceed the risk of antibiotic side effects include travel to underdeveloped rural regions for less than 3 weeks or presence of comorbidity (e.g., cardiovascular disease) in which mild dehydration may precipitate serious morbidity. Despite these recommendations, some patients may insist on receiving antibiotics. Fluoroquinolones taken once daily are highly effective at preventing bacterial enteric infection but should not be used in children or pregnant patients because of possible side effects to developing cartilage. Doxycycline also may be used, but side effects include increased skin sensitivity to sunlight; it should be avoided in pregnancy and childhood because it may cause tooth staining and has a deleterious effect on bone growth. Bismuth subsalicylate may be an acceptable compromise; two tablets 4 times/day have been shown to be highly effective in diarrhea prevention in adults.[8] At this dose mild tinnitus may be experienced, and patients should be advised against taking other aspirin-containing compounds. In addition, patients should be instructed that their stool and tongue may turn black as a side effect.

Pitfalls in Practice. Most cases of traveler's diarrhea are self-limited, and proper hydration is the cornerstone to treatment. Prolonged illness, febrile symptoms, bloody stool, and increasing pain are symptoms that require further work-up. Education about ensuring safe drinking water and avoiding uncooked foods may help to avoid unnecessary exposure to causes of traveler's diarrhea. Use of local water for brushing teeth and mouth rinsing is a frequently unrecognized potential source of causative agents.

Febrile Illness in Travelers

Differential Diagnosis. The history of fever in a recent international traveler offers a broad differential diagnosis as to the source of the fever. In addition to common domestic causes of infectious fever, the physician should consider the possibility of "foreign" pathogens in febrile patients with risk factors. Table 10 (next page) provides an abbreviated list of more common causes of infectious fever in international travelers, diagnostic aids, and treatment.

History and Physical Examination. Eliciting a history of travel or infectious exposure in an international traveler is imperative in patients with an unusual presentation of fever. Destination, length of stay, pretravel vaccinations, and possible exposures may help to focus the differential diagnosis. Remote travel history may be helpful since the length of incubation period for infectious agents is variable. In addition, onset, duration, extent of temperature elevation, and nature of fever may be helpful (e.g., malaria is a cyclical febrile state, whereas amebiasis may be more persistent). An organ system approach to complaints also may help to narrow the differential.

Physical examination is often not helpful in evaluating the source of many travel-related febrile illnesses but occasionally provides distinguishing information. Often patients are dehydrated and possibly anemic. Measurement of orthostatic vital signs, evaluation of skin turgor, or presence of dry mucous membranes may help evaluate the extent of dehydration and the need for intravenous hydration. Abdominal exam may reveal an enlarged spleen; rectal exam may be positive for occult or gross bleeding. Signs of central nervous system involvement may be present secondary to elevated temperature, shock, or encephalitis.

Diagnostic Aids. If the source of the fever is suggested by the history and physical examination, the diagnostic work-up may be tailored to confirm the diagnosis, but often this is not the case in the diagnosis of travel-related illness. A baseline complete blood count may provide information about blood loss and nature of infection (e.g., eosinophilia of parasitic illness). Electrolyte imbalances may occur with dehydration due to fever and gastrointestinal losses, and an electrolyte panel may help to guide fluid replacement. Blood, stool, and urine cultures, urinalysis and, possibly, cerebral spinal fluid analysis for cell count, differential, and culture also should be obtained. Additional specific antibody or antigen tests may be of use (see Table 10).

Management. Dehydrated patients should receive intravenous rehydration with normal saline or lactated Ringer's solution. Care should be taken to avoid aspirin or platelet-inhibiting medications in patients with a hemorrhagic component. Admission to the hospital is often necessary for completion of work-up, supportive treatment, and possibly antibiotics. Consultation with an infectious disease specialist may be appropriate. (See Table 10 for disease-specific management.)

Pitfalls in Practice. Patients with an acute febrile illness, especially if no source can be identified, should be questioned about travel history. It is possible that some of the illnesses

Table 10. **Febrile Illnesses in Travelers** *(Columns continue on next page)*

Disease	Epidemiology	Presentation
Malaria	Intracellular protozoan. Transmission: bite of *Anopheles* mosquito, blood products, shared contaminated needles, congenitally. Greatest incidence in the tropics, subtropics.	Onset: precipitous illness occurring weeks to years after the infection. Duration: acute attacks last 4–12 hr, cycling every 24–72 hr; will recur for years if untreated. Signs and symptoms: shaking, chills, rigors, elevated temperature (105° F), headache, malaise, abdominal discomfort, confusion, altered level of consciousness, hypotension.
Amebiasis	Extracellular protozoan (*Entamoeba histolytica* spp.) Transmission: ingestion of cysts in contaminated food and water. Greatest incidence in the tropics, including Mexico.	Onset: precipitous illness occurring at variable times after ingestion of cysts of various ages. Duration: variable; relapses may occur. Signs and symptoms: abdominal discomfort, alternating bloody diarrhea and constipation, fever, chills, hepatomegaly.
Hepatitis	Viral agents A, B, C worldwide distribution. Hepatitis A common in developing countries.	Onset: variable after incubation periods. Hepatitis A: 2–6 wk Hepatitis C: 6–12 wk Hepatitis B: 2–6 mo Duration: variable, clinical recovery may occur in 2–3 mo. Hepatitis B and C may enter chronic carrier state. Symptoms: low-grade fever, RUQ pain, hepatomegaly, jaundice, anorexia, nausea.
Dengue fever	Viral illness. Transmission: mosquito bite. Greatest incidence in South America, Carribean, Central America, Asia, and the Pacific.	Onset: precipitous illness following a 6–12-day incubation period. Duration: first episode lasts 2–3 days, recurrence is less severe, total duration of febrile illness approximately 6 days. Signs and symptoms: high fever, headache, altered mental status, arthralgias, macular rash starting after onset of fever, petechiae, epistaxis, bleeding gums, hypotension.
Hemorrhagic fevers	Arboviruses, multiple vectors. Greatest incidence in Africa, Asia, former Soviet Union countries, and South America.	Onset: precipitous illness occurring less than three weeks after travel to endemic areas. Duration: variable. Signs and symptoms: high fevers, myalgias, headaches, rashes, gastrointestinal bleeding, petechiae.
Typhoid fever	Transmission: ingestion of food or water contaminated with *Salmonella typhi*. Greatest incidence in developing countries, worldwide.	Onset: insidious, occurring after 4-day to 3-wk incubation period. Duration: elevated fever persists for 2–3 weeks if untreated. Signs and symptoms: fever, malaise, abdominal discomfort, transient rash, splenomegaly, headache, chills, occasionally intestinal perforation, shock.
Japanese encephalitis	Arbovirus Transmission: mosquito bite. Greatest incidence in Asia, especially in summer	Onset: precipitous illness. Duration: variable. Signs and symptoms: rigors, altered mental status, elevated temperature, neurologic symptoms.

NSAIDs = nonsteroidal anti-inflammatory drugs, PO = orally, tid = 3 times/day, IV = intravenously, qid = 4 times/day.

mentioned above may result in a chronic carrier state (e.g., hepatitis B and C, *Salmonella typhi*), and infection may have occurred by exposure to an infected person.

Education about avoidance of uncooked foods, unboiled or unbottled water, immunizations, prophylaxis, and liberal use of mosquito repellants and nets may reduce the risk of contracting a travel-related illness. Chemoprophylaxis for malaria is outlined in Table 11 (page 94), but the geography of resistance is evolving. Contacting the CDC for updated information is advised. In addition, the risk of chemoprophylaxis must be understood and weighed against the benefits of pretreatment.

Table 10. *(Columns continued)*

Diagnostic Aids	Treatment
Complete blood count (anemia), thrombo-cytopenia, elevated coagulation studies, peripheral blood smear (intracellular parasites)	Chemoprophylaxis for traveler to endemic areas (see Table 11). Treatment of acute infection: supportive. For chemotherapy see Table 11. Caution: avoid aspirin, NSAIDs.
Stool samples: look for cysts and trophozoites.	Asymptomatic and passing cysts: paromomycin 500 mg PO TID x 7 days or iodoquinol 650 mg PO tid × 20 days. Symptomatic with diarrhea/dysentery: metronidazole 750 mg PO tid x 10 days, followed by iodoquinol 650 mg tid x 20 days or paromomycin 500 mg PO tid x 7 days. Extra-intestinal infection (hepatic): metronidazole 750 mg IV/PO tid x 10 days, followed by iodoquinol 650 mg PO tid x 20 days.
Elevated liver function tests (predominantly aminotransferases), positive immuno-globulins (IGM) hepatitis antibody titers or antigenemia, bilirubinuria, elevated coagulation studies.	Prophylaxis with vaccine. Supportive if acute: fluids, antimetics. If chronic and persistent elevation of aminotransferases, consider alpha interferon, lamivudine, or famciclovir.
Elevated antibody titer, CBC may show leukopenia or neutropenia.	Care is solely supportive. May have significant hypotension with dehydration and hemorrhage. May need intensive care admission.
Viral cultures (contact CDC).	Supportive therapy; isolation.
Blood, stool cultures. Complete blood cell count may show anemia, leukopenia.	Antibiotics: ciprofloxacin 500 mg PO bid x 10 days or chloramphenicol 500 mg PO qid x 14 days or ceftriaxone 2 gm IV × 5 days. May need hospitalization for anemia, hypotension, or shock syndrome. With shock, dexamethasone 3 mg/kg loading followed by 1 mg/kg every 6 hr for 8 total doses.
Clinical diagnosis.	Supportive.

NSAIDs = nonsteroidal anti-inflammatory drugs, PO = orally, tid = 3 times/day, IV = intravenously, qid = 4 times/day.

Infectious Diseases and Health Care Delivery

The initial evaluation and treatment of blood or body fluid exposure may occur in the urgent care setting. Although many infectious diseases may be transmitted by such exposure, most attention has been paid to hepatitis B virus (HBV) and human immunodeficiency virus (HIV). Although the rate of transmission of HIV by needle puncture exposure is extremely low, seroconversion of health care workers with no other known risk factor has been documented. In 1997, the CDC reported 52 cases of HIV seroconversion

Table 11. Chemoprophylaxis and Treatment of Malaria

Species	Primary	Comment
Prophylaxis *Plasmodium falciparum,* non–chloroquine resistant	Chloroquine (CQ) 500 mg every wk starting 1–2 wk before departure, during travel, and 4 weeks after travel	Pediatric dose is 8.3 mg/kg. CQ is safe in pregnancy.
Plasmodium falciparum, chloroquine resistant	Mefloquine (MQ) 250 mg PO every wk for 1 wk before, during, and 4 weeks after travel, or Doxycycline 100 mg/day PO 1–2 days before, during, and after travel.	No MQ in first trimester of pregnancy. Doxycycline contraindicated in pregnancy, and causes photosensitivity.
Alternative prophylaxis Atovaquone-proguanil	One tablet daily for 2 days before and during travel, and for 1 wk after travel.	Fewer side effects than other drugs.
Treatment *Plasmodium vivax* or *ovale*	CQ 1 gm PO × 1, then 0.5 gm PO every 12 hr × 3 plus Primaquine (PQ) 26.3 mg/day PO × 14 days.	

PO = orally.

after occupational exposure and 114 probable cases, including needlestick exposure.[9] The risk of overt hepatitis B after needle puncture exposure to blood from persons positive for hepatitis B surface antigen (HBsAg) is about 20% in patients without immunoprophylaxis.[10]

Management decisions about prophylaxis for hepatitis B and HIV can be complex and are best handled through an institutional protocol. Figure 2 provides a sample protocol for management of needle punctures and blood and body fluid exposures.

Hepatitis B immune globulin is given intramuscularly at a dose of 0.06 ml/kg (up to 10 ml). It should be given as soon as possible and should not be delayed beyond 7 days for serologic testing. There is no harm in giving HBIG to persons who are already immune if

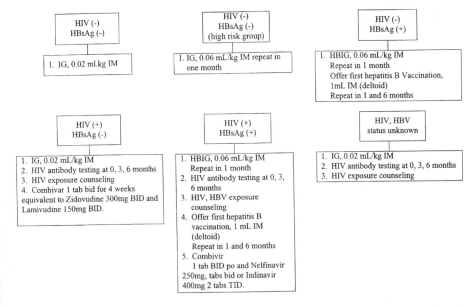

Figure 2. Strategy for the management of blood and body fluid exposure. (The source patient is health care worker exposed.)

test results cannot be obtained within 7 days. Because most needle punctures result from occupational exposure, it is recommended that the hepatitis vaccine series be initiated with the first dose of HBIG. The intramuscular dose of the hepatitis vaccine is 20 mg for adults, 10 mg for infants or children younger than 10 years of age, and 40 mg for patients on dialysis or other immunosuppressed patients.[10] The second and third doses are given 1 and 6 months after the first.

Table 12 lists body fluids that are of actual or theoretical concern in transmission of either HIV or HBV. All blood and body fluids that contain visible blood should be handled as if infected. These precautions also apply to the handling of semen and vaginal secretions, although infection in health care providers from occupational exposure to these body fluids has not been reported. The risk of infection through exposure to cerebrospinal fluid, synovial fluid, pericardial fluid, peritoneal fluid, and amniotic fluid is not known; therefore, these fluids also should be considered infected. Although of theoretical concern, the risk of transmission of HIV and HBV through infected feces, nasal secretions, sputum, sweat, tears, urine, and vomitus appears to be low if present at all.[13]

Table 12. Transmission of Human Immunodeficiency Virus and Hepatitis B Virus

Routes of documented transmission	Sexual contact
	Transfusion of infected blood or blood products
	Perinatal transfer from mother to child
Routes of theoretical transmission (virus isolated: no documented cases)	Breast-feeding
	Saliva
	Tears
	Contact lenses
	Urine
	Cerebrospinal fluid (HIV)
	Synovial fluid
	Amniotic fluid
	Peritoneal fluid (HBV)
Viruses not isolated and not transmitted	Immune globulin preparations
	Hepatitis B vaccine
	Casual, household contact
	Insect bites

In delivery of health care in the urgent care setting, the guidelines developed by the CDC should be followed. Wearing barrier protection (gloves, masks, eyewear, and gowns) reduces the risk of exposure to contaminated body fluids and should be encouraged.

Infectious Diseases and Intravenous Drug Abuse

Patients who abuse intravenous (IV) drugs are at risk of acquiring infectious diseases from blood-borne contaminants on shared needles or contaminants carried through soft tissues into the veins when the drugs are injected. In addition, the generalized debilitated state of IV drug abusers increases their susceptibility to routine infectious diseases. Patients who use IV drugs frequently delay seeing health care because of embarrassment, fear of being reported to the authorities, or altered mental status. A history of IV drug use, no matter how remote, is a positive history and should be diligently sought in all patients who present with unclear histories, unusual or nonspecific symptoms, or prior episodes of infectious diseases common to IV drug abusers.

Most IV drug abusers who develop fevers have an identifiable infectious source. Occasionally, fever is the only or first sign of a serious, potentially life-threatening infectious disease in this patient population. The presence of fever in a patient who uses IV drugs should prompt a careful history and physical examination. If the infectious source is not found, the patient should be hospitalized for observation and continued work-up. Hospitalization also is advised if the severity of the illness is unclear or if there is any question of the patient's ability or willingness to comply with scheduled follow-up.

Skin Infections

Differential Diagnosis. Patients who use IV drugs can introduce skin contaminants into veins and soft tissues when they inject drugs. Skin infections are the most common infections in this population. Local abscesses must be differentiated from trauma-induced or myocotic pseudoaneurysms. Cellulitis should be differentiated from chemical irritation due to powder or crystals injected with the drug or from deeper soft tissue infections.

Management. As described elsewhere in this handbook, local subcutaneous abscesses require incision and drainage for complete resolution. Local cellulitis with no evidence of fever or lymphangitis can be managed on an outpatient basis with antibiotics and follow-up arranged within 24–48 hours. Compliance is essential in these high-risk patients,; if it is doubtful, the patient should be hospitalized. If the skin infection is extensive, if the patient appears acutely ill, or if there is a question of involvement of underlying structures, the patient should be hospitalized for administration of IV antibiotics.

Pitfalls in Practice. Incision of a mycotic pseudoaneurysm that is mistaken for an abscess obviously can result in significant hemorrhage. Failure to detect infection that involves underlying structures or joints can result in prolonged morbidity and possibly life-threatening complications of skin infections. Intravenous drug abusers with infections cannot be treated as outpatients unless they are not acutely ill and compliance with early follow-up is likely.

Musculoskeletal Infections

Differential Diagnosis. Direct inoculation of skin contaminants and other contaminants into the tissues and structures underlying the skin can occur with IV drug abuse and result in infection of the deep tissues, vasculature, and joints. Hematogenous spread of infection from any infected site also can result in infections of the musculoskeletal system.

Infectious arthritis is described in Chapter 9. Muscle infection (pyomyositis) is usually the result of hematogenous spread of infection from distal infectious sites. The skin overlying the involved muscle may appear to be normal. The infected muscle is extremely tender and swollen and can exert enough pressure on the surrounding tissue to cause a compartment syndrome. Osteomyelitis can be a primary infection due to inoculation of bacteria into the bone, or it can result from hematogenous spread of infection. Patients complain of local pain and warmth or swelling over a bony region.

Radiographic examination of the involved areas sometimes demonstrates cortical irregularities or elevation.

Management. The management of infectious arthritis is discussed in Chapter 9. Pyomyositis is managed by surgical drainage of the muscle abscess and administration of intravenous antibiotics. Osteomyelitis is treated with long-term intravenous antibiotic therapy.

Pitfalls in Practice. Failure to suspect deep tissue infections in IV drug abusers can delay the diagnosis and increase morbidity and mortality. Failure to drain a muscle abscess can result in a compartment syndrome with subsequent ischemia of the limb.

Pulmonary Infections

Differential Diagnosis. The depressed mental status that accompanies the use of some drugs of abuse can reduce the patients' ability to handle oral secretions. IV drug abusers, therefore, are at risk of developing aspiration syndromes and aspiration pneumonia. The offending chemical or infectious agent is usually introduced in aspirated secretions from the oral cavity or gastric contents. Nonaspiration pneumonias can result from hematogenous spread of bacteria during septicemia. *Pneumocystis carinii* pneumonia is common among IV drug abusers who have AIDS. The clinical picture of drug-abusing patients with pulmonary infections or chemical pneumonitis is similar to the presentation of the disease in any other patient population.

Management. IV drug abusers who present with pulmonary infections require aggressive management. IV antibiotic therapy should be considered. Attempts to culture the causative agent should be made, and distant infections that may be responsible for bacterial seeding in the lungs should be sought.

Pitfalls in Practice. Because of their frequently debilitated or possibly immunocompromised state, pulmonary disease processes can quickly become fulminant in IV drug abusers. Outpatient management of pneumonia requires absolute compliance with follow-up, which is unlikely in most patients who abuse drugs.

Vascular Infections

Differential Diagnosis. Infection of the veins is common in IV drug abuse, and septic phlebitis is usually a well-localized infection. Infected veins are usually hard, and the overlying skin is warm and red. Occasionally the differential diagnosis is confused with chemical irritation due to injected powder or drug crystals.

Besides infection, complications of intra-arterial injection of drugs include vasospasm, occlusion of microcirculation, formation of traumatic pseudoaneurysms, and chemical endarteritis with resultant venous and lymphatic stasis. Tissue pressure may be elevated from venous stasis and result in a compartment syndrome in the involved limb.

Management. Localized infections can be managed with broad-spectrum antibiotics and local comfort measures. Early reevaluation should be arranged. In extensive infections, the patient should be hospitalized. If examination suggests tissue ischemia from an intra-arterial injection, the patient should be hospitalized. Fasciotomy is required in cases of compartment syndrome.

Pitfalls in Practice. The diagnosis of septic phlebitis as chemical irritation of veins can delay appropriate therapy and result in extension of the localized infection.

Unrecognized compartment syndrome can result in limb ischemia and subsequent loss of function.

Acquired Immunodeficiency Syndrome (AIDS)

Differential Diagnosis. Since AIDS was first reported in 1981, over 1.25 million cases have been reported worldwide. Kelen and coworkers found a 4% incidence of unrecognized HIV infection among inner city emergency department patients.[11]

It is believed that patients who are seropositive for HIV are infectious. Transmission of the virus has been documented through sexual contact, contact with infected blood or blood products, and perinatal contamination of the neonate by the infected mother. IV drug abusers acquire the infection by using needles contaminated with infected blood. Most patients who develop AIDS have no overt clinical manifestations for 6–10 years after the primary infection with HIV.[12]

According to the CDC, AIDS is formally diagnosed when the CD4 T-cell count is less than 200 cells/mm^3, or certain indicator opportunistic diseases develop in the absence of other reasons for immunosuppression.[8] The diagnosis of AIDS cannot be made in the urgent care setting, but patients with AIDS may present for routine medical care of other problems. As always, the history and physical examination should be directed toward the organ system involved in the complaint.

Various medications are currently prescribed to patients with AIDS. None can cure AIDS, but they often reduce the duration of opportunistic infections and lessen other constitutional effects of the disease. The side effects of these drugs are often significant and should be considered in the medical evaluation of the patient. Table 13 lists some drugs currently used by patients with AIDS, along with their side effects.[14,15]

Management. The management of routine medical problems is usually the same in patients with or without AIDS. If the patient presents with an unusual problem or evidence of a new opportunistic infection, an infectious disease specialist should be consulted. Additional information may be found on several websites, including the CDC Divisions of HIV/AIDS prevention at http://www.cdc.gov/nchstp/hiv_aids/dhwp.htm.com.

Pitfalls in Practice. The medical complaints of immunosuppressed patients cannot be minimized because they are at risk for development of significant morbidity and even mortality from usually nonserious infectious diseases. Contact with the primary physician caring for the patient with AIDS is essential to ensure careful follow-up and should be made as soon as possible when patients present to the urgent care center. Although the symptoms that prompt the patient with AIDS to seek medical help may be due to side effects of drugs, medications should not be stopped unless so advised by the patient's primary physician.

Hepatitis

Differential Diagnosis. The patient who uses IV drugs is at risk for acquiring viral hepatitis from blood exposure on shared needles. Hepatitis caused by acute viral infection is described in Table 14. Regardless of the infectious agent, the clinical course of acute viral hepatitis is similar among all patients. Acute hepatitis is divided into the incubation period (asymptomatic), the preicteric and icteric periods (prodrome and acute illness), and the period of convalescence (asymptomatic except for malaise). The clinical manifestations of the disease are variable, and subclinical disease is probably common.

Table 13. Some Chemotherapeutic Agents for AIDS

Drug	Uses and Characteristics	Side Effects
Nucleoside reverse transcriptase inhibitors		
Zidovudine (AZT)	Delays clinical progression in previously untreated patients. Because of modest antiviral effects when used singly, it is rarely used alone.	Suppresses myelopoiesis and erythropoiesis; headaches, nausea, CNS stimulation.
Didanosine	Because of side effects, didanosine is rarely used as an initial agent despite moderate to good antiviral activity.	Peripheral neuropathy (dose-related), which is reversible if the drug is discontinued. Rapid onset of pancreatitis, which may become life threatening.
Zalcitabine (dideoxycytidine, ddc)	Limited use as a single agent because of side effects. Used only in combination, or in patients who cannot tolerate zidovudine and didanosine or lamivudine. Often used in combination for patients with advanced AIDS.	Peripheral neuropathy (dose dependent, reversible).
Stavudine	Used in combination for moderate to advanced AIDS.	Peripheral neuropathy (dose dependent, reversible); hepatitis.
Lamivudine	Potentiate antiviral activity of zidovudine by inhibiting suppressor mutations.	Well tolerated at high doses and in advanced AIDS; may suppress bone marrow.
Abacavir	Extremely potent, but activity compromised by several viral mutations.	Well tolerated; occasionally produces headaches and nausea. Rarely can cause a shock syndrome in patients experiencing a febrile syndrome.
Nonnucleoside reverse transcriptase inhibitors		
Nevirapine	Potent, but resistance is common and rapid following initiation of therapy that does not totally suppress the virus. Provides modest but transient benefit in combination therapy.	Well tolerated; occasionally causes a maculopapular rash.
Delavirdine	If administered initially in doses that do not completely suppress viral replication, resistance is common.	Well tolerated; may cause a rash.
Efavirenz 2	In late stages of development, less viral resistance than other drugs.	Confusion, lightheadedness (dose-related).
Saquinavar	Excellent antiviral activity but limited bioavailability.	Poor oral tolerance of required doses, hepatotoxicity.
Indinavir	High antiviral activity with substantial reduction in morbidity and mortality when used in combination.	Transient hyperbilirubinemia, nephrolithiasis.
Ritonavir	Potent antiviral but use is limited by side effects.	Subjective toxicities (perioral tingling, GI side effects).
Nelfinavir	Less potent than others of its class, but better tolerated. Additive effects with reverse transcriptase inhibitors.	Well tolerated; can cause diarrhea.

CNS = central nervous system, GI = gastrointestinal.

The nonspecific prodrome, especially with HBV infection, usually cannot be distinguished from that of other viral syndromes. Most infected patients experience anorexia, nausea, fever, or weakness before the icteric period begins. The presence of myalgias, arthralgias, rashes, and fever in IV drug abusers should alert the clinician to the possibility of HBV infection as well as several other serious infectious diseases.

During the icteric phase of the disease, liver dysfunction may develop. Patients frequently present with nausea, vomiting, and diarrhea. Jaundice develops late in the clinical

Table 14. Infectious Hepatitis

Type	Epidemiology	Presentation	Serologic Tests	Prophylaxis
Hepatitis A virus (HAV)	Route: fecal-oral. Incubation: 15–50 days. Onset: abrupt. Duration: 6–8 wk. Carrier state: none.	Mild liver enlargement and tenderness; occasionally jaundice, malaise, weakness.	Positive for antibodies to HAV IgM (indicates infection within past 4 mo).	Inactivated vaccines available (Havrix, Vaqta); IG if allergy to vaccine components (Recombivax HB, Engerix-B)
Hepatitis B virus (HBV)	Route: parenteral, sexual contact, exposure to contaminated body fluids, maternal-neonatal Incubation: 45–160 days. Onset: insidious. Duration: 3–4 mo.	Mild liver enlargement and tenderness, jaundice, serum-sickness-like prodrome (fever, rash, myalgias, arthralgias, nausea, vomiting).	Positive for HBsAg (indicates infection or carrier state), HbeAg, antibodies to HbcAg (indicates acute infection)	IG, HBIG, hepatitis B vaccine.
Hepatitis C	Route: same as HBV, especially with blood products. Incubation: 40–60 days. Onset: insidious. Duration: same as HBV.	Same as HBV.	Negative serologies.	IG may be effective.

HBeAg = hepatitis B e antigen, HbeAg = hepatitis core antigen, HBIG = hepatitis B immune globulin.

course. In most cases of hepatitis A virus (HAV) infection, recovery is complete. With HBV, however, a carrier state as well as a state of chronic disease can develop.

Management. Most patients with viral hepatitis can be managed as outpatients. Supportive care includes assurance of adequate hydration and rest. Activity should be allowed as tolerated. Indications for hospitalization of patients with hepatitis include evidence of liver failure (hepatic encephalopathy, ascites, prolonged prothrombin time, and hypoglycemia), inability to maintain hydration, intractable vomiting, excessive anorexia, and nausea.

Pitfalls in Practice. Acute hepatitis can be caused by agents other than viruses; in the evaluation of patients with hepatitis, these causes (drug-induced, alcoholic, or biliary causes of hepatitis) should be considered. Physical findings of chronic liver disease are not due to acute viral hepatitis, and their presence suggests other liver pathology. IV drug abusers who present with nonspecific symptoms may have hepatitis prodrome. Other more serious diseases also must be considered, however. Patients must be carefully evaluated for other infectious diseases common to IV drug abusers.

References

1. Moffa DA, Emerman CL: Bronchitis and pneumonia. In Tintinalli JE, Kelen GD, Stapczynski JS (eds): Emergency Medicine: A Comprehensive Study Guide, 5th ed. New York, McGraw-Hill, 2000, pp 452–461.
2. Bardenheier B, Prevots DR, Khetsurian N, et al: Tetanus: Surveillance—United States, 1995–1997. MMWR 47(52):1–13, 1998.
3. Recommendations of the Immunization Practices Advisory Committee: Diptheria, tetanus and pertussis: Recommendations for vaccine use and other preventative measures. MMWR 40(RR-10):1-28, 1991.
4. Krebs JW, Smith JS, Rupprecht CE, Childs JE: Rabies surveillance in the United States during 1996. JAMA 211:1525–1529, 1997.

5. Advisory Committee on Immunization Practices: Recommendations, 1999. MMWR 48(RR-1):1–21, 1999.
6. Advisory Committee on Immunization Practices: Recommendations: Prevention and control of influenzae. MMWR 46(RR-9):1–25, 1997.
7. Weller PF: Health advice for international travelers. In Scientific American Medicine. New York, Scientific American, 2000, pp 1–12.
8. DuPont HL, Ericsson CD, Johnson PC de La Cabada FJ: Use of bismuth subsalicylate for prevention of travelers diarrhea. Rev Infect Dis Supppl 1:S64–S67, 1990.
9. Centers for Disease Control and Prevention: PHS Guidelines for the management of health care workers' exposure to HIV and recommendations for post exposure prophylaxis. MMWR 47:1–12, 1998.
10. Gitlin N: Hepatitis B: Diagnosis, prevention and treatment, Clin Chem 43:1500–1506, 1997.
11. Kelen GD, Fritz S, Quaqish B, et al: Unrecognized HIV infection in emergency department patients. N Engl J Med 31:1645–1650, 1998.
12. Schooley RT: Acquired immunodeficiency syndrome. In Scientific American Medicine. New York, Scientific American, 2000, pp 1–13.
13. Pearlmutter BL, Harris BA: New recommendations for prophylaxis after HIV exposure. Am Fam Physician 55:507–512, 515–517, 1997.
14. Weiner HR: HIV: An update for primary care physicians. Emerg Med (Sept):52–62, 1997.
15. Flexner C, Wood AJ (eds): HIV: Protease inhibitors. N Engl J Med 338:1281–1291, 1998.

Chapter 7

Common Medical Problems: Hypertension, Syncope, Anaphylaxis, and Weakness

E. Corradin Vogel, MD
David Plummer, MD
Catherine A. Ripkey, MD

Hypertension

An estimated 58 million people in the United States have hypertension (blood pressure > 140/90 mmHg), and most people older than 50 years of age intermittently have elevated blood pressure.[1] Most patients with hypertension are asymptomatic, and the diagnosis is frequently made incidentally when vital signs are routinely checked. Nevertheless, cardiovascular morbidity and mortality appear to correlate directly with the degree of blood pressure elevation over time.[2] Mortality is 2.5 times greater in 35–45-year-old men with a diastolic blood pressure of 95 mmHg and 5 times greater when the diastolic pressure reaches 100 mmHg compared with age-matched normotensive men.[3] An elevated blood pressure noted in the urgent care setting, even if the patient is asymptomatic, should not be ignored. An isolated blood pressure without evidence of end-organ damage does not alone constitute a diagnosis of hypertension. The diagnosis is confirmed only after elevated blood pressures are documented on at least two separate occasions. Based on the recommendations of the Sixth Report of the Joint National Committee, hypertension is diagnosed after two or more readings at each of two or more visits documenting elevated blood pressures.[4] Hypertension is defined as a systolic pressure greater than 140 mmHg or a diastolic pressure greater than 90 mmHg. Relative severity of long standing hypertension is classified as stage 1–3.[5]

Stage 1: Systolic 140–159 or diastolic 90–99 mmHg.
Stage 2: Systolic 160–179 or diastolic 100–109 mmHg.
Stage 3: Systolic 180–209 or diastolic 110–119 mmHg.
Stage 4: Systolic ≥ 210 or diastolic ≥ 120 mmHg.

Differential Diagnosis. Four general categories of hypertension are based on symptoms and level of aggression required for treatment: emergencies; urgencies; mild, uncomplicated hypertension; and transient hypertension.[6] **Hypertensive emergencies** occur in 1% of all patients with hypertension and are defined as increased blood pressure with evidence of end-organ damage (i.e., central nervous system, cardiac, or renal impairment). Signs and symptoms of end-organ damage may develop over hours to days. It must be stressed that the symptoms associated with elevated blood pressure—not the degree of elevation—are important in arriving at the diagnosis of a hypertensive emergency. Thus, the patient's clinical condition, not the blood pressure, should guide treatment decisions.[6]

Hypertensive urgencies are defined as dangerous degrees of blood pressure elevation (diastolic pressure typically > 115 mmHg) without signs, symptoms, or evidence of end organ damage.[6] This condition is most often due to noncompliance with medication.

Mild, uncomplicated hypertension is defined as asymptomatic blood pressure elevation of less than 115 mmHg diastolic with no evidence of end-organ damage.

Transient hypertension is seen commonly in the urgent care setting and may be caused by anxiety or "white coat hypertension," pain, alcohol withdrawal, and other conditions. Factors common in the urgent care setting include stress and anxiety from the crisis at hand as well as pain that the patient may be experiencing. It is therefore important to check the patient's blood pressure after pain and anxiety have been alleviated.

History and Physical Examination. The patient should be questioned about any history of hypertension or documented elevated blood pressure measurements (e.g., from a military or job physical examination). The remainder of the history should be directed toward the assessment of end-organ damage, presence of cardiovascular risk factors, and detection of obvious causes or reversible secondary hypertension.

Special attention should be given to central nervous system and cardiovascular symptoms suggestive of end-organ damage. Central nervous system symptoms of headache and dizziness are nonspecific unless they occur with grade 3 or 4 funduscopic changes or other signs of central nervous system dysfunction.[6] Blurred vision, diplopia, hemiparesis, aphasic episodes, and seizures as well as cardiovascular symptoms of ischemic chest pain or acute congestive heart failure establish the diagnosis of hypertensive emergency.

The presence of other major cardiovascular risk factors (advanced age, male sex, family history, cigarette smoking, hyperlipidemia, and diabetes) should alert the physician to the patient's relative risk of potential cardiovascular end-organ damage. The risk of a coronary event in any individual rises exponentially when two or more of these major risk factors are present.[7] Elements of the history that are pertinent to identifying reversible secondary hypertension include documentation of current medications as well as symptoms suggestive of certain endocrine disorders.

After alleviation of the patient's pain and anxiety, blood pressure should be measured by the physician in both arms with an appropriately sized cuff. Funduscopy is mandatory to detect retinopathic changes consistent with acute or longstanding hypertension. Pulses should be evaluated in all four extremities to exclude coarctation of the aorta. Careful examination of the heart and lungs is necessary to detect signs of congestive heart failure or murmurs. Abdominal masses and bruits alert the examiner to the presence of renal disease; renal artery stenosis is suggested by an upper, lateral abdominal bruit with a diastolic component.[5]

Diagnostic Aids. Complete blood count, urinalysis, and measurements of serum glucose, blood urea nitrogen, creatinine, and electrolytes should be performed. Microangiopathic hemolytic anemia results from shearing of red blood cells as they pass exposed subendothelial collagen and fibrin deposits in damaged vessels.[6] Hypokalemia may be observed with high-renin forms of hypertension and in patients on diuretic therapy. Blood urea nitrogen and creatinine values suggest the patient's renal function. Urinalysis may show proteinuria, red cells, and red cell casts, all of which signify kidney damage and a hypertensive emergency.

Management. Appropriate therapy begins with identifying the patient's hypertensive category. Patients with evidence of acute end-organ dysfunction, by definition, are experiencing a hypertensive emergency. Immediate transfer to a hospital by ambulance is mandatory. The goal in such patients is to lower the blood pressure in a controlled and graded manner over 30–60 minutes to a level that is normal for the patient.[6]

Patients with long-standing hypertension who run out of medication and are seen in the urgent care setting should have their prescription refilled and be referred to their primary physician. If such a patient's blood pressure is consistent with a hypertensive urgency (i.e., diastolic pressure > 115 mmHg), immediate therapy in the urgent care center is warranted. Table 1 lists appropriate medications for the treatment of hypertensive urgencies in the urgent care setting.

Table 1. Medications for Acute Hypertensive Urgencies

Drug	Mechanism of Action	Onset of Action	Dosage and Route	Duration of Action	Comments
Captopril	ACE inhibitor	15–30 min	25 mg PO	6 hr	May induce renal insufficiency in patients with bilateral renal artery stenosis.
Clonidine	Central α-2 agonist	30–60 min	0.2 mg PO initial, then 0.1 mg every 2–3 hr, total dose < 0.7 mg	6–8 hr	Watch for hypotension.
Labetalol	α-1, β-1,2 blocker	PO: 30–60 min IV: 10 min	PO: 100–200 mg every 4 hr IV: 20 mg every 10 min	6 hr	Watch for hypotension, bradycardia. Rare bronchospasm in asthma/COPD.
Metoprolol	β-1-blocker	PO: 30–60 min IV: 5–10 min	PO: 25–50 mg IV: 5 mg every 5 min × 3 prn	6 hr	Watch for hypotension, bradycardia. Rare bronchospasm in asthma/COPD.
Nitroglycerin	Vasodilator	5 min	SL: 0.4 mg every 5 min × 3 prn	20–30 min	Watch for hypotension especially in presence of sildenafil (Viagra). Consider as first-line therapy in patients with chest pain.

ACE = angiotensin-converting enzyme, PO = orally, IV = intravenously, prn = as needed, COPD = chronic obstructive pulmonary disease, SL = sublingual.

Patients with a newly discovered elevated blood pressure without symptoms may have mild, uncomplicated blood pressure, but the diagnosis is not assigned on the basis of one blood pressure reading alone. Such patients are best managed with documentation and referral to a primary care provider for further assessment. Initial management includes education about weight reduction; diet low in cholesterol and sodium, avoidance of excessive alcohol, smoking cessation, and regular aerobic exercise.[5,8]

Pitfalls in Practice. Physician complacency is the greatest pitfall in managing hypertensive patients. All too often, elevated blood pressures are either overlooked or attributed to pain and anxiety without further evaluation. A number of investigators have pointed out a general failure on the part of providers delivering acute care either to recognize hypertension or to ensure appropriate follow-up care.[2] This is tragic because hypertension is a major predisposing factor for cardiovascular disease.

Another common error is improper technique in obtaining blood pressure readings. The cuff should be deflated slowly (at a rate of about 3 mmHg/second) because rapid deflation causes a falsely elevated reading.[2] The systolic pressure is recorded when the first tapping sound is heard as the cuff is deflated. Although several endpoints have been used to define diastolic pressure, the most widely accepted is the complete disappearance of sound. Certain patients, however, may not have complete disappearance of sound; in such cases, the point of distinct muffling is a more accurate measurement.[2] Obese patients pose a special problem because the use of a standard-size cuff may result in a falsely elevated reading. The cuff should be about 20% wider than the diameter of the patient's arm for an accurate reading.[9]

Syncope

Syncope is defined as a sudden, transient loss of consciousness marked by unresponsiveness and lack of postural tone with spontaneous recovery not requiring resuscitative measures. It is a relatively common problem accounting for almost 3% of emergency department visits and up to 6% of hospital admissions.[1] The causes of syncope range from benign vasoregulatory dysfunction to life-threatening cardiac arrythmias. The goal of the urgent care evaluation is to differentiate the life-threatening causes that require hospital admission from less serious causes that can be managed on an outpatient basis.

Differential Diagnosis. Many causes of syncope must be considered when symptomatic patients present in the urgent care setting (Table 2). The most common causes of

Table 2. Causes of Syncope

Vasodepressor or Cardiovascular (Life-Threatening)	Vascular (Non–Life-threatening)	Neurologic	Miscellaneous
Ventricular tachycardia	Carotid sinus hypersensitivity	Seizures	Posttussive syncope
Supraventricular tachycardia	Subclavian steal	Transient ischemic attack	Micturition-induced
Atrial fibrillation	Orthostatic hypotension	Migraine headache	Valsalva's maneuver (defecation-induced)
Sick sinus syndrome		Tumor	Drug- or metabolic-
Bradycardia		Glossopharyngeal neuralgia	induced intoxication
Complete heart block		Hydrocephalus	(alcohol, illicit drugs),
Mobitz II arterioventricular block		Stroke	hypoglycemia
Pacemaker malfunction		Trigeminal neuralgia	Hypoxia
Congenital prolonged QT syndromes			Pain-induced
Aortic stenosis			Glossopharyngeal neuralgia
Hypertrophic cardiomyopathy			Trigeminal neuralgia
(idiopathic hypertrophic subaortic			Hyperventilation
stenosis)			Hysterical syncope
Pulmonary embolism			Takayasu's arteritis
Pulmonary hypertension			Systemic mastocytosis
Angina			Post prandial
Myocardial infarction			Sneeze induced
Dissecting aortic aneurysm			
Cardiac tamponade			

syncope, in descending order, are neurally mediated syncope, arrhythmia, neurologic causes (including seizure), orthostatic hypotension, and situational syncope.[12] A syncopal episode may result through several different pathophysiologic mechanisms. The basic mechanism of decreased cerebral blood flow can result from decreased cardiac outflow, intracerebral ischemia, and vasomotor dysfunction leading to decreased systemic vascular resistance. In addition, systemic metabolic causes, such as hypoglycemia, hyperventilation syndromes, and hypoxia/hypercapnia, can produce syncopal episodes. Finally, psychological causes must be considered, often as a diagnosis of exclusion.

History and Physical Examination. The most important aspect of the work-up for syncope includes the history and physical exam. In fact, when a diagnosis is made for a syncopal episode, the history and physical exam identify the potential cause in 49–88%.[13] When interviewing a patient for the work-up of syncope, keep in mind that the patient's recollection of events may be inaccurate. Interview witnesses to add insight to the patient's account of the episode. During the interview, try to elicit key historical points:

1. Position and activity immediately preceding syncope. Many causes require standing or sitting to cause syncope. Syncope with or abruptly after exercise strongly suggests a cardiovascular cause.

2. Precipitating factors

3. Evidence of trauma

4. Associated symptoms just before syncope. Faintness, lightheadedness, dizziness, weakness, diaphoresis, epigastric discomfort, nausea, and other gastrointestinal symptoms are common and nonspecific.

5. The estimated duration of any warning period preceding the event provides an important clue to the diagnosis.

6. The most valuable clue is the estimated duration of loss of consciousness. Brief periods of unconsciousness associated with a normal physical examination are usually benign; unconsciousness lasting more than a few minutes generally indicates serious underlying disease.[14]

7. Focal neurologic symptoms. Patients should be questioned about dysarthria, vertigo, ataxia, diplopia, hemiparesis, or focal sensory changes.

8. Postsyncopal period. The patient should be asked about the time necessary for mental clearing and any residual symptoms.

In addition, it is important to identify the patient's medical history, including previous similar episodes, psychiatric illness, and chronic medical problems. Obtain a list of the patient's medications and any history of drug or alcohol use.

Physical exam should focus on evidence of abnormal vital signs, neurologic deficits, and cardiovascular signs. The physical exam provides the objective evidence needed to direct the examiner toward a final diagnosis.

1. Vital signs should be checked for hypotension, specifically orthostatic hypotension. The blood pressure and pulse should be recorded with the patient supine for at least 5 minutes and standing for at least 2 minutes; pulse and pressure while sitting are not accurate assessments for orthostasis.[15] A systolic blood pressure drop > 20 mmHg or an increase in pulse > 20 beats/min indicates orthostatic hypotension.[16,17]

2. Findings on neurologic examination include focal deficits of cranial nerves, extremity weakness or paresthesias, and brainstem findings. Be sure to look for signs of seizure,

including minor extremity trauma, postictal confusion, tongue biting, and Todd's paralysis (a transient focal extremity weakness).

3. Cardiovascular findings include asymmetric extremity blood pressures, which indicate aortic dissection or subclavian steal syndrome. Heart murmurs and gallops can indicate intracardiac pathology, such as aortic stenosis, idiopathic hypertrophic subaortic stenosis, mitral valve prolapse, myocardial infarction, ischemia, myxomas, and pulmonary hypertension.

4. If the history or initial physical exam indicates that the patient is at risk for GI bleeding, a rectal examination should be done to test for occult blood loss.

Diagnostic Aids. The electrocardiogram is an important diagnostic tool when a cardiac arrhythmia is suspected after physical examination. Patients with increased risk for cardiovascular causes of syncopal episode (including elderly patients and those with a medical history of heart disease) should have a 12-lead ECG. In 2–11% of patients with syncope, a cause is assigned by initial ECG or rhythm strip at presentation.[13]

Routine blood tests are generally regarded as unhelpful in most work-ups for syncope.[18,19] They are justified if clinical suspicion based on the history and physical exam points to a specific diagnosis. Anemia, diabetes mellitus, hypoglycemia, hypoxia, renal failure, seizures (low bicarbonate, chloride, sodium abnormalities), or specific electrolyte disorders may be confirmed by laboratory analysis.

Other diagnostic studies used in the work-up of syncope are beyond the scope of an urgent care center but should be mentioned as important tests to consider for patients requiring further work-up in an emergency department or on hospital admission:

- Computed tomographic (CT) scans of the head are crucial studies to obtain in patients who may have had a seizure or who have a focal neurologic deficit on exam. In addition, patients with head trauma associated with syncope may require a head CT to rule out intracranial pathology.
- Electroencephalograms (EEG) for seizure work-up are not urgently available and would not be helpful in the initial syncope work-up.
- Echocardiograms are useful for evaluation of structural abnormalities within the heart. Electrophysiologic studies are used to rule out aberrant conduction pathways in the heart, which may produce arrhythmias.
- Tilt table tests are used in patients with recurrent syncope suspected of having a neurocardiogenic or vasovagal etiology. Patients are placed on a table and tilted upright for several minutes to evaluate for the reproduction of a syncopal episode.

Specific Causes of Syncope

Table 3 (next page) describes the characterizations and management of several causes of syncope.

Vasovagal Syncope

Syncope is produced through vagal-mediated parasympathetic stimulation of the cardiovascular system to cause bradycardia concurrent with vasodilation. Vasovagal syncope is considered the most common cause of syncope in the urgent care setting, accounting for 38–40% of explainable causes in two emergency department studies.[18,19]

History and Physical Examination. A prodrome of nausea, diaphoresis, lightheadedness, weakness, and pallor often immediately precedes the episode and sometimes

Table 3. Differential Diagnosis of Syncope

Cause	Etiology	Presentation	Physical Findings	Diagnostic Aids	Management
Vasodepressor (vasovagal) syncope	Decreased cerebral perfusion due to autonomic peripheral vaso- dilation and bradycardia	Age: young Onset: sudden after prodrome Precipitating factor(s): pain, fever, stress, sight of blood, lack of food or sleep, and the like Duration: seconds to a few minutes if patient is not recumbent Complaints: vague prodrome (light- headedness, nausea, vomiting) for sec- onds or minutes	Rapid mental clearing, occa- sional tonic- clonic movement, bradycardia during event	None	Avoid precipitating factors and prepare for event; place patient recumbent or sitting with head between legs; educate on management if prodrome recurs; reassure
Cardiac dysrhythmic syncope	Decreased cerebral perfusion due to decreased car- diac output	Age: usually older patients Onset: usually sudden (seconds); can be several minutes Precipitating factor(s): often history of coro- nary artery disease Duration: 10 seconds to several minutes Complaints: no warning, or brief (seconds) nonspecific prodrome (e.g., lightheadedness)	Normal cardiac examination	ECG often normal as inpatient	Prolonged cardiac monitoring, then therapy as appropriate
Obstructive cardiac syncope	Decreased cerebral perfusion due to limited ability to increase cardiac output and to decrease periph- eral resistance or due to dysrhythmia	Age: variable (depends on etiology) Onset: sudden Precipitating factor: exertion Duration: variable Complaints: shortness of breath, chest pain, nonspecific symptoms (dia- phoresis, weakness, nausea)	Midsystolic murmur (aortic stenosis, hyper- trophic cardio- myopathy)	ECG may show left ventricular hypertrophy	If older patient, ambulance transfer for hospital admission to rule out acute myocardial ischemia as cause of exertional syncope All patients require immediate work- up as inpatients
Myocardial ischemia	Decreased cerebral perfusion due to decreased cardiac output or dysrhythmia	Age: usually older than 40 years Onset: variable Precipitating factor(s): often prior cardiac disease Duration: variable Complaints: possibly chest pain	The following find- ings are suggestive of but not diagnos- tic of myocardial ischemia, tachy- cardia, tachypnea, hypotension, dia- phoresis, rales, distended neck veins, cardiac gallop	ECG normal or shows acute ischemic changes	Transfer by advanced cardiac life support (ACLS) personnel for admission to hospital

(Cont'd on next page)

Table 3. Differential Diagnosis of Syncope *(Continued)*

Cause	Etiology	Presentation	Physical Findings	Diagnostic Aids	Management
Pulmonary emboli	Decreased cerebral perfusion due to decreased cardiac output and hypotension	Age: adults Onset: sudden Precipitating factor(s): birth control pills, pregnancy, trauma, bed rest, surgery, congestive heart failure, malignancy Complaints: shortness of breath, hemoptysis, chest pain	Hypotension, hypoxia, right-sided heart failure (S3, distended neck veins, parasternal heave)	ECG normal or shows cor pulmonale (incomplete or complete right bundle branch block; S1Q3T3 pattern); arterial blood gases, ventilation-perfusion scan	Transfer by ACLS personnel for admission to medical intensive care unit
Subclavian steal	Brainstem ischemia due to blood flow redistribution from vertebral-basilar system to exercising arm	Age: older patients or those with other evidence of diffuse atherosclerosis Onset: variable Precipitating factor(s): exercise of affected arm Duration: brief Complaints: reproduction of syncope with use of arm	Supraclavicular bruit, decreased pulse or blood pressure on affected side	None	Vascular surgery referral
Neurologic seizures, transient ischemic attacks, basilar migraine		See Chapter 19, Neurology			
Orthostatic hypotension	Decreased cerebral perfusion due to hypotension	Age: usually elderly patients or those with defined underlying conditions (see Table 4) Onset: seconds to minutes Precipitating factor(s): see Table 4 Duration: usually seconds, but can be longer Complaints: faintness, lightheadedness, weakness, blurred or faded vision on standing	Systolic blood pressure drop on standing, rapid mental clearing on wakening	None	Correct identifiable cause (e.g., dehydration). If cause not apparent, refer patient to internist, primary care provider
Carotid sinus hypersensitivity	Decreased cerebral perfusion due to bradycardia and subsequent hypotension (carotid sinus is compressed)	Age: usually elderly patients Onset: abrupt Precipitating factor(s): tight collar, twisting of neck immediately before episode Duration: brief Complaints: history of hypertension, atherosclerosis	Reproductive syncope with gentle, brief (2–4 seconds) carotid sinus pressure while patient is recumbent (first auscultate to ensure that there are no carotid bruits	None	Prompt referral to internist or cardiologist

continues afterward. Usually, the event occurs when the patient is standing or experiences a stressful event, such as venipuncture, intramuscular injections, or hearing/seeing stressful events. In addition, vagal stimulation may result from Valsalva maneuvers, which occur during specific situations in which the intraabdominal or intrathoracic pressure is increased. The Valsalva maneuver is often associated with defecation, urination, and coughing. There are few physical findings during presentation, because signs have usually resolved by the time the patient arrives to the urgent care center. A thorough exam to exclude trauma associated with falling should be conducted.

Diagnostic Aids. No specific testing is definitive, although reoccurrence of the syncopal episode through reproduction of precipitating factors is highly suggestive.

Management. Patients who are young and otherwise healthy should be instructed to avoid precipitating factors, recognize the prodrome, and prepare for the event. Elderly patients require further work-up to rule out cardiogenic causes.

Cardiac Syncope

Cardiovascular causes of syncope are related to obstruction of blood flow, myocardial ischemia, or dysrythmias. All three produce syncope through a transient reduction in blood pressure, resulting in decreased cerebral perfusion.

History and Physical Examination. Cardiac syncope should be suspected in patients with a history of coronary artery disease or structural heart defects. These disorders tend to occur in older patients, but disorders such as hypertrophic cardiomyopathies (idiopathic hypertrophic subaortic stenosis) and primary pulmonary hypertension occur in adolescents and young adults. Hypertrophic cardiomyopathy is the most common cause of sudden death in young athletes.[20] Obstructive cardiovascular syncope often is associated with exertion and stressful events. Syncope secondary to dysrhythmias can occur in any position or situation and is often associated with prodromal symptoms such as lightheadedness, weakness, dizziness, nausea, epigastric distress, chest pressure, or palpitations. Diaphoresis, tachypnea, anxiety, tachycardia, irregular pulse, and frequent premature ventricular beats can be observed with dysrhythmias.

Diagnostic Aids. Electrocardiograms are often normal and cannot rule out cardiac syncope.

Management. Admission for prolonged cardiac monitoring and cardiology consultation is warranted as cardiac syncope carries significant morbidity and mortality.

Pulmonary Embolism

Syncope is produced through the reduction in cardiac and cerebral blood flow secondary to intrapulmonary obstruction by embolus. Pulmonary embolism (PE) is a rare cause of syncope but must always be considered because of the high mortality rate associated with untreated events. One study demonstrated that 13% of patients with PE had syncopal episodes.[21] The patient should be questioned about risk factors, including congestive heart failure, acute myocardial infarction, COPD, pregnancy, prolonged immobilization, previous PE or deep vein thrombosis (DVT), obesity, malignancy, estrogen use, recent surgery (past 3 months), or lower extremity trauma.

History and Physical Examination. In addition to syncope, patients may present with pleuritic chest pain, dyspnea, anxiety, and hemoptysis. Signs include an elevated respiratory rate (i.e., > 16 breaths/minute), rales, tachycardia, hypoxia, hypotension, and right-sided heart failure (S3, distended neck veins, parasternal heave) low-grade fever, wheezing, respiratory distress, and signs of lower extremity DVT.[22]

Diagnostic Aids. Pulse oximetry and arterial blood gas analysis are useful to evaluate for hypoxia and increased arterial-alveolar gradient; an ECG demonstrating S1Q3T3—a large S wave in lead I, and a Q wave and inverted T wave in lead III—is the classic finding but is seen in less than 15% of ECGs. The most common ECG findings are sinus tachycardia or a normal tracing.[23] A ventilation-perfusion scan, spiral computed tomography, and pulmonary angiogram are the most useful diagnostic tests.

Management. If PE is suspected after the history and physical exam, the patient should be transferred via ambulance to an emergency department or hospitalized for definitive diagnosis.

Carotid Sinus Hypersensitivity

Pressure on a hypersensitive carotid sinus can cause bradycardia, resultant hypotension, and subsequent syncope

History and Physical Examination. Carotid sinus hypersensitivity occurs in older patients with a history of hypertension or atherosclerosis. Loss of consciousness is abrupt, and duration is usually brief. It may occur after movement of the head and neck, especially when the patient is wearing a tight collar.

Diagnostic findings include syncope induced with a unilateral, 2–4 second carotid message. The presence of carotid bruits is a contraindication to performing this simple test.

Diagnostic Aids. As above.

Management. Cardiology referral is mandatory. Admission for cardiac monitoring is advisable if cardiac arrhythmia is suspected.

Neurologic Syncope

Neurologic disorders, which can present as syncope, include seizures, migraine headaches, stroke/cerebral vascular accidents, and transient ischemic attacks. (See also Chapter 19.)

History and Physical Examination. Generally, seizures differ from other causes of syncope by postictal confusion rather than the rapid mental clearing after syncope (e.g., a vasodepressor event). In addition, patients with seizures often demonstrate incontinence of bladder or bowel and tonic-clonic extremity movement and are amnestic to the event. Patients with a history of seizure disorder may recall a prodrome that helps to define the syncopal event as epileptic in nature.

In basilar migraines, vasospasm of the basilar artery results in brainstem ischemia. Loss of consciousness may occur. The patient first develops an aura, headache, and lightheadedness; then syncope gradually occurs. Syncope from transient ischemic attacks and seizures generally occurs abruptly.

Evidence of trauma from a fall, tongue biting, mouth lacerations, and muscle soreness are often present, and the physical examination may reveal focal neurologic deficits (Todd's paralysis).

Diagnostic Aids. Ancillary testing should be guided by the suspected cause of the neurologic syncope and often requires resources not offered in the urgent care setting.

Examples include CT scans, magnetic resonance imaging studies, electroencephalogram, and lumbar puncture.

Management. The work-up for neurogenic syncope necessitates transfer to an emergency department or hospitalization for more sophisticated management, because the etiologies described above carry significant morbidity and mortality if left untreated.

Orthostatic Hypotension

Syncope can be caused by dehydration and vasodilation resulting in hypotension and decreased cerebral perfusion (Table 4).

Table 4. Causes of Orthostatic Hypotension

Correctable Causes	Peripheral Neuropathies	Central Nervous System Disorders	Miscellaneous
Hypovolemia	Diabetes mellitus	Intracranial tumors	Advanced age
Hemorrhage	Chronic alcoholism	Wernicke's encephalopathy	Idiopathic orthostatic
Gastrointestinal loss	Amyloidosis	Brainstem lesions	hypotension
Overdiuresis	Pernicious anemia	Multiple cardiovascular	Idiopathic orthostatic
Drugs	Porphyria	accidents	hypotension with somatic
Vasodilators and other	Vincristine therapy	Syringomyelia	neurologic deficits
anti-hypertensive drugs		Tabes dorsalis	(Shy-Drager syndrome)
Psychotropic agents		Guillain-Barré syndrome	Gastrectomy
Prolonged bed rest		Traumatic and inflammatory	
Physical exhaustion		myelopathies	
Pregnancy		Familial dysautonomia	
Poor muscular tone		(Riley-Day syndrome)	
Adrenal insufficiency			
Electrolyte disturbance			

History and Physical Examination. Patients are often elderly, but syncope also occurs in younger patients with evidence of hypovolemia secondary to dehydration, anemia, or sepsis. The onset and duration of the syncopal episode is brief (seconds to minutes). Patients often complain of faintness, light-headedness, weakness, and blurred or faded vision on standing. As described earlier, orthostatic blood pressures should be checked, comparing standing and lying blood pressure and pulse. In addition, signs of anemia may be observed, including pale mucous membranes and hemoccult positive stool.

Diagnostic Testing. No specific diagnostic tests establish this diagnosis.

Management. The key to management is the correction of identifiable causes (chronic anemia, dehydration). Patients with sustained orthostatic blood pressure change even after rehydration deserve emergency department referral or hospital admission for further work-up and treatment.

Management of Syncope

The initial treatment of syncope is directed toward the specific cause if it has been determined. It may involve education to avoid precipitating factors in situational syncope, intravenous fluids for orthostatic hypotension, or discontinuation or substitution of precipitating medications. In addition, the patient should avoid precarious situations that may prove dangerous if a syncopal episode reoccurred (e.g., driving, sports).

Most urgent care patients with syncope are assigned a benign diagnosis after history, physical exam, and diagnostic testing. Such patients may be reassured and discharged home with outpatient follow-up. Other patients, however, require further work-up to define the cause of the syncopal episode.

Figure 1 provides an algorithm for the general evaluation of syncope. Hospital admission is necessary when a specific cardiac or neurologic etiology for the syncopal event is discovered. Patients who are not assigned a diagnosis, whether benign or malignant, present a disposition dilemma. In general, patients > 60 years old with risk factors for pulmonary emboli, with a history or suspicion of cardiovascular disease, medication-related syncope, or exertional syncope associated with chest pain, and patients with multiple episodes require hospital admission or referral to an emergency department for further work-up. Patients with orthostatic syncope unresponsive to IV fluid replacement also should be transferred for further management and assessment. To ensure their safety, such patients should be transferred via ambulance with cardiac monitoring.

Pitfalls in Practice

Failure to obtain a detailed history and complete physical examination in patients presenting with syncope can result in misdiagnosis and delay in the diagnosis of a potentially

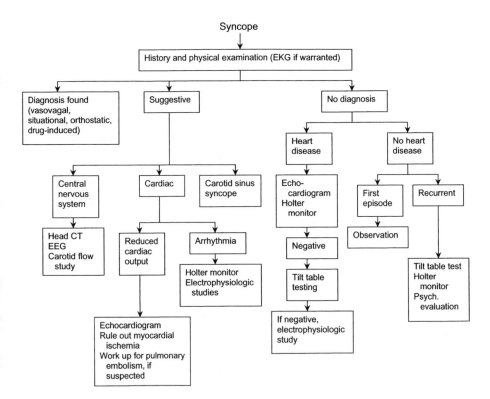

Figure 1.   Algorithm for the work-up of syncope. (Adapted from Hart GT: Evaluation of syncope. Am Fam Physician 51:1941–1948, 1995.)

serious medical illness. Vasovagal syncope is the most common type of syncope; the physician should be wary of this diagnosis if the syncopal event appears atypical or the patient reports no history of a prodrome before loss of consciousness.

Convulsions and urinary or fecal incontinence are not diagnostic of seizures because they are at times found with loss of consciousness caused by ventricular dysrhythmia or heart block.[14,24] Brief tonic-clonic movements have been observed with vasovagal syncope and posttussive syncope.[14,18] The history and physical examination must assess for these potential causes as well as for seizures.

All patients with syncopal events need evaluation for possible trauma caused by a fall in addition to the evaluation for the cause of syncope. Conversely, patients who present with injuries from a fall should be assessed to determine if the fall resulted from a syncopal episode.

Anaphylaxis

Anaphylaxis is a systemic, immediate hypersensitivity reaction. Anaphylactic reactions are immunoglobulin E–mediated, whereas anaphylactoid reactions are clinically similar reactions that occur through non–IgE-mediated mechanisms. The term anaphylaxis generally includes both IgE- and non–IgE-mediated reactions, because they are indistinguishable in their acute clinical presentation. Onset and progression are rapid with multisystem involvement. Anaphylaxis is occasionally immediately life-threatening because of airway obstruction or hypotension, but lesser reactions are usually uncomplicated. As many as 500–1000 anaphylaxis-related deaths occur annually in the United States with peak incidence in the summer.[35] Differentiation of life-threatening from uncomplicated reactions, with rapid intervention if necessary, is the goal of the urgent care physician.

Differential Diagnosis. Anaphylaxis is a clinical diagnosis. No immediately available ancillary studies confirm the diagnosis in the short time within which treatment is necessary. Although several important and potentially life-threatening conditions present like anaphylaxis, a careful history and a focused physical examination aid in the diagnosis.

Exposure to an offending antigen initiates anaphylaxis. The most common offending agents include drugs (penicillins, NSAIDs, angiotensin-converting enzyme inhibitors), insect (bee, wasp) stings, radiocontrast dye, foods (peanuts, fish, dairy products), and more recently, latex.[35,36] The multisystem involvement in anaphylaxis accounts for the wide spectrum of signs and symptoms. The most important systems are respiratory, cardiovascular, and cutaneous. The gastrointestinal and genitourinary systems are also commonly involved. The development of symptoms within minutes of exposure to a known antigen all but confirms the diagnosis.

Urticaria, the most common symptom of anaphylaxis, is present in 88% of patients.[36] The most important respiratory manifestations of anaphylaxis are laryngeal edema and airway obstruction, which account for 75% of fatal cases.[37] Angioedema of the upper airway may occur anywhere from the tongue to the subglottic structures. Hoarseness and stridor are early signs of impending obstruction. More commonly, patients present with shortness of breath and wheezing related to bronchospasm in the lower airways. Although small airway obstruction is not as immediately life-threatening as upper airway obstruction, it may rapidly progress to respiratory failure if left untreated.

Anaphylactic shock occurs secondary to diffuse vasodilatation and increased vascular permeability. The resulting hypotension accounts for 25% of deaths from anaphylaxis. Patients are usually warm, dry, and flushed, with a wide pulse pressure and a low diastolic blood pressure. Crucial watershed areas that require a high diastolic blood pressure for adequate perfusion can become compromised. After successful management of hypotension, the physician should specifically seek evidence of secondary ischemic cerebrovascular accidents or myocardial ischemia.

Management. The ABCs of basic life support must first be assessed in any patient presenting with symptoms of acute anaphylaxis. Supplemental oxygen, intravenous access, and cardiac and oxygen saturation monitoring are recommended. Patients with impending airway obstruction require a secure airway via intubation. Hypotension needs to be aggressively managed with isotonic crystalloid infusion through large bore IVs.

The medical treatment of choice is epinephrine. Patients with progressive symptoms without airway compromise or hypotension may benefit from an initial dose of 0.2–0.5 mg (0.2–0.5 ml of 1:1000) subcutaneous epinephrine. Impending airway obstruction or hypotension requires 0.5–1.0 ml of 1:10,000 epinephrine IV, as needed, every 5–10 minutes. Complications of epinephrine therapy include rebound hypertension, myocardial ischemia, and myocardial dysrhythmias. A history of ischemic heart disease and the presence of tachycardia are not contraindications to the use of epinephrine; it is mandatory in treatment of life threatening cardiovascular collapse. Patients on beta-blocker antihypertensive agents may be resistant to epinephrine. Glucagon, 1 mg IV, is an alternative in such patients. Table 5 outlines the different routes and doses for epinephrine.

Table 5. Epinephrine Administration

Route	Dose
Subcutaneous	0.2–0.5 mg (0.2–0.5 ml of 1:1000)
Endotracheal	0.1–0.2 mg or twice IV dose (1.0–2.0 ml of 1:10,000)
Intravenous	0.5–0.1 mg (0.5–1.0 ml of 1:10,000)

Other classes of useful medications include antihistamines (H_1 and H_2 receptor blockers), steroids, beta-sympathomimetics, and vasopressors. Steroids and antihistamines decrease the incidence and severity of delayed reactions. Beta-sympathomimetics are useful in bronchospasm that is not immediately responsive to epinephrine. Vasopressors (dopamine, norepinephrine, phenylephrine) should be used when hypotension is unresponsive to epinephrine and fluid resuscitation. Table 6 (next page) outlines additional medications that can be used in anaphylaxis.

Additional interventions, such as military antishock trousers (MAST), are helpful in blood pressure maintenance in hypotensive patients who are not immediately responsive to epinephrine. Trendelenburg positioning is useful to maintain cerebral perfusion in persistent hypotension.

Patients should be isolated from further antigenic exposure. This may require removal of contaminated clothing or retained insect stingers.

Table 6. Additional Medications Used to Treat Anaphylaxis

Class	Medication	Dose for Standard Adult
Antihistamines	Diphenhydramine (H$_1$ antagonist)	25–50 mg IM/IV
	Cimetidine (H$_2$ antagonist)	300 mg IV
Steroids	Hydrocortisone	100 mg IV
	Methylprednisolone	125 mg IV
	Prednisone	20 mg/day × 4 days
β-Sympathomimetics	Albuterol	5 mg/ml nebulized
	Terbutaline	0.25 mg SQ
Vasopressors	Dopamine	5–20 µg/kg/min IV
	Norepinephrine	2–4 µg/min IV
	Phenylephrine	40–180 µg/min IV

IM = intramuscularly, IV = intravenously, SQ = subcutaneously.

Uncomplicated cases (i.e., resolved urticaria, resolved bronchospasm) may be managed on an outpatient basis. Any patient with airway obstruction, hypotension, or recurrence of symptoms during observation requires hospitalization. Admission also should be considered for any patient who is unable to avoid reexposure to the offending antigen. Patients without significant symptoms may be discharged only after a short period of observation (30–60 minutes). Such patients require specific instructions about the identification of anaphylaxis and activation of the emergency medical system. All patients should be educated about antigen identification (ie, keeping an allergy diary) and antigen avoidance. Discharge medications include antihistamines and steroids (see Table 6). A self-administering epinephrine device (Epi-Pen) should be supplied to high-risk patients. Patients should be referred for long-term evaluation and care to a primary care physician or allergist for consideration of RAST testing to identify potential allergens.

Pitfalls in Practice. Failure to rapidly recognize and aggressively treat anaphylaxis in patients presenting with hypotension or airway compromise can be a fatal error. Patients with complications require immediate therapy and stabilization before ambulance transfer for medical intensive care hospitalization. Proper observation for progression of symptoms is necessary in mildly symptomatic patients because symptoms develop over 5–60 minutes after antigen exposure. Biphasic anaphylaxis (symptom onset over 1–8 hours) may require prolonged observation and education in high-risk patients.[36]

Weakness and Fatigue

Weakness and fatigue are often encountered in the urgent care patient population. Because of the subjective signs and symptoms associated with these conditions, the work-up can be frustrating for both patient and physician. The terms *weakness* and *fatigue* are often misunderstood by patients and thus misinterpreted by examining physicians. *Fatigue* refers to tiredness, lack of energy and enthusiasm, feeling of being run down, or lessened ability to perform or think as before. *Weakness* includes more objective findings and presents as generalized or focal neuromuscular disorders resulting in decreased strength. It is important to differentiate between the two because underlying causes may carry significant morbidity and mortality and are treated in very different manners. For example, acute weakness may place patients at risk of respiratory failure due to respiratory muscle compromise, where as fatigue may be a symptom of major depression and, if left unrecognized, may result in suicide.

Differential Diagnosis: Weakness. When weakness presents in the urgent care setting, the physician must make a concerted effort to rule out the presence of life-threatening causes. The initial history, physical exam, and directed lab testing separate life-threatening disorders from benign or chronic disorders that can be managed by the primary care provider. Specific neuromuscular disorders that may result in weakness are listed in Table 7.

Table 7. Etiology, Diagnosis, and Management of Weakness

Disorder	Signs and Symptoms	Diagnosis	Management
Hypercalcemia	Diffuse and bilateral weakness, increased DTRs, spasticity. Seen in malignancy, hyperparathyroidism, thiazide diuretic use.	ECG (flattened T, P waves, shortened QT) Serum calcium	Cardiac monitoring, IV fluid rehydration, calcitonin
Hypocalcemia	Diffuse and bilateral weakness, tetany, decreased DTRs, altered mental status. Seen in chronic pancreatitis, hypoparathyroidism, renal failure.	ECG (prolonged QT with decreased QRS) Serum calcium	Cardiac monitoring, calcium replacement
Hyperglycemia	Subjective weakness, altered mental status. Seen in diabetes, acute stress.	Serum glucose, urine analysis, look for associated diabetic ketoacidosis	Fluid resuscitation, insulin, monitor pH, potassium
Hypoglycemia	Subjective weakness, altered mental status, sweating, tremors. Seen in diabetics, malnutrition, alcohol abuse.	Serum glucose	1 amp D50 or oral replacement if mild
Hyperkalemia	Weakness is often ascending and symmetric. DTRs are decreased. Predisposed by medications, chronic illnesses, renal failure, rare family history; muscle injury including burns, crush injury, excessive exercise.	ECG (peaked T waves, pronged QRS, decreased P waves, sine wave), serum K+	Cardiac monitoring, Kayexalate, calcium chloride, bicarbonate, dialysis
Hypokalemia	Diffuse and symmetric weakness, DTRs are decreased, confusion, paresthesias. Seen in malnutrition, profuse diarrhea, diuretic use.	ECG (flattening of T waves, ST depression U waves), serum K+	Cardiac monitoring. If K+ is less than 3.0, IV/oral replacement
Hypermagnesemia	Generalized weakness, nausea, vomiting, arrhythmias, decreased DTRs, respiratory distress, history of chronic illness.	ECG, serum magnesium	Cardiac monitoring, calcium gluconate, dialysis
Hypomagnesemia	Diffuse and symmetric weakness, increased DTRs, altered mental status, muscle fasciculations. Seen in alcoholics, renal disease, malnutrition.	ECG (bradycardia, prolonged PR, QRS, QT intervals), serum magnesium	IV replacement
Hypophosphatemia	Distal paresthesias, weakness, respiratory distress.	Serum phosphorus	Replacement
Botulism	GI symptoms, descending motor weakness starting with diplopia, dysarthria, dry mouth, dysphagia, mydriasis becoming generalized with history of contaminated food ingestion, honey in infants.	Serum, stool, and food cultures, diagnosis is clinical	Respiratory support, two vials of ABE antitoxin
Diphtheria	Ascending weakness, decreased DTRs with remote history (1–3 mo) of pharyngitis.	History of immunizations, throat cultures	Respiratory support, antitoxin

(Cont'd on next page)

Table 7. Etiology, Diagnosis, and Management of Weakness *(Continued)*

Disorder	Signs and Symptoms	Diagnosis	Management
Tetanus	Muscle spasms exemplified by lockjaw, neck stiffness, risus sardonicus (facial muscle contraction), opisthotonos (back muscle contractions producing extension), History of wound infection in patients lacking adequate tetanus prophylaxis.	Clinical suspicion	Respiratory support, antibiotics, human tetanus immune globin
Guillain-Barré syndrome	Ascending paralysis +/- sensory deficits, decreased DTRs with history of recent viral illness.	Clinical suspicion, CSF analysis, EMG, pulmonary function testing	Respiratory support, plasmapheresis, immune globulin
Myasthenia gravis	Weakness begins in facial muscle muscles with ptosis predominating, increases with repetitive use.	Tensilon test, EMG	Respiratory support, pyridostigmine, thymectomy
Polymyositis	Ascending proximal muscle weakness.	Clinical suspicion elevated ESR, CPK, muscle biopsy	Corticosteroids
Organophosphates and carbamates	Paralysis, miosis, GI symptoms, sweating, bradycardia, pulmonary edema, respiratory distress. History of insecticide exposure.	Clinical suspicion	Respiratory support, atropine, 2-PAM (pralidoxime)
Tick paralysis	Ascending symmetric flaccid paralysis, decreased DTRs, ataxia, paresthesias.	Dog or wood tick exposure	Respiratory support, tick removal

DTRs = deep tendon reflexes, K+ = potassium, CSF = cerebrospinal fluid, EMG = electromyography, ESR = erythrocyte sedimentation rate, CPK = creatine phosphokinase.
Adapted from LoVecchio F, Jacobson S: Approach to generalized weakness and peripheral neuromuscular disease. Emerg Med Clin North Am 15:605–623, 1997; and Biros MH: Special medical conditions. In Biros MH, Sterner S: Handbook of Urgent Care Medicine. Rockville, MD, Aspen, 1990, pp 169–171.

History and Physical Examination. The interview should elicit basic historical features of the patient's weakness, including onset, duration, progression, weakness with repetitive use, and effects on activities of daily living. Attempt to differentiate between proximal and distal muscle weakness (stair climbing, fine motor skills, dysphagia). In addition, search for probable causes, including trauma, drug exposures (prescription and illicit drugs, alcohol), and family history of inherited diseases (metabolic and neuromuscular).

Explore the patient's medical history for prior episodes of similar weakness and any work-up conducted at that time. In addition, ask the patient about any recent viral or bacterial illness, immunizations, or toxic exposures. Travel history should be discussed to determine infectious exposures. Also consider ingestions including alcohol and illicit drug use. Ask about living quarters to explore possible exposures to lead paint in children.

All patients examined for neuromuscular weakness need to be assessed immediately for potential respiratory compromise. Start with the ABCs of the primary survey; airway and breathing are assessed first. Patients demonstrating confusion, broken speech, or tachypnea may be hypoxic and in respiratory distress. In addition, look for tachycardia and hypotension, which may be due to toxin exposure, infection, endocrine disorders, or primary pulmonary or cardiac disease. Further assessment with pulse oximetry or arterial blood gases can aid in detecting the degree of respiratory distress.

Initial maneuvers include placing the patient on oxygen and securing the airway. If the examining physician is not qualified or resources are unavailable, 911 should be called in order to transfer the patient to a facility where a secure airway can be provided.

The secondary survey should include a detailed physical exam. Concentrate on the head and neck exam for evidence of facial paralysis and ptosis (i.e., smaller muscles, which are the first to demonstrate weakness in some disorders). The pulmonary exam should look for respiratory distress demonstrated by use of accessory muscles of respiration or tachypnea. Include a rectal exam to assess rectal tone and hemoccult to rule out gastrointestinal bleeding and anemia. Skin should be inspected for lesions and rashes suggestive of infections, drug reactions, and animal bites. The mental status examination should determine the patient's level of consciousness. Examine extremities for evidence of trauma, which may contribute to focal weakness. Look for focal neurologic deficits. Assess cranial nerves, deep tendon reflexes, and proximal and distal muscle groups. Muscle strength should be graded on a 0–5 point scale (Table 8), and it should be determined whether the weakness is bilateral. A partial listing of the differential diagnosis of bilateral diffuse muscle weakness is presented in Table 9. In addition, determine if fasciculations, atrophy, hyper- or hypotonia, or tenderness exists.

Table 8. Grading of Muscle Strength

Grade	Assessment of Muscle Strength
5	Normal muscle strength/movement
4	Movement against gravity and resistance
3	Movement against gravity
2	Movement when gravity is eliminated
1	Trace muscle movement
0	No muscle movement

Table 9. Partial Differential Diagnosis of Bilateral Diffuse Muscle Weakness

Distal muscle weakness	Proximal muscle weakness
• In the presence of fever Bacterial infections (diphtheria, botulism, tetanus) Viral infections (polio) • In the absence of fever Intoxication (metals, carbon monoxide, organic compounds) Metabolic disorders (electrolyte disturbances) Systemic disturbances (endocrine disease, anemia) Insect envenomations (ticks, spiders) Postinfectious syndromes (Guillain-Barré syndrome)	• Positive Tensilon response Myasthenia gravis • Negative Tensilon response with muscle tenderness Polymyositis, alcoholic myositis • Negative Tensilon response without muscle tenderness Periodic paralysis

After completion of the physical exam, attempt to classify the weakness according to the location of injury. True muscle weakness results from injury to the central nervous system (including brain and spinal cord), peripheral nervous system, neuromuscular junction, and muscles themselves. Some lesion-dependent characteristics of weakness are listed in Table 10. To differentiate between injury to the central and peripheral nervous systems, determine whether the physical findings represent upper or lower motor neuron injury. Injury to upper motor neurons produces spastic paralysis characterized by increased deep tendon reflexes and increased muscle tone without evidence of atrophy. Traumatic, ischemic, and hyperplastic lesions in the brain and spinal cord produce focal neurologic deficits, depending on the neural topography affected by the lesion.

Table 10. Some Lesion-dependent Characteristics of Weakness

Site of Lesion	Weakness	Reflexes	Sensation	Bowel and Bladder Function
Spinal cord	Usually lower limb involved	Absent lower limb reflexes	Sensory deficit at specific level	Abnormal
Peripheral nerve	Generalized	Absent	Glove-stocking sensory deficits	Normal
Neuromuscular junction	May be generalized, may involve ocular muscles	Usually normal	No sensory deficits	Normal
Muscle	Generalized, patient may have muscle tenderness	Decreased	No sensory deficits	Normal

Lower motor neuron injury demonstrates decreased deep tendon reflexes with muscular flaccidity and atrophy. Termed neuropathies, lesions involving lower motor neurons in the spinal cord and peripheral nervous system demonstrate these characteristic findings. Examples include Guillain-Barré syndrome, toxic neuropathies such as heavy metal poisonings, and even diabetic neuropathies. Guillain-Barré syndrome is an immune-mediated disorder involving the demyelination of the peripheral nervous system and is believed to be an autoimmune response to viral infections.[25] Characteristic findings include progressive loss of motor function in an ascending pattern, often originating in the lower extremities; occasional sensory involvement (some reports demonstrate sensory dysfunction in up to one-third of cases[26]); decreased deep tendon reflexes; and, in some cases, progression of weakness to include cranial nerves and respiratory muscles. Toxins producing peripheral neuropathies include lead, mercury, arsenic, thallium, and hexacarbon solvents.[27] Characteristically, these neuropathies involve the lower extremities, producing a generalized weakness with increased distal muscle weakness. Patients with such physical findings must be identified and observed closely for evidence of respiratory distress.

Disorders affecting the neuromuscular junction produce periodic muscle weakness, eventually leading to progressive, generalized muscle weakness and decreased strength on physical exam. These findings are characteristic of myasthenia gravis, the most common neuromuscular junction disorder. In this autoimmune disorder, the body produces antibodies against acetylcholine receptors, resulting in decreased postsynaptic motor neuron stimulation.[27] Characteristic findings secondary to muscle fatigue of small facial muscles include ptosis, diplopia, and visual changes. Stress, including surgery, infection, heat, and even pregnancy, precipitates episodes of weakness. Diagnosis is made by the Tensilon test. Intravenous injection of 2 mg of Tensilon (edrophonium) causes increased stimulation of postsynaptic acetylcholine receptors, decreasing weakness temporarily.

Toxins also cause weakness by affecting neural transmission along the nerve axon or at the neuromuscular junction. Botulism is caused by ingestion of toxin produced by *Clostridium botulinum*, which is found in contaminated foods, including canned goods and honey. Diffuse life-threatening weakness is produced because the toxin prevents acetylcholine release at the presynaptic membrane. Treatment involves respiratory support and infusion of a trivalent antitoxin. Other toxins, including tetanus and diphtheria, also produce generalized muscle weakness and/or spasticity (see Table 7).

Myopathic disorders directly affecting muscles are associated with generalized muscle weakness of proximal muscles more than distal muscles. Patients may complain of muscle tenderness on exam. Lack of sensory deficits is characteristic for myopathy. Myopathy may be secondary to infection, inflammation, metabolic disorders, trauma, burns, or ischemia. When a myopathic disorder is suspected, careful review of history including toxic exposure, trauma, family history of similar complaints, and current medication use is important.

Diagnostic Aids. Diagnostic testing should be directed by history and physical findings to rule out suspected life-threatening causes of weakness and to rule in suspected diagnoses. Suspicion of anemia warrants checking the hemoglobin. Suspicion of malignancy warrants evaluation of the complete blood count and electrolyte screening, including calcium, magnesium, and phosphate. Creatinine phosphokinase is elevated in patients with myopathy or rhabdomyolysis. Patients suspected of having Guillain-Barré syndrome or other pathology known to affect respiration should have peak flow or pulmonary function testing to assess respiratory capacity.[27] Refer to Table 7 for further recommendations.

Differential Diagnosis: Fatigue. Patients presenting to the urgent care setting with fatigue often describe a feeling of decreased energy, increased tiredness, feeling run down, and other similar complaints. They often suffer from psychosocial problems but must be evaluated to rule out physical ailments. Fatigue is differentiated from other disorders in that it is not relieved by rest or sleep and is not associated with prolonged or vigorous exercise.[28] Fatigue is a common complaint of patients presenting to the primary care setting. In one study, 41.2% of patients had complaints of persistent fatigue in a select general practitioner's patient population with several reports demonstrating an increased incidence among women.[28–30] Other risk factors include depression, chronic medical illness, HIV/AIDS, pregnancy or postpartum state, sleep disturbances, and stress.[28,31,32] The broad spectrum of causes makes the diagnosis of fatigue, let alone the specific cause, a challenge in an isolated urgent care visit. Patients must be made aware that a primary care physician, who can follow the patient through time, is best suited for the work-up of fatigue. Some common causes of fatigue are listed in Table 11 (next page).

History and Physical Examination. After determining that the patient's chief complaint truly represents fatigue, it is important to derive a few key historical points. The duration of symptoms is an important characteristic. Chronic fatigue, represented by symptoms lasting longer than 6 months, is rarely diagnosed or treated in the urgent care setting. The syndrome does not represent an immediate threat to the patient and requires long-term health maintenance not available in the urgent care setting.

New onset of symptoms consistent with fatigue demands a thorough history to determine length and frequency of symptoms, prior episodes, current sleeping patterns, recent viral illness, and signs of depression, including weight gain, anhedonia, increased sleep, and feelings of isolation. Both psychological and physiologic causes of fatigue exist. Psychological causes include depression, anxiety, panic disorder, adjustment disorder, and stress. An estimated 40–50% of patients with complaints consistent with chronic fatigue suffer from depression.[33,34] Clues to psychologic fatigue include age (depression has a mean age of onset at age 40), sex (depression is twice as common in women), family history of psychologic disorders, and recent life-changing events. Physiologic causes of fatigue include pregnancy, metabolic disorders (diabetes, anemia,

Table 11. Frequent Characteristics of Some Causes of Fatigue

Cause	History	Presentation	Daily Course	Sleep Patterns	Associated Symptoms
Psychosocial	Stressful daily life, recurrent or long-standing symptoms, possible prior functional problems	Depressed, anxious, possibly lethargic	Fatigue is worst in morning, improves during the day; physical activity improves symptoms; emotional stress worsens symptoms	Disrupted	Nonspecific, multiple
Before or after acute infection	Possible suggestive history; frequently young patients, recent onset	Possible appearance of illness, lethargy, signs and symptoms of infection	Fatigue improves with rest, worsens with activity	Normal	Possibly specific
Cardiovascular or pulmonary	Significant prior history; frequently older patients, recurrent episodes, multiple medications; fatigue usually secondary complaint	Possible appearance of illness; physical examination suggests underlying disease	Fatigue improves with rest, worsens with activity	Variable (depends on underlying disorder)	Specific
Drugs	History of multiple medications or changed dose; usually elderly patients, gradual onset	With depressants: often lethargic. With stimulants: often hyperactive	Variable, usually worse with activity; little relief with rest	Variable	Nonspecific
Endocrine	Possible prior history, recurrent episodes; fatigue usually secondary complaint	Often appearance of illness, usually lethargic	Fatigue worsens as day progresses, with activity; improves with rest	Normal	Specific
Metabolic	Usually prior history; usually elderly patients, gradual onset; fatigue may be primary complaint	Possible appearance of illness, usually lethargic	Fatigue worsens as day progresses, with activity; improves with rest	Normal or	Specific
Miscellaneous chronic diseases (anemia, cancer, acquired immuno-deficiency syndrome (AIDS), tuberculosis, rheumatoid arthritis)	Usually prior history, gradual onset; fatigue usually secondary complaint	Possible appearance of illness, lethargy	Fatigue worsens as day progresses, with activity; improves with rest	Normal	Specific
Normal	History of unusual exertion, grief, recent illness, injury, inadequate rest; recent onset	Patient appears to be well, not lethargic	Fatigue worsens with exertion, improves with rest	Normal	Nonspecific

hypothyroidism, malignancy), infections, sleep disturbances, medication side effects, and illicit drug use.

Physical examination includes general appearance, vital signs (e.g., temperature, head and neck exam for evidence of infection or thyroid masses), cardiopulmonary exam for evidence of pneumonia or congestive heart failure, skin for evidence of dry skin or myxedema, rectal exam for evidence of occult blood loss, muscle strength testing for evidence of focal neurologic deficits, and a brief mental exam. Ancillary testing is directed by history and physical findings only; no test reliably diagnoses fatigue.[33]

Management of Weakness and Fatigue. Initial management of weakness and fatigue in the urgent care center requires the identification of immediate life threats. Patients who present in respiratory distress or with an acute neurologic event require a secure airway and primary survey to look for any impairment of the ABCs. If the patient's condition requires resuscitation efforts beyond the capabilities of the urgent care center, 911 should be called immediately for transfer to a referral center. Patients with toxic or metabolic abnormalities should have treatment to correct these abnormalities. Patients with severe abnormalities associated with life-threatening sequelae should be transferred.

Pitfalls in Practice. Although many abnormalities associated with fatigue and weakness are chronic conditions that are unlikely to be identified during a short urgent care visit, every patient with such complaints necessitates a thorough work-up. Underlying conditions may have potential life-threatening or permanently disabling sequelae. Even patients with subjective complaints can have life threatening conditions. Assess every patient with a complaint of weakness with a primary survey that includes evaluation of airway, breathing, circulation, and neurologic deficits. Patients with complaints of fatigue may be reaching out for help in dealing with major depression. It is important to differentiate between the two disorders, because underlying causes may carry significant morbidity and mortality and are treated in different manners. Acute weakness may place patients at risk of respiratory failure due to respiratory muscle compromise, whereas fatigue may be a symptom of major depression and, if left unrecognized, may result in suicide. After ruling out life-threatening conditions, patients should be reassured and referred to primary care physicians for further work-up. Contacting the primary physician ensures follow-up.

References

1. Roccella EJ, Bowler AE, Horn M: Epidemiologic considerations in defining hypotension. Med Clin North Am 71:785–802, 1987.
2. Jenkins JL, Los Calzo J: Manual of Emergency Medicine: Diagnosis and Treatment. Boston, Little, Brown, 1987, pp 153–155.
3. Fine RH, Schofferman J: Hypertension. In Diamond N, Guze PA, Schofferman J, et al (eds): Ambulatory Care for the House Officer. Baltimore, Williams & Wilkins, 1982, pp 164–171.
4. Sixth Report of the Joint National Committee on Detection, Evaluation, and Diagnosis of High Blood Pressure (JNC VI). Arch Intern Med 157:2413, 1997.
5. Kaplan NM, Rose BD: Hypertension: Who should be treated? Definitions and recommendations. Up to Date 7(2):1–4, 1998.
6. Jackson RE: Hypertension emergencies. In Tintinalli JE, Krome RL, Ruiz E (eds): Emergency Medicine: A Comprehensive Study Guide, 2nd ed. New York, McGraw-Hill, 1988, pp 222–232.
7. Heger JW, Nieman JT, Boman KG, et al (eds): Cardiology for the House Officer. Baltimore, Williams & Wilkins, 1982, pp 89–92.
8. Kaplan NM: Long-term effectiveness of nonpharmacologic treatment of hypertension. Hypertension 18(3 Suppl): 1153, 1991.
9. Bates B, Hoekelman RA: A Guide to Physical Examination, 2nd ed. Philadelphia, J.B. Lippincott, 1979, pp 178–180.

10. Kaplan NM, Rose BD: Initial therapy in essential hypertension. Up to Date 7(2):1–8, 1999.
11. Thach AM, Schultz PJ: Non-emergent hypertension: New perspectives for the emergency medicine physician. Emerg Med Clin North Am 13:1009–1025, 1995.
12. Hayes OW: Evaluation of syncope in the emergency department. Emerg Med Clin North Am 16:601–615, 1998.
13. Kapoor WN: Workup and management of patients with syncope. Med Clin North Am 79:1153–1170, 1995.
14. Wayne HH: Syncope: Pathophysiological considerations and analysis of the clinical characteristics in 510 patients. Am J Med 73:15–23, 1982.
15. Hart GT: Evaluation of syncope. Am Fam Phys 51(8):1941–1948, 1995.
16. Atkins D, Hanusa B, Sefcik T, Kapoor W: Syncope and orthostatic hypotension. Am J Med 91:179–185, 1991.
17. Rosen P, Barkin R: Emergency Medicine: Concepts and Clinical Practice. St. Louis, Mosby, 1998, p 1575.
18. Martin GJ, Adams SL, Martin HG, et al: Prospective evaluation of syncope. Ann Emerg Med 13:499–504, 1984.
19. Day SC, Cook EF, Funkenstein H, Goldman L: Evaluation and outcome of emergency room patients with transient loss of consciousness. Am J Med 73:15–23, 1982.
20. Maron BJ, Roberts WC, McAllister HA, et al: Sudden death in young athletes. Circulation 62:218–229, 1980.
21. Thames MD, Alpert JS, Dalen JE: Syncope in patients with pulmonary embolism. JAMA 238:2509–2511, 1977.
22. Cline D, Ma OJ, Tintinalli JE, et al: Emergency Medicine: A Comprehensive Study Guide Companion Handbook. New York, McGraw-Hill, 1996, pp 212–214.
23. Stein PD, Dalen JE, McIntyre KM, et al: The electrocardiogram in acute pulmonary embolism. Prog Cardiovascular Dis 17:247–257, 1975.
24. Schott GD, McLeod AA, Jewitt DE: Cardiac arrhythmias that masquerade as epilepsy. BMJ 1:1453–1454, 1977.
25. Loffel NB, Rossi LN, Mumenthaler M, et al: The Landry-Guillian-Barré syndrome: Complications, prognosis, and natural history in 123 cases. J Neurol Sci 33:71–79, 1977.
26. Moore P, James O: Guillain-Barré syndrome: Incidence, management, and outcome of major complications. Crit Care Med 9:549, 1981.
27. LoVecchio F, Jacobson S: Approach to generalized weakness and peripheral neuromuscular disease. Emerg Med Clin North Am 15:605–623, 1997.
28. Cahill CA: Differential diagnosis of fatigue in women. JOGNN 28:81–86, 1999.
29. Fuhner P, Wessely S: The epidemiology of fatigue and depression: A French primary care study. Psychol Med 25:895–905, 1995.
30. Stewart D, Abbey S, Meana M, Boydell M: What makes women tired? A community sample. J Women's Health 7:69–76, 1998.
31. Libbus K, Baker JL, Osgood JM, et al: Persistent fatigue in well women. Women Health 23:57–72, 1995.
32. Perkins DO, Leserman J, Stern RA, et al: Somatic symptoms and HIV infection: Relationship to depressive symptoms and indicators of HIV disease. Am J Psychiatry 152:1776–1781, 1995.
33. Jarrett WA: Lethargy in general practice. Practitioner 225:731–737, 1981.
34. Montgomery GK: Uncommon tiredness among college undergraduates. J Consult Clin Psychol 51:517–525, 1983.
35. Neugut AI, Ghatak AT, Miller RL: Anaphylaxis in the United States: An investigation into its epidemiology. Arch Intern Med 161:15–21, 2001.
36. O'Dowd LC, Zweiman B. Anaphylaxis. Up to Date 7(2):1–6, 1998.
37. Delage C, Irey NS: Anaphylactic deaths: Clinicopathologic study of 4333 cases. J Forensic Sci 17:525, 1972.

Chapter 8

Minor Surgical Trauma

Michelle H. Biros, MS, MD
Brian Isaacson, MD

Minor traumatic injuries of the soft tissues and their complications are frequent occurrences that prompt visits or calls to health care professionals. The urgent care physician must carefully assess the patient for associated unrecognized injury, significant medical illness that may have precipitated the minor trauma (e.g., syncope or seizures), and mechanisms that suggest a more significant injury than is apparent on initial examination (e.g., a chin laceration in a patient whose injury could have resulted in cervical spine injury). Once the patient has been fully evaluated, proper minor wound management can be initiated.

The goals of acute wound care are to restore continuity of tissue, to preserve viable tissue, to develop maximum wound strength, and to reduce the risk of excessive wound inflammation, infection, and scarring.

General Approach to Minor Soft Tissue Trauma

Physical examination of soft tissue injury requires sufficient light and instruments, gentle handling, and a comfortable and cooperative patient. Adequate examination of a painful injury may require sedation, analgesia, and local anesthesia (only after the neurologic exam is completed). It is advisable for the patient to lie down during the examination. All jewelry must be removed from injured extremities. Sterile technique should be used to assess location and depth of the wound, degree of contamination, and presence of debris, foreign bodies, and devitalized tissue. Deformity, additional injury, and possible injury to underlying structures also should be evaluated. The range of motion and neurovascular status of the injured part should be determined.

Certain wounds that appear to be benign are at great risk for complications. Examples include roller or wringer injuries, high-pressure injection injuries, high-voltage electric shock, prolonged compression injuries from heavy objects, and human bites. The importance of a careful history cannot be overemphasized.

Wound Preparation

After examination and before any intervention, the area of injury and surrounding skin should be cleansed. It is essential to prevent additional contamination of the area, and surgical masks, gloves, and hats should be worn. Visualization of the wound is enhanced in some areas by removing a small amount of hair. Clipping is better than shaving surrounding hair because it does not injure the surrounding skin as much; in either case, it usually is necessary to remove hair from only a small area (i.e., 3–5 mm) surrounding the edges of the wound for good visualization. Removing hair at any interface between the hair and skin, such as at the hairline of the scalp, results in loss of landmarks in laceration repair and should be avoided if possible. This principle also applies to repair of lacerations that involve the eyebrow; in addition, regrowth of eyebrow hair is extremely slow and unpredictable and can lead to cosmetically poor results. For these reason, eyebrow hair should not be removed during wound care.

The area around the injury should be scrubbed with a circular motion for 2–3 minutes, with the radius of each circle increasing away from the edges of the wound to carry skin contaminants from the wound. There are several available scrubbing solutions; nonirritating soaps and povidone-iodine (Betadine) solution are commonly used agents. Soaking wounds may loosen debris but is no substitute for adequate scrubbing and wound irrigation.

After the surrounding skin is scrubbed, the wound is cleaned. Scrubbing the wound itself is controversial. Some authorities hold that scrubbing adds injury to potentially viable tissues, whereas others believe that it may further debride the wound and remove embedded foreign particles. In general, most authorities advise that scrubbing should be considered only for heavily contaminated wounds.[1]

The most commonly used method for wound cleansing is irrigation. High-pressure pulsatile delivery of the irrigating solution can be achieved with the use of a large syringe and an attached plastic catheter. This system is effective for removing loose debris from the wound and should be used to deliver at least 200–300 ml of irrigating solution to minor wounds or until all visible particles are removed. The most commonly used irrigating solution is normal saline. Lactated Ringer's solution is advocated by some authorities because its pH is close to neutral; 1% povidone-iodine solution is also effective and may reduce the risk of wound infection. Recent studies suggest that irrigating the wound under flowing tap water also may provide effective cleansing. The investigators suggest that the key to successful cleaning of wounds is high-pressure irrigation, regardless of the solution used.[2,3]

Debridement of the wound is then performed to remove nonviable tissue or contaminated tissue that cannot be cleaned. The tissue is removed with a blade or scissors. If the wound is a laceration with ragged edges that require repair, the edges are trimmed to make closure easier. It is difficult to determine acutely the extent of tissue injury; therefore, as little tissue as possible should be removed during debridement, especially for wounds of the face.

Wound Dressing

After the general preparation of the wound, specific management is performed. Following management, most wounds require wound dressing. Dressings lessen the likelihood of wound contamination from surrounding skin, which can occur until healing reepithelialization takes place (usually 2–3 days). Dressings also serve to absorb secretions (which can macerate healing skin), to immobilize the wound and thus promote healing, to exert a slight pressure on the wound and thus prevent painful exposure of nerve endings to air, to add comfort, and to prevent wound dehydration.

The dressing begins with a nonadherent layer that is in direct contact with the wound. Many commercial products are available, and all are equally effective. An absorbent gauze layer is applied over this layer and held in place by an outer dressing layer of gauze. The outer layer can be wrapped around the extremity to hold the dressing in place and should consist of an expansible material applied distally to proximally on the extremity. Circumferential dressings should not be applied to digits because tissue ischemia can develop if the digit swells and the dressing cannot expand. Occasionally, pressure dressings are needed to prevent excessive hematoma formation (e.g., in ear wounds and sutured wounds with dead space). All patients with dressed wounds should be instructed to return for reevaluation if they develop signs and symptoms of decreased circulation distal to the dressing or if the injury becomes more painful with time.

Wounds that are heavily contaminated or located across joints should be immobilized with a bulky dressing or with a splint incorporated into the outer dressing layer. Immobilization reduces lymph fluid flow in the area of injury and thus can reduce contamination. It also protects fragile, newly forming capillaries and therefore can promote healing.[1]

The initial wound dressings should be left in place for 48 hours. Subsequent wound dressings should be applied as long as there is serous drainage from the wound. If the location of the wound makes application of a dressing impractical (e.g., on the face and scalp), careful wound cleansing should be followed by application of a thin layer of antibiotic ointment. Patients should wash such wounds with water and reapply the antibiotic ointment 3 times daily.

Wound Aftercare

The injured part should be kept elevated for the first 48 hours after injury to reduce edema formation, enhance healing, and reduce pain. The timing of follow-up examination depends on the degree of injury and the potential for contamination; if complications arise, they usually manifest by 48 hours.

Abrasions

Abrasions are skin disruptions caused by shearing forces that remove the superficial layers of the skin. Such injuries are common, especially in children and especially during the summer months.

Differential Diagnosis. Abrasions due to minor trauma and the circumstances of the injury are usually recalled by the patient. Because the dermal nerve endings are exposed after injury, the lesions are painful. They are usually dirty, and embedded foreign bodies, such as particles of dirt and road tar, are common. Occasionally, abrasions are deep enough to extend into the subcutaneous tissue.

Management. A thorough initial cleansing is necessary to reduce the risk of subsequent wound infection and tattooing (discoloration of the healed skin from retained pieces of road tar or dirt). The use of local anesthesia, such as infiltrated lidocaine, is possible only with small wounds. Large wounds are difficult to anesthetize locally. TAC solution (0.5% tetracaine, 1:2,000 epinephrine, and 11.8% cocaine) applied on sterile gauze with pressure to the wound for 5–10 minutes may be helpful in achieving anesthesia. Recent studies suggest that the tetracaine component of this solution does not contribute to its effectiveness and may be eliminated.[4] Sterile gauze impregnated with 4% lidocaine and applied to the wound with pressure for 5–10 minutes occasionally produces adequate local anesthesia to permit wound cleansing. If local measures are ineffective in providing pain relief required for proper wound cleaning, parenteral analgesia may be necessary.

The initial cleaning should remove obvious loose dirt and can be accomplished by irrigation with water or normal saline. If road tar is embedded in the wound, Neosporin or Bacitracin ointment can be used to dissolve it. Both ointments are water-soluble and can be washed off once the road tar has been removed. Any embedded foreign bodies should be removed. Often the pointed end of a number 11 blade is helpful in dislodging embedded particulate matter; obviously, this procedure should be done gently to avoid further tissue damage. Debridement of devitalized tissue is also important to promote wound healing.

Home care instructions should emphasize the signs and symptoms of infection. The patient should be advised to return if any of these develop and to wash the abrasion daily with soap and water. If the wound is kept moist with application of an antimicrobial ointment such as Neosporin or Bacitracin, 3 or 4 times per day, it should heal within 7–10 days. Loose dressings should be applied to abrasions located on weight-bearing surfaces or surfaces that are rubbed by clothing; all others may be left open to heal. Appropriate tetanus prophylaxis should be given (Fig. 1).

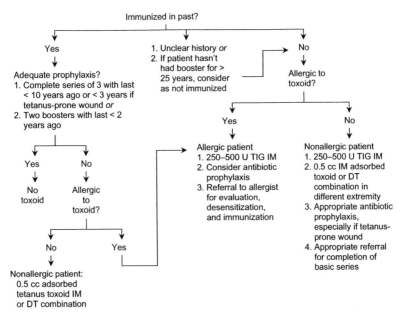

Figure 1. Guidelines for tetanus immunization. (Adapted from Mathews J: Tetanus. In Markovchick VJ, Pons PT (eds): Emergency Medicine Secrets, 2nd ed. Philadelphia, Hanley & Belfus, 1999, pp 232–235.)

Pitfalls in Practice. Healing is delayed and risk of infection increased if foreign material is retained in the wound. A careful inspection, therefore, is essential to avoid these potential problems. Failure to cleanse an abrasion adequately can result in infection or unacceptable cosmetic results (i.e., tattooing).

Puncture Wounds

Puncture wounds are extremely common. The most common sites of injury are the feet and hands, and the most frequently reported offending objects are nails, needles, and splinters.

History and Physical Examination. Patients who present with puncture wounds usually can relate the time and circumstances of the injury. It is essential to determine whether the wound was made by a "clean" (i.e., never used) or "dirty" (i.e., potentially contaminated) object, how deeply the injured site was penetrated, and the likelihood of retained foreign material in the wound. Punctures through clothing or shoes have an increased risk of foreign material in the wound. As with all minor trauma, the patient's tetanus and allergic status must be determined.

On examination, the wound should be assessed for potential damage to underlying structures. The location of the injury, vascular status, and neurologic assessment are important. After the surface of the involved area has been cleansed, the wound should be anesthetized and gently probed to assess its depth and to search for foreign bodies. Pieces of glass frequently can be seen on plain films, as can metallic chips or slivers.

Management. After anesthesia is accomplished, the edges of the wound should be circumferentially trimmed back approximately 2–3 mm so that they will remain open and allow drainage from the wound. Additional exploration can be done at this time. High-pressure irrigation should be performed with normal saline delivered through a plastic intravenous catheter attached to a syringe or with a commercial irrigation device. The end of the catheter should not be placed within the wound because normal saline delivered under high pressure may cause ballooning of the surrounding tissues with trapping of contaminants under the tissue.

If it is determined by history and examination that the wound is "clean," bandage dressings are applied daily for 3–4 days and the patient can be instructed to return if signs and symptoms of infections occur. "Dirty" wounds are similarly dressed and should be examined again in 2 days. Although controversial, a short course of broad-spectrum antibiotics (e.g., dicloxacillin or a cephalosporin) is usually considered in puncture wounds to the foot, especially if bits of torn clothing or footwear may have been introduced into the wound.[1] Immunocompromised patients should receive close follow-up and antibiotics for treatment of "dirty" puncture wounds. The first dose of antibiotic should be given parenterally at the time of examination. A foot with a "dirty" puncture wound that has potentially penetrated a bone or joint should be kept elevated during rest, and the patient should avoid weight bearing for 4 days. Tetanus prophylaxis should be given when indicated.

Pitfalls in Practice. Given their relatively minor presentation, puncture wounds often are treated casually because their seriousness is underestimated. Complications of puncture wounds are frequent, however, especially in the children, and are predominantly bacterial infections. Cellulitis resulting from puncture wounds usually develops within 1–4 days after injury, and osteomyelitis can present 6 days to 16 months later. Infectious complications are seen in up to 15% of foot wounds, and the presence of a retained foreign body markedly increases the risk of infection.[5] Failure to appreciate the extent and dangerous potential of such wounds can lead to substantial subsequent morbidity.

Retained Foreign Material

The presence of foreign material in soft tissues can be a serious problem. Even in cases in which the embedded material is inert and does not promote tissue inflammation or infection, the patient presenting with a retained foreign body may worry about the immediate and long-term consequences. Although any material can be embedded within soft tissues, the most commonly retained foreign materials are wood, glass, and metal.

In some circumstances, a retained foreign body can be removed easily in the urgent care setting. In other situations, the foreign body can be safely left in place or requires specialized equipment to locate and remove it. The goals of urgent care management are to determine which foreign bodies must be removed, when they should be removed, and where the procedure should be done. A true emergency involving retained foreign material is a high-pressure injection injury. This entity must be recognized and treated immediately to prevent significant morbidity.

Retained Soft Tissue Foreign Bodies

Differential Diagnosis. Most patients who relate a history of a possible retained foreign body recall the circumstances of the injury. The history can give clues to the nature of the retained material; if the patient states that it feels as if the material is still embedded, it probably is. The nature of the material determines the need for and timing of removal. The possibility of contamination introduced with the foreign material also influences the decision to remove it.

Inert material does not decompose or change in composition; therefore, it is not always necessary to remove the foreign material in an urgent manner. Long-term retention of inert material may result in chronic pain, however, and it is recommended that only the smallest inert fragments be left in place and then only if they are in a noncrucial area. Noninert material, such as wood, has the potential to cause significant tissue reaction and to harbor bacteria and fungi; therefore, it is more likely to cause infection than inert material.

In addition to the circumstances surrounding the injury, the patient's tetanus status, medication allergies, and general state of health should be determined. If the foreign body became embedded during a blast or as a missile, it is important to ascertain that no additional injuries have occurred.

Once it has been determined that a foreign body is retained, the clinician must decide whether to remove it. The decision depends on the type, location, and size of the foreign body. Materials that promote tissue inflammation or infection need prompt removal. A retained piece of wood, for example, must be removed promptly.

Occasionally, superficial foreign bodies can be seen or palpated directly under the skin. If no foreign body is seen, anteroposterior (to suggest location) and lateral (to suggest depth) plain films may help to locate the object. The site of entry should be marked to facilitate orientation when retrieval is begun. Most pieces of glass are visible on plain films; most organic substances (e.g., wood) are not.[1] Wood that has been embedded for more than 24 hours absorbs water, so that its density is lowered to nearly that of soft tissue; it thus becomes difficult to visualize on plain films.[6] Air is often introduced with the foreign object, and examining air patterns on plain films may help locate the object. If a patient presents with a prolonged history of a retained foreign body not visible on plain films, a computed tomography (CT) scan may be useful, although expensive. Ultrasonography is also useful in identifying most retained foreign bodies.[6,7]

Management. In retrieving the foreign body, it is often wise to set a time limit for exploration; most clinicians do not have the time or patience to continue searching for the object for more than 20 minutes. A pre-exploration film may be helpful in cases in which the object is seen; postexploration films should be taken to ensure that removal is complete. The results of pre-exploration and post-exploration physical examinations should be documented, especially with regard to the neurovascular status of the involved part. In general, embedded foreign bodies are easier to remove if local or regional anesthesia is used.

If the object is protruding from the skin and will not splinter, it should be grasped firmly and pulled out in a line parallel to its skin track. If the object can be seen under the skin, an incision immediately adjacent and parallel to it should be made, the object rolled out of its track, and the track irrigated with normal saline. If the object can be seen on plain films but is deeper than subcutaneous, the entrance wound should be enlarged and the wound probed with a closed pair of hemostats. Often the object can be felt on gentle probing before it can be seen. No attempts to remove a retained object should be made unless the object is visualized. If the material is lodged perpendicular to the skin but not protruding from it, a small elliptical incision should be made and the edges of the skin pushed slightly downward. Often the retained object bulges out of the center of the wound and can be grasped and pulled out. Metal detectors with small probes may facilitate localization of an embedded metal object; it is essential, however, that the probes be sterile or covered with a sterile glove before they are introduced into the wound. If the foreign body is not visible on plain films, the entrance site should be enlarged and the wound explored.

If material is embedded under the fingernail or toenail, a digital block may facilitate retrieval. A small-gauge needle (no. 25) with the end bent can be run parallel to an embedded splinter, and the curved end can then be used to hook the distal end of the splinter and drag it from under the nail. If this technique does not work, it is necessary to cut a small wedge from the overlying nail so that the foreign object can be removed.

Once the foreign body is removed, the track should be copiously irrigated under pressure with normal saline or 1% povidone-iodine. Contaminated tissue should be debrided. With highly contaminated wounds, it may be necessary to remove a small block of surrounding tissue to ensure that the area is appropriately cleansed.

Foreign body removal cannot be accomplished effectively unless the field is bloodless and the object directly visualized. The entrance wound and any additional incisions that are made during retrieval should be left open to drain. The patient should be given tetanus prophylaxis if indicated. Antibiotics (e.g., a cephalosporin) are frequently given if the wound appears to be contaminated or if the foreign material is organic, although they have not been shown to be necessary. Follow-up examinations should be scheduled for 2 days after removal, and in the interim the patient should be instructed to elevate the involved part.

When the foreign object is embedded in the face or hands, no attempt should be made to remove it unless the clinician is confident of the anatomy of the area and the object is easily seen. Because of the delicate neurovascular structures in these areas, probing within the wound is extremely dangerous and is best left to a specialist. Foreign bodies in the foot, even if they are seen on plain x-rays, are usually difficult to retrieve. The risk of tissue destruction from vigorous exploration should be carefully considered; these situations are often best managed by specialty consultation. Exploration under fluoroscopy can then be used.

Whenever an embedded foreign object impairs function of the involved, part, it must be removed expeditiously (i.e., < 72 hours). Conversely, embedded foreign bodies have a remote possibility of migrating if left in place. If retrieval is difficult or contraindicated, the specialist often may elect to leave an inert foreign body where it is.

Pitfalls in Practice. Recurrent abscesses or cellulitis after removal of a foreign body suggests the presence of retained materials. Organic material is prone to cause infection and tissue reaction; organic material should not remain embedded. When physicians attempt to remove an embedded foreign object, it is essential that careful exploration be done; overly vigorous probing can cause significant neurovascular damage.

Embedded Fishhooks

Differential Diagnosis. Embedded fishhooks are a common occurrence. Usually the angler has unsuccessfully attempted to remove the embedded hook before visiting the urgent care setting.

Management. If the barb of the hook is small or embedded superficially, it is sometimes possible to back it out of the skin by pulling it perpendicular to the site of entry. Occasionally, extending the puncture site slightly will aid this process. If the hook is large or deeply embedded, however, pulling directly backward causes the barb to become impinged or hooked on the inferior aspect of the skin. The easiest method of removal is to push the barb forward completely through the skin. The skin around the hook should be scrubbed and anesthetized. The hook is then pushed forward through the skin. Once the barb has pierced the skin, it is cut off with a heavy scissors or wire cutter, and the shaft can be pulled back from the site of entry. The principles of management after removal of the hook are similar to those for any puncture wound.

If the hook is embedded in the eye, it should be left in place until it can be removed by a specialist. The eye should be shielded with a metal eye-guard taped securely in place; no pressure dressings should be applied. The patient should be referred emergently.

If the fishhook is embedded over a joint and may have penetrated the joint capsule, an x-ray may define its location more precisely or determine whether there is air in the joint space, which could have accumulated when the hook pierced it. A fishhook that has penetrated the joint capsule or joint space should be emergently removed by a specialist. Because it is often impossible to determine whether the joint space has been entered when deep penetration in the region of a joint has occurred, specialty consultation should be considered.

Pitfalls in Practice. The use of pressure over a fishhook embedded in the eye may cause extrusion of intraocular contents from the puncture wound. Attempting to remove a hook that has penetrated a joint capsule by pulling it out rather than pushing it through may break off the end of the barb into the joint itself.

High-Pressure Injection Injuries

Differential Diagnosis. High-pressure injection injuries are usually work-related and involve the hand. The patient gives a history of sustaining the injury while using a high-pressure system such as a spray gun for painting, fuel injection apparatus in engines, high-pressure grease guns, or hydraulic systems of heavy equipment. The damage is caused by injection of a foreign chemical into the soft tissues. Most often the initial complaint is a painless stinging sensation of the hand. Occasionally a small puncture wound can be seen. If the injection has been under very high pressure or of a large volume, swelling may be significant and immediate. Within about 1 hour, the affected part becomes swollen, pale, and exquisitely tender. Sensation may be increased or decreased, and the patient experiences throbbing pain.

Management. High-pressure injection injuries are surgical emergencies. The time interval between the injury and surgical decompression is directly related to outcome. If the tissue is not decompressed, venous and arterial flow is compromised, and tissue ischemia, damage, and death may result. Foreign material is forcefully introduced under high pressure, resulting in serious deep contamination as well as tissue ischemia and necrosis from the deposited material that has increased tissue pressure. Plain films may be used to track the route of deposition of the material or air tracks within the soft tissues. Because such wounds are tetanus-prone, the tetanus status of the patient should be determined. All patients with high-pressure injection injuries should receive parenteral antibiotics while awaiting transfer to a facility where the injury can be surgically decompressed. Digital blocks may increase tissue pressure and should be avoided.[8]

Pitfalls in Practice. Failure to diagnose a high-pressure injection injury can result in serious morbidity because tissue survival depends on the speed at which surgical decompression can be done. A careful history is often of more use in the initial diagnosis than the physical examination.

Bites

Animal bites occur frequently and are estimated to account for over 1% of all visits to emergency care facilities annually. The true incidence of bites is difficult to determine because many patients do not seek care for injuries that they judge to be inconsequential and because the reporting of bites is often not mandatory. Dog bites are the most commonly seen (60–90% of all bites), followed by cat bites (5–15%); rodents account for 7% and other species for approximately 2% of all recognized bites.[9] Human bites are often the sequelae of assaultive behavior and contribute to between 1% and 2% of all reported bites.[9]

Animal bites are complicated injuries, and some aspects of their management are controversial. Most bites are a combination of blunt and penetrating injuries. Wound infection is a major concern because bites are contaminated with the oral flora of the offending animal. The animal also may harbor a systemic illness such as rabies, which can be transmitted through the bite.

Dogs have strong jaws, but their teeth are often not very sharp. Bites therefore are often an obvious combination injury, which may include puncture wounds and skin tears from the animal's teeth, crush injury from the forceful closure of its jaws, and avulsion of tissue (if the animal shook its head or if the patient tried to escape). Most dog bites in adults occur on the lower extremities. Bites to the face, neck, and scalp are much more common in children and involve the potential for skull and facial bone fracture. The microorganisms found in dog bites are numerous and the overall incidence of infection is 5–10%.[10]

A recent study isolated *Pasteurella* sp., a highly virulent gram-negative pathogen, from one-half of dog bites, contradicting the view that is uncommon.[11]

Up to 30% of cat bites become infected, with potential sequelae of septic arthritis, meningitis, septic shock, and endocarditis.[10] The long slender teeth of cats and other small animals typically produce puncture wounds, which can be deep and are inoculated with the animal's oral flora. Most cat bites occur on the hand. *Pasteurella* sp. is found in up to 75% of cat bites.[9]

Human bites of the hand, in particular the commonly encountered "fight bite" or closed-fist injury to a metacarpophalangeal (MCP) region, are associated with a high incidence of infectious complications. Often patients are too embarrassed to seek medical attention for such injuries, or the injury is not initially painful. As a result, patients often present 2–3 days after the injury because of the development of infectious complications. Simple human bites elsewhere on the body rarely become infected.

The goals of urgent care management of bites are (1) proper, meticulous wound care to reduce the risk of infection, disfigurement, and disability; (2) determination of the need for antibiotics and, with animal bites, rabies prophylaxis; (3) determination of the patient's tetanus status; and (4) determination of the need for and type of additional therapy (directed by the nature of the wound). The urgent care physician also must ensure that no additional trauma occurred at the time of attack and that the patient is able to assist in his or her own aftercare.

History and Physical Examination. A proper history is essential in the evaluation of a patient presenting after an animal or human bite. Specific details of the incident are important, including whether the animal attack was provoked, the type of animal involved, whether the animal is known or accessible, and the immunization status of the animal. In many communities the local health department can aid in capturing the animal. For all bites the patient's immunization status and medical history should be considered in subsequent wound management.

All patients who have been attacked by an animal have the potential for serious injury, and initial assessment should proceed in the routine manner for patients sustaining major trauma. After ensuring patient stability and ruling out associated injuries, evaluation of the wound may proceed. Neurovascular status, position of wound relative to joints and underlying structures, obvious bony deformities, and the presence of gross contamination and devitalized tissue should be determined. Local anesthesia may be necessary to facilitate wound exploration and subsequent management.

Diagnostic Aids. Plain radiographs are useful to help determine the presence of underlying bony injury, joint capsule violation, or a retained foreign body. If a bite has entered a joint or if there is injury to the bone or other underlying structures, the patient should be referred to an emergency department. Infants and toddlers who have sustained dog bites to the skull or face are at risk for cranial penetration, and if interruption in bony cortex is discernible, the patient has sustained an open fracture. Potential complications include brain lacerations, intracranial abscess, and meningitis.[10] Admission for intravenous antibiotics and neurosurgical consultation is mandated. Initial Gram stain and culture rarely yield the pathogen ultimately responsible for a wound infection and are not routinely obtained. However, as a guide to therapy it is advisable to obtain cultures of established infections in immunocompromised patient and in patients for whom empiric therapy has failed.

Management. Initial first aid of bite wounds, regardless of source involves rinsing or washing the skin and application of a clean dry dressing. Direct pressure is best for control of bleeding and an involved extremity should be elevated. Patients should then be instructed to seek medical attention. Attempts to locate or capture the animal should be made. Public health authorities or the police should be contacted for further instructions regarding the disposition of the animal.

Urgent care treatment of bite wounds involves thorough cleansing and pressure irrigation with either normal saline or 1% povidone-iodine solution to dislodge foreign particles and bacteria. This procedure is best accomplished using a syringe with a Zerowet splash shield or 19-gauge intravenous catheter. Between 200 and 500 ml of irrigating solution should be used. Most studies demonstrate that soaking bite wounds or irrigating them with low pulsatile flow is not effective in reducing the incidence of wound infections; high-pressure irrigation is preferred.[2] Foreign bodies should be sponged (not scrubbed) from the wound, and debridement of devitalized and grossly contaminated tissue should be prudently performed, retaining enough tissue to preserve function and provide closure. Sharp and straight wound edges promote wound healing.

Adequately cleaned and low-risk bites can be closed primarily.[10] Closing the wound increases slightly the risk of infection but decreases the time to full function of the extremity. Deep suture should be avoided because it can serve as a nidus for infection. Higher-risk bites should be left open after cleansing, irrigation, and debridement (Table 1). They may be covered with normal saline-soaked dressings and wrapped with dry gauze, then reevaluated in 48–72 hours for signs and symptoms of infection. Delayed primary closure may then be performed if the wound is free of infection. The edges of the wound will have dried and contracted and may need some additional debridement to allow good closure. Bite wounds to the face and scalp from any species may be sutured after meticulous wound preparation.[10] Bite wounds that are difficult to irrigate and debride adequately, such as puncture wounds, bites to the foot, and human bites to the hand, should not be closed.[11,12]

Table 1. Animal and Human Bites with Low and High Risk for Infectious Complications

Low-Risk Bites	High-Risk Bites
Human bites to the torso	Human bites to the hand
Dog bites	Primate or unusual animal bites
Rodent bites	Cat bites and scratches
Large lacerations (easy to clean)	Small bites, foot bites, or punctures
Scalp and face bites	Bites in poorly vascularized areas
Early presentation of any bite	Delayed presentation (more than 6 hours) of any bite
	Head or face bites in children
	Bites in patients with chronic illness or immunosuppression
	Bites in patients at extremes of age (< 2 and > 50 years)
	Extensive crush injury
	Bites over joints

In the presence of high-risk factors prophylactic antibiotic therapy is recommended, including all bite wounds to hands and all cat bites or other puncture wounds. Guidelines for administration of antibiotics, including recommended choices, dosages, and duration are suggested in Table 2. Empiric therapy depends on the nature and location of the injury. The first dose of antibiotic should be given intravenously or intramuscularly to achieve adequate blood levels quickly in the presence of high-risk factors. Outpatient therapy is usually effective for local cellulitis, but patients must be monitored closely and re-evaluated within 1–2 days. If patients fail outpatient therapy, have systemic signs of toxicity, or are immunocompromised, unable to provide continued local wound care, or of questionable reliability, admission for intravenous antibiotics is warranted. Significant bites to the hand and bites that violate a joint space, disrupt underlying structures, or penetrate bone should be referred to an emergency department where surgical consultation may be obtained for hospitalization for intravenous antibiotics and possible operative debridement.

Table 2. Suggested Antibiotics for Prophylaxis of High-risk Bite Wounds

Type or Time of Injury	Antibiotic Choices
Cat bite or scratch	Cefuroxime Amoxicillin-clavulanate Penicillin VK + dicloxicillin
Dog bite	Dicloxacillin Cephalexin
Human "fight" bite (clenched fist injuries)	Cefuroxime Amoxicillin-clavulanate (Augmentin)
Human bite (not fight bites)	Dicloxacillin Cephalexin Amoxicillin-clavulanate
Less than 12 hours (probably *Pasteurella multocida*)	Penicillin VK Oral cephalosporins Erythromycin (if patient is allergic to penicillin)
Greater than 12 hours (probably mixed flora)	Dicloxacillin Amoxicillin-clavulanate Oral cephalosporins

Tetanus immunization status must be established and proper vaccination performed. Tetanus results twice as frequently from bite injuries as from other wounds,[13] and up to 4% of all tetanus cases occur after bites. Tetanus is especially common in adults older than 50 years and immigrants, who may not have received a complete immunization series.

In the United States human rabies is extremely rare. One or two deaths are reported per year on average, usually in patients who acquired the disease in another country. More than 90% of all cases of rabies in the U.S. are in wild animals, especially raccoons, skunks, and bats (Table 3). Dogs are the principal reservoir worldwide, including Mexico and Latin America.[10] Rabies is almost nonexistent in rabbits and rodents. To assist in determining whether a patient who has sustained an animal bite should receive a rabies vaccination series, local or state public health departments should be contacted for information about rabies presence in the area. The Centers for Disease Control and Prevention (CDC) may be contacted at 404-639-3311. The decision to treat depends on several factors, including the biting animal and location of the incident. Generally, most authorities start the rabies vaccination series if the bite was inflicted by a wild carnivore;. If the bite was incurred by a domestic animal, the animal should be isolated and observed for any behavior changes before starting the vaccine.[10] The actual transmission rate of rabies from a rabid animal is variable, and the closer the site of entry is to the patient's brain, the shorter the incubation period.

Table 3. Bites with High and Low Risk for Rabies

High-Risk Bites	Low-Risk Bites
Wild carnivores	Rodents
Bats	Rabbits
Raccoons	Casual contact (petting, playing)
Skunks	
Foxes	
Unprovoked attacks	
Salivary exposure (open skin)	
Air-borne exposure (laboratories, caves)	

Rabies virus is killed readily by soap, drying, and sunlight. Wound care is a critical component of postexposure rabies prophylaxis. Current CDC recommendations include thorough and immediate cleansing of bite wounds with soap and water. Actual swabbing of the wound is essential. It should be rinsed with water or normal saline afterward. In wounds at high risk for rabies, 1% benzalkonium chloride (Zephiran) can be applied to the wound. It is viricidal for rabies but irritating to the wound and should be rinsed out with normal saline. Rabies immunoprophylaxis is effective in preventing the disease and requires both active and passive vaccination (Table 4). With high-risk bites, most physicians start the immunization series regardless of when the bite occurred; the usual incubation period for the rabies virus ranges from 30 to 90 days, but there have been confirmed incubation periods of up to 7 years.[10] Bites on the head and neck have a shorter incubation time than bites to the trunk or extremities. The first day of treatment is considered day 0. To ensure that the drug is delivered to muscle, it should be administered to the deltoid region. The vaccines do not have adverse fetal effects and prophylaxis should not be withheld from pregnant patients.

Table 4. Postexposure Primary Vaccinations for Rabies

Immunization	Dose	Route	Timing	Exceptions
Passive (HRIG)	50 IU/kg	Infiltrate half of dose at bite site if anatomically possible, half intramuscularly at distant site	Day 0	Previous immunization with HRIG and HDCV or with measurable titer
Active (HDCV)	1 ml	Intramuscular	Days 0, 3, 7, 14, and 28	Previous immunization (give boosters at days 0 and 3)

HRIG = human rabies immunoglobulin, HDCV = human diploid cell vaccine.

Adverse reactions to rabies vaccination occur frequently; local reactions, such as erythema and pruritus, are seen in 30–40% of recipients. Systemic reactions such as headache, nausea and myalgias are also common. Anaphylaxis and neurologic sequelae are rare.

Pitfalls in Practice. Injuries over the MCP joint should be considered close-fist injuries and treated as human bites. All patients attacked by large animals should be examined carefully for multiple trauma. All children bitten about the face and head should be considered to have penetrating skull wounds until proved otherwise. Bites are tetanus-prone wounds and need tetanus prophylaxis. Patients who have sustained a bite should be examined for signs of infection 24–48 hours after receiving treatment.

A wide variety of other communicable diseases has been transmitted through bites. Patients who sustain human bites are at risk for acquiring other communicable diseases, such as hepatitis; if indicated, appropriate prophylactic therapy should be initiated.

Insect and Spider Bites and Stings

Insect and spider stings and bites can cause a wide variety of symptoms ranging from local pain and irritation to severe allergic and anaphylactic response. In most circumstances, the goal of urgent care management is to provide symptomatic relief and local wound care. Recognition of diseases and syndromes that can develop after exposure to various insects and spiders facilitates proper treatment and reduces morbidity from insect-borne infectious diseases.

The reactions following stings and bites are due to the actions of biochemicals, mainly proteins, found in the venom or saliva of the offender. The composition of these fluids varies from species to species. Generally, local irritants can produce local inflammatory reactions, proteins can induce allergic reactions, proteolytic enzymes can cause local skin breakdown, and neurotoxins may cause neurologic symptoms.

Differential Diagnosis. Table 5 lists the differential diagnosis and management of various insect bites and stings. Stings of wasps, bees, and other hymenopterans are frequent and in sensitized patients can cause severe and anaphylactic responses. They are encountered frequently, and the normal response to a venomous exposure consists of pain, local erythema, edema, and pruritus. However, several more serious reactions may occur, usually within a few minutes of the sting. For unsensitized patients, sequelae depend on location (a local reaction in the mouth or throat can cause airway obstruction), number of stings (and therefore amount of venom injected), type of insect, and body size and health status of the patient. Multiple stings may produce a toxic reaction. Symptoms of a toxic reaction include gastrointestinal disturbance, headache, fever, lightheadedness or syncope, muscle spasms, edema, and seizures (rare). Sensitized patients may experience a generalized systemic response, which may range from mild symptoms of generalized urticaria, pruritic eyes, and dry cough to rapidly progressive and fatal respiratory failure and cardiovascular collapse. In general, the shorter the interval to onset of symptoms, the more severe the reaction. Honeybees have barbed stingers, which may become embedded in wounds. If present, they should be scraped or pulled but not squeezed from the wound, because they can continue to release venom.

Black widow spiders venom consists of a neurotoxin that causes release of neurotransmitters producing protracted muscle contractions. Symptoms begin at the site of the bite and gradually spread to involve large muscle groups. Classically, involvement of abdominal musculature can mimic an acute abdomen. Severe cases may progress to respiratory failure due to compromise of chest wall function by muscle paralysis. Treatment includes narcotics for pain relief and benzodiazepines for muscle relaxation. Patients should be transferred to an emergency department. The diagnosis of a brown recluse spider bite is often complicated by the innocent appearance of the spider and the patient's inability to recall exposure. Manifestations range from a firm erythematous lesion to severe pain

Table 5. Differential Diagnosis of Insect Bites

Insect	Characteristics	Patient Presentation		Acute Management	Disposition
		Local Symptoms	Systemic Symptoms		
Mosquito	Found spring through fall, especially in moist areas Offending agent: saliva deposited during blood feeding	Local pain, itching swelling	Urticaria (rare), lethargy, headache, nausea	Consider transmission of other diseases (e.g., malaria)	Follow-up as needed
Deer fly, sand fly, black fly	Found spring through fall Offending agent: saliva deposited during blood feeding	Intense local pain, swelling, itching, nausea	Urticaria (rare), lethargy, headache	Local wound care, topical anti-inflamma-tory cream, oral steroids if systemic reaction	Follow-up as needed
Caterpillar (gray furry)	Offending agent: chemical irritant on body spines	Gridlike lesions, intense pain, local swelling, regional adenopathy, skin desquamation (hours to days)	Respiratory irritation if spines inhaled; nausea, fever, muscle cramps, headache, numbness	Remove spines with adhesive tape. In severe reactions: calcium gluconate, antihistamines	Follow-up as needed
Blister beetle	Offending agent: chemical irritant in released hemolymph	Cutaneous blisters	Nephrotoxicity if toxin ingested	Topical magnesium sulfate	Follow-up needed
Scorpion (bark)	Large, spider-like Environment: warm climate (e.g., south-eastern U.S.); tree bark, rotted trees Offending agent: neurotoxin	No local signs; local discomfort	Paresthesia, motor hyperkinesis, central nervous system dys-function, dysphagia, facial paresthesia, opisthotonus, hyper-tension, salivation Symptoms subside in 24 to 48 hr	Ice, local wound care, tetanus prophylaxis Immobilize involved limb Supportive care (oxygen, IV fluids) Antivenin (serious en-venomation), atropine (to counteract para-sympathetic effect) Avoid opiate analgesia (may potentiate symptoms)	Admit acutely ill patients, children, adults with hypertension
Black widow spider	12–18-mm long spider with dark body, hour-glass marking on ventral surface Environment: dry, dark, temperate, tropical Offending agent: neurotoxin	Minimal (no pain, or pinprick sensation and numbness) Small red puncture wound	In 10–60 min: muscle cramping and spasms Additional symptoms: paresthesia, headache, dysphagia, nausea, vomiting, fever, edema, tachypnea, seizures, hypertension or hypo-tension, severe abdominal pain, respiratory distress In 24–36 hr: diaphoresis, salivation, hypertensive crisis Symptoms subside in 48 hr	Ice packs, wound care, tetanus prophylaxis Reduce muscle spasms; diazepam (Valium; adults, 5–10 mg IV over 10 min; children, 0.02–0.05 mg/kg IV up to 5 mg) Treat other symptoms as needed (antiemetics, antihypertensives, narcotics)	Observe patient for at least 8 hr Admit children, pregnant women, elders, those with severe reactions

(Cont'd on next page)

Table 5. Differential Diagnosis of Insect Bites *(Continued)*

Insect	Characteristics	Patient Presentation		Acute Management	Disposition
		Local Symptoms	*Systemic Symptoms*		
Brown recluse spider	9–14-mm long spider with violin mark on dorsal surface Environment: dry, dark (e.g., south central U.S.) Offending agent: destructive enzymes, vaso-constrictor	No pain; minimal burning at bite site, increasing by 3–4 hr At 1–4 hr: bull's-eye lesion (central red bleb surrounded by white area of vasoconstriction and erythematous periphery) Eventual tissue necrosis	Fever, chills, rash, nausea, vomiting, weakness, malaise, intravascular hemolysis seizures, congestive heart failure	Ice packs, wound care, tetanus prophylaxis Avoid local heat Treat symptoms as needed (antiemetics, narcotics, etc.) Local excision some-times advised Plastic revision may be required	Long-term: schedule follow-up to determine extent of tissue
Centipedes	Many appendages Environment: warm climate (e.g., south-eastern U.S.) Offending agent: destructive enzymes	Extreme pain, swelling; occa-sional suppuration	Regional lymphadenopathy	Local nerve block	Follow-up as needed
Millipedes	Many appendages Environment: warm climate Offending agent: chemical irritant	Local discomfort	Usually none	Decontaminate skin	Follow-up as needed
Hymenop-terans (bees, wasps, hornets, yellow jackets, fire ants)	May sting and bite Environment: fire ants, south-eastern U.S; others, widespread	Immediate pain, swelling, redness, itching; sterile pustule (fire ant)	Mild: hives, cough, wheezing, nausea, vomiting, fever, weakness Severe: diffuse urticaria, laryngeal edema, bronchospasm, cyanosis, abdominal pain, cardiovascular collapse	Ice, local wound care, tetanus prophylaxis Remove stinger if still embedded For severe reactions (allergic): oxygen, IV fluids; support airway; epinephrine (adults, 0.3–0.5 ml 1:1,000 subcutane-ously; children, 0.1 ml/kg subcu-taneously every 20–30 min) plus diphenhydramine (adults, 50 mg intra-muscularly; children, 1 mg/kg) or epi-nephrine, 1:1,000 IV (adults, 0.1 mg [1 ml] in 10 ml over 10 min) then infusion of 1:1,000 (1–4 mg/min [1 ml in 250 ml]); steroids	For allergic reactions, observe pa-tient for 1 hr If no symptoms administer antihistamine; bee sting kit; refer to allergist For severe symptoms, admit, refer for desensi-tization Admit if mul-tiple (> 10) stings, intractable vomiting, persistent facial swelling

with erythema, blister formation, and bluish discoloration, with progression to necrosis over 3–4 days. Systemic involvement may occur, generally within 1–2 days of the bite, and includes fever, chills, gastrointestinal upset, myalgias, hemolysis, and seizures. Necrotic wounds should be referred for possible surgical treatment.

Mosquito and fly bites are common but rarely produce systemic responses. Mosquitoes are vectors for many diseases such as encephalitis and malaria. In endemic areas, patients should be advised of the signs and symptoms of such diseases and prophylactic measures should be taken if indicated. The local health department can provide advisement if necessary.

Fleas, lice, and scabies are ectoparasites and especially common in children. Diagnostic cues and treatment are discussed in Table 6. Spread occurs easily through close personal contact with an infested person, infected personal articles and clothing, and bedding.

Table 6. Bites of Ectoparasites

Insect	Characteristics	Local Symptoms	Acute Management	Follow-up
Lice	Gray, crablike parasites		Shampoo (Kwell, Eurax), comb	As needed
Body		Itching, excoriation, pustules	out, boil clothing; refer close	
Head		Nits on scalp hair, excoriations, pustules, posterior cervical adenopathy	contacts for treatment	
Pubic		Itching, excoriations, bluish macular eruptions on thighs, trunk, near pubis		
Bed bugs	Nocturnal blood feeders	Itching, erythematous wheals	Palliative	As needed
Kissing bugs	Nocturnal blood feeders	Hemorrhagic papules, bullae, urticarial lesions	Palliative	As needed
Mites			Topical astringents (camphor,	As needed
Chiggers	In green vegetation, hot areas	Papular disruption; itch often on wrist	phenol), oral antihistamines Shampoo (Kwell) initially; repeat	
Itch mites	Epidemic outbreaks	Raised, pruritic, linear lesion	in 1 week Clean clothes, sheets Refer contacts	
Fleas	Especially seen in children during summer months	Small, raised, pruritic, red lesions	Bathe thoroughly	As needed

Tick bites are usually harmless and cause few local reactions. Ticks harbor a great number of significant infectious diseases, however, that produce morbidity and mortality if not appropriately treated (Table 7; see also chapter 6).

Management. Initial pain and swelling from insect bites can be reduced if ice is applied and the involved extremity elevated. Because venom may contain enzymes that are activated by heat, local heat should not be applied to the bite site. Wounds from stings and bites should be washed with soap and water, and the patient should receive tetanus prophylaxis if immunization status is not current.

Some caterpillars release an irritant through body spines that become embedded when a person comes in contact with the insect. Spines can be removed with adhesive tape and the irritant washed from the skin with soap and water. Millipedes also release a chemical irritant that must be washed from the skin. In such circumstances, the fingernails of the

Table 7. Differential Diagnosis of Diseases Transmitted by Tick Bites

Syndrome	Characteristics	Skin Symptoms	Systemic Symptoms	Acute Management	Disposition
Tick paralysis	Pregnant female hard ticks; neurotoxin	Attached tick for 2–3 days	Progressive ascending motor paralysis, impaired coordination, areflexia, possible respiratory failure	Remove tick; recovery in hours to days Supportive therapy	Admit all cases
Rocky Mountain spotted fever	South Atlantic, southwestern U.S., dog tick; wood tick; reportable disease (see also chapter 6)	2–4 days after bite: blanching small macules that become petechial Starts at wrist or ankles, spreads	2–12 days after bite: headache, fever, nausea, vomiting, abdominal pain, meningismus	Adults: doxycycline, 100 mg 2 times/day (5–7 days); tetracycline, 500 mg 2 times/day (5–7 days); chloramphenicol, 50 mg/kg/day in 4 doses (5–7 days) Children: doxycycline, chloramphenicol	Outpatient treatment for reliable patients, mildly ill patients; inpatient treatment for systemically ill patients or if diagnosis not clear
Lyme disease	New England, Midwestern and western U.S. (see also chapter 6)	Stage 1: expanding maculopapular lesion with red border and clear center (erythema chronicum migrans)	Stage 1: fever, headache, malaise, lethargy Stage 2: cardiac, neurologic symptoms Stage 3: arthritis	Stage 1: amoxicillin, doxycycline or cefuroxime Stage 2: amoxicillin, doxycycline, ceftriaxone, cefotaxime Stage 3: penicillin, cefotaxime	Outpatient treatment for stage 1; inpatient suggested for stages 2 and 3
Ehrlichiosis	Dog ticks	None	Sudden-onset fever, rigors, headache, myalgia, nausea, vomiting	As for Rocky Mountain spotted fever	Outpatient treatment unless patient is severely ill
Relapsing fever	Rocky Mountains Ticks do not remain attached Also spread by body lice (see also chapter 6)	None, or ill-defined macular, papular, or petechial rash	7 days after bite: sudden-onset rigors, headache, fever, myalgia; relapses	Tetracycline, chloramphenicol, erythromycin; complete recovery even without antibiotics	Outpatient treatment unless patient is severely ill
Tularemia	South-central U.S.; also transmitted by infected animals (e.g., rabbits) (see also chapter 6)	Painful skin ulcer at bite site	5–9 days after bite: sudden-onset fever, chills, malaise, fatigue, regional adenopathy	Streptomycin 7.5–10 mg/kg intramuscularly 2 times/day for 14 days	Outpatient treatment unless patient is severely ill

patient should be cleaned carefully to prevent the spread of the irritant to other regions of the body.

When patients present with tick bites, it is essential to remove attached ticks to prevent local infections and, in the case of tick paralysis, to prevent life-threatening complications of the bite. Application of petroleum jelly, mineral oil, isopropyl alcohol, or fingernail polish to smother the tick has been described, but actual success with such methods is questionable.[14] Anecdotal reports of success described the use of 10% potassium hydroxide or ethyl chloride on the body of the tick or a suture needle to try to pry the tick off the skin. Holding a lighted match to the tick's body also has been suggested but may cause a burn to the patient. Careful removal of the tick by means of forceps and a gloved hand and slow, steady, upward pressure is usually successful and does not cause trauma to the patient. Thorough washing of the bite site should follow removal of the tick. In the rare instance when the tick cannot be entirely removed, mouthparts that remain embedded may need to be excised.

Prophylactic antibiotics are usually not recommended for stings and bites, but a broad-spectrum antibiotic should be prescribed in the presence of an established local infection.

Pitfalls in Practice. Patients who are hypersensitive to bites and stings can develop systemic signs and symptoms requiring rapid diagnosis and treatment to prevent such serious complications as respiratory and hemodynamic compromise. Emergency therapy should be started in the urgent care setting and the patient transported to an emergency department. Often patients who have sustained bites or stings develop a local tissue reaction with an area of redness around the bite site. This local reaction resolves spontaneously but must be differentiated from local cellulitis, which requires antibiotic therapy.

Minor Burns

Appropriate initial care for minor burns are essential to restore full function to the injured part and to reduce the risk of cosmetic defect at the site of injury. Up to 90% of all burns are caused by thermal injury; chemical burns account for 5% of burns and electrical injuries for 2%.[15]

Thermal Burns

Differential Diagnosis. The severity of burns, regardless of their cause, is determined by depth, size, and body location. Outcome depends on the patient's age, overall medical status, and ability to care for the wound as well as on the severity of injury. Essential historical points include the timing of the injury, the patient's tetanus status, the potential risk of simultaneous smoke inhalation or other injury, and medication and medical history.

The depth of a burn is determined by how much of the skin is injured. First-degree burns affect the epidermis and result in redness, pain, tenderness, and swelling. An example is sunburn. About 7 days after insult the burned epidermis may peel off, with new, healed epidermis beneath. Second-degree (partial-thickness) burns result in blister formation beneath injured epidermis. If the second-degree burn is superficial, the surface under the blister is red, with intact sensation and capillary refill. Healing occurs spontaneously in about 2–3 weeks. The surface of a deep second-degree burn is a mixed red-and-white color, and sensation and capillary refill may be somewhat impaired. On examination, such burns have evidence of blister formation, but often the blisters have ruptured. Pressure sensation is often intact, but two-point discrimination may be impaired.[15] Deep second-degree burns usually heal spontaneously in about 3–6 weeks. Third-degree or full-thickness burns destroy the dermis, epidermis, and germinal cells. The involved tissue is white, nonblanching, or bronze and feels leathery. Sensation and perfusion of the area are lost. The eschar that forms usually pulls off in about 1 week. If the third-degree burn is small (< 1.0 cm in diameter), it may undergo spontaneous healing, with contraction and granulation from the periphery of the wound. Otherwise, skin grafting is necessary to resurface the injured area.

The total body surface area (TBSA) of burn is best estimated by the "rule of the nines," which assigns parts of the body a percentage of TBSA on the basis of the number nine. Despite the widespread availability of burn charts and graphs, the size of burns is often overestimated. An accurate estimate is important because the management and disposition of the patient are influenced by the amount of body surface involved. To aid in estimating the area of the burn, comparison of the area of the burn to the size of the patient's flattened palm is helpful. The size of the patient's palm is approximately 1% to 1.5% of the TBSA.[15] The TBSA of infants is calculated slightly differently because of their proportionally larger head than and proportionately smaller lower extremities compared with adults.

The physical examination should include evaluation of the burn, a search for occult injury that may have occurred at the time of the burn, and an evaluation of the patient's pulmonary status. Soot in the nares, carbonaceous sputum, and a smoky smell on the patient's skin or clothing suggest smoke inhalation.

Management. In general, patients with large burns present to an emergency department. If a patient presents to the urgent care setting with more than a 10% second- or third-degree burn or burns involving the hands, face, feet, perineum, or genitalia, the burns should be covered with a sterile sheet and the patient transferred by ambulance to a burn center for further evaluation and possible admission. Burns over joints and all circumferential burns should be seen immediately by a burn specialist. Intravenous morphine can be administered for pain relief in small incremental doses (2–3 mg); larger doses may compound the hypotension already possible from fluid loss. Patients with significant burns (typically > 20% TBSA) need fluid replacement. The intravenous fluid of choice is lactated Ringer's solution; the rate of administration depends on the patient's clinical status.

First aid to small burns begins with immersion of the burned part in cool water, which is effective in relieving pain and may enhance wound healing if done immediately after injury. This is good telephone advice, and most patients instinctively apply this remedy after injury. Cool, wet towels can be applied over the burn, or the injured part can be bathed in cool tap water or normal saline. Care must be taken to avoid application of ice to burns, which can lead to frostbite injury and delayed healing. First-degree burns are treated with cleansing and analgesia. The patient should avoid further injury to the involved skin. Ointments and burn dressings are not necessary.

The treatment of second-degree burns with intact blisters is controversial. Some authorities believe that the blister fluid is protective for the new epithelial layer and prevents its desiccation. Others have suggested that the prostaglandin content of the blister fluid can cause local vasospasm, which may convert the burn to a deeper injury, or that blister fluid is a good culture medium and therefore increases the risk of wound infection.[15] Usually the blister should be left intact unless it is in a region where it is bound to break open (i.e., the dorsum of the foot under a shoe) or unless it contains harmful chemicals (see below). The burn should be cleaned carefully with soap and water and dressed with a bulky dressing to avoid breaking of the intact blister. If the blister has ruptured spontaneously, the dead skin should be removed with an iris scissors and the wound irrigated with normal saline. Before the application of a bulky dressing, an antibiotic ointment such as silver sulfadiazine (Silvadene) or Neosporin is applied to the area in a sterile fashion. The dressing should be changed daily for the first 2 or 3 days. Residual ointment should be removed before fresh ointment is applied. Patients unable to attend to dressing changes should be instructed to follow up with their primary care physician or to return to the urgent care center for dressing changes. Unless complications develop, after the first 2 or 3 days the patient can be seen on a weekly basis until the wound is healed. Early mobilization is essential to avoid joint stiffening. The overall infection rate for second-degree burns is low; in general, patients do not require prophylactic antibiotics. Open therapy of second-degree burns is usually reserved for the face.[15] Such burns should be covered with Bacitracin ointment. Gentle cleansing should be performed every 6 hours, followed by reapplication of the ointment

Third-degree burns usually require skin grafting. The initial therapy is similar to that for second-degree burns, but early referral (1–2 days) to a plastic or burn surgeon is essential.

If a burn patient requires transfer to another facility, it is best not to apply ointment to the affected area, because it may obscure subsequent examinations. Instead, the burn should be covered with a sterile dressing. Patients should be immunized for tetanus if indicated. Even minor burns can be quite painful, and oral analgesics should be administered. Certain high-risk patients, such as those unable to care for themselves, alcoholics, diabetics, immunosuppressed patients, the very old, and the very young, may need hospitalization for relatively minor burns to ensure adequate care.

Pitfalls in Practice. Patients who sustain burns should be questioned carefully and examined for other injuries that occurred simultaneously but are unnoticed because the patient is distracted by the pain of the burn. The potential for edema formation after burns is great and should be considered in all patients, especially those with facial burns and possible airway injury. If the potential for respiratory compromise or airway obstruction exists, the patient needs admission, regardless of the size or depth of the injury.

Any child who presents with an unusual distribution of burn injury, such as buttock and heel burns, patterned burns, or cigarette burns, should be considered abused until proved otherwise. If abuse is suspected, hospitalization with subsequent social service and child protection investigation is advised.

Parents often have difficulty in providing adequate burn care to their child because they feel that they are hurting the child when they change dressing. Wound care should be done by the primary care physician, or the child should return to the urgent care center.

Patients should be advised that scars may form after burn healing and that the final configuration of the scar may not appear for several months. In addition, pigment changes in the healed tissue will occur. Undesirable pigment changes can occur after sun exposure. Sun block should be applied over the healed area for at least 6 months after healing to prevent color changes.

Chemical Burns

Differential Diagnosis. Chemical burns can occur under a wide variety of circumstances but are usually work-related. Many chemicals cause burn when they come in direct contact with skin through chemical reaction with the tissue, direct thermal injury, or thermal injury resulting from chemical reactions at the exposed skin surface. Common chemical substances that can burn on contact are listed in Table 8.

Table 8. Chemicals that Cause Burns

Chemical	Source	Toxic Activity	Presentation	Management
Hydrofluoric acid	Rust removers, semiconductors, glass, etching chemicals, dyes, plastics	Fluoride ion produces soft tissue liquefaction necrosis and decalcification and erosion of bone	Erythema; possible blisters; tough surface coagulum; painful, deep ulcerations	Copious water wash; remove nails if involved No blisters: bulky dressing soaked with calcium gluconate or magnesium oxide ointment Blisters: regional nerve block; debridement; 10% calcium gluconate, local injection (0.5 ml/cm² of involved skin); reevaluate in 24 hr
Gasoline	Fuel	Direct skin irritant; can occasionally cause epidermal necrolysis	Erythema; possible blisters; pneumonitis secondary to fume inhalation; neurologic, gastrointestinal, cardiovascular symptoms if gas is absorbed through skin	Copious water wash If systemic toxicity, ambulance transfer for hospitalization
Lyes (corrosive alkali metals)	Cleaning agents, paint removers	Solubilize protein and collagen to liquefy skin; also dehydrate tissue cells	Soft, friable, brownish eschars	Copious water wash
Sodium hypochlorite	Disinfectants, bleaches, deodorizers	Free chloride released, which coagulates tissue protein	Erythema; possible blisters; mucous membranes reddened, irritated	Copious water wash; apply demulcent pastes (starch paste, aluminum hydroxide gel, magnesium trisilicate gel)
Phenols	Deodorants, sanitizers, disinfectants	Protein denaturation of surface tissue cells	White or brownish stains; soft, white coagulum; deep necrotic lesions May be painless (phenols demyelinate or destroy nerve fibers) Central nervous system, cardiovascular effects if absorbed through skin	Copious water wash (polyethylene glycol solutions may be more effective than water) If systemic toxicity, ambulance transfer for hospitalization
Tar and asphalt	Construction or road surfacing materials	Thermal injury to skin	Adherent tar material overlying thermal burn	Cool material; once solidified, remove with solvents; copious water wash of underlying burn

The classification of the degree and involved area of chemical burns is similar to that for thermal burns. In addition, the type and concentration of the chemical and the duration of exposure influence the severity of injury. Systemic complications from chemical exposure occasionally result from absorption of the substance through the skin or inhalation of toxic fumes.

Physical characteristics of the exposed area may be identical to those seen in thermal burns. Occasionally, chemically injured skin shrivels or puckers if the agent desiccates cells. Discoloration is common with some chemicals. The injured area may feel hot to touch, be painful, and have soft or colored eschar or early ulceration. As with other burns, the possibility of other injuries should be evaluated. Because many chemicals can cause systemic effects, a careful and complete physical examination should be performed, including an ophthalmologic evaluation to ensure that liquid chemicals have not splashed into the eyes.

Management. The management of chemical burns starts with removal of the chemical contaminant. If the chemical is a solid material, it should be brushed gently off the skin, and irrigation should be begun. If the chemical was a solution, irrigation should be started. Irrigation flushes the chemical from the area and dilutes the chemical. In general, water and normal saline are appropriate irrigating solutions. If the area of exposure is large and if the patient can tolerate it, water wash can be done in a shower. The irrigation should not involve high pressure, which may cause the chemical to splash into the eye or mouth and cause further damage. Irrigation of the eye is necessary if chemical splash is suspected, and contact lenses must be removed immediately. Contaminated clothing should be removed as soon as possible; if the patient's hair was splashed, it should be rinsed. Precautions such as gloves, mask, gowns, and protective eyewear decrease the risk of contamination of medical personnel who are working with the chemically exposed patient.

Some chemical burns have specific antidotes; common examples are listed in Table 8. For the most part, the key is copious irrigation with subsequent wound care as described for thermal burns. Some chemicals concentrate in the blister fluid of second-degree burns. For this reason, it is frequently advised to rupture blisters associated with chemical burns with subsequent copious irrigation of the underlying wound.[16]

The removal of solidified asphalt or tar can be difficult. A large number of commercial solvents are available. Other reportedly successful agents include Polysporin or Neosporin ointment, mineral oil, cold cream, lard, and mayonnaise.

Patients with extensive exposure or any sign of systemic toxicity require ambulance transfer to a burn care center. Indications for pain medications and intravenous fluid therapy are the same as for thermal burns.

Pitfalls in Practice. Systemic toxicity due to skin absorption and inhalation injury from toxic fumes are frequently delayed complications of chemical exposure. Careful follow-up is essential, and the patient should be advised to return for evaluation immediately with the appearance of any suspicious symptoms. Caregivers should be aware of the risk of contamination in caring for chemically exposed patients, regardless of how trivial the exposure appears to be.

Electrical Burns

Differential Diagnosis. Damage due to electrical burns depends on the amperage of the current, resistance to current flow, duration of contact, and site of contact. Resistance depends on the thickness of the skin; the thicker the skin, the greater the resistance to electric current delivery to underlying tissues. Electrical injury to the skin results from the generation of heat as the current passes through tissues. If the resistance is high, less current is internalized, and the skin is more damaged than if the resistance were low. When the skin is moist, the resistance to electrical current drops. Patients with high-voltage (> 1,000 V) electrical injuries usually have associated severe injuries and do not present to the urgent care setting. Low-voltage (< 1,000 V) injuries may appear to be insignificant, but as little as 25 V has been associated with clinically significant injury.[17]

Often accidents with household electricity (110–220 V) do not even cause skin burns; occasionally, however, injury or complications may result. Children most often sustain electrical injuries in the home, and the most common sites of involvement are the hands (from playing with poorly insulated electrical cords) and mouth (from sucking electrical cords and sockets). In hand wounds, entrance and exit sites are usually discernible. If the electric current that produces a mouth wound enters the mouth, an exit wound (most often in the hand) will be found. In most mouth injuries, however, the current arcs between the source and the person through the saliva to an external ground; thus, exit wounds are not found.

The entrance wound in hands is usually small and deep with a central blanched area surrounded by a well-demarcated zone of edema and erythema. The wound may be crater-like with a coagulated center. Such wounds are usually dry and painless. Oral wounds are most commonly found on the corner of the mouth, involving both the upper and lower lips and the commissure. The wound is grayish-white with a depressed center and hyperemic margin. Within a few hours, edema may increase to the point of causing problems with mouth closing and swallowing of saliva. In rare cases, the tongue, palate, or teeth may be injured. The eschar that forms on such wounds sloughs off between 7 and 21 days after injury; in 10% of patients, exposure of the labial artery results in significant bleeding.[17]

Management. Because even low voltages have been associated with significant complications involving the cardiac, neurovascular, ophthalmologic, and central nervous systems, it is essential to screen for such injuries as well as to treat any skin injury associated with exposure to low-voltage electricity. Therefore, if indicted by symptoms or the clinical status of the patient, electrocardiography should be done to determine the presence of dysrhythmias, and urine analysis should be done to determine the presence of released muscle myoglobin. Patients with chest pain, palpitations, altered mental status, significant thermal burns, or muscle pain after an electrical exposure should be transported by ambulance with cardiac monitoring to a burn center for hospitalization. The burn should be covered with a sterile sheet and an intravenous line should be established.

Skin burns from an exposure to electrical current should be treated like thermal burns. The burn should be cleaned and debrided, antibiotic ointment should be applied, and the wound should be dressed. Follow-up is on a daily basis until healing has begun. Electrical burns are tetanus-prone, and the tetanus immunization should be brought up to date. The burned extremity should be elevated and immobilized to reduce edema formation in the first 24 hours.

Oral burns should be cleaned and debrided. A petroleum-based antibiotic ointment (not soluble in water) should be applied in a thin layer. Bulb-syringe feedings may be necessary to avoid further trauma to the injured area. It may be necessary to immobilize the child's hands to keep them away from the injured site. If such measures are impossible in the home setting, the patient may need to be admitted to a burn center for supportive care. All parents should be advised to obtain early follow-up (in 5–7 days) with a burn specialist. Often a mouth splint is applied early to prevent contraction and scarring. Parents should be told of the possibility of delayed bleeding from the wound and be instructed to apply pressure to the bleeding site if the eschar falls off and exposes the labial artery. If the bleeding is not controlled with pressure, parents should bring the child to an emergency department as soon as possible. Some burn centers prefer to admit children with oral burns; management should be initiated according to the preferences of the local center involved in the patient's long-term care.

Pitfalls in Practice. Oral burns in children are usually not a sign of child abuse. Parents should not be accused of neglect but educated about prevention of future injury.

Electrical injury can appear to be benign when in fact it is significant. It is important to evaluate the patient carefully for multisystem injury and, when in doubt, to treat conservatively. It is difficult to differentiate between burns caused by electricity and burns caused by thermal injury. Both have potential delayed complications, and both can occur simultaneously. A good history is essential to ensure evaluation for the associated complications of each type of injury.

Early follow-up is essential to prevent cosmetic deformity from electrical burns and to ensure proper healing. The neurovascular system can be re-evaluated at this time.

Frostbite

Frostbite is the tissue damage that results from cold exposure. The degree of injury is determined by the duration of exposure and, to a lesser extent, the temperature of the exposure. Cold, windy, humid weather conditions aggravate the problem. In most civilian settings, frostbite occurs when self-protective natural defenses are impaired, such as during states of altered mental status, extreme exhaustion, drug intoxication, acute injury, or entrapment during cold weather. Predisposing factors that contribute to development of frostbite include peripheral vasoconstriction (i.e., from smoking or peripheral vascular disease), vasodilation resulting in increased heat less, or previous frostbite injury resulting in vascular instability.

The direct effect of cold exposure on tissues causes ice crystals to form in the extracellular space. Intracellular water is drawn in the extracellular space because of the resultant osmotic gradient, and the ice crystals enlarge and cause mechanical tissue damage. The cell is left dehydrated, and intracellular electrolytes are concentrated at levels that interfere with normal cell processes. Damaged endothelial cells leak fluid, and local edema develops. As the damage continues, thromboxane and other prostaglandins are released, resulting in platelet aggregation, sludging from increased leukocyte adherence, and vasoconstriction. Progressive dermal ischemia occurs.

Initial appropriate therapy can reduce the amount of tissue damage that results from frostbite, although the true extent of tissue damage may not be obvious for several weeks to months after the injury.

Differential Diagnosis. Chilblains is cold hypersensitivity and may be confused with frostbite. The affected area has been directly exposed to cold and is red, warm, and swollen in a patchy distribution. Passive or active rewarming returns the area to nearly normal conditions; with repeated exposures, however, the skin can become chronically inflamed or insensitive. No underlying tissue damage occurs.

The severity of frostbite injury is classified in degrees, much like burns. The physical findings and history of exposure assist in making the diagnosis and initiating therapy, even though the full extent of injury is not known acutely.

The frostbitten area initially appears as a whitened, waxy, nonblanching patch of skin that may feel burning, itchy, or painful. Sensation may be decreased in the area, and capillary refill may be delayed. The underlying tissue remains soft and resilient. As the area thaws, it becomes painful, flushed, and swollen. Blisters may develop between 1 and 24 hours after exposure; if left intact, they will spontaneously resolve. Eschar formation occurs in 4–10 days with sloughing of the eschar in 3–4 weeks.[18] Hemorrhagic fluid indicates injury to the subdermal vascular plexus and represents a more significant injury than if clear fluid is present in the blister. In mild injuries, the new skin under the eschar is initially pink, tender, and temperature sensitive.

In severe frostbite injuries, the tissues underlying the skin are involved and feel hard, woody, or solid. Even after rewarming, the area remains mottled and gray with persistent swelling. If blisters develop, they contain hemorrhagic fluid; the absence of blister formation is a poor prognostic sign.[19] A distinct demarcation of viable and nonviable tissue is obvious with the development of the eschar, and as the eschar sloughs off, partial amputation of nonviable tissue can occur.

Management. Patients who call for telephone advice about possible frostbite injury should be instructed to elevate the affected part and to avoid rubbing the affected area to prevent additional tissue damage. Rewarming should not be started unless it can be controlled and completed; tissue damage is increased more with thawing and refreezing than with prolonging the first episode of freezing for the time it takes to transport the patient. Thermal injury is a possibility if rewarming is not done carefully.

Immediate rewarming reverses the direct effects of ice crystals within the affected tissue. Rewarming should be performed by warm water immersion of the affected part at a temperature of 38°–42°C. The end point of therapy is flushing of the area when it is removed from the bath. This procedure may take up to 1 hour and can be extremely painful; when possible, the patient should be given narcotic analgesics and sedation. If it is not possible to submerge the affected part, warm, wet towels should be applied to the area until flushing of the skin is obvious.

Subsequent therapy is directed toward prevention of progressive dermal ischemia caused by thromboxane and prostaglandin release. Clear blisters contain thromboxane; although controversial, it is generally recommended that such blisters be opened and debrided. Hemorrhagic blisters should remain intact, because secondary desiccation of deep dermal layers may extend the injury.[18] The affected area should be treated topically with a prostaglandin inhibitor, such as aloe vera (Dermaide) every 6 hours, until the thromboxane-releasing phase of the injury is over (about 96 hours). Aspirin (325 mg every 6 hours for 96 hours, 125 mg every 6 hours for children) also is prescribed for its antiprostaglandin activity. Ibuprofen also limits the accumulation of products of arachidonic acid breakdown and may be preferable to aspirin, because it also produces fibrinolysis. Penicillin (500,000 U every 6 hours for adults and 50,000 U/kg for children) is recommended until the edema resolves (usually 48–72 hours).[18] Tetanus prophylaxis should be done if the patient's immunization status is not current, and the patient should avoid any pressure to the damaged part.

Patients with chilblains or minor small areas of frostbite may be treated as outpatients, but most patients who have had significant cold exposure require transfer to a facility equipped to rewarm frozen body parts and hospitalized to determine the full extent of their injury.

Pitfalls in Practice. It is impossible to predict the extent of final tissue damage that will result from the frostbite when the patient is acutely evaluated. Patients should be informed of the natural history of frostbite injuries so that they will expect the changes that may occur at the site of the injury over the several weeks to months after cold exposure. The acute injury should not be rubbed vigorously or with snow (as once advocated); these manipulations increase mechanical damage from the ice crystals formed in the tissues.

Lacerations

The goal of management of lacerations in the urgent care setting is to provide adequate wound care to reduce the risk of subsequent infections and to promote the best possible healing of injury. Simple, uncomplicated lacerations with straight edges can be closed easily in the urgent care setting after appropriate wound cleansing, preparation, and local anesthesia. Because patients sometimes judge the medical care that they receive by the appearance of the scar that results after laceration repair, it is essential that the urgent care physician feel confident about the procedure before starting a surgical repair. Lacerations that injure underlying structures, or are extensive, located in difficult anatomical locations, grossly contaminated, or not recent are complicated lacerations, and closure in the urgent care setting depends on the experience and confidence of the physician. If the laceration is complicated or if the urgent care physician has limited time to attend to it, it is probably best to refer the patient to an emergency department for laceration repair.

Differential Diagnosis. Lacerations can be simple, stellate (i.e., with multiple lacerated skin lines emerging from a single central wound), or avulsions (i.e., with a portion of tissue completely detached from its base). The patient also can present with partial or complete amputations of distal body parts (fingers, toes, nose, ears).

In evaluation of the wound, it is necessary to know the timing, mechanism of injury, and instrument that caused the laceration. The condition of the involved site before injury determines whether complete neurovascular function is to be expected on examination. The medical history and tetanus status of the patient determine the need for tetanus and antibiotic prophylaxis. The patient also should be asked whether other injuries occurred simultaneously.

Physical examination includes visual inspection of the laceration site and surrounding areas to assess the degree of contamination, the nature of the injury itself, and the potential for injury to underlying structures. A complete musculoskeletal and neurovascular examination distal to the laceration is essential. Adequate examination requires knowledge of the local anatomy and testing of each component muscle, nerve, and major vascular structure independently from one another. Sensation should be tested by determination of two-point discrimination, and vascular status should be assessed by evaluation of pulses and capillary refill. Integrity of underlying tendons and joint capsules also must be ensured. If any dysfunction is found, injury to underlying structures must be assumed. The presence of embedded foreign bodies can sometimes be determined by plain films, as can presence of bony cortical disruption or fracture or possible joint violation.

Once the wound has been cleaned, additional physical examination determines the complexity of the injury, the need for simple or deep closure, the presence of nonviable tissue, and, in old lacerations, the presence of an established infection. The characteristics of nonviable and infected tissue as well as factors that put wounds at risk for subsequent infection and tetanus are listed in Table 9.

Table 9. Evaluation of Lacerations

Nonviable tissue	*Infectious risk*	*Tetanus-prone wounds*
Persistent, abnormal, darkened color	More than 6 hours old before wound care	Highly contaminated
Does not bleed when cut	Associated crush injury	More than 24 hours before
Will not contract when electrically	Obvious contamination	wound care
stimulated	Embedded foreign materials	Cannot be adequately debrided
	Lacerations of the lower extremities	Contains much devitalized tissue
Infected tissue	Immunosuppressed patients	Injury occurred in dirty
Warm	Debilitated patients	environment (barnyard, sewer)
Tender	Hematoma formation after repair	
Erythematous	Epinephrine use with local anesthetic	
Indurated	Reactive suture material (braided,	
Purulent drainage	chromic, silk)	
Wound breakdown after repair	Lacerations due to bites or punctures	
Regional lymphadenopathy		
Systemic signs of infection		

The results of the physical examination determine whether the laceration can be managed in the urgent care setting or whether referral is most appropriate. A decision about the need for surgical closure of the laceration must be made. Although there are no absolute guidelines, gaping lacerations that involve more than the superficial layers of skin probably need to be closed, especially in cosmetic or highly exposed or used anatomic areas. Lacerations that are allowed to heal without closure have more inflammation, scar formation, and skin contraction than those that are closed.[1] Nevertheless, in some circumstances laceration repair is difficult or contraindicated. Wounds at high risk for infection usually should be left open or repaired by a specialist. In some anatomic positions, such as the pretibial area, the skin is immobile; completely closing a large laceration may be extremely difficult and is best done by a specialist.

If the laceration appears to be deep and involves tissues below the epidermis (subcutaneous fascia or dermis), it may qualify for deep sutures as well as superficial skin closure. Deep sutures eliminate potential dead space, which can increase infection risk and hematoma formation and interfere with wound healing. If the laceration is deeper than it is wide, it may be due to a puncture or stab wound. Such injuries are difficult to cleanse adequately, and it is often best to leave these injuries open. If the wound has occurred on the hand, it is essential to determine that it is not a human bite or "fight bite." If a bite is suspected, hand lacerations should not be repaired.

Management. Table 10 summarizes the management of lacerations. Special issues to be considered when treating lacerations in particular anatomical positions are listed in Table 11. Each patient and clinical circumstance should be handled individually. Physician judgment is often the best method for determining whether a wound should be treated in an open or closed manner. In general, most wounds more than 12 hours old are at significant risk of infection if they are sutured closed. Some clinicians are comfortable with certain exceptions to this time guideline if the laceration can be adequately cleaned, if the patient is reliable, and if the laceration is in an anatomic position that requires closure for cosmetic or functional reasons. One study suggests that the healing of clean, simple wounds involving the head is not affected by the time interval from injury to repair.[19] The timing of closure must balance the likelihood of infection against the possibility of promoting favorable conditions for wound healing.

Table 10. Summary of Management of Acute Lacerations

Initial evaluation	*Wound repair*
Wash away dried blood and dirt	Explore wound visually
Remove patient's jewelry	Palpate underlying structures to ensure continuity
Assess neurovascular and musculoskeletal	Excise nonviable tissue
function	Debride contaminated tissue
Control bleeding	Sharpen jagged wound edges
	Select suture material
Wound preparation	Place deep sutures (absorbable, interrupted)
Remove obvious contaminants	Place skin sutures (nonabsorbable, interrupted)
Irrigate wound with 1% povidone-iodine solution	
or normal saline	*Wound aftercare*
Clean surrounding skin with povidone-iodine	Apply wound dressing
solution	Administer tetanus prophylaxis if indicated
Clip surrounding hair (do not clip eyebrows	Consider antibiotics
or hair-skin interfaces)	Educate patient regarding drainage, scarring, infections
Drape area	Arrange wound check
Anesthetize locally or with regional block	Arrange suture removal

All patients who require wound care should be placed in a comfortable supine position in a well-lighted area. The area surrounding the laceration should be scrubbed with 1% povidone-iodine solution or another detergent scrub. Hair that may interfere with the surgical repair should be clipped away from the area unless it is the eyebrow (where the hairline serves as a landmark for alignment of the wound). It is usually not necessary to trim more than a few millimeters away from the edges of the wound to allow effective closure. If it is undesirable to clip the hair, loose strands can be plastered away from the edges of the wound with a sterile gel-like antibiotic ointment or a thin layer of petroleum jelly. The prepared area should be draped with sterile towels.

It is impossible to explore, clean, and repair a laceration adequately unless bleeding is controlled. In addition, if a hematoma develops beneath the sutured laceration, the risk of bacterial infection is increased as well as the likelihood of separation of wound edges and impaired healing. Table 12 compares methods of controlling hemorrhage. In most cases, simple compression of the bleeding site is effective. Once the bleeding is controlled, the wound should be irrigated under high pressure with normal saline. This procedure can be effectively done using a 35-ml or 65-ml syringe with a Zerowet splash shield or 19-gauge needle or intravenous catheter. Pressure irrigation of simple lacerations with tap water may be equally efficacious.[3]

It is sometimes helpful to anesthetize the wound before irrigation. Local anesthesia infiltration or appropriate regional blocks should be used. Local infiltration through the wound itself is less painful than subcutaneous injection around the site. Lidocaine (1–2%) is frequently used. Onset of action is immediate if it is locally infused and between 4 and 10 minutes if used in a regional block. Lidocaine causes a burning sensation as it is infused; this sensation can be reduced if the infusion is buffered immediately before injection by mixing nine or ten parts lidocaine with one part sodium bicarbonate

Table 11. Special Considerations for Specific Lacerations

Location	Key Points on Physical Examination	Key Points on Surgical Repair	Follow-Up Issues
Face	Function of facial nerve (five branches); integrity of parotid duct and gland; integrity of lacrimal system, canthus movement of globe; visual acuity	Test facial nerve before anesthesia. Do conservative debridement; do not shave eyebrows or eyelashes. Meticulously align hairlines with first stitch. Do layered closure with deep lacerations; muscle must be repaired if involved.	Immediate consultation if any underlying structure is damaged
Ear	Evidence of perichondrial hematoma	Must drain accumulated hematoma. Use small needle (no. 27) for local anesthetic infiltration; do not use epinephrine. Repair lacerated cartilage with 5-0 or 6-0 absorbable material. Exposed cartilage must be covered.	Apply pressure dressing to prevent hematoma formation
Nose	Evidence of nasal septal hematoma; evidence of associated nasal fracture	Use small needle for local anesthetic infiltration; do not use epinephrine. Do conservative debridement. Cartilaginous repair usually not necessary. Meticulous alignment of ala, nostril rims required.	Antibiotics (penicillin) occasionally recommended if associated fracture
Oral cavity	Integrity of vermillion border and commissure; size of intraoral defect and possibility of food trapping; presence of trapped or embedded foreign bodies	Copious irrigation required for cleaning. Meticulous alignment of lip landmarks required. Local infiltration of anesthetics will distort landmarks. Close through-and-through lacerations in three layers (skin-muscle-skin). Intraoral lacerations less than 2 cm long probably do not need repair. Use absorbable suture for intraoral and tongue lacerations. Use nonabsorbable sutures for extraoral lacerations.	Antibiotics (penicillin) recommended for through-and-through lacerations and tongue lacerations
Scalp	Continuity of underlying bone; presence of clotted blood	Remove hematomas. Clip hair that interferes with repair; do not clip at hair-skin interfaces (will obscure landmarks). Layered closure if extensive laceration to avoid dead space and hematoma formation. Leave ends of sutures long for ease of removal.	Apply pressure dressing if bleeding was extensive
Hands	Independent function of all underlying nerves, vessels, tendons, joints, muscles; integrity of underlying structures; evidence of human bite (closed-fist injury)	Assume underlying injury until demonstrated otherwise. Cover exposed tendons with skin closures while awaiting repair. Do not close suspicious wounds that may be human bites.	Immediate consultation if dysfunction seen on examination
Nails	Presence of subungual hematoma; presence of nail bed lacerations	Drain subungual hematomas with nail drill, heated paper clip; if hematoma larger than 25% of visible nail, remove fingernail and repair nail bed laceration (absorbable suture). Lift cuticle away from nail bed with gauze, or replace nail to prevent adhesion. Nail bed repair can also be done without removal of nail; nonabsorbable sutures are placed through nail on each side of laceration	Tetanus prophylaxis indicated with hematoma drainage, even if no nail bed laceration seen

in a syringe and then infiltrating. Lidocaine comes with or without epinephrine. Epinephrine solutions are sometimes useful to reduce bleeding from highly vascular areas such as the scalp, but they should never be used in locations supplied with distal vasculature (nose, ears, digit, penis, and tissue flaps). Epinephrine is useful in overcoming the

Table 12. Methods to Control Hemorrhage from Lacerations

Method	Indication	Technique	Pitfalls and Drawbacks
Direct pressure	Briskly bleeding lacerations of all sizes	Elevate involved extremity; apply direct pressure to bleeding site with gloved hand and sterile gauze for 5–10 minutes.	Time-consuming
Compressive dressing	Briskly bleeding lacerations of all sizes if unable to apply direct pressure while attending to other problems	Elevate involved extremity; apply sterile gauze over laceration and hold securely in place with elastic dressing.	Too much sterile gauze with too little compression can absorb much blood. If elastic is applied too tightly, can cause neurovascular damage.
Vessel repair	Vascular bleeding from small to moderate-sized vessels	Clip end of bleeding vessel with hemostat; tie off end with absorbable 5-0 or 6-0 suture with at least three knots; cut end of suture as short as possible.	Time consuming and difficult to do in bloody field. Blind application of hemostat can damage underlying structure. Any tissue included in suture will become necrotic.
Electrical	Vascular bleeding from small	Isolate end of bleeding vessel with hemostat; apply cautery either directly to vessel or to top of hemostat.	Requires appropriate equipment and dry field.
Topical agent	Small lacerations with slow to moderate bleeding.	Soak gauze with 1:100,000 epinephrine and apply with pressure to site with sterile gauze.	Increased infection risk with prolonged vasoconstriction near wound. Reduces total blood flow, which can jeopardize survival of marginally viable tissue.
Foams or gelatins	Small lacerations with slow to moderate bleeding	Apply foam or gelatin directly into bleeding wound; apply gentle pressure to site with sterile gauze.	Brisk bleeding rinses applied agent away from site.
Tourniquets	Briskly bleeding lacerations of all sizes	Elevate bleeding extremity and apply tourniquet proximal to injury. With tourniquet, use wide bands, apply tightly, and limit use to 1 hr (20–30 min for digits). With blood pressure cuffs, inflate to pressure greater than patient's systolic blood pressure. Use lowest pressure that stops bleeding.	Extended duration of use can cause tissue ischemia and jeopardize survival of marginally viable tissue. Prolonged compression can damage underlying structures and is uncomfortable.

vasodilation effects of lidocaine and prolongs the anesthetic effect by slowing the clearance of lidocaine from the site. It also causes vasoconstriction around the edges of the wound, however, and can reduce blood flow to marginally viable tissue. The decrease in blood flow can cause delays in healing and increase the risk of wound infection.

Once the laceration is irrigated and anesthetized and a sterile preparation has been performed, it is explored for the presence of embedded foreign bodies and adherent contamination. The status of underlying structures also can be determined by local exploration, as can the depth of the wound. Any nonviable tissue must be debrided; grossly contaminated tissue that cannot be cleaned also should be excised. If the edges of the wound are jagged, they may be straightened by removal of small amount of tissue with a number-11 blade scalpel or iris scissors. It is desirable to preserve as much tissue as possible during debridement, but wounds heal better and have less risk of infection if the edges are sharp, straight, healthy, and clean.

Deep sutures are placed to allow approximation of underlying tissues and to reduce tension on skin sutures. They are generally placed with absorbable materials and an interrupted simple suture. Acceptable types, sizes, and recommended length of time until suture removal are listed in Table 13.

Table 13. Suturing Guidelines

Wound Location	Suture for Deep Closure	Suture for Superficial Closure	Timing of Suture Removal (Days)
Face	5-0 PGA	6-0 nylon*	3–5
Scalp	4-0 PGA	4-0 or 3-0 nylon	7–10
Trunk	4-0 PGA, 3-0 in high-tension area	5-0, 4-0, or 3-0 nylon	7–10
Arm	4-0 PGA	5-0 or 4-0 nylon	8–10
Hand	5-0 PGA	5-0 nylon	8–12
Leg	4-0 PGA, 3-0 in high-tension area	5-0, 4-0, or 3-0 nylon	12–14
Foot	4-0 PGA	5-0 or 4-0 nylon	12–14
Oral mucosa		5-0 chromic gut	

PGA = polyglycolic acid (Dexon).
* Ethilon or Dermilon.
From Trott A: Principles and Techniques of Minor Wound Care. New York, Elsevier Science, 1984, with permission.

The tissue adhesive octyl cyanoacrylate (Dermabond) was approved for commercial use in the United States in 1998. Dermabond works by polymerizing with the layers of water on the skin to form a strong bond. It works best on lacerations that are short (< 6–8 cm), under low tension (< 0.5 cm separation of wound edges), clean-edged, and straight or curvilinear and do not cross joints or creases. Wounds are prepared in the usual manner, but anesthesia is often unnecessary. The plastic container holding the adhesive is broken, the applicator tip is saturated, the approximated edges of the wound are coated with adhesive, and the edges are held together for 30–60 seconds of drying. Dressings are not necessary, and the manufacturer does not recommend ointments, creams or tape strips across the adhesive. The adhesive flakes off with sloughing epidermis in 7–14 days. Advantages to the use of tissue adhesives include no need for local anesthesia (unless extensive cleaning or debridement is necessary), a reported antibacterial effect, less time required for the repair, no return visit for suture removal, and elimination of needlestick risks to the health care provider.[20] Care should be taken to avoid drip or run-off of adhesive to uninvolved areas by properly positioning the patient and avoiding excessively heavy application, especially with facial lacerations. The eye also should be protected with a gauze pad. Long-term cosmetic results have compared favorably with conventional suturing. Detailed information and a guide for application can be found at the manufacturer's website: www.ethicon.com.

Other types of closure materials include wound tapes (Steri-Strips) and staples. Superficial small lacerations may be taped closed after appropriate wound care if the skin is not under tension and if the wound is not gaping. The tape strips should be evenly spaced to approximate the wound edges and allow drainage between the strips. Tapes should be left in place until they fall off spontaneously. If a strong risk of infection prevents suturing, taping the laceration closed may be an alternative. Tapes can be used to provide additional wound support after suture removal and may be technically easier to apply to the fragile skin of elder patients. Tapes do not adhere well to oily or sweaty skin and are not suitable for lacerations with ragged edges. Staples are useful in noncosmetic areas for quick repair of large lacerations. Care must be taken to space the staples evenly and avoid inverting the edges of the wound. Staples are left in place as long as sutures are in the area.

To allow healing and to keep the wound clean, most wounds are dressed after the application of a thin layer of antibacterial ointment. Dressings should remain on the wound for 2 days. By this time an epithelial layer has formed, and the wound is impregnable to water. A serosanguinous discharge from the laceration is frequently seen; the patients should be told that discharge is likely and educated to distinguish it from a purulent discharge. Patients can wash sutured lacerations carefully with water after 2 days. If the wound was dirty, at risk for hematoma formation, or at other risk for infection, the patient should be seen for a wound check 2 days after repair. Wounds over joints or in areas of increased skin tension sometimes heal better if a splint is incorporated into the dressing.

The timing of suture removal depends on the anatomic location of the laceration, the tensile strength of the skin at that site, the possibility of scar widening, and whether suture track marks are cosmetically unacceptable. Guidelines are included in Table 13.

Healing lacerations undergo their most rapid phase of reepithelialization within the first 7 days after repair. Slower healing then begins and may continue for as long as 1 year. Because the scar can change significantly in appearance during the entire time of healing, it is advisable to tell patients that the appearance of the scar will not be final until at least 1 year after repair; if a revision is desired, it should not be done before this time.

Tetanus prophylaxis should be done when indicated. The usefulness of prophylactic antibiotics for prevention of infection after lacerations is not well established. Nevertheless, most clinicians consider broad-spectrum antibiotic therapy in certain high-risk lacerations. If antibiotics are to be effective, they must be delivered to attain therapeutic blood levels by 4 hours after injury.[1] In general, decontamination is more important that antibiotics. Indications for antibiotics include intraoral lacerations, open fractures, exposed joints or tendons, and bites (as discussed earlier).[21]

If repair of the laceration is not possible in the urgent care setting, the wound should be covered with a sterile dressing and the patient referred to an appropriate facility. If an amputation has occurred, the amputated part should be placed in dry sterile gauze and then in a plastic bag. The plastic bag should be placed on ice and the patient referred for possible replantation. The injured extremity should be cleansed with normal saline and covered with saline dressings.

Repair of tendons is beyond the capabilities of the urgent care setting. If a laceration has resulted in partial or complete severing of a tendon that is now exposed, a specialist should be consulted to determine the timing of the repair. If the repair cannot be done immediately, the specialist may ask that the skin over the exposed tendon be temporarily closed to avoid desiccation and infection of the tendon. Subsequent repair can then be arranged.

Pitfalls in Practice. Failure to perform a complete neurovascular and musculoskeletal examination of the involved extremity can result in a delay in the diagnosis of serious underlying injuries and subsequent significant dysfunction. The extent of injury can be underestimated. Injury to underlying structures should be assumed until meticulous exploration shows otherwise. Inadequate wound preparation and examination increase the risk for wound infection. Tetanus prophylaxis is mandatory if the patient's immunization status is not current or unknown and if the wound is tetanus-prone. Failure to remove jewelry from injured extremities can result in compromised distal circulation due to subsequent edema formation.

Local anesthetics can be systemically absorbed, and attention must be paid to the total amount injected. Too much local anesthesia can distort important landmarks and make repair difficult. It is essential to aspirate backward with the syringe before delivering local anesthesia to avoid an intravascular injection.

If nonabsorbable suture material is used for deep sutures, a foreign body reaction may result in chronic inflammatory reactions, chronic wound infections, and draining fistulas. If absorbable sutures are used for skin closure, they may break off prematurely, and the wound may gape open.

Tissue adhesive run-off due to improper patient positioning or heavy application can result in inadvertent bonding of uninvolved tissues, including eyelids, fingers of health care providers, or instruments. Improperly applied adhesive can produce unacceptable healing.

Patients often judge the adequacy of medical care by the appearance of the resultant scar after repair of a laceration. They should be informed that all repaired lacerations result in scar formation and that, if desired, revision can be done at a later date once scar remodeling is complete.

Cutaneous Abscesses

An abscess is a localized infection of the skin or its appendages, usually caused by local skin flora. Abscesses develop after folliculitis, cellulitis, or minor trauma that results in a break in the skin. Immunocompromised or chronically ill patients have increased risk of bacterial abscess formation. Sterile abscesses, from which no bacteria can be isolated, develop as a result of injected chemical irritants and are common in intravenous drug abusers.

Differential Diagnosis. Acute abscesses present as well-localized areas of induration that are tender, erythematous, and warm and may be surrounded by areas of cellulitis. A discrete area of fluctuance usually can be palpated but is not always present or may be deep within the area of edema and therefore difficult to appreciate on physical examination. If an abscess is suspected but no fluctuance appreciated, the diagnosis can be confirmed if pus is aspirated from the center of the suspicious-looking area. Aspiration can be done with a sterile 19-gauge needle attached to a 12-ml syringe.

Abscesses can form at any anatomic site and usually occur singly. If appropriately treated, simple abscesses do not recur. Certain specific abscesses can cause repeated or chronic problems. Infected sebaceous cysts are common in the area of the head and neck and are filled with thick, cheesy material. They are surrounded by a thick white capsule. Such cysts can become acutely infected and are treated like other cutaneous abscesses. Unless they are eventually completely excised, however, they recur. Pilonidal abscesses are formed when the pilonidal sinus tract occludes and infection develops. An acutely infected pilonidal cyst is managed in the same manner as other abscesses, although a more prolonged period of packing usually is necessary. Hydradenitis suppurativa is abscess formation due to occluded apocrine glands and usually occurs in the axilla or groin regions. Even after appropriate acute drainage, such abscesses tend to recur, and a wide surgical excision of the apocrine glands of the area may be necessary to cure the problem.

Although the diagnosis of cutaneous abscess is generally straightforward, it is important to realize that abscess formation may indicate other serious medical problems, such as diabetes, immunocompromise, or intravenous or parenteral drug abuse.

Management. As stated above, the presence of pus can be confirmed by needle aspiration of the suspicious-looking area. If no pus is aspirated, the patient should be directed to apply warm compresses to start warm soaks to the area. Local heat reduces pain at the site and may help speed localization of the infection. Antibiotics covering the predominant local skin flora can be started, and the patient should be seen for follow-up in 24–48 hours. If fluctuance has developed, the abscess can be treated definitively with incision and drainage.

If the needle aspiration yields frank pus or if a defined area of fluctuance is present, the area should be cleaned gently in preparation for incision and drainage. This procedure is painful. Ethyl chloride sprays produce variable and short-term numbness of the skin of the abscess dome and generally are not effective for anesthesia unless the procedure is done during or immediately after the spray is applied. Local infiltration of anesthesia agents is technically difficult, and the low pH of the infected area makes most agents ineffective. Field blocks to the base of the abscess have variable success; the increased blood flow to the region results in rapid clearing of any injected drug. In addition, excessive pressure caused by the volume of injected anesthetic agent can increase the pain. Regional blocks are effective but not applicable in many anatomic areas. Because of the difficulty in achieving effective local anesthesia, patients should be given parenteral narcotics or sedation before the procedure begins.

An incision through the skin and abscess capsule is made along the entire length of the abscess, with care taken not to enter the abscess cavity itself with the scalpel. A number-11 blade allows a nick to be made through the capsule, and the incision can be made with upward motion of the blade. Some clinicians recommend removing a small wedge of tissue at the incision site to ensure that the edges of the wound do not close on themselves; others do not recommend this approach because the wound edges under such circumstances may become necrotic and do not heal as well.[22]

Once the incision has been made and the purulent contents of the abscess are drained, a hemostat or other blunt instrument is used to break loculations within the abscess cavity. The abscess is then loosely packed with sterile gauze wick. Because iodoform gauze occasionally stings when it comes in contact with healthy tissue, many clinicians prefer to use plain gauze for packing. The purposes of packing are to stop bleeding (which is usually brisk after drainage), to keep the wound edges open and allow further drainage of the abscess, and to promote formation of granulation tissue within the abscess cavity. A wick of packing material is left protruding from the incision site to serve as a track for further drainage and to facilitate packing removal. An absorbent dressing is then applied, and the patient is advised to elevate the involved part, if possible. Healing is promoted if the area that has been drained is immobilized. Packing is removed in 48 hours. If a significant amount of drainage is present, the abscess is irrigated and repacked at this time. Re-evaluation should take place in another 48 hours. Once the abscess has stopped draining, the area should be soaked in warm water 2–4 times daily, or warm compresses may be applied.

For abscesses on the face, the smallest skin incision that allows adequate drainage should be used. The incision line should follow natural skin folds, and packing material should be removed in 24 hours. Facial abscesses above the upper lip and below the eyebrow are particularly worrisome because they drain into the cavernous sinus and, if not properly treated, may cause cavernous sinus septic thrombosis. Patients with abscesses in this area should receive prophylactic antibiotics. For other simple abscesses, the definitive therapy is incision and drainage; antibiotics are not indicated. In such cases, Gram stain and cultures do not direct therapy and therefore are not necessary.

Most patients with subcutaneous abscesses are treated as outpatients. If the abscess is large or in a difficult anatomic position, the patient may require conscious sedation or general anesthesia for adequate incision and drainage. In addition, immunocompromised patients and patients with signs of systemic toxicity, significant overlying cellulitis, or questionable medical compliance also may need hospitalization. Patients who have had an abscess drained should be immunized for tetanus, if indicated.

Pitfalls in Practice. If an abscess is not treated, cellulitis, lymphadenitis, and regional adenopathy can develop. Failure to attempt needle aspiration for pus in an abscess with no definite area of fluctuance can delay definitive therapy and prolong pain and discomfort. If incision and drainage are attempted before localization of pus, the infection can extend, and bacteremia may result. Too vigorous a manipulation of the abscess during the drainage procedure also can result in bacteremia.

If the abscess is packed too tightly, no further drainage is possible, and healing will be delayed. If the packing is removed too soon, the edges of the incision can close on themselves, and the drainage may reaccumulate. If the packing is continued beyond the time that drainage continues, healing is delayed. Recurrent abscesses suggest an underlying medical problem, embedded foreign body, chronic fistula formation, underlying osteomyelitis, or unusual pathogens.

References

1. Simon R: Principles of wound management. In Rosen P, Barkin R (eds): Emergency Medicine: Concepts and Clinical Practice, 4th ed. St. Louis, Mosby, 1998, pp 382–396.
2. Walsh AP: A comparison of wound irrigation solutions used in the emergency department. Ann Emerg Med 19:704, 1990.
3. Moscoti RM, Reardon RF, Lerner EB, Mayrose J: Wound irrigation with tap water; Acad Emerg Med 5:1076–1080, 1998.
4. Bonadio WA: Efficacy of tetracaine adrenaline: Cocaine topical anesthetic without tetracaine for facial laceration repair in children. Pediatrics 86:856–857, 1990.
5. Inaba AS, Zukin DD, Perro ML: An update of the evaluation and management of plantar puncture wounds and pseudomonas osteomyelitis. Pediatr Emerg Care 8:38–44, 1992.
6. Steele MT: Retained soft tissue foreign bodies. Crit Decis Emerg Med 3:2–8, 1998.
7. Banerjee B: Sonographic detection of foreign bodies of the extremities. Br J Radiol 64:107–112, 1991.
8. Antosia RE, Lyn E: The hand. In Marx J, Hockberger R, et al (eds): Emergency Medicine: Concepts and Clinical Practice, 5th ed. St. Louis, Mosby, 2002, pp 493–534.

9. Stewart C: Skin and soft tissue infection update: Presentation, diagnosis, and syndrome specific antibiotic management. Emerg Med Rep 21:35–44, 2000.

10. Weber EJ: Rabies. In Marx J, et al (eds): Emergency Medicine: Concepts and Clinical Practice, 5th ed. St. Louis, Mosby, 2002, pp 1834–1841.

11. Talan DA, Citron DM, Abrahamian FM, et al: Bacteriologic analysis of infected dog and cat bites. N Engl J Med 340:85–91, 1999.

12. Kizer KW: A new look at managing mammalian bites. Emerg Med Rep 5:53–60, 1984.

13. Callahan MC: Human and animal bites. In Callahan ML (ed): Current Theory in Emergency Medicine. Toronto, B.C. Decker, 1987, pp 895–899.

14. Rudnitsky GS, Barnett RC: Soft tissue foreign body removal. In Roberts JR, Hedge JR (eds): Clinical Procedures in Emergency Medicine, 3rd ed. Philadelphia, W.B. Saunders, 1998, pp 631–634.

15. Edlich RF, Bailey TL, Bill TJ: Thermal burns. In Marx J, et al (eds): Emergency Medicine: Concepts and Clinical Practice, 5th ed. St. Louis, Mosby, 2002, pp 801–813.

16. Edlich RF, Bailey TL, Bill TJ: Chemical injuries. In Marx J, et al (eds): Emergency Medicine: Concepts and Clinical Practice, 5th ed. St. Louis, Mosby, 2002, pp 813–821.

17. Cooper MA: Electrical injury. In Callahan ML (ed): Current Therapy in Emergency Medicine. Toronto, B.C. Decker, 1987, pp 928–930.

18. Danzl DF: Frostbite. In Marx J, et al (eds): Emergency Medicine: Concepts and Clinical Practice, 5th ed. St. Louis, Mosby, 2002, pp 1972–1979.

19. Berk W, Osbourne DD, Taylor DD: Evaluation of the golden period for wound repair: 209 cases from a third world emergency department. Ann Emerg Med 17:496–500, 1988.

20. Knapp JF: Updates in wound management for the pediatrician. Pediatr Clin North Am 46:1202–1213, 1999.

21. Hollander JE, Singer AJ: Laceration management, Ann Emerg Med 34:356–367, 1999.

22. Blumstein H: Incision and drainage. In Roberts JR, Hedges JR (eds): Clinical Procedures in Emergency Medicine, 3rd ed. Philadelphia, W.B. Saunders, 1998, pp 640–641.

Chapter 9

Orthopedic Problems in Urgent Care

Scott Freiwald, MD
Travis Heining, MD
Steve Sterner, MD
Michelle H. Biros, MS, MD

Orthopedic injuries are commonly seen in the urgent care setting. Because of subsequent swelling and pain, the earliest examination after injury is often the most accurate. Therefore, the initial evaluation should be thorough and carefully documented.

Evaluation of an orthopedic injury begins with a detailed history. The mechanism of injury and the patient's symptoms can be the key to diagnosis. The history should include (1) time from injury to presentation; (2) mechanism of injury; (3) first aid measures already performed, including medications or other therapies; (4) handedness if an upper extremity injury is involved; and (5) the patient's medical history, medications, and allergies.

The orthopedic physical examination begins with general inspection for swelling, discoloration, and deformity. Active and passive range of motion should be assessed at the injury site and in the joints proximal and distal to the injury. Palpation of the injury may reveal tenderness or a more subtle deformity. Lastly, the neurovascular status of the injury site should be carefully assessed. Sensation, motor function, and peripheral pulses distal to the site of injury should be examined early and before any significant manipulation or reduction maneuvers.

The most common orthopedic problems in primary care are sprains and strains, which can be cared for in the urgent care setting. On occasion, serious orthopedic trauma may present. Orthopedic emergencies include open fractures, joint dislocations, and injuries associated with a neurovascular deficit. An open fracture is a fracture exposed to the outside environment by an overlying soft tissue injury. These injuries require emergent referral because of the risk of infection. Dislocated or subluxed joints require emergent treatment because of the risk of permanent neurologic or circulatory compromise. In general, the sooner a joint is relocated the better. Any injury associated with neurovascular compromise must be treated immediately; the longer a deficit goes untreated, the more likely it will be irreversible.

Nearly all displaced fractures will need to be reduced. The urgent care setting may not be ideal for such procedures since conscious sedation or intravenous narcotic pain medication may be required to accomplish the reduction. Referral to an appropriate facility is recommended after consultation with an orthopedic or emergency physician.

Soft Tissue Injuries: Sprains and Strains

Differential Diagnosis. Soft tissue injury accompanies almost all injuries to the musculoskeletal system. Sprains are ligamentous injuries of the joints and range from tearing of ligamentous fibers to gross ligamentous disruption. Strains range from muscular fiber tearing to full muscular disruption. Soft tissue injury causes microcirculation injury with local hemorrhage, increased capillary permeability, and swelling. Common soft tissue injuries are described in Table 1.

Table 1. Common Soft Tissue Injuries

Injury	Mechanism of Injury	Physical Examination	X-ray	Management	Follow-Up
Shoulder dislocation	Anterior: fall on abducted and hyperextended arm. Posterior: direct blow, fall on flexed arm.	Soft tissue swelling, decreased range of motion. Check axillary nerve sensation (lateral proximal forearm and deltoid area).	Anteroposterior (AP) lateral, transscapular axillary views; postreduction series.	Reduction (anterior: internal rotation, hanging weight method; posterior: traction method), sling and swathe or shoulder immobilizer.	Orthopedic follow-up in 3–7 days.
Acromioclavicular (AC) separation	Direct blow to distal clavicle, falls.	Pain over AC joint; distal clavicle may be elevated.	AP shoulder, AP clavicles with AC joints.	Arm sling.	Orthopedic follow-up in 3–7 days.
Thigh contusion	Direct blow	Swelling and tenderness in quadriceps muscle.	None required.	Ice, rest from vigorous exercise.	Orthopedic follow-up in 1 wk. Late complication: myositis ossificans.
Knee ligament strains	Twisting, quick change of direction, direct blow.	Palpate joint line; valgus and varus stressing; look for anterior or posterior drawer sign; ask for history of locking (indicating meniscus tear).	AP, lateral, oblique views.	Ice, elevation, rest non–weight-bearing with crutches, knee immobilization.	Orthopedic follow-up in 1–2 days.
Knee dislocation	Direct blow.	Check popliteal artery and distal pulses; check peroneal nerve.	AP, lateral, oblique views.	Immediate orthopedic consultation. Transfer to an ED.	
Patella dislocation	Lateral malalignment with medial retinaculum tearing.	Usually spontaneously relocates before examination; patella subluxed laterally.	Sunrise views of patella.	Reduction by straightening leg, place slight medial pressure on patella, apply ice, keep knee immobilized, rest, no weight-bearing.	Orthopedic follow-up in 1–2 days.
Chondromalacia	Seen after recurrent trauma.	Pain under patella with stair climbing, mild effusion, tenderness at patellar margin.	Knee: AP, lateral, oblique views.	Quadriceps strengthening, nonsteroidal anti-inflammatory drugs (NSAIDs).	Orthopedic follow-up within 2 wk.

(Cont'd on next page)

Table 1. Common Soft Tissue Injuries *(Continued)*

Injury	Mechanism of Injury	Physical Examination	X-ray	Management	Follow-Up
Shin splints	Overuse syndrome, direct trauma.	Tender over pretibial region.	Usually no findings; bone scan may be positive.	Rest, ice, NSAIDs; decrease vigorous activity.	Orthopedic follow-up within 2 wk.
Achilles tendon rupture	Severe or quick dorsiflexion of foot.	Loss of plantar flexion, palpable mass in calf, positive Thompson's test (plantar flexion not elicited with calf squeezed).	None indicated.	Robert Jones splint, ice, elevation.	Orthopedic consultation immediately.
Ankle sprains	Inversion injury typical.	Swelling, ecchymosis, tender malleoli; check fibular head.	Ankle: AP, lateral, mortise, OK views. (Apply Ottawa ankle rules to decide if x-rays should be done).	Air or gel cast, Robert Jones splint, crutches.	Orthopedic follow-up for ankle retraining.
Hamstring strain	Rapid start of motion from resting position.	Tenderness of posterior thigh mass, decreased range of motion, painful passive or active movement.	Normal, or soft tissue swelling.	No weight-bearing; ice, elevation, NSAIDs.	Orthopedic follow-up within 2 wk.
Iliopsoas strain	Sudden hip flexion against resistance.	Severe groin pain with radiation to upper thigh, lumbar region, in abdomen; painful active movement; possible decreased sensation over anterior thigh and medial lower leg; possible decreased knee jerk reflex.	Normal or enlarged iliopsoas shadow.	Bed rest for 3–5 days if moderate-to-severe pain; NSAIDs.	Orthopedic follow-up in 5–7 days; urgent orthopedic consultation in presence of neurologic symptoms.

History and Physical Examination. As with all orthopedic injuries, neurovascular function must be evaluated and documented. All major nerve groups and tendons should be evaluated separately, especially in hand injuries.

Diagnostic Aids. Radiologic examination should be used to support the clinical diagnosis. Occasionally a radiograph may identify a fracture that was not suspected.

Management. The specific management of common soft tissue injuries is outlined in Table 1. Appropriate primary care includes elevation to reduce the hydrostatic forces causing swelling, ice to diminish blood flow by vasoconstriction, and supportive dressings to prevent any further injury.

Pitfalls in Practice. Failure to document neurovascular status at the time of initial presentation may confuse postmanipulation examination and follow-up care. Because bleeding and subsequent swelling within muscle groups create the potential for compartment syndrome, such injuries require appropriate and timely follow-up evaluation.

Joint injuries may not be isolated. Any joint injury necessitates examination of the entire extremity to ensure that no other injury is missed. For example, proximal fibular head fractures (Maisonneuve's fracture) are occasionally seen with ankle fractures or sprains.[1] Therefore, the fibular head must be palpated to avoid missing this associated fracture. The patient should be warned that recovery may be disabling and painful even in the absence of a fracture.

Common Fractures

Differential Diagnosis. Common fractures are described in Table 2. Patients who sustain fractures usually give a history of trauma involving the injured part that is followed by pain, swelling, and occasionally numbness.

Table 2. Common Fractures

Bone	Common Mechanism of Injury	X-ray	Acute Management	Precautions	Follow-up
Clavicle fracture (distal third)	Fall, direct trauma	AP view	Sling	Check sternoclavicular joints	Orthopedic follow-up in 3–7 days
Humerus fracture (surgical neck)	Fall, direct blow	AP, lateral views	Sling and swathe	Check neurologic status	Orthopedic follow-up in 1–3 days
Humerus fracture (shaft)	Fall, direct blow	AP, lateral views	Sugartong splint and sling	Check radial nerve function	Orthopedic follow-up in 1–3 days
Monteggia's fracture (radial head dislocation)	Fall	AP, lateral views: forearm, elbow	90° dorsivolar splint with sling	Urgent orthopedic consultation	
Radial head fracture	Fall	AP, lateral views: forearm, elbow	Long arm splint with sling	Urgent orthopedic consultation	
Forearm bones Ulna and radius (midshaft)	Fall	AP, lateral views: forearm, elbow	Long arm splint with sling	Urgent orthopedic consultation	
Distal radius and ulna (Colles' fracture)	Fall	AP, lateral views: forearm, elbow	Closed reduction if simple extra-articular fracture	Urgent orthopedic consultation if intra-articular comminuted fracture or poor closed reduction	Orthopedic follow-up in 1–3 days
Carpal bone fractures, scaphoid, lunate, trapezium, and trapezoid	Fall, direct compression	AP, lateral views: wrist, carpal series (may be normal)	Short arm thumb spica splint	Always splint if snuff box tenderness present	Orthopedic follow-up in 3–7 days
Metacarpal fractures	Blow, crush	AP, lateral oblique views	MC II-V: depends on fracture (quite variable); ulnar/radial gutter splint, thumb splint	Discuss with orthopedist; check for abnormal rotation of distal pieces	Orthopedic follow-up in 3–5 days
Triquetrum, pisiform hamate, capitate	Blow, crush	AP, lateral oblique views	Dorsal volar wrist splint		Orthopedic follow-up in 3–7 days

(Cont'd on next page)

Table 2. Common Fractures *(Continued)*

Bone	Common Mechanism of Injury	X-ray	Acute Management	Precautions	Follow-up
Tibia or fibula	Twisting blow	AP, lateral views: tibia, fibula, and knee	Robert Jones splint	Urgent orthopedic consultation	
Ankle	Inversion, eversion, twisting	AP, lateral, oblique views	Robert Jones splint	Discuss with orthopedist; check for dislocation	Orthopedic follow-up in 1–3 days
Toes	Direct trauma	AP, lateral, oblique views	Buddy-taping, crutches with gradual weight-bearing	Hard-soled shoe	Orthopedic follow-up for complex fractures

Physical Examination. Inspection reveals swelling and often deformity of the injured part. The joint above and below the fracture must be evaluated for function and associated injury. The functional assessment includes sensation, two-point discrimination, and capillary refill. Range of motion and individual flexor-extensor tendon function must be evaluated.

Diagnostic Aids. In addition to clinical examination, the diagnosis of fracture is made by x-ray examination of the injured part. The x-ray views depend on the area of injury. Table 2 lists the x-ray views that are most helpful in diagnosing these common fractures. Table 3 describes terms that are used to characterize fractures. These terms are useful to know when discussing the case with a consultant.

Table 3. Important Features of Descriptions of Fractures

Involved bones
Open or closed
Location of fracture along bone (anatomic land marks, midshaft, distal, proximal: distance from end of bone)
Presence of dislocation/subluxation
Description of fracture: transverse, spiral, and oblique
Extension into joints
Angulation of fragments (% of width of bone; direction of distal fragment related to proximal)
Overriding of fracture fragments (cm or mm); displacement of fracture fragments
Involvement of epiphysis in young adults, children

Management. The management of specific fractures is constantly evolving and therefore often controversial. General principles can be applied in fracture management. Open fractures (those open to the outside environment through a break in the skin) should be meticulously irrigated and debrided before reduction. This goal is best accomplished in an operating room. Intravenous antibiotics should be administered early. Fractures that are not displaced should be splinted acutely, followed by definitive casting in a few days.

Fractures that are displaced should be reduced. A displaced fracture is one in which the normal anatomical alignment of the bone has been lost. Reduction of a fracture includes manipulating bone into a normal or nearly normal anatomic position and then holding it in that position. A closed reduction is done by simple manipulation of the part. An open reduction is performed surgically, allowing the use of orthopedic hardware to fix the fracture in good anatomical position. In the treatment of many fractures, there is no clear consensus about whether open or closed reduction is superior. When treating a specific fracture, an inexperienced physician should consult an experienced physician.

Splinting and Casting Concepts

Splinting provides comfort to the patient and mechanical support for fractures, sprains, and soft tissue injuries. Splints are typically noncircumferential to allow for swelling of an acute injury. As swelling subsides over a few days, it becomes safe to apply a circular cast, which provides more secure support and protection. Casts also provide pain relief and stability to an extremity injury but are more commonly applied after the majority of swelling has resolved. A circumferential cast applied to an acute injury may lead to marked discomfort and pressure sores and even circulatory compromise of the distal extremity. Fiberglass or plaster may be used for both splints and casts, depending on the physician's preference.

The first step in splinting an injured extremity is wrapping the extremity in cotton batting or sheet-type padding (Webril). The padding should be several layers thick, and particular attention should be paid to bony prominences. The length of the splint should be sufficient to fully immobilize the injured joint. For midshaft fractures, the splint should immobilize the joint above and below the fracture. Splint strength for the upper and lower extremity injuries should consist of 12–15 layers of plaster. Additional layers may be added to reinforce children's splints, because children usually remain very active despite the injury and may disrupt or crack a thinner splint. The plaster strips should be cut or torn to length before wetting. After excessive water is squeezed out, the layers should be massaged together until they fuse. The plaster then can be applied in a lengthwise fashion and molded into position over the extremity. The splint is secured with elastic bandages, wrapped distally to proximally. Bends, wrinkles, and indentations should be molded out of the plaster before the elastic bandage is applied. While the plaster is setting, the joint should be held in the desired position. Once the splint has dried, it should be checked for tight areas, unpadded corners, and general comfort. Commonly used splints are illustrated throughout this chapter.

Hand Disorders

Physical Examination and Diagnostic Aids. The examination of hand injuries begins with inspection for deformity, swelling, or bruising. Palpation of bony structures should include assessment of snuffbox tenderness. Grip strength and individual finger strength through normal ranges of motion should be carefully evaluated. Radial, ulnar, and median nerve function should be assessed as well as regional pulses and capillary refill. Radiographs should include posteroanterior, lateral, and oblique views of the hand or focused digits.

Fractures

Differential Diagnosis and Management. Some common fractures of the hand are described in Table 2. Carpal bone fractures are often difficult to diagnose. Treatment should be based on clinical suspicion if a fracture is not seen on radiographs.

Metacarpal fractures often result from a direct blow with a closed fist. Associated lacerations from a "fight bite" must be treated with aggressive wound irrigation and antibiotics. Metacarpal II–V fractures generally can be treated with ulnar (Fig. 1) or radial gutter splints (Fig. 2) with the wrist extended 20°, the metacarpophalangeal (MCP) joints flexed to 90°, and the proximal interphalangeal (PIP) and distal interphalangeal (DIP) joints in no more than 20° of flexion.[2] Thumb metacarpal fractures can be placed in a thumb spica splint.

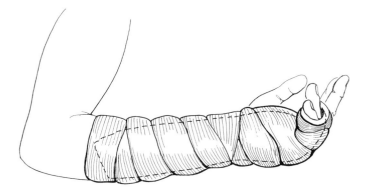

Figure 1.   Ulnar gutter splint.

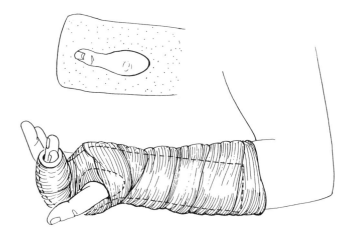

Figure 2.   Radial gutter splint.

Phalanx fractures should be assessed for angulation and rotational deformities. Proximal and middle phalanx fractures that are nondisplaced and stable can be immobilized with "buddy taping." Fractures that are unstable or reducible may be splinted from the forearm to the DIP in the position described above for metacarpal fractures. Distal phalanx fractures are treated with protective splinting. Follow-up with a hand surgeon should occur within 5 days. Splints commonly used in finger and hand fractures are illustrated in Figure 3.

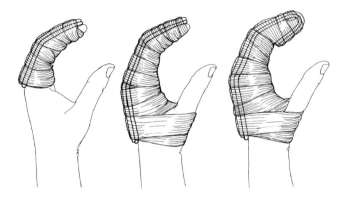

Figure 3. Finger splints.

Pitfalls in Practice. Acute fractures may be diagnosed on clinical grounds alone; radiographs can be negative despite the presence of a fracture. In cases in which clinical examination or history suggests that a fracture is likely, it is best to treat the patient as if a fracture is present. Failure to assess for neurovascular function distal to the injury can result in missing the diagnosis of an orthopedic emergency and substantial morbidity.

Evaluation of children for fractures can be difficult because of ongoing changes in their musculoskeletal system. If x-ray examination is difficult to interpret, comparative views of the opposite side may be useful. When doubt exists, the affected limb should be splinted. Caretakers and parents should be warned that certain fractures in children have the potential to cause growth abnormalities. All children who present with a limp must be evaluated both for traumatic injury and septic arthritis. Child abuse should be considered in children presenting with fractures and must be suspected if the reported mechanism of injury is inconsistent with the physical examination.

Soft Tissue Injuries

Diagnosis and Management. Tendon injuries of the hand most often result from a hand laceration. Suspected flexor tendon injuries must be evaluated for the integrity of both the flexor digitorum profundus and flexor digitorum superficialis (full finger flexion, distal finger flexion). Each finger must be tested individually. All flexor tendon lacerations should be referred to a hand surgeon within 12 hours. If a consultant is not immediately available, lacerations can be irrigated, loosely closed, and splinted in a position of function (wrist, 30° of extension; MCP, 70° of flexion; interphalangeal (IP) joints, 15° of flexion) before referral. Treatment with prophylactic antibiotics is often recommended. Extensor tendon lacerations also should be promptly referred. The affected finger should be splinted in extension.

Dislocations and ligament injuries of the carpal bones most often result from a fall on an outstretched hand. Carpal injuries tend to occur sequentially, starting with scapholunate ligament instability and ending with perilunate and lunate dislocations.[2] Scapholunate dissociation produces pain and swelling on the radial aspect of the wrist with focal tenderness over the scaphoid. The posteroanterior (PA) radiograph reveals widening of the scapholunate joint space (Terry Thomas sign). Treatment consists of a radial gutter splint and orthopedic follow-up in 3–5 days. Triquetrolunate ligament instability presents with tenderness on the ulnar aspect of the wrist just distal to the ulna. The PA radiograph may reveal a widened triquetrolunate joint space. Treatment with an ulnar gutter splint and orthopedic follow-up in 3–5 days is sufficient. Perilunate and lunate dislocations usually result from a higher-energy injury. Most often swelling and tenderness are present in the region. In a perilunate dislocation, the capitate is displaced posteriorly to the lunate on the lateral radiograph. The "spilled teacup" sign characterizes the lateral radiograph in a lunate dislocation. The lunate is dislocated off of the radius in a volar direction, resembling a teacup spilling in the direction of the palm.[3] Perilunate and lunate injuries require immediate consultation.

Dislocations and ligament injuries of the hand often result from a direct blow that causes an axial load or hyperextension. Distal and proximal IP joint dislocations are usually dorsal. Examination reveals a deformed joint that is tender and swollen. Reduction usually can be accomplished with longitudinal traction, hyperextension, and direct dorsal to volar pressure on the base of the phalanx. A digital block can facilitate reduction. The affected joint should be splinted in 30° of flexion for 3 weeks.[4] Follow-up with primary care is sufficient. MCP dislocations are also usually dorsal. They are reduced by applying pressure over the base of the proximal phalanx in a distal and volar direction. The affected joint then should be splinted in flexion. Thumb IP dislocations are reduced much like those in other fingers, whereas thumb MCP dislocations are reduced with direct pressure on the base of the proximal phalanx with the metacarpal flexed and abducted.[4] Gamekeeper's thumb (skier's thumb) is a tear in the ulnar collateral ligament during excessive abduction of the thumb MCP joint. Stress testing of the MCP joint reveals laxity in a partial or complete tear. Such injuries should generally be managed with splinting (thumb spica; Fig. 4, next page) and orthopedic follow-up within 1 week. Dislocations that are unstable or nonreducible require orthopedic follow-up in 1–2 days.

Pitfalls in Practice. Rings must be removed early in the evaluation of hand and finger injuries. Delay makes removal more difficult as swelling increases. If the ring cannot be removed, it must be cut off. Failure to remove a ring before splinting may lead to compromised circulation and ischemic necrosis.

Overuse Injuries

Diagnosis and Management. Carpal tunnel syndrome is an overuse injury caused by repeated flexion and extension of the wrist. Edema within the carpal tunnel results in compression of the median nerve, which then causes paresthesias or pain in the median nerve distribution. Tapping on the carpal tunnel often reproduces pain. In addition to pain in the wrist and hand, the pain from carpal tunnel syndrome may migrate to the forearm and shoulder.[5] Initial management consists of a wrist splint (neutral position) and nonsteroidal anti-inflammatory drug (NSAID). Follow-up with primary care is sufficient. Surgical management may be necessary for recurrent symptoms.

Tendinitis of the flexor or extensor tendons of the hand results in tenderness to palpation along the tendon sheath and pain with flexion or extension of the finger. It is crucial to exclude infection as the source of the pain. Treatment consists of splinting in a position of function and NSAIDs. Follow-up in 2–3 days with primary care is recommended. DeQuervain's tenosynovitis is tenosynovitis of the extensor pollicis brevis and abductor

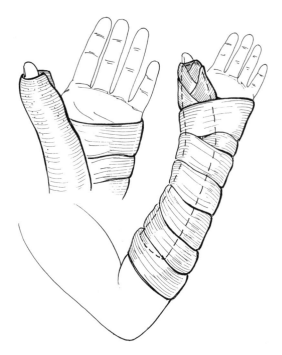

Figure 4. Thumb spica splint.

pollicis tendons. It is an overuse injury of the thumb that presents with pain over the radial aspect of the wrist and forearm. Treatment consists of splinting (thumb spica, see Fig. 4) and NSAID. Follow-up is again with primary care with referral to a hand specialist in recurrent cases.

Pitfalls in Practice. The diagnosis of overuse syndromes relies heavily on history. It is essential to consider first other pathologies (e.g., infections) as the source of pain. Patients with carpal tunnel syndrome should be referred for medical evaluation. Some significant medical illnesses may cause carpal tunnel syndrome.

Hand Infections: General Principles

Hand infections usually result from a skin laceration. Because hand infections can lead to significant morbidity, accurate diagnosis and treatment are essential. It is important to determine whether the infection involves the skin, subcutaneous tissues, fascial spaces, tendon, joint, or bone. Deep infections involving tendon sheaths, the deep palmar space, or the bone mandate emergent consultation with a hand or orthopedic surgeon. Minor local infections can be treated in the urgent care setting with incision and drainage of discrete local infections (paronychia and felons), elevation, immobilization (position of function), and broad-spectrum antibiotics. Early and repeated follow-up is essential.

Table 4 lists the differential diagnosis of specific hand infections. As with any infection, the source for the contamination must be found and removed. In the hand, this involves removing any foreign bodies and identifying the exact site and extent of the infection. Treatment of sprains, strains, and fractures of the hand is described elsewhere in this chapter.

Table 4. Common Infections of the Hand

Type	Cause	Diagnosis	Management	Follow-Up
Paronychia	Usually from hangnail or nail biting; causes infection of area next to fingernail.	Skin next to nail or eponychium, including nail matrix, is red, swollen, tender and fluctuant.	Cephalexin or amoxicillin-clavulanate if cellulitis is present; incision into paronychia next to nail; if pus under entire nail, remove nail.	Wound check in 2 days.
Felon	Infection in pulp of finger tip; due to puncture wound; or minor trauma to finger-tip; staphylococcal or streptococcal organisms most common infections.	Tender, red, swollen fingertip; may have draining sinus.	Early incision and drainage; immobilize; elevate; consider antistaphylococcal antibiotics	Follow-up as arranged by consultant.
Herpetic whitlow	Herpes simplex; common in dentists and others with oral secretion contact.	Recurrent episodes; begins as tender, red finger pad, then clear vesicles.	Keep lesions clean and dry; instruct patient about in-fectious cause and methods to prevent spread to others.	No follow-up needed; resolves in 1–2 wk; self-limited disease.
Tenosyno-vitis	Infection of flexor tendon sheath; due to penetrating or hematogenous spread.	Kanavel's four signs: pain on passive extension, resting in flexed position, swelling along sheath, tender on palpation along sheath.	Hospitalization, with IV antibiotics (broad-spec-trum). Early infection: elevation immobilization, and compression. Late infection: operative de-compression, irrigation.	Follow-up as arranged by specialist, physical therapy to prevent adhesions and loss of function.
Palmar space infection	Puncture wound or spread from tenosynovitis into deeper spaces of hand.	Localized severe pain and swelling over palmar space.	Urgent hospitalization, IV antibiotics and drainage if abscess has formed. Leave incision open. May require continuous indwelling catheter irrigation.	Follow-up as arranged by specialist, physical therapy to prevent adhesions and loss of function from scarring of overlying tendons.
Septic arthritis	Puncture wound or bite into joint space or hematoge-nous spread (especially gonorrhea).	Circumferential joint redness and swelling, extreme pain with passive motion.	Urgent hospitalization, IV antibiotics, surgical irri-gation and debridement; may require continuous indwelling catheter irrigation.	Follow up as arranged by specialist, physi-cal therapy to pre-vent loss of function from scarring of joint capsule.
Closed-fist injury	Striking an object with closed fist; may result in open fracture; may have human oral flora inoculated into wound (fight-bite).	Suspect whenever injury overlies metacarpo-phalangeal joints (espe-cially on dominant hand); requires x-ray of hand to rule out fracture or foreign body.	Immobilization, ice if acute, irrigation and debridement if skin is penetrated. Amoxicillin-clavulanate for bites.	Follow-up next day for wound check; refer to specialist if more than minor injury, to check for delayed infection.

General Treatment Principles. Once the infection has been diagnosed, the four mainstays of therapy are immobilization, elevation, antibiotics, and drainage. Once the wound has been cleaned, the area surrounding the site of infection should be immobilized. Immobilization allows good penetration of antibiotics and cell-mediated immune factors and helps prevent the local spread of infective organisms. A plaster or aluminum splint can be used to achieve immobilization. Once the splint has been placed, the patient must understand that the wound can no longer be seen but that the infection can still progress. The patient must be cautioned to return if the pain markedly increases or if fevers, chills, or any proximal swelling or erythema develops. Dressings should be changed at least daily—if not by the patient, then at the urgent care center. The splint should be left in place for 1–3 days. Once the swelling and erythema have resolved, the hand should undergo early mobilization to prevent contractures.

Along with immobilization, elevation aids in the removal of the edema and infected fluid surrounding the site. Elevation reduces extravasation of intracapillary fluid into the interstitial space around the infection. By removing this excessive fluid, much of the pain associated with tissue tension is also relieved. The goal of elevation is to keep the hand higher than the heart; for example, the hand can be propped on pillows when the patient is supine or carried on top of the head when the patient is upright.

Antibiotics are the third modality for treating hand infections. Drug selection should be based on the most likely pathogen causing the infection and on culture results, when available. Wounds should be cultured whenever possible to allow a specific antibiotic to be initiated if the empiric choice fails. *Staphylococcus aureus* is the most common infecting organism, and a penicillinase-resistant drug (e.g., dicloxacillin, cephalosporins, or clavulanate-containing antibiotics) is indicated.

If an abscess is present, incision and drainage are indicated. Successful and safe incision and drainage of infections in the hands require knowledge of where and how to make the incision and of the underlying anatomy (nerves, arteries, and tendons). There is no margin for error in the hand because of the complexity and proximity of the underlying structures.

To drain an abscess, a wedge of overlying skin should be removed to allow free drainage of the pus and to prevent its reaccumulation.[6] Another method to keep the wound open is to insert a drain into the abscess after incision and drainage. Because the hand is highly vascular, it is important to achieve a bloodless field during this procedure. A digital tourniquet can be used with caution; pressure necrosis of the finger can occur if the tourniquet is used for prolonged periods of time. Digital or wrist regional block with 1% lidocaine without epinephrine should be used for anesthesia.

Specific Hand Infections

Paronychia

Differential Diagnosis. Paronychia is an infection of the lateral nail fold. It may extend to the cuticle or involve the entire nail bed. It is a relatively common hand infection, most often due to *S. aureus*.

Management. If only the lateral fold is involved, drainage may be accomplished by inserting a scalpel blade into the fluctuant area, entering from above the nail at an oblique angle away from the nail matrix. A digital block is effective anesthesia. If the paronychia has extended into the eponychial fold and if pus is present under the proximal nail, this part of the nail should be removed to allow adequate drainage. Antibiotics are necessary if cellulitis is present. Drainage of paronychia is illustrated in Figures 5 and 6.

Pitfalls in Practice. Complications of paronychia are nail bed scarring and nail disfiguration if the nail bed and eponychium are involved. If the drainage is not complete, the

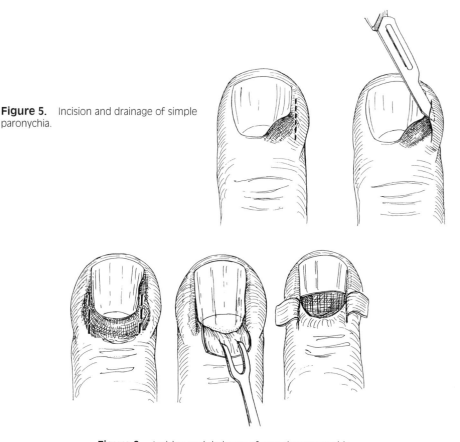

Figure 5. Incision and drainage of simple paronychia.

Figure 6. Incision and drainage of complex paronychia.

infection can progress down to the finger pad septa to form a felon and from there into the distal phalanx to form a chronic osteomyelitis.

Felons

Differential Diagnosis. Felons are infections of the digital pulp matrix. The infection spreads through the septa of the finger pad, forming multiple individual abscesses. Felons usually result from minor trauma to the finger pad. Examination reveals a tender, red, and swollen fingertip.

Management. Bacterial felons must be widely incised to allow drainage of the infection from between the fibrous septa of the fingertip pad. There is no clearly superior method of drainage. A good method involves drainage through a unilateral longitudinal incision on the side of greatest fluctuance. Another good method involves longitudinal incision of both sides of the distal pad with blunt dissection through the septa and a drain passed through and through and left in place for 2 or 3 days. The patient must be treated with antibiotics. Felons should be incised and drained only by an experienced physician who is knowledgeable about finger anatomy.

Pitfalls in Practice. If a felon is not surgically drained, ischemia and tissue loss may develop in the distal pad. Care must be taken to open up the septa in the distal pad without opening the flexor tendon sheath or injuring the flexor tendon insertion.

Tenosynovitis

Differential Diagnosis. Tenosynovitis is an infection of the flexor tendon sheath resulting from a penetrating injury or hematogenous spread of a separate infection. The middle three fingers are most commonly involved. Examination reveals (1) pain on passive extension of the digit, (2) a resting flexed position, (3) swelling along the flexor tendon sheath of the digit, and (4) tenderness on palpation along the sheath. The differential diagnosis includes simple cellulitis of the skin and subcutaneous abscesses of the fingers or midhand.

Management. Treatment of tenosynovitis is described in Table 4. If the infection is without abscess formation, conservative treatment with intravenous broad-spectrum antistaphylococcal antibiotics, immobilization, and elevation may be sufficient. If an abscess forms, operative decompression, irrigation and packing, or continuous irrigation is necessary.

Pitfalls in Practice. Tenosynovitis is an infectious disease emergency, and delay in diagnosis and management can result in devastating complications. The flexor tendons can become scarred and immobile.

Palmar Space Infections

Differential Diagnosis. Palmar space infections usually are caused by a puncture wound or bites into the deep soft tissues or expansion of a tenosynovitis into the closed spaces of the hand. There are four locations for infections in the hand: the web, thenar, midpalmar, and hypothenar spaces. Infections at these sites appear as pain and swelling over the respective spaces. Thenar infection forces the thumb into abduction. Midpalmar infection causes the hand to lose its palmar concavity and limits motion of the middle and ring fingers. Hypothenar infection causes hypothenar tenderness.

Management. Patients presenting with palmar space infections require emergent specialty consultation. Treatment requires admission for intravenous antibiotics and surgical drainage.

Pitfalls in Practice. Failure to diagnose these infections may result in life- and limb-threatening complications, including extension of infection into the arm, sepsis, and loss of the use of the tendons as they cross over the palm.

Closed-Fist Injuries

Differential Diagnosis. Closed-fist injuries occur during fights and usually are seen over the MCP joints of the dominant hand. The teeth of the person who is struck pierce the hand over the knuckles, resulting in lacerations, fractures, and deep infections of the MCP joints (septic arthritis). Radiographs can reveal fractures, foreign bodies (teeth) or air within the joint.

Management. These wounds must be irrigated, scrubbed, and debrided as necessary. The patient is placed on antibiotics (cephalexin and penicillin; amoxicillin or clavulanate) to cover common oral bacteria.[6] The hand should be immobilized and the patient told to return on the following day for reevaluation. If there is an open fracture, a specialist should be contacted for possible open irrigation and reduction. If the joint is grossly infected at the time of presentation, it may be prudent to hospitalize the patient for treatment with intravenous antibiotics and intermittent joint irrigation.

Pitfalls in Practice. Inadequate therapy can lead to septic arthritis and loss of function of the injured joints. Embedded teeth or other foreign bodies must be identified and removed, or therapy will fail. This injury should be suspected in all patients who present with injury over the MCP joints, even if the patient denies a history of fighting. It is, in effect, a human bite and therefore requires aggressive therapy.

Joint Sepsis

Differential Diagnosis. Like the other deep infections of the hand, septic arthritis usually begins from a puncture wound; in rare cases, it may result from hematogenous spread from a separate infection (most commonly disseminated gonorrhea).[7] Radiographs are essential to rule out open fractures, osteomyelitis, and foreign bodies. Local cellulitis and abscess can be difficult to differentiate from septic arthritis. Key findings are circumferential swelling and tenderness and extreme pain with minimal passive movement of the involved joint.

Management. Patients with suspected septic arthritis require hospital admission for intravenous antibiotic therapy, possible arthrotomy for irrigation, and possible intermittent catheter irrigation.

Pitfalls in Practice. Complications may include loss of function at the joint and chronic osteomyelitis if therapy is not initiated early.

Shoulder Injuries

Physical Examination and Diagnostic Aids. The shoulder complex consists of the clavicle, scapula with acromion and coracoid processes, and proximal two-thirds of the humerus. Physical examination begins with observation for evidence of swelling, discoloration, deformity, or asymmetry compared with the contralateral shoulder. Palpation of the bony surfaces and articulations is useful to detect tenderness, bony crepitus, or instability. Active and passive range of motion also should be tested, including abduction/adduction, flexion/extension, and internal/external rotation. Specific maneuvers may assist in differentiating among various clinical entities. For example, a positive Hawkin's sign (shoulder pain with forward flexion and internal rotation of the arm) suggests impingement syndrome.[8]

Suspicion of fracture or dislocation warrants radiography. Anteroposterior (AP) and lateral images are standard, and scapular Y-views are helpful in discerning direction of glenohumeral dislocation. A simple AP chest film may be sufficient (to rule out associated hemothorax or pneumothorax) if clavicular fracture is clinically obvious.

Fractures

The clavicle is the most frequently fractured bone in childhood; injury often results from a fall or direct blunt trauma.[9] The diagnosis frequently can be based on the physical examination, but an AP chest confirms the extent of the injury and helps rule out associated injuries, such as pneumothorax. Most clavicular fractures respond well to conservative management with a sling (see Table 1). Significantly displaced fractures involving the lateral third require orthopedic consultation for possible surgical repair.

Fractures of the proximal humerus are common in elders, often resulting from a fall. Humeral shaft fractures are seen across a wide spectrum of ages and are frequently associated with radial nerve damage. Many humeral fractures can be managed with splinting, slinging, and orthopedic evaluation in a few days (Figure 7). Fractures involving neurovascular compromise, comminution, associated dislocation, articular involvement, or a particularly young patient warrant orthopedic consultation.

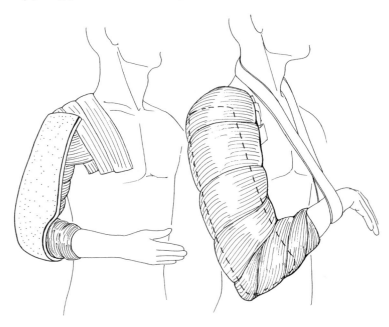

Figure 7. Sugartong splint, humerus.

Dislocations

The glenohumeral joint is the most frequently dislocated joint in the body.[10] Most cases result from blunt trauma, but dislocations may occur spontaneously, especially in patients with a history of recurrent instability. Most glenohumeral dislocations are anterior and can be successfully reduced via various closed methods (see Table 1). If the dislocation is reduced, slinging and orthopedic evaluation in a few days are adequate. Posterior dislocations account for a small minority of cases. Posterior dislocations tend to be more difficult to manage in the urgent care setting. Closed reduction may be attempted, but open reduction is often necessary.

Acromioclavicular (AC) dislocations are also quite common and tend to occur in young active males. Management of acromioclavicular joint dislocations depends on their severity. Conservative management with ice and slinging yields positive outcomes for simple AC injuries (see Table 1). Operative repair is recommended when the clavicle is displaced posteriorly into or through the trapezius muscle, gross disparity exists between the acromion and clavicle, or the clavicle is displaced inferior to the acromion or coracoid process.[11]

Overuse Injuries

The shoulder is also subject to pain from chronic disorders; the most common is impingement syndrome. The subacromial space (between the acromion and the greater tuberosity of the humerus) contains numerous soft tissue structures, including the rotator cuff tendons, long head of the biceps tendon, and subacromial bursa. Impingement syndrome is a spectrum of disease ranging from simple inflammation to complete disruption of these structures secondary to chronic mechanical trauma. In general, acute management of the chronic causes of shoulder pain consists of rest, ice, anti-inflammatory medications, and activity modification. Local anesthetic and steroid injections also may be beneficial.

Rotator cuff tears are infrequently caused by acute trauma. Patients may present with strains, partial-thickness tears, or full-thickness tears. Most rotator cuff tears result from impingement.[3] Definitive management of the different rotator cuff injuries can vary greatly. Full-thickness tears generally require surgical repair, whereas strains and partial thickness injuries do well with conservative management. Since it may be impossible to make the exact diagnosis without magnetic resonance imaging, patients with suspected rotator cuff lesions should undergo orthopedic evaluation within 7 days. In the meantime, slinging, ice, and early range of motion are recommended.

Adhesive capsulitis (frozen shoulder) is a chronic condition that manifests as gradual loss of active and passive motion of the glenohumeral joint. The cause is unknown, but risk factors include female gender, age > 40 years, trauma, diabetes, prolonged immobilization, thyroid disease, stroke or myocardial infarction, and autoimmune disease. Up to one-third of patients have eventual involvement of the contralateral shoulder.[12] Therapy for adhesive capsulitis in the acute setting is mainly conservative; nonurgent orthopedic referral is recommended.

Pitfalls in Practice. Scapular fractures and sternoclavicular dislocations are rarely seen in the urgent care setting, but must be ruled out when patients present after trauma to the shoulder complex. Significant force is required to produce such injuries, which often result from motor vehicle accidents or sports injuries. In many cases, these injuries are not isolated. Scapular fractures are associated with severe injuries to the neck, shoulder, kidney, and thoracic structures in up to 98% of cases.[11] Sternoclavicular dislocations, especially those displaced posteriorly, also have a high incidence of associated life-threatening injury. Evidence for these orthopedic problems should prompt immediate consultation and probable transfer to an institution capable of ruling out other life threats. Failure to evaluate for neurovascular status after an injury to the shoulder can result in missing an orthopedic emergency and lead to substantial morbidity and mortality.

Elbow Injuries

Physical Examination and Diagnostic Aids. The elbow is the site of articulation of the distal humerus with the olecranon process of the ulna and the proximal radius.

Physical examination begins with observation for signs of swelling, discoloration, or deformity. Palpation of the olecranon process, radial head, and medial and lateral humeral epicondyles is helpful in detecting point tenderness or bony crepitus. Deformity, swelling, and point tenderness are common with fractures but atypical of radial head subluxation.

Flexion/extension and pronation/supination should be tested both actively and passively. These tests are especially helpful in differentiating olecranon bursitis from arthritis. A painless, full range of motion with pronation and supination makes bursitis more likely.

Injured patients often maintain the elbow in a certain position based on the specific injury. For example, the classic presentation of radial head subluxation involves decreased use of the arm and posturing with the limb held close to the body, elbow partially flexed and forearm pronated. Manipulation of these patients typically reveals pain with supination of the forearm or motion of the elbow.

Pain secondary to overuse injuries often can be reproduced on physical examination as well. Symptoms of medial epicondylitis can be reproduced by forearm pronation with simultaneous resisted dorsiflexion of the wrist. Lateral epicondylitis (pain at the tendinous insertion of the forearm flexor muscles) can be exacerbated by a similar maneuver which substitutes resisted volar flexion for dorsiflexion.[13]

Standard elbow series roentgenograms include at least AP and lateral views; sometimes oblique images are added. Attempts should be made to achieve true lateral views, which is necessary to delineate the extent of injury with an olecranon fracture and accurately identify fat pad signs. Anterior and posterior fat pad signs are suggestive of radial head injury.

Fracture Management

Supracondylar humeral fractures tend to be common in childhood; 95% of cases include anterior displacement secondary to an extension injury.[14] Such injuries are associated with a high frequency of complications, including neurovascular deficits. Supracondylar fractures with signs of neurovascular compromise warrant immediate transfer to an emergency department for orthopedic surgery. Other supracondylar fractures should be splinted and the patient admitted for observation of developing complications.

In adults, distal humeral fractures tend to be intercondylar rather than supracondylar. Undisplaced intercondylar fractures generally can be treated with splinting and referral for subsequent casting. Fractures with displacement, rotation, or comminution require consultation for probable open repair.

The subcutaneous position of the olecranon makes it susceptible to injury from direct trauma. The radial head is also prone to fracture, often due to a fall on an outstretched hand. Undisplaced olecranon or radial head fractures can be treated with splinting and orthopedic referral in a few days. Displaced fractures generally require consultation for operative repair. In cases of radial head fracture, aspiration of hemarthrosis with injection of local anesthetic may reduce pain and facilitate early range of motion, but improved outcomes have not been demonstrated.[15]

Pitfalls in Practice. Supracondylar fractures in children can result in devastating neurovascular complications and always warrant at least admission and observation. The most serious complication is Volkmann's ischemic contracture, which can lead to tissue necrosis and fibrosis.[14] Early signs of Volkmann's ischemia include refusal to open the hand, forearm tenderness, and pain with passive finger extension. Failure to identify supracondylar fractures or signs of neurovascular compromise can result in significant morbidity.

Dislocations

Despite the inherent stability of the elbow, elbow dislocations are not rare. A fall on an outstretched hand is the usual mechanism; the majority of dislocations are posterior. Elbow dislocations generally can be reduced by gentle wrist traction with downward pressure on the proximal forearm.[13] After reduction, posterior splinting provides stability pending orthopedic evaluation in a few days.

In childhood, radial head subluxation (nursemaid's elbow) is a frequent cause of elbow pain or refusal to use the upper extremity. The typical mechanism is axial traction of the affected arm. Reduction of radial head subluxation can be accomplished simply by performing a few simultaneous maneuvers. With the patient's arm in extension and pronation, quickly apply downward pressure to the radial head with a thumb, passively supinate the forearm, and flex the elbow.[13] A brief period of observation should reveal a return to normal usage of the limb. No further management is necessary, but caretakers should be informed that recurrences are frequent.

Overuse Injuries

Lateral epicondylitis (tennis elbow) is a condition marked by pain at the origin of the extensor muscles of the lower arm. The common name is derived from the frequency of the syndrome among tennis players with one-handed backhand strokes that are fundamentally unsound. Medial epicondylitis is a similar disorder, known commonly as golfer's elbow or little league elbow. Acute management of both medial and lateral epicondylitis consists of activity modification and anti-inflammatory medications. Orthopedic referral may be indicated if symptoms persist.

Olecranon bursitis is often caused by repetitive motion but also may result from acute trauma or infection. Typical presentation includes pain and swelling over the olecranon. Septic bursitis commonly is associated with a puncture wound or overlying cellulitis. Treatment of olecranon bursitis depends on the etiology. Suspicion of infection necessitates drainage, although aspiration may help alleviate symptoms in other cases as well. Ice, anti-inflammatory medications, and activity modification are appropriate management for noninfectious bursitis.

Pitfalls in Practice. As with fractures of the elbow, dislocation can cause neurovascular compromise. Dislocations should be reduced as quickly as possible to avoid ischemic complications.

Wrist Injuries

Physical Examination and Diagnostic Aids. Physical examination of the wrist should include visual assessment of any swelling or discoloration. Diagnosis may be based on obvious deformity, such as the classic "dinner fork" appearance of the Colles' fracture. Systematic palpation of the distal portions of the radius and ulna as well as their articulations with the carpal bones is essential. The individual carpal bones also should be palpated, and snuffbox tenderness should be assessed.

Range of motion at the wrist includes dorsiflexion and volar flexion as well as radial and ulnar deviation. Complete neurovascular assessment at and distal to the affected area is necessary. Standard AP, lateral, and oblique x-rays are a valuable tool, but many injuries of the wrist must be diagnosed clinically because they are not apparent radiographically.

Fractures

Colles' fracture is the most common wrist fracture seen in adults, and is defined as a transverse fracture of the distal radial metaphysis, which is dorsally displaced. Most Colles' fractures are amenable to closed reduction, with a finger trap apparatus being a helpful tool. The Smith's fracture is similar to the Colles' but involves volar displacement. Special care must be taken to rule out associated median nerve or flexor tendon injury. General management guidelines are provided in Table 2. A sandwich splint (Fig. 8) can be used for immobilization).

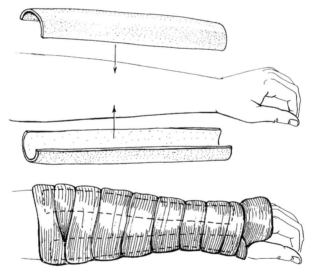

Figure 8. Sandwich splint.

Lateral force, dorsiflexion, rotatory stress, or forced radial/ulnar deviation may result in fracture of either the radial or ulnar styloid. Radial styloid fractures are associated with scapholunate disassociation and radiographs must be scrutinized closely. Undisplaced fractures can be splinted with a radial-ulnar sugartong splint (Fig. 9) and referred, while displaced injuries (especially involving the radial styloid) may necessitate open reduction with internal fixation (ORIF).

Pitfalls in Practice. In evaluating orthopedic injuries in children, the possibility of physeal involvement must be considered. Diagnosis is largely clinical, based on history and the presence of point tenderness over a physis. The Salter-Harris classification of

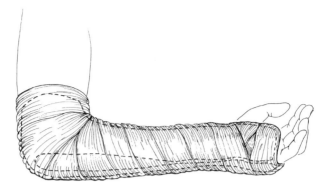

Figure 9. Sugartong splint, radioulnar.

physeal injuries (Table 5) describes the five variations of fracture involving the growth plate. Diagnosis of type I injuries requires a high index of suspicion, because roentgenograms may be normal. Salter-Harris type I fractures should be managed with splinting and orthopedic referral in a few days. Failure to identify physeal injuries can lead to inadequate bone growth and significant future disability.

Table 5. Salter-Harris Classification of Physeal Injuries

Type I	Fracture line through the physis only
Type II	Fracture line through the physis and metaphysis
Type III	Fracture line through physis and epiphysis
Type IV	Fracture line through physis, metaphysis, and epiphysis
Type V	Crush injury to physis

Failure to examine the snuffbox region can result in missing the diagnosis of a scaphoid fracture. This fracture is prone to malunion if not properly treated. A thumb spica splint should be applied to patients with snuffbox tenderness, even if x-rays do not reveal a fracture. Radiologic reassessment at a later date can confirm or refute the tentative diagnosis.

Knee

Physical Examination and Diagnostic Aids. Physical examination of the knee begins with inspection for swelling, bruising, redness, or deformity. The patient's gait should be observed, if possible, along with assessment of range of motion of the joint. Palpation should include the patella, popliteal fossa, medial and lateral joint lines, and tibial and femoral condyles. Knee stability is assessed by applying stress across the joint. Varus, valgus, anterior, and posterior stability should be examined. McMurray's test (flexing and extending the knee while simultaneously internally and externally rotating the tibia on the femur) is used to demonstrate meniscal injuries. As with all orthopedic physical examinations, assessment of neurovascular status is crucial. AP, lateral, and oblique radiographs may be helpful in diagnosing knee injuries. Guidelines, such as the Ottawa knee rules (Table 6), may be helpful in determining the need for x-rays.[16]

Table 6. Ottawa Knee Rules

A radiograph is indicated if a patient with knee pain meets any of the following criteria:
1. Patient older than 55 years
2. Tenderness at the head of the fibula
3. Isolated tenderness of the patella
4. Inability to flex the knee to 90°
5. Inability to transfer weight for four steps both immediately after the injury and in the emergency department

Adapted from Stiell IG, Wells GA, Hoag RH, Sivilotti ML: Implementation of the Ottawa Knee Rules for the use of radiography in acute knee injuries. JAMA 278:2075, 1977.

Fractures

Distal femur and tibial plateau fractures are often caused by an axial loading force from a fall. Any degree of fracture displacement or joint incongruity requires open reduction and internal fixation; thus, immediate orthopedic consultation is mandated. The leg should be splinted and the patient should avoid weight-bearing until definitive management is provided.

Fractures of the patella generally result from a direct blow to the knee. It is important to assess the integrity of the extensor mechanism by having the patient straighten the injured leg against gravity. Displaced fractures and loss of the extensor mechanism require early orthopedic consultation for open reduction and internal fixation, wheras less severe fractures may be treated with a knee immobilizer, ice, elevation, NSAIDs and orthopedic follow-up within 3–5 days.

Pitfalls in Practice. Radiographs can be negative despite the presence of a fracture. If the history and clinical examination suggest that a fracture is present in the knee or any other location, it is prudent to treat the injury as if a fracture is present. Repeat radiographs at follow-up may confirm a suspected fracture.

Soft Tissue Injuries to the Knee

Physical Examination and Diagnostic Aids. The ligaments of the knee include the lateral and medial collateral ligaments and anterior and posterior cruciate ligaments. These ligaments, along with the joint capsule and surrounding muscles, provide support for the knee joint. Ligament injuries may range from mild sprains to complete tears and may involve a combination of structures.

The medial and lateral collateral ligaments can be tested for injury by applying varus and valgus stress to the knee. Pain during these maneuvers suggests a sprain, whereas laxity of the joint suggests partial or complete tears.

The anterior and posterior cruciate ligaments can be tested for injury by performing the anterior and posterior drawer test. Abnormal anterior displacement, compared with the uninjured knee, suggests injury to the anterior cruciate ligament. Posterior displacement is seen with posterior cruciate ligament injuries. Most cruciate ligament injuries present with joint effusion (hemarthroses) that develops within minutes to hours of the injury. Plain radiographs in ligamentous injuries are usually normal but may reveal an effusion. Anterior cruciate ligament ruptures may be associated with an avulsion fracture on the lateral tibial condyle, whereas an avulsion fracture of the medial tibial plateau is associated with tears of the posterior cruciate ligament.

Medial and lateral meniscus injuries also may occur in combination with other ligamentous injuries. Locking of the knee joint during flexion and extension suggests meniscal injury. Definitive diagnosis requires either MRI or arthroscopy.

Patella dislocations can result from relatively minor trauma. The mechanism is usually a twisting motion on an extended knee. Lateral displacement of the patella is most common. Reduction is performed by pushing the patella back into place with a flexed hip and extended knee. Intravenous narcotic pain medicine or conscious sedation may be required to perform the reduction. After reduction, radiographs should be obtained to rule out a fracture.

Knee dislocations are high-energy injuries with a high incidence of associated arterial (popliteal) and nerve (peroneal) injuries. Immediate orthopedic consultation is required for early reduction (most often under conscious sedation). A dislocated knee that has spontaneously reduced is usually extremely unstable because of extensive ligamentous disruption and also requires immediate consultation.

Management. Management of most soft tissue knee injuries consists of ice, NSAID, and knee immobilization or partial weight-bearing with crutches. Orthopedic follow-up within 1 week is suggested. A locked knee from a meniscus injury may require conscious sedation to reduce. More immediate orthopedic consultation or transfer to a facility capable of conscious sedation should be arranged for this injury.

Pitfalls in Practice. Patients who are diagnosed with a stable knee injury and treated with a knee immobilizer are at risk for muscle contracture, quadricep atrophy, and loss of joint mobility. Such patients should be instructed to perform daily range-of-motion exercises to maintain mobility. These exercises simply involve flexing and extending the knee several times 3 or 4 times/day.

Overuse Injuries of the Knee

Patellofemoral pain syndrome (often called chondromalacia patellae) is caused by changes in the patellofemoral articulation.[17] Malalignment and tracking abnormalities of the patella lead to pain in the anterior knee while climbing stairs, kneeling, or rising from a chair. This syndrome is most common in women and athletes. An apprehension test (pushing the patella laterally on a relaxed leg to elicit quadriceps muscle contraction in anticipation of pain) may help diagnose this disorder.

Patellar tendinitis, also known as "jumper's knee," is most common in athletes who repetitively jump, run, or cut. Physical exam findings include tenderness over the quadriceps tendon at the upper pole of the patella or tenderness over the patella tendon at the lower pole or at the tibial tuberosity.

Iliotibial band syndrome is an overuse injury most commonly seen in long distance runners.[18] It is characterized by pain in the lateral aspect of the knee during repetitive knee movement, as in running or cycling. The iliotibial band is a strip of fascia that serves as a lateral knee stabilizer. Overuse can cause inflammation of the underlying bursa at the lateral femoral epicondyle. Physical exam findings consist of tenderness over the lateral femoral epicondyle.

Bursitis of the knee is the inflammation of one or more of the many bursae located around the joint. Bursitis may result from overuse, trauma, crystal deposition, infection, or other inflammatory processes. Prepatellar bursitis is characterized by swelling and tenderness over the lower pole of the patella. It is usually caused by repetitive kneeling on hard surfaces.

Osteoarthritis results from chronic degenerative changes in the knee and other joints. It is most common in elders, obese patients, and people with previous knee trauma. The pain of osteoarthritis is typically worsened with activity and relieved by rest. Physical exam may reveal angular deformities at the knee as well as tenderness along the joint line. AP radiographs (weight-bearing) often demonstrate joint space narrowing with osteophyte formation and subchondral sclerosis.

Management. Management of overuse injuries to the knee consists of rest, NSAID, and quadriceps strengthening (particularly the vastus medialis oblique). Treatment of iliotibial band syndrome includes rest, ice, NSAID, stretching, shoe changes, and decreased distances for running or cycling.

Pitfalls in Practice. Rest of the involved joint is the major key to treatment of any overuse injury. Active patients, such as athletes, are often reluctant to rest the knee long enough for complete resolution. Suggesting alternative exercises (e.g., swimming instead of running) may help improve compliance.

Lower Leg Injuries

Physical Examination and Diagnostic Aids. Physical examination of the lower leg includes inspection (for swelling, bruising or deformity) and palpation of the entire length of the extremity. Sensory examination should include the web spaces, lateral heel, and sole of the foot. The popliteal, dorsalis pedal, and posterior tibial pulses must be assessed, along with motor function of the ankle (plantar flexion, dorsal flexion, inversion, and eversion). AP and lateral radiographs of the tibia and fibular, which include the ankle and knee joints, are often sufficient for initial imaging.

Fractures

Fibula fractures may result from a direct blow to the lateral leg or from rotational forces during exercise or a fall. Patients with fibula fractures are generally able to walk because the fibula is a minimal weight-bearing bone. Examination usually reveals swelling and tenderness over the fracture site.

Tibia fractures typically result from higher-energy trauma than isolated fibula fractures. Both direct trauma (e.g., automobile accident) and indirect trauma from a rotational or compressive force (e.g., skiing, falling) can cause tibia fractures. Because the tibia and fibula are so tightly bound to each other, displaced fractures of one bone are often associated with fracture or ligamentous injury to the other bone. Physical examination may reveal deformity, bruising, and swelling with tenderness to palpation. Distal neurovascular status must be well documented.

Management. Treatment of fibula fractures consists of immobilization (knee immobilizer or Robert Jones splint [Fig. 10] for proximal fractures, elastic wrap for distal fractures), ice, elevation, and pain medicines. The patient should avoid weight-bearing for a few days until partial weight-bearing can be tolerated. Orthopedic follow-up within 1 week is suggested. Immediate orthopedic consultation should be sought for nearly all tibia fractures. A long-leg posterior splint, with the knee flexed at 10–20° may be placed for transport.

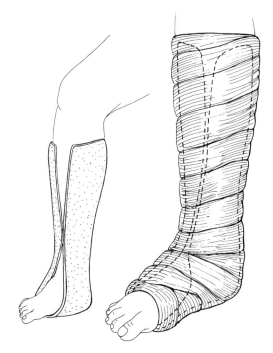

Figure 10. Robert Jones splint.

Pitfalls in Practice. Compartment syndrome is a potential complication of tibia fractures. It also may be seen in soft tissue injuries without associated fractures. Increased tissue pressure within an enclosed fascial space leads to inadequate perfusion within the compartment and ischemic necrosis of muscle and nerve. The clinical hallmark of compartment syndrome is pain out of proportion to the injury or physical exam findings. Pain with passive movement of the muscle groups in the compartment is also common. Pallor and pulselessness are late findings. If compartment syndrome is suspected, immediate orthopedic consultation is required. The treatment for compartment syndrome is fasciotomy.

Soft Tissue Injuries

Achilles' tendon rupture can occur during forceful plantar flexion. The patient typically has difficulty with ambulating and experiences pain in the region. Examination may reveal a palpable defect in the tendon with associated tenderness and swelling. The diagnosis is primarily made clinically with the Thompson test (squeezing the calf produces plantar flexion with an intact tendon[19]). Gastrocnemius strain or rupture also can occur during forceful plantar flexion. Ambulation usually is painful, and the region is tender and swollen on exam. The pain and tenderness are more proximal than in an Achilles tendon rupture, and the Thompson test is negative.

Shin splints is a term for an overuse injury that produces pain over the anterior and lateral tibia. The pain, usually exertional, is common in runners. Physical examination may reveal tenderness to the anterior or lateral tibia.

Osgood-Schlatter disease is most commonly seen in teenaged athletes. Partial separation of the tibial tuberosity at the insertion of the patellar tendon results from repetitive microtrauma. The tibial tuberosity is often tender and indurated on examination. Radiographs are generally not helpful in diagnosing Osgood-Schlatter disease but may rule out other pathology.

Management. Urgent care treatment of Achilles tendon rupture consists of ice, elevation, NSAID, splinting (Robert Jones splint in neutral position [see Fig. 10]) and orthopedic follow-up in 2–3 days. Management of gastrocnemius injury includes immobilization with a posterior splint, ice, elevation, and NSAID. Orthopedic follow-up should occur within 1 week. Shin splints are treated with rest and NSAIDs. Initial management of Osgood-Schlatter disease includes rest, ice, and analgesics. Orthopedic follow-up may be necessary if the initial treatment fails.

Pitfalls in Practice. It is essential to assess for distal neurovascular compromise after any leg injury. Immobilization of the lower extremity is accompanied by a rash of deep venous thrombosis. Patients should be encouraged to mobilize as soon as possible.

Ankle

Physical Examination and Diagnostic Aids. The ankle joint has three major articulations: The medial malleolus with the medial talus, the tibial plafond with the talar dome, and the lateral malleolus with the lateral talus. The syndesmotic ligaments, the lateral collateral ligaments, and the medial collateral ligaments provide structural stability to the joint.

The physical examination of ankle injuries includes inspection and palpation for swelling, tenderness, and deformities. Joint stability should be assessed in the anteroposterior plane as well as inversion and eversion planes. Most importantly, a thorough neurovascular exam should be documented. A standard radiographic series includes an AP, lateral, and mortise views. Guidelines, such as the Ottawa ankle rules (Table 7), may be helpful in determining the need for x-rays but should not supplant clinical judgment.[20]

Table 7. Ottawa Ankle Rules

A radiograph is indicated if a patient with ankle pain meets any of the following criteria:
1. Tenderness at the posterior edge or tip of the lateral malleolus
2. Tenderness at the posterior edge or tip of the medial malleolus
3. Inability to bear weight on the ankle both immediately and in the clinic or emergency department

Adapted from Stiell IG, McKnight RD, Greenberg GH: Implementation of the Ottawa Ankle Rules. JAMA 271:827, 1994.

Fractures

Physical Examination and Diagnostic Aids. Ankle fractures occur more often after inversion or eversion injuries. Patients present with deformity, swelling, pain, and bruising and usually are unable to bear weight. Fractures with dislocations are generally grossly deformed.

Management. The treatment goal of all ankle fractures is to restore anatomic relationships. The urgency with which orthopedic consultation is obtained depends on the overall stability of the fracture. All open fractures, fracture dislocations, and injuries with associated neurovascular compromise require immediate consultation. Any displaced or unstable ankle fracture also requires prompt consultation. Only stable, extra-articular, unilateral fractures can be initially managed with immobilization, non–weight-bearing, and delayed follow-up.

Pitfalls in Practice. Unimalleolar fractures with associated ligamentous disruption can result in an unstable or displaced joint. Unstable unimalleolar, isolated posterior malleolar, bimalleolar, and trimalleolar fractures require immediate consultation.

Soft Tissue Injuries

Physical Examination and Diagnostic Aids. Most ankle sprains result from an inversion and plantar-flexion mechanism. Sprains can be classified into three grades. Grade I consists of ligamentous stretching without joint instability. Grade II consists of a partial ligament tear with moderate joint instability. A grade III injury involves a complete tear with severe joint instability.[21]

Lateral ligament sprains are the most common ankle sprains and usually involve the anterior talofibular ligament. More extensive sprains also involve the posterior talofibular and calcaneofibular ligaments. Physical examination reveals swelling, tenderness, and bruising over the involved ligaments.

Medial ligament sprains are much less common than lateral ankle sprains. These injuries most often result from an eversion mechanism. The sprain may be isolated to the deltoid ligament, but associated fractures (fibula) and syndesmosis tears are often seen. Physical examination reveals tenderness around the medial malleolus with swelling and ecchymosis.

Management. Patients with an unstable joint should be splinted and receive orthopedic follow-up in 1–3 days. Stable lateral ankle sprains can be managed with ice, elevation, rest, and NSAID. An ankle brace and crutches with partial weight-bearing as tolerated may be prescribed for the first 2–3 days. Progressive weight-bearing and mobilization should follow. Patients with minor ankle sprains can follow-up with their primary physician or orthopedist if symptoms do not improve over the course of 1 week.

Pitfalls in Practice. Joint injuries may not be isolated. Any joint injury necessitates examination of the entire extremity to ensure that no other injury is missed. For example, proximal fibular head fractures (Maisonneuve's fracture) are occasionally seen with medial ankle sprains or fractures.

Splints must be properly padded to avoid pressure sores. Bony prominences are particularly susceptible to this complication. Excessive pressure from a splint or cast may contribute to the development of compartment syndrome, particularly if the splint or cast is circumferential. Splints that are painful should be removed and redone after a thorough examination of the extremity.

Foot Disorders

Because the foot bears the entire weight of the body, it is not surprising that many people present to the urgent care center with foot pain. Most foot conditions are chronic and require follow-up care with a podiatrist or orthopedic surgeon. The goals of urgent care evaluation are to initiate appropriate therapy and to identify serious diseases and injuries.

Physical Examination and Diagnostic Aids. The foot is made up of 28 bones and is often divided anatomically into the hindfoot (talus and calcaneus), midfoot (navicular, cuboid, and cuneiforms), and forefoot (metatarsals, phalanges, and sesamoids). Physical examination begins with observation of gait (if the patient is able) and the position of the foot at rest. Swelling, deformity, and discoloration also should be observed. Because blood often tracks through tissue planes, however, the location of ecchymosis may not indicate the actual site of injury. Palpation of bony landmarks helps identify point tenderness, and special attention should be given to the navicular bone and base of the fifth metatarsal. Lastly, the foot contains 57 joints, and range of motion should be tested in joints that are relevant to the chief complaint.

Standard foot radiography consists of three views, including AP, lateral, and oblique. Foot films tend to be difficult to interpret because of the numerous structures, potential for overlap, tendency for fractures to be undisplaced, and high frequency of normal variants. Additional views may be necessary to identify specific injuries.

Fractures

The calcaneus is involved in roughly 60% of all tarsal fractures; the majority result from falls and compression injury.[22] Because calcaneal fractures are difficult to reduce and often heal poorly, emergent orthopedic consultation is recommended. For undisplaced fractures, however, posterior splinting with orthopedic referral may suffice.

Talus fractures are the second most common foot fracture. Because of its tenuous blood supply, the talus has a propensity to develop avascular necrosis when injured. Simple undisplaced chip or avulsion fractures may be amenable to splinting and evaluation by an orthopedist in a few days. More complex fractures or fractures with associated dislocation require immediate consultation.

The midfoot is susceptible to direct trauma because of its lack of mobility. Fractures of the midfoot tend to involve multiple bones or associated dislocation/subluxation. The navicular is the only bone commonly fractured in isolation. Undisplaced fractures can be treated with immobilization and conservative management, whereas others should prompt orthopedic consultation.

The metatarsals are subject to injury from direct trauma, twisting-type forces, and repetitive stress. The second and third metatarsals are especially prone to stress fracture in runners and other athletes. The Jones fracture involves transverse disruption of the proximal metaphysis of the fifth metatarsal. Jones fractures are noteworthy because they are the most common metatarsal fracture and have a high incidence of nonunion.[21] Most metatarsal fractures can be managed with splinting and referral for casting in a few days. The exceptions that require consultation involve significant displacement, comminution, or associated injuries.

Management. Simple fractures of the phalanges generally can be treated conservatively with buddy taping. However, special care must be given to injuries of the great toe because it bears considerably more weight than the other toes. Open fractures and associated dislocations occur commonly with phalangeal injuries. If possible, dislocations should be reduced and then managed conservatively. Consultation should be considered for complex fractures, open fractures, and dislocations that cannot be reduced.

Pitfalls in Practice. Calcaneal fractures typically result from a significant mechanism of trauma, and associated injuries are common. Specific attention should be given to the back, hips, pelvis, and knees. If thorough evaluation for associated injuries cannot be completed in the urgent care setting, the patient should be transferred to a facility capable of such management.

Disruption of the tarsal-metatarsal joint (Lisfranc injury) is uncommon and typically results from a motor vehicle accident. Radiographic signs are sometimes subtle and easily missed.[23] Fracture at the base of the second metatarsal, decreased range of motion at Lisfranc's joint, or a concerning history should arouse suspicion. Management of such injuries is complex, and early orthopedic consultation is essential. Failure to recognize associated articular injury can lead to improper healing and loss of function.

Soft Tissue Injuries

The dense plantar fascia arises from the calcaneus and inserts into the forefoot at the metatarsal heads. This strong band of fascia supports the internal convex arch of the metatarsal bones. Overuse of the foot leads to inflammation. Plantar fasciitis presents as tenderness at the medial tubercle of the calcaneus and in the bottom of the foot medially.

Morton's neuroma arises from compression of the interdigital nerve between two metatarsal heads. Pain is burning or sharp between the two involved heads and worsens with activity. Palpation at the site should elicit pain and may detect crepitus from local adhesions.

Any condition that causes inflammation within or near the tarsal tunnel can lead to compression of the posterior tibial nerve. The result is tarsal tunnel syndrome, analogous to carpal tunnel syndrome in the hand. Symptoms include medial malleolar pain that radiates to the heel, sole, or calf. Sensory changes also may be present.

Bunions arise from the anatomic disorder of lateral deviation of the great toe (hallux valgus). Patients develop an exostosis over the first metatarsal head, which becomes painful.

Corns (calluses) are formed by chronic friction over a bony prominence of the foot or between the toes. Corns may ache at rest or cause pain with palpation or pressure. Corns can be differentiated from plantar warts by removing the top with a scalpel. Warts typically demonstrate core lesions with pinpoint bleeding, whereas corns show only heaped keratin layers.

Ingrown toenails are characterized by hypertrophy, pain, and redness at the lateral edges of the toenail, where the nail has become embedded in hypertrophied granulation tissue. The cause is usually pressure on the lateral aspect of the great toe from a shoe.

Management. Management of plantar fasciitis consists of activity modification, ice, and anti-inflammatory medications. Heel cups and orthotic supports also may help distribute weight on the foot and prevent recurrence. Treatment of Morton's neuroma includes arch supports, metatarsal pads, and shoes with greater width. Severe or persistent cases eventually may require surgical excision. Acute management of tarsal tunnel syndrome consists of rest, ice, anti-inflammatory medications, and possibly local steroid injection. Referral for orthopedic evaluation should be considered in cases that prove recalcitrant to conservative therapy. Treatment of bunions includes insoles, metatarsal arches, and shoes that fit properly. Prevention is the key to management of corns and is aided by well-fitted shoes, arch supports, and foam pads over symptomatic areas. Keratolytic agents or removal with a scalpel also may be beneficial. Management of ingrown toenails may require removal of a portion of the nail. Careful trimming, local wound care, and soaks may prevent recurrence.

Pitfalls in Practice. Patients with peripheral neuropathy may present late in the course of a soft tissue injury. They should be followed carefully to ensure that the problem is resolving. Bunions can become infected and have the potential to develop osteomyelitis. Suspicion of infection warrants early, aggressive management.

Joint Disorders

Swollen and Tender Joints

The urgent care physician sees many patients with the chief complaint of joint pain. The goals of urgent care evaluation of joint disease are to diagnose and treat patients who need urgent therapy and to initiate therapy and referral for patients with chronic disease.

Swollen and tender joints may be due to traumatic or nontraumatic causes. An accurate history is crucial. Even in the absence of a traumatic history, occult or forgotten trauma must be considered and fractures searched for. The key diagnostic test is joint aspiration with analysis of the joint fluid aspirate. Table 8 lists characteristics of joint fluid in health and disease.

Table 8. Characteristics of Joint Fluid in Health and Disease

Type of Fluid	Appearance	Clot	Glucose	White Blood Cells/mm³ (% Segs)	Gram Stain
Normal (type 1)	Clear	Firm	Near serum level	100–200	Clear
Inflammatory (type 2)	Turbid	Less firm	May be low	1,000–300,000	Clear
Traumatic (type 3)	Bloody	Firm	Near serum level	> 200	Blood cells
Purulent (type 4)	Turbid	Friable	Much less than serum level	> 75,000	Bacteria probable

The first step in the differential diagnosis of arthritis is deciding whether it is monarticular (simple isolated joint) or polyarticular (multiple joints).

Monarticular Disease

Table 9 lists common causes of monarticular pain and/or swelling. Even though the patient may complain of only one painful joint, careful questioning about other joint pain is essential. Monarticular complaints also may be early polyarticular disease. Table 10 lists the differential diagnosis and management of monarticular disease.

Table 9. Common Causes of Monarticular Disease

Infectious	Traumatic	Metabolic	Inflammatory	Degenerative
Bacterial	Fracture	Gout	Rheumatoid arthritis	Osteoarthritis
Lyme disease	Ligamentous injury	Pseudogout	Reiter's syndrome	Osteochondritis dissecans
	Contusion	Bleeding disorders		

Table 10. Differential Diagnosis of Monarticular Complaints

Cause	Presentation	Physical Findings	Diagnostic Aids	Joint Fluid (see Table 8)	Management
Nongono-coccal infection	Rapid onset. Primary joint involved: children, hip; adults, knee; IV drug users, sacroiliac, sternocla-vicular. 85% of cases are monarticular. Predisposing factors: prior joint damage, prosthesis, and immunocompromised status.	Warm, swollen, tender; amount of joint effusion; elevated temperature.	White blood cell count (WBC) > 10,000/mm^3 in 50% of cases, posi-tive blood culture in more than 50% of cases. X-rays: subchondral bone erosion or osteo-myelitis. Radio-nuclide scan can be helpful.	Purulent (type 4); positive Gram stain in 50–75% of cases, positive culture in 90% of cases; lactate > 1,000 mg/dl, low glucose level.	Urgent hospitalization, for IV anti-biotics, surgical drainage, immobilization.
Lyme disease	In areas with deer ticks; knee affected most often; arthritis lasts 1 wk and tends to recur; usually mon-articular; occurs in summer and fall; flu-like symptoms initially.	Erythema chronicum migrans present at stage 1; rash begins at bite site and lasts 3 wk; neurologic and cardiac disturbances at stage 2 ; large joint effusion at stage 3.	*Borrelia burgdorferi* is causative organism; electrocardiogram may show heart blocks; positive immunofluorescent assay or enzyme-linked immuno-sorbent assay.	Inflammatory (type 2)	Doxycycline 100 mg PO 2 times/day for 20–30 days.
Gout	90% of cases are mon-articular; family history in 10–50% of cases; acute onset; recurrent episodes usually; men affected more often than women.	Metatarsal-phalanx of great toe; ankle and knee often affected; fever 101–103° F; effusion in large joints.	WBC and erythrocyte sedimentation rate elevated; hyperuri-cemia. Radiographs: if chronic, punched-out lesions near joints.	Inflammatory (type 2): urate crystals with negative birefringence.	Indomethacin (75–150 mg 4 times/day), phenylbutazone (300–400 mg twice daily for 1 day, then 300 mg 4 times/day, colchicines (1 mg IV), allo-purinol (100–300 mg 3 times/day, for prevention).
Osteo-arthritis	Pain with activity, relief with rest. Involved joints: weight-bearing (e.g., knee or hip).	No signs of inflammation; crepitus frequent.	Laboratory examina-tion normal. Radiographs: cysts, spurs, decreased joint spaces.	Normal (type 1)	Rest, salicylates, indomethacin (50–100 mg 4 times/day, other NSAIDs as needed if no response to indomethacin.
Osteo-chondritis dissecans	Ages 10–25 yr; males affected more often than females; knees affected most often.	Gritty sensation on movement.	Radiographs: tunnel view of knee shows subchondral defects on femoral condyle.	Normal (type 1)	NSAIDs

Polyarticular Disease

Diagnosing the patient with complaints of polyarticular pain is often a perplexing process; causes are listed in Table 11. Many causes of polyarthritis often present like monarthritis, es-pecially in the early phase of the disease. A careful history, physical examination, and selective laboratory tests narrow the diagnostic possibilities. Table 12 describes the differential diagnosis of polyarticular disease.

Table 11. Common Causes of Polyarticular Disease

Infectious	Metabolic	Inflammatory	Degenerative
Bacterial	Gout	Rheumatoid arthritis	Osteoarthritis
Subacute endocarditis	Pseudogout	Reiter's syndrome	
Rheumatic fever	Bleeding disorders	Behçet's disease	
	Gaucher's disease	Enteritis or colitis	

Table 12. Differential Diagnosis of Polyarthritis

Cause	Presentation	Physical Findings	Diagnostic Aids	Joint Fluid (see Table 8)	Management
Gonococcal infection	Most common bacterial arthritis; women affected more often than men; history of sexually transmitted disease; often occurs during menses; genitourinary complaints.	Fever in more than 90% of cases, dermatitis (e.g., papules, purpura, vesicles), tenosynovitis in wrists and ankles, joint effusions.	Positive blood culture in less than 10% of cases, positive genital gonococcal culture in 80% of cases.	Purulent (type 4), lactic acid < 50 mg/dl, positive culture in less than 25% of patients; no organisms on Gram stain.	Penicillin (10^7 U/day IV) or ceftriaxone (1 gm every 24 hr), frequent joint aspiration, immobilization.
Rheumatic fever	Follows group A β-hemolytic streptococcal infection; 75% of cases have polyarticular and migratory arthritis; knees and ankles most often affected.	Fever, arthritis pain greater than physical findings, new heart murmur, chorea, erythema marginatum.	Positive streptococcal culture and elevated antistreptolysin-O titer.	Inflammatory (type 2).	Admission for cardiac monitoring, IV antibiotics.
Pseudogout	Patient older than 50 yr; less painful than gout; polyarthritis in more than 50% of cases.	Large joints affected in more than 50% of cases; low-grade fever; red, warm tender joints with effusion.	Elevated white blood cell (WBC) count, elevated erythrocyte sedimentation rate (ESR); radiographs: fine calcium in fibrocartilage in knee, wrist.	Inflammatory (type 2), crystals with weak positive birefringence.	Indomethacin (75–150 mg 4 times/day), phenylbutazone (300–400 mg twice daily for 1 day, then 300 mg 4 times/day).
Rheumatoid arthritis	Females affected more often than males; morning stiffness; knee worse than hands worse than wrists worse than feet.	Rheumatoid nodules, fever, lymphadenopathy in 25% of cases, splenomegaly in Felty's syndrome.	Elevated or decreased WBC, positive rheumatoid factor. Radiographs: subluxation of cervical spine (especially C1–2), periarticular osteoporosis.	Inflammatory (type 2), rheumatoid cells possible.	Salicylates, NSAIDs, rest with therapeutic exercise, splint to immobilize during rest.
Reiter's syndrome	Polyarticular arthritis in more than 90% of cases; most frequent causes of arthritis in young men; urethritis, conjuncitivits.	Keratoderma blennorrhagicum; urethritis appears first; fever, prolonged PR interval on ECG.	Elevated WBC, ESR; radiographs: periostitis and new bone formation, calcaneal spurs, os calcis periostitis.	Inflammatory (type 2).	Splint, salicylates; resolves spontaneously.

Physical Examination and Diagnostic Aids. Examination of a joint begins with a thorough inspection. It is important to note swelling, deformity, asymmetry, skin changes, and evidence of trauma. Particular attention should be paid to evidence of penetrating trauma or signs of overlying infection. Attention also should be paid to involvement of other joints in the body and any pattern of joint involvement that may be present.

Palpation is necessary to identify subtle effusions as well as to determine location and degree of tenderness. Evaluation of active and passive range of motion is necessary and may be helpful in differentiating problems such as bursitis from true articular involvement.

Radiographs may be helpful in diagnosis but often only confirm findings obvious on physical examination. Films typically demonstrate soft tissue swelling and effusion, although may suggest specific causes. Radiographic signs of osteoarthritis include nonuniform joint space narrowing, osteophytes, subchondral sclerosis, and, with advanced disease, bony cysts. Rheumatoid arthritis manifests as uniform joint space narrowing, bony erosions, and loss of periarticular bone density. Gout is rarely associated with the appearance of radiolucent bony tophi near joint spaces. The calcium pyrophosphate crystals associated with pseudogout may be radiopaque and appear as linear deposits within the joint space.

The definitive diagnostic test in the management of the undifferentiated swollen, painful joint is arthrocentesis. If septic arthritis is a possibility, it is necessary to obtain synovial fluid. If the urgent care physician cannot perform this procedure, immediate orthopedic consultation is necessary. Relative contraindications to joint aspiration before orthopedic consultation include overlying cellulitis or involvement of the hip or glenohumeral joint.[7] Arthrocentesis of these joints often requires fluoroscopic guidance. Fluid should be evaluated for gross appearance, culture and sensitivity, Gram stain, cell count and differential, glucose level, and presence of crystals (see Table 12).

Differential Diagnosis. Traumatic causes of joint pain and swelling are typically evident from the history. Patients often complain of an acute injury followed by rapid onset of pain and swelling. Swelling is generally due to hemarthrosis and may be related to associated fractures, ligamentous injuries, cartilaginous injuries, or capsular injuries. Without a history of acute injury, such joints may be clinically indistinguishable from the atraumatic problems listed below.

Infection is not the most common cause of joint pain and swelling but it is probably the most serious. Joints previously affected by trauma or arthritis are more susceptible to sepsis. Also at risk are patients who use intravenous drugs or have indwelling catheters. Various causative organisms have been implicated. The development of severe pain over a period of a few hours is characteristic of gram-positive bacteria such as streptococci and staphylococci. Gram-negative infections tend to develop less rapidly, and are associated with immunosuppressed patients. Gonococcal and meningococcal infections often have unique clinical presentations, involving a prodrome of migratory arthritis. Although much less common, mycobacterial and fungal infections tend to affect immunosuppressed hosts and typically have indolent courses.

Degenerative joint disease (osteoarthritis) is an extremely common cause of painful, swollen joints. The knee, cervical and lumbar spine, MCP, and DIP joints are classically affected. Risk factors include obesity, increased age, and history of severe or chronic articular injury. As suggested by the name, degenerative joint disease typically develops gradually over time, although acute flares often lead to presentation for pain relief.

Rheumatoid arthritis (RA) is a chronic systemic disorder that includes a vast array of clinical problems. The specific cause is uncertain but is thought to involve an autoimmune process. Articular involvement is generally symmetrical, with the wrist, knee, ankle, metatarsophalangeal, MCP, and PIP joints most commonly affected. Women are affected more often than men, with peak incidence in the third and fourth decades of life. RA can involve numerous extra-articular organ systems, including the eyes, skin, vasculature, and pleural and pericardial membranes. A plethora of less-common autoimmune disorders also may present with articular involvement, including systemic lupus erythematosus, ankylosing spondylitis, and progressive systemic sclerosis. Definitive diagnosis of these syndromes is generally impossible in the urgent care setting, although history and physical examination may help identify associated symptoms and signs.

Gout is characterized by elevated blood levels of uric acid and deposits (tophi) of urate crystals in various tissues, usually including the joints. Gout may occur as a primary inherited metabolic disorder or secondary to renal failure, diuretic use, or disease of the bone marrow. Patients are generally at least middle-aged and tend to be male. Acute attacks classically occur at night, involve the first MCP joint (podagra), and are excruciatingly painful.[7] Pain may be progressive, generally with resolution of symptoms in a few days.

Pseudogout (chondrocalcinosis) is another crystalline arthropathy similar to gout, except the crystals are calcium pyrophosphate.[7] Anatomic predilection is one of the few differences in the clinical presentation; pseudogout prefers the knee (gonagra) to the metatarsophalangeal joint. Pseudogout tends to affect elders and to run in families. Patients often have associated diseases, including hyperparathyroidism, hemachromatosis, and gout.

Bursitis, either acute or chronic, can be a source of pain and swelling near a joint. The knee is commonly affected, given the multiple bursae (prepatellar, superficial infrapatellar, deep infrapatellar). Other joints commonly affected include the elbow and shoulder. Inflammation may be secondary to acute trauma or chronic friction. Swelling and pain may be severe, although diagnosis often can be made with physical examination. Bursitis generally should not affect range of motion in contrast to swelling within the joint capsule.

Occasionally, a Baker's cyst may lead to a painful and swollen knee. Chronic inflammatory arthritis (classically RA) can lead to articular fluid dissecting into the potential popliteal space. These fluid collections may persist for a long period and then experience acute rupture, leading to pain. Rupture also may mimic deep venous thrombosis with pain and swelling of the calf.

Management. The primary goal in the acute management of joint pain and swelling is to differentiate between septic arthritis and all other causes. Septic arthritis is a medical emergency. If septic arthritis can be excluded, more specific diagnosis is generally unnecessary because management consists of symptomatic relief in most other cases.

History and physical examination alone are often insufficient to exclude septic arthritis. Acute onset of a painful, warm, swollen joint is consistent with multiple etiologies. A medical history of osteoarthritis or RA may point toward a recurrence, but it is important to remember that previously damaged joints are at increased risk for septic arthritis. Penetrating wounds in proximity to the joint, overlying cellulitis, or associated fevers and chills are especially worrisome and mandate exclusion of infection via arthrocentesis.

Once synovial fluid is obtained, empiric intravenous antibiotics should be started. *Staphylococcus* and *Streptococcus* spp., and *Neisseria gonorrhoeae* are the most common causes of acute bacterial arthritis.[7] Host factors must be considered because the incidence of gram-negative, mycobacterial, and fungal infections is increased in certain populations. Antibiotics can be discontinued or the choices refined once fluid analysis provides definitive diagnosis. If an infectious etiology cannot be ruled out by the initial fluid analysis, admission for continued parenteral antibiosis is recommended.

Acute management of osteoarthritis exacerbations consists mainly of rest, ice or heat, anti-inflammatory medications, and analgesics. Temporary immobilization may be beneficial. Urgent care management of RA should include NSAIDs; aspirin is classically the drug of choice. Intra-articular steroid injections also have been used effectively. Specific pharmacologic therapies for RA tend to be complex and have numerous toxicities; a rheumatologist or primary provider should handle their dispensation in the long-term care of the patient.

Suspicion of autoimmune disease other that RA should prompt symptomatic treatment and referral. Gout and pseudogout flares are best managed with NSAIDs and analgesics. Disease-specific medications for gout depend on the underlying abnormality, which should be determined through further testing by a primary care provider.

Pitfalls in Practice. The primary goal in the approach to the swollen, painful joint must always be exclusion of intraarticular sepsis. History and physical examination may be suggestive, but arthrocentesis is the gold standard in such cases. Once synovial fluid is obtained, empiric antibiotics should be given parenterally until analysis is definitive. Intra-articular injection of a steroid should never be attempted if sepsis is a possibility. Missed diagnosis or improper management of a septic joint can be devastating, leading to joint destruction and severe disability.

References

1. Antosia RE, Lyn E: Knee and lower leg. In Marx JA, Hockberger RS, Walls RM (eds): Rosen's Emergency Medicine Concepts and Clinical Practice, 5th ed. St. Louis, Mosby, 2002, pp 674–706.
2. Meulleman RL: Injuries to the hand and digits. In Tintanelli JE, Kelen GD, Stapczynski SJ (eds): Emergency Medicine: A Comprehensive Study Guide, 5th ed. New York, McGraw-Hill, 2000, pp 1753–1763.
3. Chin HW, Vehara DT: Wrist injuries. In Tintanelli JE, Kelen GD, Stapczynski SJ (eds): Emergency Medicine: A Comprehensive Study Guide, 5th ed. New York, McGraw-Hill, 2000, pp 1772–1783.
4. Ritchie JV, Munter DW: Emergency department evaluation and treatment of wrist injuries. Emer Med Clin North Am 17:823–842, 1999.
5. Wang MM: Acute peripheral neurologic lesions. In Tintanelli JE, Kelen GD, Stapczynski SJ (eds): Emergency Medicine: A Comprehensive Study Guide, 5th ed. New York, McGraw-Hill, 2000, pp 1471–1476.
6. Lester B: Hand infections. In The Acute Hand. Stanford, CT, Appleton & Lange, 1999, pp 409–438.
7. Burton JH: Acute disorders of the joints and bursae. In Tintanelli JE, Kelen GD, Stapczynski SJ (eds): Emergency Medicine: A Comprehensive Study Guide, 5th ed. New York, McGraw-Hill, 2000, pp 1892–1899.

8. Neer CS: Anterior acromioplasty for chronic impingement syndrome in the shoulder. J Bone Joint Surg 54:41–50, 1972.
9. McQuillen KK: Musculoskeletal disorders. In Rosen P, Barkin R (eds): Rosen's Emergency Medicine Concepts and Clinical Practice, 5th ed. St. Louis, Mosby, 2002, pp 2370–2373.
10. Riebel GD, McCabe JB: Anterior shoulder dislocation. Am J Emerg Med 9:180–188, 1991.
11. McKoy BE, Benson CV, Hartstock LA: Fractures about the shoulder. Orthop Clin North Am 31:205–216, 2000.
12. Hannafin JA, Chiaia TA: Adhesive capsulitis. Clin Orthop Rel Res 372:95–109, 2000.
13. Geiderman JM: Humerus and elbow. In Rosen P, Barkin R (eds): Rosen's Emergency Medicine Concepts and Clinical Practice, 5th ed. St. Louis, Mosby, 2002, pp 555–575.
14. Harris IE: Supracondylar fractures of the humerus in children. Orthopedics 15:811–817, 1992.
15. Gutierrez G: Management of radial head fracture. Am Fam Physician 55:2213–2216, 1997.
16. Stiell IG, Wells GA, Hoag RH, Sivilotti ML: Implementation of the Ottawa jbee rules for use of radiography in acute knee injuries. JAMA 278:2075–2079, 1997.
17. Zappala FG, Taffel CB, Senderi GR: Rehabilitation of patellofemoral joint disorders. Orthop Clin North Am 23:555–566, 1992.
18. Barber FA, Sutker AN: Iliotibial band syndrome. Sports Med 14:144–148, 1992.
19. Thompson TC, Doherty DH: Spontaneous rupture of tendon of Achilles: A new clinical diagnostic test. J Trauma 2:126, 1962.
20. Stiell IG: Implementation of the Ottawa ankle rules. JAMA 271:827–832, 1994.
21. Ho K, Abu-Laba RB: Ankle and foot. In Marx JA, Hockberger RS, Walls RM (eds): Emergency Medicine: Concepts and Clinical Practice, 5th ed. St. Louis, Mosby; 2002, pp 706–737.
22. Koval KJ, Sanders R: The radiologic evaluation of calcaneal fractures. Clin Orthop 290:41–46, 1993.
23. Englandoff G, Anglin D, Hutson HR: Lisfrance fracture dislocation: A frequently missed diagnosis in the emergency department. Ann Emerg Med 26:229–233, 1955.

Chapter 10

Ophthalmologic Disorders in the Urgent Care Center

Douglas D. Brunette, MD
Rodney L. Thompson, MD

Ophthalmologic Evaluation

Ophthalmologic diseases constitute an important group of clinical problems encountered in the urgent care setting. The goal of urgent care management is to separate vision-threatening problems that need emergent specialty management from urgent ophthalmologic problems.

Obtaining an accurate history is crucial in the initial diagnosis of ophthalmologic conditions. The chief complaints most frequently presenting to the urgent care setting are pain, redness, loss of vision, or double vision. The onset, nature, and course of the symptoms should be explored in detail. Specific questions should be asked about photophobia, visual loss, diplopia, pain, and discharge. Medication and allergy history should be obtained as well as a complete ophthalmologic and medical history.

Visual acuity is the best single test for evaluation of the eye. Every patient must undergo a careful visual acuity examination that is clearly documented in the medical record. Visual acuity should be tested by both distant (Snellen's chart) and near (pocket chart) methods. The examination should be performed with and without glasses, one eye at a time. If the patient's vision is 20/30 or less in either eye, pinhole vision should be tested. The use of a pinhole helps to correct for any uncorrected refractive errors. When visual loss is severe, the patient should be assessed for the ability to count fingers, recognize hand movements, and perceive light. Visual field testing should be conducted.

Simple inspection is also an important part of any eye examination. The periocular tissues and lids should be inspected for abnormalities. The anterior surface of the sclera and cornea should be examined for conjunctival and surface irregularities. Extraocular movements should be tested in the six cardinal positions of gaze. The anterior chamber and iris are examined for abnormalities such as hyphema or change in shape. Pupillary size, equality, shape, reaction to light, and accommodation are noted. In addition, the swinging flashlight test is invaluable in detecting afferent visual pathway disruption. This test is best conducted in a dimly lit room. The patient is asked to look into the distance, and the examiner shines a flashlight in one eye and then quickly swings it across to the other eye. The light should be alternated from eye to eye every 3 seconds, allowing each pupil to stabilize before the light swings back. In the normal patient, both pupils constrict briefly each time the flashlight is moved, with a subsequent slight oscillation before a stable pupil diameter is established. When an afferent (retinal or optic nerve) defect in one eye is present, both pupils are large when the defective eye is stimulated and small when the normal eye is stimulated.

Direct ophthalmoscopy is an important and sometimes diagnostic portion of the exam. If the proper equipment is available, slit-lamp exam and intraocular pressure (IOP) assessment provide valuable information. Normal IOP is less than 20 mmHg.

Specific Ophthalmologic Problems

Red Eye

Tables 1 and 2 list the major causes of the symptomatic red eye. These disorders must be considered in any patient presenting with conjunctival injection and ocular symptoms, such as pain or change in vision.

Table 1. Differential Diagnosis of the Red Eye

Cause	Presentation	Examination	Etiology and Epidemiology	Therapy	Follow-Up Issues
Conjunctivitis	Onset: gradual Complaints: foreign body sensation, itching (allergic reaction), pain, ocular drainage, eyelid matting in morning; involves one or both eyes	Ocular discharge: purulent Visual acuity: normal Conjunctiva: hyperemic and edematous diffusely Cornea: clear Pupils: normal Intraocular pressure: normal	Etiology: toxins, allergy, virus bacteria Route of spread: direct contact (e.g., finger) Communicability: certain viruses and bacteria highly contagious	Viral: warm compresses 4–6 times/day Bacterial: topical antibiotics, warm compresses 4–6 times/day Hospitalize if gonococcal Allergic: 4% cromolyn sodium 4 times/day	Prophylaxis: contact avoidance, proper hygiene Follow up with ophthalmologist in 3–4 days if not improved
Anterior uveitis	Onset: acute Complaints: ocular pain, photophobia, blurred vision Symptoms are unilateral; no discharge	Visual acuity: normal or slightly decreased Conjunctiva: injected, especially around limbus; ciliary flush appearance Cornea: clear Pupils: miotic, consensual photophobia Anterior chamber: flare present	Etiology: herpes simplex, herpes complex, sarcoidosis, tuberculosis, syphilis, toxoplasmosis, ankylosing spondylitis, ulcerative colitis, post-traumatic iritis, Reiter's syndrome, frequently idiopathic	Cycloplegic agent, oral analgesics as needed, antibiotics Ophthalmologic consultation: ophthalmologists frequently prescribe topical corticosteroids	Post-traumatic iritis seen within 24 hr by specialist All other uveitis seen as soon as possible
Acute glaucoma	Onset: abrupt. Complaints: ocular pain, decreased vision, headache, nausea and vomiting, abdominal pain, halo effect, photophobia	Visual acuity: decreased Conjunctiva: injected diffusely Cornea: cloudy Pupils: midposition and may be fixed	Etiology: narrowed filtration angle with decreased aqueous drainage; generally anatomic predisposition	Topical timolol 0.5% Topical pilocarpine 2% (every 15 min), acetazolamide (500 mg IV), mannitol 20% solution (1 gm/kg IV over 1 hr)	Immediate consultation necessary Definitive treatment is surgical iridotomy
Corneal disease	See Table 2				

Table 2. Corneal Disorders

Disorder	Presentation	Examination	Management	Follow-Up Issues
Corneal foreign body	Onset: acute Complaints: ocular pain, photophobia, foreign body sensation, red eye	Discharge: excess lacrimation Visual acuity: normal Conjunctiva: hyperemic diffusely Cornea: may visualize embedded foreign body Eyelids: blepharospasm	Slit-lamp examination, topical anesthesia, removal of foreign body Postremoval: cycloplegic agent, topical antibiotics, oral analgesics	Tetanus prophylaxis; reexamine daily until healed
Corneal abrasion	Onset: acute Complaints: foreign body sensation, red eye, pain	Discharge: excess lacrimation Visual acuity: normal Conjunctiva: hyperemic diffusely Cornea: defect on slit-lamp examination Eyelids: blepharospasm	Rule out foreign body, especially upper lids; cycloplegic agent; topical antibiotics; oral analgesics If contact lens related, avoid eye patches and cover *Pseudomonas* topically with gentamicin or tobramycin	Tetanus prophylaxis; reexamine daily until healed
Keratitis	Onset: gradual to acute Complaints: variable (pain, red eye)	Discharge: possible lacrimation Visual acuity: normal to decreased Conjunctiva: hyperemic Cornea: epithelial defects	Exposure keratitis: artificial tears eye patch Ultraviolet radiation: treat like corneal abrasion Infectious: topical antibiotics and consult	Follow-up in 24 hr if noninfectious, follow-up with ophthalmologist within 24 hr

Conjunctivitis

Differential Diagnosis. Conjunctivitis, an inflammation of the conjunctiva, is caused by various viral, bacterial, allergic, and toxic agents. The most common cause is viral infection. Causative bacterial organisms include *Streptococcus pneumoniae, Hemophilus aegyptius* and *H. influenzae, Staphylococcus* organisms, and *Neisseria gonorrhoeae.*

Table 1 lists signs and symptoms of conjunctivitis. Bacterial conjunctivitis is associated with a more copious and purulent discharge than viral or allergic conjunctivitis. Conjunctivitis caused by *N. gonorrhoeae* is suspected clinically by noting a copious, thick, and purulent discharge.[2]

Cultures should be obtained when clinical findings are insufficient to diagnose the cause of the inflammation, when previous therapy is ineffective, or when the inflammatory reaction is severe. A Gram stain and culture are needed for any patient with suspected gonococcal conjunctivitis.

Trachoma, an insidious form of *Chlamydia trachomatis* conjunctivitis, waxes and wanes over years. Trachoma is a major cause of blindness around the world. Ophthalmologic referral for extended topical and systemic antibiotic treatment is recommended. Tetracycline and erythromycin, topically and systemically, are the antibiotics of choice.[8]

Management. With the exception of suspected or demonstrated gonococcal conjunctivitis, treatment is usually conducted on an outpatient basis. Patients with suspected or demonstrated gonococcal conjunctivitis should be admitted to the hospital and treated with high-dose systemic penicillin and topical antibiotics because of the aggressive nature of the infection. Other obvious aggressive infections also need specialty consultation. When an allergic etiology is suspected, cromolyn sodium ophthalmic solution (4%), 4 times/day, may provide relief.

Pitfalls in Practice. Failure to recognize an aggressive and invasive infection can result in substantial morbidity. Avoid eye patches, contact lenses and topical steroids. Misdiagnosis of conjunctivitis when glaucoma, uveitis, or corneal disease is actually present can lead to permanent vision loss.

Corneal Disease

Corneal disease is any process that interferes with the primary function of the cornea (ie, providing protection of global contents with a transparent and optically uniform surface). Common causes of corneal functional disruption are listed in Table 2.

Corneal Foreign Bodies. Diagnosis. A corneal foreign body is any foreign material embedded in the superficial or deeper layers of the cornea. Common substances include metal, wood, and glass. Patients may or may not recall the exact moment at which the foreign body was introduced. Signs and symptoms are listed in Table 2. It is important to ask for historical clues that may suggest global penetration of the foreign body, such as the recent use of a high-speed drill, grinder, or sander.

A light shone tangentially on the cornea often reveals the foreign body. Slit-lamp examination is invaluable in both detection and determination of the degree of corneal penetration. Foreign bodies that have penetrated the cornea are surgical emergencies. Clues that the cornea has been perforated include flattening of the anterior chamber, hyphema, herniation of the iris through the injury, or flow of anterior chamber fluid from the injury. Consult an ophthalmologist immediately if cornea perforation is suspected.

Management. Treatment starts with removal of the object. After topical anesthesia is applied, many superficial foreign bodies can be removed with a fine stream of sterile fluid. A moistened cotton swab should not be used because of inadvertent additional corneal abrasion. A 25-gauge needle on a tuberculin syringe can be used in cooperative patients to remove a small superficial corneal foreign body. A "spud" is a surgical instrument ending in a small, flat triangle. When available, spuds are an ideal alternative to sharper needles for foreign body removal. The procedure is best accomplished with the use of a slit lamp. Deep or multiple foreign bodies require ophthalmologic consultation.[3]

Treatment after the foreign body is removed consists of instilling a cycloplegic agent and applying antibiotic ointment. Eye patching is controversial. Most ophthalmologists agree that, in general, eye patches should be avoided. Eye patches increase patient comfort but also increase the risk of infection. Always avoid eye patches in patients who wear contact lenses or have foreign bodies that are soiled or wooden. Reliable patients with large corneal abrasions (> 50%), tremendous discomfort, and a relatively low risk of infection can be managed with eye patching for comfort. Commercially available soft eye pads are used to facilitate eye patching. At least two eye pads are used.[3] The first is folded in half and placed on the patient's closed eyelids. The second, unfolded eye pad is placed on top of the first pad, and both are secured in position by several pieces of cloth adhesive tape. The tape should be fastened securely and directed from the patient's midforehead, across the eye pads, and down onto the ipsilateral facial cheek. Care should be taken to ensure that both eyelids are and will remain closed. Oral analgesics may be needed for comfort. Tetanus vaccination should be provided, when indicated. In general, the physician should discourage eye patching and reserve this treatment for large, painful corneal abrasions in reliable patients requesting an eye patch.

Patients with a corneal foreign body should be reevaluated within 24–48 hours of removal.

Pitfalls in Practice. Central corneal foreign bodies located in the visual axis and those penetrating into deeper layers of the cornea should be removed by a specialist to avoid additional injury. Metallic foreign bodies cause rust rings that form around the object. These rings also must be removed; removal is best accomplished 24–48 hours later, when the surrounding cornea softens and can be removed as a plug with a special drill. Do not prescribe corneal topical anesthetics because repeated dosing delays corneal healing.[3]

Corneal Abrasions. Diagnosis. Corneal abrasions are focal defects in the corneal epithelium. They are most often associated with contact lens misuse, foreign bodies, or trauma. The signs and symptoms of corneal abrasions are described in Table 2. Patients present in various degrees of distress. Often, because of the pain and accompanying blepharospasm, it may be difficult to examine the eye adequately. Topical corneal anesthesia facilitates examination. The corneal defect is best seen on slit-lamp examination with the cobalt blue filter after fluorescein dye has been applied.[3] If a slit lamp is not available, a Wood's lamp can be used after fluorescein staining of the cornea. In all patients with a corneal abrasion, a careful search for a foreign body must be undertaken, including eversion of the eyelids.

Management. The therapy for corneal abrasions is the same as that after removal of a corneal foreign body (see Table 2).

Pitfalls in Practice. Any corneal abrasion that involves more than 50% of the corneal surface must be evaluated by an ophthalmologist. Such lesions have a great tendency for significant complications, including delayed healing, infection, and scarring. A corneal foreign body that is missed on initial examination can continue to abrade the corneal surface. The importance of a thorough examination for foreign bodies in patients with corneal abrasions or foreign body sensation cannot be overemphasized.

Keratitis. Diagnosis. Keratitis is any inflammation of the corneal epithelium. Noninfectious causes include exposure, ultraviolet radiation, and keratoconjunctivitis sicca. The keratitis seen with Bell's palsy (exposure) and keratoconjunctivitis sicca are similar in appearance, resulting generally from local desiccation. Sources of ultraviolet radiation-induced keratitis include the sun, welding arcs, and tanning lamps. Infectious causes of keratitis are numerous and include bacterial, herpes simplex, herpes zoster, adenoviral, chlamydial, and fungal infection.

The signs and symptoms of keratitis are presented in Table 2. Because of the large number of causes of keratitis, the historical presentation may differ greatly from patient to patient. Slit-lamp examination reveals the diagnosis in most cases. The lesions range from punctate epithelial defects to large ulcerations. Certain etiologies have fairly specific characteristics. Diffuse punctate epithelial lesions are commonly seen in exposure keratitis, ultraviolet radiation-induced keratitis, and virally induced keratitis. Frank ulceration is seen in bacterial and fungal infection. Both herpes simplex and herpes zoster can present with frank ulceration or the characteristic dendritic lesion. Patients with herpes zoster typically have facial skin involvement, which suggests the diagnosis.

Management. The management of keratitis is described in Table 2.

Pitfalls in Practice. The major danger is misdiagnosis. Because keratitis has many causes and many possible manifestations, a conservative approach is best. Any patient who presents with keratitis that is not fully explained by a noninfectious cause should be evaluated by an ophthalmologist as soon as possible. In addition, any patient with frank ulceration of the cornea needs immediate referral. Patients with herpes simplex or herpes zoster infection need immediate ophthalmologic referral for definitive therapy.

Uveitis

Diagnosis. Uveitis is any inflammatory process involving the uveal tract. The uveal tract is the middle layer of the eye, including the choroid and ciliary body posteriorly and the iris anteriorly. Uveitis can be divided into posterior or anterior types, depending on the focus of inflammation.[4] Anterior uveitis or iritis produces redness and pain, whereas posterior uveitis does not. Table 1 lists the various causes as well as the signs and symptoms of uveitis.

The conjunctival injection is greatest immediately adjacent to the limbus, giving the typical ciliary flush appearance. In using the slit lamp, the beam of light should be reduced vertically and horizontally to form a narrow point of light and shone through the anterior chamber at an acute angle to facilitate viewing of the flare effect. The numerous cells in the anterior chamber that are present as a result of the inflammatory process cause the beam of light to be visualized as it courses through the anterior chamber. The flare effect is like the effect seen when a flashlight beam is projected through a dusty and completely darkened room. Consensual photophobia (discomfort when a light is shown on the contralateral pupil) is another suggestive physical exam finding.

Management. Symptomatic treatment consists of cycloplegic medication for pain relief and prevention of posterior synechiae formation. The need for further therapy, such as antibiotics or corticosteroids, should be determined by a specialist. Patients with posttraumatic iritis should be seen by an ophthalmologist within 24 hours after urgent care evaluation and treatment. Iritis that is not clearly related to trauma should be evaluated by an ophthalmologist as soon as possible.

Pitfalls in Practice. Posttraumatic iritis is the only form of anterior iritis that can be initially managed by a nonophthalmologist. The consequence of missing another form of uveitis may be significant visual loss. Misdiagnosis of uveitis as conjunctivitis is common. Consensual photophobia, pain unrelieved by topical anesthetics, anterior chamber cells, and ciliary flush favor a diagnosis of uveitis.

Acute Glaucoma

Diagnosis. Acute glaucoma is a sudden increase in intraocular pressure. It is usually caused by closure of the filtration angle in the anterior chamber in patients at risk because of an anatomically narrow angle. Once this filtration angle is closed, drainage of the aqueous humor is markedly decreased, leading to an increase in intraocular pressure. The signs and symptoms of acute glaucoma are presented in Table 1.

The increase in intraocular pressure, when severe, can be palpated digitally. Tonometry with either a Schiotz tonometer or a tonopen is diagnostic. The cornea and conjunctiva should be anesthetized with a topical anesthetic (proparacaine 0.5%) prior to tonometry. Intraocular pressures in acute glaucoma are generally greater than 40 mmHg. If a 5.0- or

7.5-gm weight is used on the Schiotz tonometer in a patient with an intraocular pressure above 40 mmHg, the reading is zero. The tonopen displays the average of three tonometry readings. Normal intraocular pressures are less than 20 mmHg.

Management. The immediate therapy is aimed at decreasing intraocular pressure as quickly as possible. Definitive management is listed in Table 1. Immediate ophthalmologic consultation is needed for further medical therapy and consideration of an emergent iridotomy.

Pitfalls in Practice. Misdiagnosis of acute glaucoma occurs frequently because of the occasional dramatic systemic or referred complaints, such as headache and chest or abdominal pain. A second concern is the administration of several dehydrating agents; care must be taken to ensure against significant iatrogenic hypovolemia. The main consequence of untreated acute glaucoma is vision loss. Be vigilant for adverse systemic effects of timolol in patients with asthma or CHF.

Eye Trauma

The categories of trauma include chemical burns, intraocular foreign bodies, optic nerve injury and contusion injuries to the anterior segment.

Chemical Burns

Diagnosis. Chemical burns cause injury to the eye as a result of direct contact of tissues with caustic substances. Acid burns, as from battery acid, are commonly encountered injuries. Acids cause damage in the first few minutes to hours. Acidic substances coagulate the superficial proteins of the eye, which in turn limits the amount of penetration and deep injury. Alkali burns, as from lye, are more severe than acidic burns because they rapidly penetrate the cornea and anterior chamber, causing extensive damage. In addition, tissue destruction may continue for days as a result of retention of the basic compounds within the tissues. Mace burns are fairly common. In general, they do not result in major injury or complication.

Chemical burns are the most urgent of ophthalmologic conditions and require immediate therapy. Often, immediate therapy precedes complete history taking. It is important to ascertain the chemical involved to judge the seriousness of the accident. Injuries can be initially classified as mild, moderate, or severe, depending on the degree of corneal opacity and blanching of the sclera (white eye).

Management. Immediate therapy includes manual separation of the lids and copious irrigation with any readily available source of water (e.g., shower, drinking fountain, hose, bathtub). This irrigation should last at least 10 minutes, at which time the patient should be taken immediately to a medical care facility. The patient then should have instillation of a topical anesthetic solution and undergo irrigation with 2 L of normal saline over 1 hour. Application of the topical anesthetic may be repeated every 20 minutes as necessary. Any particulate matter should be removed from the fornices by a cotton swab. Irrigation should be continued until the pH of the tears is 7.3–7.7.[5] Once a normal pH is obtained, it needs to be rechecked 5, 15, and 60 minutes after irrigation. An ophthalmologist should be contacted as soon as possible for all significant chemical burns. Minor corneal injuries from chemical exposure can be handled in the same manner as corneal abrasions.

Mace burns generally do not result in major injury or complication, but there have been case reports of permanent loss of vision. Therefore, these injuries should be treated similarly to other chemical burns.[5]

For apparently minor chemical injuries a physical examination must be done before the patient is discharged, including visual acuity and slit-lamp examination. Often a corneal abrasion is present.

Pitfalls in Practice. The need for rapid treatment for significant chemical injuries cannot be overemphasized, and the immediate treatment should precede most of the history taking and physical examination. Adequate irrigation of alkali burns may take as long as 24 hours.

Optic Nerve Injury

Diagnosis. Optic nerve injury may occur if the optic nerve is impinged by bony fragments, the vascular supply is jeopardized, or excessive traction occurs. Suspicion is warranted after blunt or penetrating trauma, in patients with an afferent pupil defect, decreased visual acuity, or decreased color sensation.

Management. Consult an ophthalmologist for suspected nerve injury or diminished visual acuity after blunt trauma. High-dose steroids may be beneficial in optic nerve injury. Surgical interventions may be indicated if structural abnormalities are impinging the optic nerve.

Pitfalls in Practice. Always consider significant globe and optic nerve injury when victims of trauma report visual abnormalities.

Globe Perforation or Intraocular Foreign Body

Diagnosis. Globe perforation can occur with penetrating or blunt trauma to the eye and causes disruption of the integrity of the anterior or posterior chamber of the eye (or both). Most often the patient presents with an accurate and obvious history revealing the diagnosis. Certain injuries can be historically subtle, however, such as high-speed grinding or drill-related accidents. Patients can present with various complaints, depending on the degree of damage already incurred. Pain, decreased vision, and foreign body sensation are the most common presentations.

Signs suggestive of globe perforation include decreased visual acuity, decreased intraocular pressure, flattening of the anterior chamber, alteration in pupil size or shape (teardrop sign), obvious corneal or scleral laceration, prolapse of intraocular contents, marked conjunctival edema, subconjunctival hematoma, hyphema, and vitreous hemorrhage.

Intraocular foreign bodies can sometimes be located by orbital radiography, ophthalmoscopy, and slit-lamp examination.

Management. Emergency treatment includes avoiding manipulation of periocular tissues, covering both eyes with a metal or plastic shield to minimize global movements, and ophthalmologic consultation. Care should be taken to avoid any increase in global pressure or movement. Any nausea or vomiting should be suppressed by immediate administration of an antiemetic, and the patient may be given a sedative or analgesic as needed. Tetanus prophylaxis (if needed) and parenteral antibiotics should be given. Any patient suspected of having a globe perforation on the basis of either history or physical examination must be evaluated immediately by an ophthalmologist.

Pitfalls in Practice. No medications should be placed in the eye except by an ophthalmologist. Globe perforation may be present despite an entirely normal examination.

Anterior Segment Injury

Direct blows to the orbit can produce hyphema, traumatic pupillary mydriasis or miosis, dislocated lens, or subconjunctival hemorrhage.

Hyphema. Diagnosis. Hyphema is blood in the anterior chamber. Patients generally present with a history of receiving a blunt blow to the orbit. The anterior chamber may be completely filled with blood or partially filled and layered in the inferior portion. Direct inspection generally reveals the diagnosis.[6]

Management. Treatment traditionally includes hospitalization and bed rest with sedation, as needed. The use of eye patches, cycloplegic agents, and steroids is controversial. Approximately 20% of patients bleed again between hospital days 3 and 5.[5] Complications include blood staining of the cornea with opacification, which requires months or years to clear. Glaucoma may develop if anterior chamber outflow is inadequate. Immediate ophthalmologic consultation is required once the diagnosis has been made. Small hyphemas are sometimes managed on an outpatient basis, but this decision should be made by an ophthalmologist.

Pitfalls in Practice. Blood in the anterior chamber settles into a layer over time. If the eye is examined shortly after injury, the blood may be dispersed throughout the aqueous humor. Slit-lamp examination may be necessary to appreciate the hyphema. Avoid NSAIDs and aspirin to limit the risk of rebleeding.

Traumatic Mydriasis or Miosis. Diagnosis. Abnormal mydriasis (dilated pupil) or miosis (constricted pupil) may be present immediately after blunt trauma to the eye. If no globe perforation or neurologic deficits exist, the deformity may be attributed to mechanical dysfunction of the iris sphincter. Traumatic mydriasis or miosis should be distinguished from an afferent pupillary defect by normal consensual constriction with the swinging flashlight test.

Management. The condition may be transient or permanent. No specific therapy is needed.

Pitfalls in Practice. A dilated pupil can cause acute glaucoma in susceptible patients. The patient should be instructed to return immediately in the event of increased pain or decreased vision in the eye. The eye should be reexamined within 24 hours in any case.

Dislocated Lens. Diagnosis. A dislocated lens is caused by disruption of the zonular fibers that attach the lens to the ciliary body. If more than 25% of these fibers are damaged, subluxation can occur. Iridodonesis (tremulousness of the iris) is seen when the eyes are moved back and forth. This injury is more common in patients with Marfan's syndrome or rheumatoid arthritis.

Management. Unless secondary glaucoma develops as a result of pupillary block, a dislocated lens does not require immediate therapy. Ophthalmologic consultation is nonetheless needed on diagnosis.

Pitfalls in Practice. A dislocated lens will not be identified unless a thorough examination is performed. If thorough examination is not possible because of severe swelling of the periorbital tissues, timely ophthalmologic consultation is advisable.

Subconjunctival Hemorrhage. Diagnosis. Subconjunctival hemorrhage occurs spontaneously or traumatically, appearing as a flat, deep, red hemorrhage beneath the conjunctiva. If enough blood is present, chemosis with a "bag of blood" appearance inferiorly may be present.

Management. Treatment is conservative, with reassurance to the patient that the blood will clear in 2–3 weeks

Pitfalls in Practice. Serious ocular injuries may be accompanied by subconjunctival hemorrhage. A thorough examination must be performed on patients with subconjunctival hemorrhage.

Sudden Visual Loss

There are a number of causes for a sudden loss of vision (Table 3, next page). In general, the more acute the onset of decreased visual acuity and the worse the visual acuity, the more urgent the problem. It is quite important to distinguish a decrease in vision that actually just occurred from a decrease in visual acuity that in reality occurred some time ago but has just been recognized by the patient. It is essential to assess and document visual acuity, visual fields, and afferent pupillary response in all patients reporting visual changes.

Central Retinal Artery Occlusion

Diagnosis. Central retinal artery occlusion results from rapid occlusion of the central retinal artery and represents an ischemic stroke of the retinal tissue. Atherosclerosis or embolization is the most common cause. Table 3 lists the signs and symptoms of central retinal artery occlusion. The cherry red spot at the fovea represents an unaffected choroidal blood supply (Fig. 1).

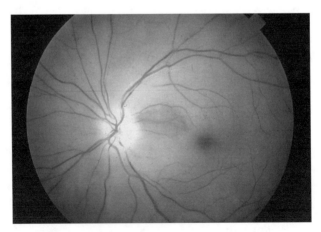

Figure 1. Typical appearance of a central retinal artery occlusion. Note the ischemic retinal whitening with cherry-red spot. (From Vander JF, Gault JA (eds): Ophthalmology Secrets, 2nd ed. Philadelphia, Hanley & Belfus, 2002, with permission.)

Management. The mainstays of therapy are aimed at dislodging or dissolving the clot, dilating the artery to promote blood flow, and reducing intraocular pressure to allow an increase in the perfusion gradient. Initial therapy, as described in Table 3, should be

Table 3. Sudden Visual Loss

Cause	Presentation	Examination	Treatment
Central retinal artery occlusion	Onset: sudden Complaint: painless visual loss	Discharge: none Visual acuity: decreased Conjunctiva: normal Cornea: normal Pupils: dilated on affected side Retina: cherry red fundus Retinal arteriole "boxcarring"	Digital massage of globe, inhalation of 5% carbon dioxide or paper bag rebreathing, immediate ophthalmologic consultation, oral glycerol, timolol maleate 0.5%, acetazolamide (500 mg IV), possible anticoagulation
Central retinal vein occlusion	Onset: acute Complaint: decreased vision	Discharge: none Visual acuity: decreased Conjunctiva: normal Cornea: normal Pupils: normal Retina: venous enlargement, tortuosity, hemorrhages	Immediate ophthalmologic consultation
Temporal arteritis	Onset: acute Complaints: headache, jaw pain, fever, decrease of vision, scalp pain, polymyalgia rheumatica	Discharge: none Visual acuity: decreased Conjunctiva: normal Pupils: afferent defect Retina: pale; swollen disc	Immediate ophthalmologic consultation, high-dose systemic corticosteroids
Vitreous hemorrhage	Onset: sudden Complaint: decrease vision without pain	Discharge: none Visual acuity: decreased Conjunctiva: normal Pupils: Possible afferent defect Retina: reddish haze in posterior chamber obscuring the retina	Ophthalmologic consultation as soon as possible
Retinal detachment	Onset: acute Complaint: flashes of light with subsequent decrease in vision, "black curtain" across visual field, floaters.	Discharge: none Visual acuity: decreased to normal Conjunctiva: normal Pupils: possible afferent defect Retina: possible grayish elevation on retina.	Follow-up with ophthalmologist arranged
CMV retinitis	Onset: acute to subacute Complaint: scotoma, painless visual loss, blind spots	Discharge: none Visual acuity: decreased to normal Conjunctiva: normal Cornea: normal Pupils: possible afferent defect Retina: white patches with or without adjacent hemorrhage	Antivirals with prompt ophthalmologic follow-up

started before consultation with an ophthalmologist. Additional therapy may be requested by the ophthalmologist, and patients should be transferred emergently to the care of an ophthalmologist.

Pitfalls in Practice. This is an ophthalmologic emergency that needs prompt recognition and treatment if there is to be any salvage of vision. The diagnosis needs to be entertained in any patient who presents with a sudden loss of vision.

Central Retinal Vein Occlusion

Diagnosis. Central retinal vein occlusion results from sudden obstruction of the central retinal vein. It most often occurs in patients with hypertension, diabetes mellitus, or glaucoma. The signs and symptoms of central retinal vein occlusion are presented in

Table 3. The historical presentation can vary widely, depending on the degree of obstruction. In the most severe cases, vision can deteriorate to recognition of hand movement only. Severe retinal changes induced by uncontrolled hypertension or diabetes mellitus can appear funduscopically similar. A key point in the appropriate diagnosis is comparing the results of both the funduscopic and the visual acuity examinations of each eye.

Management. No medical therapy has been shown to be useful in reversing existing retinal damage. Any patient suspected of having central retinal vein occlusion should be seen immediately by an ophthalmologist.

Pitfalls in Practice. Inadequate funduscopic examination is the usual cause of misdiagnosis.

Temporal Arteritis

Diagnosis. Temporal arteritis is an idiopathic inflammation of the temporal and ophthalmic arteries. The signs and symptoms of temporal arteritis are presented in Table 3. The disease usually occurs in patients older than 50 years. One-third of patients develop severe visual loss if untreated, and loss of vision is frequently abrupt. One eye is affected first, but the second eye becomes involved in a high percentage of cases within hours to days.[7] The erythrocyte sedimentation rate (ESR) is greater than 50 mm/min in 90% of patients and is frequently much higher. C-reactive protein (CRP) also is elevated. The definitive diagnosis can be made with a temporal artery biopsy.

Management. An immediate specialty consultation is mandatory when temporal arteritis is suspected. If the history, physical examination, and ESR point toward the diagnosis, therapy should be started before a temporal artery biopsy is performed. Early administration of high-dose corticosteroids is of great benefit. The route and amount of the dose should be determined by the specialist. Recovery of lost vision is rare, but treatment prevents progression of visual loss, especially in the second eye.

Pitfalls in Practice. Temporal arteritis is an ophthalmologic emergency. Failure to recognize the disease and to institute therapy with high-dose corticosteroids can result in further visual loss.

Vitreous Hemorrhage

Diagnosis. Vitreous hemorrhage is any acute bleeding into the posterior chamber of the eye. The most common cause of vitreous hemorrhage is diabetic retinopathy. Other causes include trauma, previous vascular occlusion, sickle cell disease, retinal detachment, and hypertensive retinopathy. The signs and symptoms are presented in Table 3.

Management. Treatment consists initially of bed rest. Ultrasonography is used to determine whether the retina is attached. Further therapy depends on the cause of the hemorrhage and may consist of vitrectomy, retinal surgery, or photocoagulation. Any patient with vitreous hemorrhage should undergo specialty consultation as soon as possible.

Pitfalls in Practice. Prompt diagnosis is important because surgical therapy may be warranted.

Retinal Detachment

Diagnosis. Retinal detachment is a separation of the two layers of cells of the retina. There are many causes of retinal detachment. Primary retinal detachments are caused by posterior vitreous detachment and trauma-related injuries. Secondary retinal detachments can result from numerous diseases, including hypertension, glomerulonephritis, diabetes, and vasculitis. The signs and symptoms of retinal detachment are listed in Table 3. Large retinal detachments are clearly visible with direct ophthalmoscopy, but small, peripherally located defects require the use of indirect ophthalmoscopy. A bulging, folding, and discolored retina with serpentine arterioles and venules is diagnostic.

Management. Retinal detachment is an ophthalmologic emergency warranting immediate consultation. A variety of surgical options exist.

Pitfalls in Practice. Frequently, retinal detachment is not seen with routine direct ophthalmoscopy. Patients suspected of having a retinal detachment on historical grounds should be referred to an ophthalmologist.

Cytomegalovirus Retinitis

Diagnosis. Cytomegalovirus (CMV) retinitis afflicts immunocompromised people. The diagnosis should be suspected with rapid progression of visual symptoms in susceptible patients.

Management. Antivirals and prompt ophthalmologic referral are indicated.

Pitfalls in Practice. CMV retinitis is a common infection in patients with AIDS. Clinicians should consider this diagnosis and have a low threshold for treatment. Once CMV retinitis is diagnosed in an AIDS patient, lifetime suppressive therapy is indicated.

Neuro-ophthalmologic Visual Loss

Diagnosis. Neuro-ophthalmologic visual loss is caused by lesions posterior to the retina and can be divided anatomically into three groups (prechiasmal, chiasmal, postchiasmal). Common causes of prechiasmal visual loss include optic neuritis and optic neuropathy (ischemic, compressive, toxic, and metabolic). The most common cause of chiasmal visual loss is tumor, specifically pituitary tumor, craniopharyngioma, and meningioma. Common causes of postchiasmal visual loss include infarction, tumor, arteriovenous malformation, and migraine disorders.

Neuro-ophthalmologic visual loss often presents as poor visual acuity without an obvious precipitating cause. A careful visual acuity and visual field examination will reveal the presence of most significant lesions. **Prechiasmal** visual loss presents as decreased visual acuity that is uncorrected with pinhole testing. The swinging flashlight test reveals an afferent pupillary defect. Visual field testing by confrontation methods reveals a nonhemianopic defect. Visual field testing is crucial in the proper diagnosis of **chiasmal** visual loss. The classic visual field loss is bitemporal hemianopsia. If the visual field loss respects the vertical meridian, chances are excellent that the lesion is chiasmal or postchiasmal. Patients with **postchiasmal** lesions generally present with normal visual acuity, but careful visual field testing reveals a defect that respects the vertical meridian, classically a homonymous hemianopsia.

Management. Neurologic visual loss is treated by the ophthalmologist and often by the neurosurgeon or neurologist, depending on the cause of the lesion. Immediate consultation with the specialist is needed.

Pitfalls in Practice. Neuro-ophthalmologic visual loss can be subtle in presentation and thus easily missed if a careful examination is not performed. Patients are frequently aware of problems only in the eye experiencing temporal field deficits.

Complications of Ophthalmologic Surgery

Diagnosis. The urgent care physician may encounter patients with ophthalmologic complaints after recent or distant surgical interventions.

Management. Each surgical procedure has a different set of possible complications. It is important to have a low threshold for consultation with the surgeon. Any procedure involving the vitreous chamber places the patient at some risk for endophthalmitis. Endophthalmitis occurs when the vitreous chamber is infected, and presents with scleral erythema, pain, hypopyon (leukocytes in the anterior chamber), and diminished visual acuity. Systemic and topical antibiotics are indicated. Endophthalmitis is an ophthalmologic emergency requiring immediate ophthalmologic consultation. In rare cases, it can complicate cataract surgery.

Laser in situ keratomileusis (LASIK surgery) is a popular keratorefractive surgical technique to improve vision. The procedure is generally well tolerated. Abruptly decreased visual acuity and ocular pain after the procedure can result from a slipped flap of corneal tissue. This complication can occur after minor trauma 24 hours to several months postoperatively.

Pitfalls in Practice. The urgent care physician should consult the appropriate ophthalmologic surgeon whenever a postoperative complication is suspected.

Eyelid Problems

Hordeolum

Diagnosis. Hordeolum is a localized acute infection of one of the eyelids that is generally due to staphylococci. External hordeolum perforates anteriorly through the skin, and internal hordeolum perforates posteriorly through the conjunctiva. Patients complain of tenderness of the lid. Physical examination reveals diffuse lid swelling and erythema during the initial stages with a subsequent red, indurated area that usually ruptures spontaneously.

Management. Treatment consists of warm compresses applied for 15 minutes 4–6 times/day. Topical antibiotic drops or ointment may be used. All patients should have ophthalmologic follow-up in 1 week.

Dacrocystitis

Diagnosis. Dacrocystitis is an acute bacterial infection of the lacrimal sac causing local induration and purulent drainage. Causative agents include *Streptococcus pneumoniae*, *Staphylococcus aureus*, and *Hemophilus influenzae*. Purulent drainage from the puncta may aid diagnosis.

Management. Warm compresses with topical and oral antibiotics covering *Staphylococcus aureus* are advised. Gram stain and culture should be obtained. Ophthalmologic referral is indicated.

Chalazion

Diagnosis. A chalazion is a chronic inflammatory process involving one of the lids. The patient complains of a nontender, slowly growing, firm nodule in the lid.

Management. Treatment is the same as for hordeolum. Nodules can be excised if bothersome symptoms persist.

Pitfalls in Practice. Hordeolum, dacrocystitis, and chalazion are confined to the lids and must be differentiated from orbital cellulitis. Orbital cellulitis is a serious infection involving the soft tissues of the orbit (see Chapter 12).

Eyelid Lacerations

Diagnosis. It is essential to assess which structures are involved by thorough examination.

Management. Suspected involvement of the globe, levator muscle, nasolacrimal system, or eyelid margin should prompt immediate ophthalmologic referral. A simple laceration without involvement of these structures can be closed primarily with careful attention to cosmesis. Nasolacrimal involvement can be assessed by injecting fluorescein into the punctum with a blunt canula and inspecting for fluorescein drainage from the wound.

Pitfalls in Practice. Failure to recognize injury to the globe or other ocular structures may result in permanent deficit.

Ophthalmologic Medications

Anesthetics

Topical anesthetics are necessary for urgent evaluation of ophthalmologic problems. Topical anesthetics should not be prescribed for home use, however, because of masking of symptoms, delayed healing of a corneal abrasion, loss of the protective blink reflex, and hypersensitivity reactions causing iritis.

Proparacaine hydrochloride (0.5%) is an excellent choice of topical anesthetic. Two drops produce adequate anesthesia to eliminate blepharospasm, facilitating complete examination and even procedures such as corneal foreign body removal. Duration of action is generally less than 30 minutes. Allergic reactions are rare.

Steroids

Prescribing steroids should be left to the ophthalmologist. Topical steroids have many ophthalmologic complications that can be quite serious, including secondary bacterial infection, masking of serious underlying disorders, exacerbation or reactivation of herpes simplex infection, increasing intraocular pressure, and formation of cataracts. Many combination drugs, such as antibiotics and steroids, are available. Nonophthalmologists should be careful not to prescribe such a combination inadvertently.

Nonsteroidal Anti-inflammatory Drugs

Ketorolac tromethamine 0.5% ophthalmic solution, 2 drops 4 times/day, is highly effective therapy for allergic conjunctivitis.[11] Ketorolac is also useful in the treatment of discomfort related to corneal abrasions. NSAID ophthalmologic drops are generally well tolerated without apparent side effects.

Cycloplegics

Cycloplegics are useful for allowing complete examination of the fundus as well as for treatment of many ophthalmologic conditions. One must exercise caution in dilating the pupils of any patient with a history of angle closure glaucoma or an intraocular lens implant.

Homatropine hydrobromide (5%) has a duration of action of about 6 hours, and tropicamide (1.0%) has a duration of action of 1–2 hours. Duration, however, is quite variable.

Antibiotics

Topical ophthalmologic antibiotics are used to treat various conditions. The urgent care physician uses this class of drugs for minor infectious conditions such as conjunctivitis and for prophylaxis against infection in treating corneal abrasions. All serious ophthalmologic infections, such as corneal ulcers, need to be handled by an ophthalmologist. Sulfacetamide sodium, polymyxin, polytrim, gentamicin, and tobramycin are the commonly used topical ophthalmologic antibiotics for superficial ocular infectious processes.

References

1. Weinstein IM, Zweifel TJ, Thompson HS: The clinical diagnosis of pupil disorders. J Clin Exp Ophthalrnol 41:1–26, 1979.
2. Howes DS: The red eye. In Mathews J, Zun LS (eds): Emergency Medicine Clinics of North America. Philadelphia, W.B. Saunders, 1988, pp 43–56.
3. Samples JR, Hedges JR: Ophthalmologic procedures. In Roberts JR, Hedges JR (eds): Clinical Procedures in Emergency Medicine, 3rd ed. Philadelphia, W.B. Saunders, 1998, pp 1089–1118.
4. Tessler HH: Uveitis. In Callaham ML (ed): Current Practice of Emergency Medicine, 2nd ed. Philadelphia, B.C. Decker; 1991, pp 282–285.
5. Pavan-Langston D: Burns and trauma. In Pavan-Langston D (ed): Manual of Ocular Diagnosis and Therapy. Boston, Little, Brown, 1980, pp 31–46.
6. Brunette DD, Ghezzi KT, Renner GS: Ophthalmologic disorders. In Rosen P, Barkin R, et al (eds): Emergency Medicine: Concepts and Clinical Practice, 4th ed. St. Louis, Mosby, 1998, pp 2698–2719.
7. Keltner JL: Giant-cell arteritis. Ophthalmology 89:1101–1110, 1982.
8. Newell FW: Ophthalmology: Principles and Concepts, 8th ed. St Louis, Mosby, 1996, pp 233–254.
9. Seiff SR: High dose corticosteroids for treatment of vision loss due to indirect injury to the optic nerve. Ophthalmol Surg 21:389–394, 1990.
10. Scott JL, Ghezzi KT (eds): Emergency Medicine Clinics of North America. Philadelphia, W.B. Saunders; 1995, pp 521–581.
11. Schultz N, et al: Double-masked paired-comparison clinical study of ketorolac tromethamine 0.5% ophthalmologic solution compared with placebo eyedrops in the treatment of seasonal allergic conjunctivitis. Surv Ophthalmol 38:133–139, 1993.

Chapter 11

Urgencies of the Ears

Cheryl Adkinson, MD
Mitchell Palmer, MD

Otologic Examination

Diseases of the ear account for a significant number of urgent care visits. The tasks of the urgent care physician are to diagnose and treat appropriately processes that are amenable to simple work-up and outpatient therapy and to identify the patient with serious disease requiring hospitalization or prompt specialty consultation.

The basic otologic history should include the nature, onset, duration, and severity of otologic symptoms as well as any associated illness or symptoms. Toxic or traumatic exposure, drug ingestion, and medication use should be included. Past surgical and medical history is frequently pertinent, as is family history of otologic and neurologic disease.

Examination of the patient with an ear complaint should include inspection of the nose, paranasal sinuses, oral structures, and pharynx. Examination of the neck for masses, adenopathy, and bruits should be performed as well as palpation of the mandible, maxilla, and temporomandibular joint (TMJ). Cranial nerves should be tested and spontaneous nystagmus sought. Examination of the ear itself includes a crude test of hearing such as the ability to hear a normal voice, whisper, or finger rubbing. The preauricular and postauricular areas, auricle, and external auditory canal (EAC) should be inspected. Careful removal of cerumen may be necessary for adequate visualization of the EAC and tympanic membrane (TM). The TM should be examined for perforations, granulomas, tumors, and inflammation. TM mobility should be tested with a pneumatic otoscope. If hearing is subjectively or objectively impaired, Weber's and Rinne tuning fork tests should be performed.

Specific Otologic Problems

Ear Pain

Patients with ear pain commonly present to the urgent care setting. Careful examination of the ear reveals the inciting cause in most cases. Most frequently the problem is inflammatory, as in external otitis, otitis media, or bullous myringitis. It is important to review vital signs and to assess for systemic toxicity even when the painful process can be easily identified.

Differential Diagnosis. History and physical examination generally localize the problem to either the external or middle ear. Pain on touching or manipulation of the pinna or tragus points to a problem of the external ear, including the EAC, whereas shooting or aching pain deep in the ear suggests a middle ear process. Signs, symptoms, and treatment recommendations for the more common painful diseases of the external ear are detailed in Table 1. Signs, symptoms, and treatment for the more common painful diseases of the middle ear are noted in Table 2.

In some cases, however, the ear examination is normal despite the patient's complaint of ear pain. In this case, disorders of any region supplied by cranial nerves V, VII, IX, or X or the second or third cervical nerves must be considered, because pain from these areas may be referred to the ear. Careful examination of the nose, face, oropharynx, and neck must be undertaken. Causes of ear pain in the presence of a normal ear examination include arthralgia, dental disease (impacted teeth, caries, abscesses), sinusitis, pharyngitis, laryngeal and pharyngeal tumors, neuralgias (glossopharyngeal, sphenopalatine, trigeminal), and deep space infections of the neck. One of the most common etiologies of pain referred to the ear is TMJ arthralgia or TMJ syndrome. Characteristics and treatment of this disorder are noted in Table 3.

Table 1. Painful Diseases of the External Ear *(Columns continue on next page)*

Etiology	Pathology	Presentation
Swimmer's ear	Diffuse inflammation of EAC; *Pseudomonas aeruginosa* or *Staphylococcus* organisms	Moderate-to-severe pain, progressive over a few hours, frequently initiated by moisture.
Impetigo	Inflammation of auricle: usually *S. aureus*	Serum-filled vesicles on erythematous base, amber crusts; common in young children; other sites involved; mildly painful
Fungal infection	Inflammation of EAC; *Candida albicans*, *Aspergillus niger*, yeast-like fungi	Moderate-to-severe pain
Erysipelas	Streptococcal infection of skin	Intense erythema, edema of pinna, extension to face, well-defined edge; systemic illness with fever, tachycardia
Malignant external otitis	*P. aeruginosa*	Serious infection with high mortality; elderly diabetic and immunocompromised patients; insidious onset; progressive pain and purulent drainage from EAC; infection spreads to deep tissues
Furuncle of EAC	Staphylococcal infection	Marked pain out of proportion to size of furuncle in EAC
Perichondritis	Infection of perichondrium with pus forming between it and cartilage of auricle; usually P aeruginosa	Follows trauma, surgery, burns, frostbite; red and tender, then swollen, then subperichondrial abscess formation

There is no substitute for careful visualization of the external ear, EAC, and TM and gentle palpation of the pinna and mastoid in the diagnosis of the painful ear. Pneumatic otoscopy is essential for the accurate diagnosis of middle ear infection. Indirect laryngoscopy and nasopharyngoscopy are useful in the examination of the patient with no apparent ear pathology, but such patients may be referred to an ear, nose, and throat (ENT) specialist on follow-up.

Management. Antibiotics, analgesics, and scheduled follow-up are adequate for the management of most cases of painful ear. Acute mastoiditis, malignant external otitis, and established perichondritis require admission and parenteral antibiotics.[1,2] Specific treatment recommendations for painful diseases of the external and middle ear are found in Tables 1 and 2.

In some diseases, water precautions may be needed. In addition to instructing the patient to keep all materials and liquids out of the ear, the patient should be told to fashion a water barrier by applying petroleum jelly to a cotton ball and placing it in the outermost

Table 1. Painful Diseases of the External Ear *(Columns continued)*

Findings	Treatment	Follow-up and Precautions
Exquisite pain on manipulation of auricle or tragus, canal lumen narrowed by edema; if visible, TM may be injected	Clean ear by gentle suction and irrigation; water precautions for 4 wk; otic combination antibiotic-steroid drops (e.g., Corticosporin otic suspension, hydrocortisone 1%-non-aqueous acetic acid, 2% polymyxin B hydrocortisone), 3 drops 3 times/day for 10 days; analgesics (potency of codeine or greater); ear wick if lumen narrowed more than 50%; systemic antibiotics for 10 days if wick needed or fever, adenopathy present	Follow up with otolaryngologist (ENT) in 7–10 days
Inflammation spares EAC	Gentle soap and water washing twice a day, oral antibiotics with staphylococcal coverage for 10 days (e.g., dicloxacillin, erythromycin)	ENT follow-up in 7–10 days
Exquisite pain on manipulation of pinna or tragus, EAC lumen narrowed by edema; exudate of various colors, hyphae	As for swimmer's ear	As for swimmer's ear
Moderate-to-marked local discomfort, leukocytosis	Penicillin intramuscularly or orally for 10 days (erythromycin also acceptable), antipyretics, analgesics, rest	Systemically improved in 24–48 hr, skin improves after several days; follow-up in 7–10 days, sooner if increased pain or systemic symptoms persist more than 2 days
Active granulation tissue in EAC, TMJ pain or tenderness on palpitation below EAC; facial nerve palsy is ominous sign; rarely fever and leukocytosis	Hospitalize for debridement and intravenous antibiotics	May progress to chondritis and osteomyelitis of temporal bone and skull, meningitis, death
Generally visualized with careful otoscopy; otherwise localized by gentle exploration of canal wall with cotton tip applicator	Incision and drainage	Diagnosis easy to miss; pain underestimated; follow-up as needed
Erythema and tenderness of auricle; fluctuance may be palpable	Broad-spectrum antibiotic; if infection well established, consultation recommended	If not controlled, may result in extensive cartilage necrosis and deformity

Table 2. Painful Diseases of the Middle Ear *(Columns continue on next page)*

Etiology	Pathology	Presentation
Bullous myringitis	Middle ear aspirates usually involve *S. pneumoniae* and *H. influenzae*.	Severe pain secondary to serous or hemorrhagic blebs on TM and adjacent canal walls.
Serous otitis media	Middle ear effusion: secondary to poor eustacian tube function; adenoid obstruction; barotrauma	Most frequent in ages 3–7 years; bilateral with mild-to-moderate fluctuating conductive hearing loss; intermittent ear aches and "plugged" sensation; no fever
Aero-otitis media	Sudden pressure changes causing negative pressure in middle ear, drawing serous fluid and blood from capillary rupture into middle ear	Associated with scuba diving, plane travel; painful with conductive hearing loss
Acute suppurative otitis media	Bacterial infection of middle ear usually secondary to *S. pneumoniæ*, *H. influenzae*, and *M. catarrhalis*	Acute, progressive unilateral ear pain, fever, systemic toxicity; often occurs after upper respiratory tract infection (URI)
Acute mastoiditis	Infection of mastoid antrum and air cells, usually by *Streptococcus pyogenes* or *Staphylococcus aureus*; *H. influenzae* rare	Rare but still most common complication of suppurative otitis media; perfuse, foul otorrhea; pain; low-grade fever

portion of the EAC. This technique is useful for keeping water out of the ear during bathing and showering but is not sufficient protection to allow swimming.

An ear wick may be placed in the EAC in cases of external otitis in which the canal lumen is narrowed more than 50% to facilitate penetration of therapeutic eardrops into the canal. Commercial wicks are available, but an acceptable version may be fashioned of cotton twisted into a cylindrical shape that is long enough to reach just past the isthmus when placed in the EAC. The drops are then applied to the outermost portion of the wick. The wick should be removed in 48 hours.

Pitfalls in Practice. Failure to recognize a suppurative otitis media that has extended into the mastoid, a malignant infection of the external ear, or a brewing perichondritis may result in increased morbidity or even mortality. Systemic toxicity and patient reliability should be taken into consideration when planning therapy and follow-up to avoid unnecessary progression of the disease. Analgesia must be adequate for the moderate-to-severe pain often accompanying disease processes of the ear.

Sudden Loss of Hearing

Sudden loss of hearing as an isolated complaint is uncommon but is likely to prompt a patient to seek urgent medical care. More commonly, sudden loss of hearing is associated with other symptoms that assist in correct diagnosis and determination of treatment.

Differential Diagnosis. In evaluating the patient with acute hearing loss, it is important to determine whether the loss is unilateral or bilateral. It is also important to note whether the loss occurred over seconds, minutes, or hours; whether it was accompanied at the onset by "popping"; whether it is associated with pain, tinnitus, or vertigo; and whether there is a coincidental viral exposure, noise exposure, head injury, or altitude change. Drug and medication history is also pertinent.

It is helpful to determine whether the loss is conductive, sensorineural, or mixed. Conductive losses result from dysfunction in the mechanical transmission of sound waves.

Table 2. Painful Diseases of the Middle Ear *(Columns continued)*

Additional Findings	Treatment	Follow-up and Precautions
No fever; may have mild, temporary hearing loss	Analgesics at least as potent as codeine. Antibiotics same as for acute suppurative otitis media	Follow up in 7–10 days
Normal canal: retracted TM, amber to pink color; may see amber-colored bubbles of fluid in the middle ear	Improve eustacian tube function with antihistamine-decongestant medications (e.g., Dimetapp, Actifed, Triaminic), humidity; specific treatment for local disease such as bacterial tonsillitis	Follow up in 10–14 days; chronic indolent course harmful to academic performance in school-aged children
TM may be injected or hemorrhagic; amber to blue to black fluid in middle ear; impaired TM mobility	As for serous otitis	As for serous otitis
Bulging, injected TM; pus in ear if TM ruptured; decreased TM mobility on insufflation	Analgesics. Amoxicillin or TMP-SMX considered first-line antibiotics. Some cephalosporins and various macrolides considered second line	Follow up in 2–3 weeks
Edema, erythema, tenderness over mastoid; x-ray shows clouding of mastoid air cells	Admit for surgical drainage of mastoid; x-ray shows clouding of mastoid air cells	

Effective sound transmission depends on a patent EAC, an intact and mobile TM, continuity and mobility of the ossicular chain, and normal middle ear pressure. Acute conductive hearing loss is frequently a treatable problem and usually can be diagnosed by history and physical examination in the acute care setting. The common cases are related to EAC obstruction, acute diseases of the TM and middle ear, and eustachian tube dysfunction.

Sensorineural hearing loss results from damage to or dysfunction of the cochlear structures or the neural structures central to the cochlea. Most sensorineural hearing losses are untreatable medically or surgically, but when they can be treated, proper diagnosis is imperative because their course may be progressive or malignant. The most important condition to consider in sudden sensorineural hearing loss without apparent cause is a cranial nerve VIII tumor.

Conductive and sensorineural hearing loss can be distinguished by Weber's and Rinne tuning fork tests. A tuning fork of 512 Hz or more should be used; the fork is tapped lightly to activate it. For Weber's test the stem of the activated fork is placed on the patient's forehead or upper incisors, and the patient is asked to indicate in which ear he or she hears it. For the Rinne test, the stem of the activated fork is placed firmly on the mastoid until the patient indicates that the sound has disappeared; then it is moved to a position 1 inch in front of the EAC, and the patient is instructed to indicate when the sound disappears. The test is then performed in reverse order. Results of Weber's and Rinne tests are interpreted as indicated in Table 4.

Table 3.   TMJ Arthralgia (TMJ Syndrome)

Symptoms	History	Examination	Treatment	Follow-up
TMJ, ear, neck mastoid or vertex pain	Often bruxism mal-fitting dentures, recent dental work	Tenderness of TMJ on palpation while patient opens and closes mouth	Symptoms usually resolve in 5 days with conservative treatment (soft diet; mild analgesia, anti-inflammatory medication, heat 4 times/day)	Oral surgeon or ENT if not resolved in

Table 4. Interpretation of Tuning Fork Tests

Test	Normal Hearing	Conductive Loss	Sensorineural Loss
Weber's	Not lateralized	Lateralizes to poorer ear	Lateralizes to better ear
Rinne	Positive (air > bone)	Negative (bone > air)	Positive (air > bone)

Management. The common causes of conductive hearing loss as well as the mechanism of loss, presentation, and treatment are detailed in Table 5. In most cases the diagnosis is straightforward and the treatment specific.

Table 5. Acute Conductive Hearing Loss

Etiology	Mechanism	Presentation	Findings	Treatment	Follow-up and Precautions
Cerumen impaction or foreign body in EAC	Obstruction of EAC or dampening of TM by direct contact	Unilateral or bilateral hearing loss, onset sudden or gradual over few days; possible vertigo, tinnitus	See foreign bodies in external auditory canal, below	Cerumen removal may be facilitated by instilling Colace liquid into the canal for 10–15 min, followed by irrigation	
External otitis	Edematous occlusion of EAC	Unilateral painful ear with hearing loss, gradual over 12–36 hours; possible tinnitus		See ear pain, above	
Serous otitis media	Dampening of TM and ossicular chain by middle ear fluid	Bilateral mild-to-moderate hearing loss, usually in in patients 3–7 years old; insidious onset with fluctuating hearing loss and intermittent pain; "plugged" sensation; no fever; possible tinnitus		See ear pain, above	
Acute suppurative otitis media	Dampening of TM and ossicular chain by purulent middle ear fluid and inflammatory debris	Usually unilateral hearing loss, moderate pain, fever, possible tinnitus		See ear pain, above	
Bullous myringitis	Dampening of TM motion by edema and blebs	Unilateral or bilateral hearing loss; very painful, no fever		See ear pain, above	
Eustachian tube dysfunction	Impaired free flow of air from nasopharynx to middle ear; abnormal pressure in middle ear; impaired TM and ossicular chain mobility	Unilateral or bilateral hearing loss; frequent association with otitis media, URI, allergic rhinitis tonsillitis, barotrauma	Retracted TM; often middle ear fluid (see serous otitis and acute otitis)	Systemic decongestants or antihistamines, antibiotics if coexisting infection	Follow-up with ENT if persistent or recurrent symptoms.
TM perforation	Impaired sound transmission by TM	Unilateral hearing loss in setting of direct trauma, acoustic trauma, barotraumas, minimal hearing loss with small perforation; moderate hearing loss with total TM disruption; possible tinnitus		See ear trauma, below	

(Cont'd on next page)

Table 5.   Acute Conductive Hearing Loss *(Continued)*

Etiology	Mechanism	Presentation	Findings	Treatment	Follow-up and Precautions
Basilar skull fracture	Eustacian tube dysfunction; secondary edema or collection of fluid in middle ear	Unilateral conductive hearing loss; sensorineural if fracture affects labyrinth	Bluish TM (hemotympanum), possible associated signs of basilar fractures, such as periorbital ecchymosis (raccoon eyes), mastoid ecchymosis (Battle's sign)	Thorough assessment for other complications of head trauma; search for cerebrospinal fluid; otorrhea or rhinorrhea; neurosurgical consult	ENT referral for thorough hearing evaluation

The etiology of acute sensorineural hearing loss is more difficult to determine, and specialty consultation is often necessary. The common causes of sensorineural hearing loss, with their mechanisms, presentation, and treatment, are detailed in Table 6. A partial list of ototoxic drugs is presented in Table 7.

Table 6.   Acute Sensorineural (SN) Hearing Loss

Etiology	Mechanism	Presentation	Findings	Treatment	Follow-up and Precautions
Round or oval window rupture (perilymph fistula)	Fistulous opening to cochlea with disruption of fluid wave transmission	Profound unilateral sensorineural hearing loss occurring over seconds, often associated with tinnitus and vertigo; onset during exertion, straining, scuba diving, or with acoustic trauma such as blast; onset frequently associated with popping sensation	Normal ear, or associated middle ear pathology as with barotrauma of scuba diving	Avoid further straining or exertion; immediate otolaryngologic consult; may require immediate surgical exploration and repair of fistula	Prepare for admission
Acoustic neuroma	Nerve VIII compressed in internal auditory meatus by tumor	Sensorineural hearing loss; usually gradual onset but sudden in 10–15% of cases; may be associated with tinnitus and vertigo; any age	Normal ear examination	Surgical	Prompt referral for otologic work-up; any case of unilateral sensorineural hearing loss and uniunilateral tinnitus without obvious cause deserves thorough tumor work-up
Ménière's disease	Increased endolymph production causes rupture of membrane separating endolymph and perilymph, allowing abnormal electrolytes to bathe hair cells and causing sudden vertigo and hearing loss	History of intermittent unilateral sensorineural hearing loss; associated with tinnitus and vertigo; often feelings of pressure in involved ear; severe attacks associated with nausea, vomiting	Directional nystagmus during acute attack of ataxia	Bed rest; symptomatic treatment with sedatives,	ENT to follow up

(Cont'd on next page)

Table 6. Acute Sensorineural (SN) Hearing Loss *(Continued)*

Etiology	Mechanism	Presentation	Findings	Treatment	Follow-up and Precautions
Impulse noise exposure	Explosion or blast injury; secondary temporary hearing threshold shift, mechanical damage to cochlea; may rupture TM or disrupt ossicles or round window	Unilateral or bilateral sensorineural hearing loss; onset related to history of exposure; if TM, ossicles, or round window damaged, will also have conductive hearing loss, often with tinnitus and vertigo	Normal examination, or evidence of TM rupture or congestion	Avoid further exposure if TM ruptured; keep ear dry	If there is TM damage or conductive loss, ENT referral If round or oval window rupture suspected, immediate ENT consultation
Ototoxic drugs	Cochlear or vestibular damage	Unilateral or bilateral sensorineural hearing loss or tinnitus, dizziness, imbalance; transient or permanent, insidious or sudden onset	Normal ear examination	Remove inciting drug	ENT follow-up Effects may continue after stopping drug
Functional hearing loss	Hysterical, psychogenic, malingering	Most probably in setting of high stress, pending litigation, other psychiatric problems	Suspect when there is lack of confirming medical evidence, no response to any level of stimuli in poor ear, exaggerated use of good ear, normal voice quality despite claim of profound hearing loss	Reassurance	ENT follow-up
Concussion	Accumulation of fluid in cochlea	Sensorineural hearing loss; immediate onset with injury but may initially go unnoticed	Normal ear, or other signs of trauma	Thorough assessment for other signs of head injury; neurosurgical consultation	ENT referral for thorough hearing assessment

Table 7. Partial List of Ototoxic Drugs

Chemicals	Antibiotics		Others	
Alcohol	Chloramphenicol	Tetracycline	Antipyrine	Methotrexate
Aniline dyes	Colistin (polymyxin E)	Doxycycline	Atropine	Vincristine
Arsenic	Dihydrostreptomycin	Minocycline	Barbiturates	Lidocaine
Benzene vapors	Gentamicin	Erythromycin	Caffeine	Bupivacaine
Camphor	Kanamycin	Streptomycin	Chlordiazepoxide	Carbamazepine
Carbon monoxide	Neomycin	Amikacin	Ergot drugs	Valproic acid
Chloroform	Polymyxin B	Netilmicin	Morphine	Diazoxide
Hydrocyanide	Vancomycin	Chloroquine	Nitrogen mustard	Enalapril
Iodine	Danamycin	Tobramycin	Procaine (Novocain)	Cimetidine
Lead			Quinine	Famotidine
Tobacco			Strychnine	Omeprazole
			Cisplatin	

Pitfalls in Practice. Failure to recognize and remove an ototoxic drug, failure to recognize and hospitalize a patient with acute round or oval window rupture, or failure to arrange timely work-up of a possible acoustic neuroma constitute the major pitfalls in managing the patient with acute loss of hearing.

Vertigo

Vertigo is the illusion of motion—either a sensation of turning or a sensation of falling. The patient experiencing vertigo may feel that he or she is moving, that the environment is moving, or both.

Vertigo results from a disturbance of the statokinetic system, which includes the semicircular canals, utricle, vestibular division of cranial nerve VIII, and vestibular nuclei. The cause of this disturbance may be simple enough to permit definitive diagnosis and cure in the urgent care setting (e.g., foreign body or cerumen impacted against the TM) or serious enough to necessitate admission and timely surgical intervention (e.g., cerebellopontine angle abscess).

Differential Diagnosis. The patient who complains of dizziness should be asked what he or she means by "dizzy"; that is, what happens when he or she gets dizzy. Only a definite illusion of motion points to vertigo. Feelings of lightheadedness, fainting, floating, sinking, drunkenness, or any other vague, nondirectional sense of motion suggest a nonvertiginous etiology. Other pertinent questions include onset, duration, frequency, severity, warning signs, circumstances, and associated symptoms. History of previous ear, eye, or gait problems, medication and drug use, and toxic exposures is also pertinent.

Physical examination of the patient complaining of dizziness should include a cardiovascular, pulmonary, neurologic, ophthalmologic, and thorough otologic examination. If a vertiginous etiology is not clear by history and physical examination, then basic laboratory studies should be considered, such as complete blood count; measurements of serum electrolytes, blood urea nitrogen, and creatinine; urinalysis; chest x-ray; and electrocardiography.

If the history and examination suggest true vertigo, an attempt should be made to distinguish between a peripheral and central cause of this vertigo. As detailed in Table 8, central and peripheral vertigo differ in onset, character, duration, associated symptoms, type of nystagmus, and presence of neurologic abnormalities.[3] Peripheral vertigo is generally the more benign process, although it may be more debilitating acutely. Of patients presenting with vertigo, 85% have a peripheral cause.[4] Disease processes of the external auditory canal, middle ear, and labyrinth are responsible for peripheral vertigo. Central causes of

Table 8. Central and Peripheral Vertigo and Nystagmus

Central	Peripheral
Gradual onset	Sudden onset
Symptoms continuous	Symptoms intermittent
Lasts weeks to months	Lasts seconds to days
Vertigo is mild (sense of unsteadiness)	Vertigo is severe (spinning or whirling sensation)
Rarely associated with autonomic dysfunction	Often associated with autonomic dysfunction (e.g., nausea and vomiting)
Usually no auditory symptoms	Hearing loss and tinnitus often present
Not affected by head positions (generally present in several positions)	Usually affected by changes in head position (often one position is worst)
Spontaneous nystagmus may be horizontal, vertical, or rotary; enhanced by visual fixation; may not be associated with vertigo	Spontaneous nystagmus never diagonal or vertical; suppressed by visual fixation; unilateral or bilateral; associated with vertigo
Direction of positional nystagmus changes; does not abate or fatigue; no latency	Positional nystagmus fixed in direction (usually rotary); latency of several seconds; abates in 30–40 seconds; fatigues with repetitive testing; associated with vertigo

vertigo are generally more serious than peripheral causes, although on initial presentation the symptoms may be less severe. Central nervous system or systemic disease affecting the central portions of cranial nerve VIII or the vestibular nuclei are responsible.

Nystagmus is the objective finding accompanying the symptom of vertigo. Nystagmus is the alternating involuntary movement of both eyes that is characterized by a slow component to one side and a corrective quick component to the other side. By convention, nystagmus is named by the direction of the quick component. Nystagmus may be horizontal, vertical, diagonal, or rotary. It is caused by stimulation of the semicircular canals and depends on the interaction of the oculovestibular system with the cerebral cortex.

Thorough examination for nystagmus is the key to evaluating the vertiginous patient and helps in distinguishing peripheral from central disorders of the vestibular system. The urgent care physician is generally limited to assessment of spontaneous or positional nystagmus, but this is frequently sufficient to establish peripheral or central etiology. More elaborate tests such as electronystagmography, optokinetic response, and caloric response can be administered by a specialist at a later time.

Spontaneous horizontal nystagmus is usually peripheral. Spontaneous vertical, rotary, or diagonal nystagmus is usually of central nervous system origin. Positional direction changes in nystagmus without apparent vertigo are usually of central nervous system origin, as is extremely active nystagmus without vertigo. The role of nystagmus in differentiating central and peripheral causes of vertigo is detailed in Table 8.

Spontaneous nystagmus is assessed by asking the patient to look straight ahead, then 30° to the left, then 30° to the right. Lateral gaze beyond 45° is not reliable because normal persons may have nystagmus at this angle. If nystagmus is noted, attention should be directed to latency, duration, direction, and associated symptoms.

Positional nystagmus is assessed by using the Dix-Hallpike maneuver (Fig. 1).[5] The patient is placed in a sitting position with the legs extended on the examining cart. The examiner stands beside the bed. The head is then held firmly in the examiner's hands and turned toward the examiner. The patient is admonished to keep the eyes open and to look at the examiner's forehead. The examiner rapidly lays the patient back into the supine position with the head tilted 30° below horizontal over the end of the cart. This position is maintained for at least 30 seconds, during which the patient's eyes are observed for nystagmus. The maneuver is repeated with the patient's head turned to the opposite side.

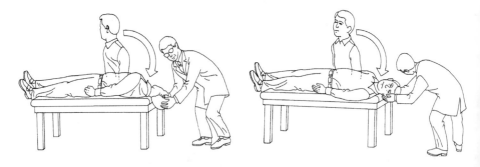

Figure 1. Dix-Hallpike maneuver. (From Cummings CW, et al (eds): Otolaryngology–Head and Neck Surgery. St. Louis, Mosby, 1986, p 2751, with permission.)

Nystagmus provoked by this positional test is always abnormal and is most prominent when the head is turned to the side of the affected ear. Its characteristics help to distinguish peripheral from central vestibular lesions (see Table 8).

Management. In most cases, the treatment of vertigo is symptomatic. Sedatives such as diazepam as well as antiemetics and antihistamines are frequently effective in controlling symptoms; bed rest may be required for marked vertigo. Specialty follow-up is indicated for precise diagnosis. Vertigo resulting from suppurative infections, acute labyrinthine fistula, and most central causes requires specialty consultation and usually acute hospitalization for specific diagnosis and therapy.

In patients who present with benign positional vertigo, a particle-repositioning maneuver, described by Epley, can alleviate the symptoms in many patients when carried out correctly.[6] The Hallpike maneuver must first be performed to identify the affected ear (see above). The particle-repositioning maneuver begins with the patient in the sitting position. The head is rotated 45° toward the affected side. The patient is then quickly moved into the supine position with the head extended 20° and maintaining its 45° rotation. The head is slowly rotated through extension until the opposite ear is down (45° rotation). The patient is then turned onto the unaffected side with the head rotated 45° in the direction of the unaffected side. The patient then slowly returns to the sitting position with the head rotated toward the unaffected side. Lastly, the head is rotated back to the midline with the neck flexed forward 20°. Pause at each position until induced nystagmus approaches termination or for around 30 seconds if no nystagmus. Immediately after the treatment, patients are advised to avoid significant head extension and flexion for 48 hours. This procedure is repeated as necessary at weekly intervals until vertigo symptoms have cleared. This procedure is not recommended for patients with significant hypertension, cervical spine disease, or possible retinal detachment. All patients who undergo this procedure should follow-up with an ENT physician within 2–3 days.

The common causes of peripheral and central vertigo are presented in Tables 9 and 10, respectively, along with their presentations, examination findings, and considerations for management.

Pitfall in Practice. Failure to distinguish disequilibrium from vertigo can lead to oversight of treatable but life-threatening cardiac, neurologic, or metabolic disease. Failure to recognize a suppurative etiology or acute labyrinthine fistula as the cause of peripheral vertigo can lead to delay in treatment with increased morbidity. Failure to recognize the central etiology of vertigo and to arrange for timely precise diagnosis and intervention can result in increased morbidity. The particle-repositioning maneuver and Dix-Hallpike maneuver should not be performed on patients with significant back or neck problems or patients with a history of vertebral-basilar insufficiency.

Tinnitus

Tinnitus is the sensation of sound (e.g., ringing, humming, clicking, or roaring) in the absence of a relevant external auditory stimulus. When sound can be heard by an observer other then the patient, it is objective tinnitus. Objective tinnitus is rare and is due to myoclonic contractions of the palate, tensor tympani, or stapedius muscle or to vascular abnormalities such as glomus jugulare, aneurysms, or arteriovenous fistulas.[7]

Table 9. Peripheral Causes of Vertigo *(Columns continue on next page)*

Etiology	Mechanism	Presentation
Foreign body in ear canal	Asymmetric stimulation of labyrinth	Complaints of vertigo, full sensation in ear; may have tinnitus, hearing loss
Acute and middle ear infection	Interference with TM and ossicular chain mobility, labyrinthine dysfunction	Mild vertigo if infection confined to middle ear; severe vertigo suggestive of mastoiditis or labyrinthitis
Otosclerosis	Genetic disease of stapedial immobilization	Vertigo and sensorineural hearing loss
Ménière's disease	Unknown, possibly osmotic disturbance at blood endolymph barrier	Vertigo, unilateral tinnitus, sensorineural hearing loss; episodic, usually lasting several hours; abrupt onset usually with nausea and vomiting, variable frequency; first attack at age 30–60, normal between attacks; 75% of patients with peripheral vertigo have Ménière's disease
Benign positional vertigo	Displaced canaliths in the semicircular canals	15–20-sec episodes of vertigo brought on by changes in head position; latency of a few seconds
Labyrinthitis	Infection or inflammation of the cochlea or vestibule (or both) secondary to bacteria, fungi, virus, allergy, toxin	Vertigo; possible hearing loss; signs of infection
Labyrinthine hemorrhage	Acute hemorrhage into perilymph of cochlea causing structural damage to cupula; secondary to vascular accident, poisoning, leukemia	Severe, sudden vertigo; nystagmus, sensorineural hearing loss, tinnitus; seen in patients with probable vascular disease
Labyrinthine fistula	Leakage of perilymph secondary to trauma such as penetrating injury to TM, disruption of ossicles into labyrinth with infection, secondary chronic ear infection, middle ear surgery	Vertigo, sensorineural hearing loss, tinnitus
Vestibular neuronitis	Viral infection of vestibular ganglion or labyrinth	Spontaneous attack of vertigo without hearing loss or tinnitus; resolves in 6–12 weeks
Motion sickness	Repetitive stimulation of semicircular canals from motion	Vertigo, nausea, vomiting with history of motion exposure during episodes
Vestibulogenic seizures	Sensory stimulation of labyrinth results in excessive stimulation of brainstem reticular nucleus and subsequent seizure activity	Seizures with early prominent vestibular symptoms (e.g., vertigo, nausea, vomiting)

Subjective tinnitus, on the other hand, is quite common and can be heard only by the patient. It is usually accompanied by hearing loss and may precede, follow, or appear at the same time as the hearing loss.

Differential Diagnosis. Careful history taking and physical examination should reveal any cause of tinnitus that is treatable in the urgent care setting. Because hearing loss is frequently an associated symptom, elements of the history and physical examination that are pertinent to the evaluation of hearing loss are also pertinent to the evaluation of tinnitus (see sudden loss of hearing, above). Conductive and sensorineural lesions frequently associated with tinnitus are listed in Table 11. It is useful to distinguish between

Table 9. Peripheral Causes of Vertigo *(Columns continued)*

Examination	Treatment	Follow-up and Precautions
Foreign body visible in ear canal	Removal; symptoms should resolve immediately	ENT if symptoms do not resolve
	See ear pain, above	
Normal-appearing ear	Symptomatic for vertigo; surgical stapedectomy for underlying disease	ENT follow-up in 7–10 days for evaluation
Normal TM, normal neurologic examination; no nystagmus, sensorineural hearing loss	Symptomatic with sedatives, antihistamines antiemetics, bed rest if necessary	ENT follow-up in 7–10 days for definitive diagnosis and long-term care
Normal ear, normal neurologic examination; vertigo, nystagmus (typically peripheral) (see Table 9)	Symptomatic with antiemetics, sedatives, antihistamines Particle repositioning maneuver (see text, Fig. 1)	ENT follow-up in 7–10 days for further work-up and therapy. If central positional vertigo suspected, immediate neurologic consult should be sought
If contiguous suppurative infection, will have obvious signs (see ear pain, above); otherwise normal ear examination and normal neurologic examination	Admission, antibiotics, debridement for suppurative infection; search for and withdraw drug, allergen, or toxin along with symptomatic treatment with antiemetics, antihistamines	ENT follow-up in 3–5 days
May have no associated findings	Symptomatic	Refer for work-up of vascular system
Evidence of middle ear trauma, infection, or recent surgery	Hospitalization, bed rest, possible surgical repair, prompt otologic consultation required	ENT follow-up
Normal	Symptomatic with sedatives, antiemetics, antihistamines	ENT follow-up in 7–10 days
Normal	Remove from environment; prevent with anticholinergic drug (promethazine, scopolamine, meclizine)	As needed if failure to resolve with removal from environment. Note: delayed onset of vertigo after air travel suggests perilymph fistula
No ear of focal neurologic signs	Antiepileptics under direction of neurologist	Neurologic consult

associated conductive and sensorineural hearing loss in the initial work-up of the patient with tinnitus, as outlined above for sudden loss of hearing.

Management. Tinnitus is an important symptom and should not be dismissed. Characteristics and treatment of specific disease processes associated with tinnitus are noted in Tables 5 and 6. Frequently the cause is not apparent even after careful examination, however. The patient with unexplained tinnitus must be referred for thorough otologic examination.

Pitfalls in Practice. Failure to recognize that tinnitus may be the first and only warning sign of serous disease such as nerve VIII tumor, cerebellopontine angle tumor,

Table 10. Central Causes of Vertigo *(Columns continue on next page)*

Etiology	Mechanism	Presentation
Vertebrobasilar insufficiency	Drop in blood flow to vestibular nuclei or surrounding structures	Common cause of central vertigo in patients older than 50 years with cerebrovascular disease; various constellations of vertigo, hemiparesis, visual changes, dysarthria, headache, vomiting Drop attacks without loss of consciousness common; tinnitus and hearing loss rare
Subclavian steal	Diversion of blood from posterior cerebral circulation to arm	Vertigo with possible lightheadedness, visual changes, facial paresthesias, loss of consciousness associated with exercise of ipsilateral arm
Multiple sclerosis	Central nervous system demyelination	Multiple transient neurologic symptoms; vertigo in 10% of cases; part of symptom complex in 30% of cases; most common symptoms are weakness, diplopia, decreased, vision, tremor, ataxia, paresthesias
Vertiginous epilepsy (cortical vertigo)	Tumor, infarction, atrioventricular malformation causing temporal lobe seizures	Vertigo may be only signs of temporal lobe seizure and may be accompanied by typical psychomotor seizures; usually associated with hallucinations of music or sound
Cerebellopontine angle lesions	80% are acoustic neuromas; others are meningiomas, cholesteatomas, metastatic carcinomas, papillomas, gliomas, cysts, or aneurysms Cause nerve VIII compression, later brainstem compression	First symptom is tinnitus and hearing loss; later ataxia, headache
Geniculate herpes zoster (Ramsay-Hunt syndrome)	Infection involving nerves VII and VII	Vertigo with nausea, vomiting, tinnitus, hearing loss, facial paralysis
Cervicogenic vertigo	Dysfunction of vertebrobasilar circulation, sympathetic vertebral plexus, or sensory afferent nerve input to vestibular nuclei often secondary to disease	Vertigo with headache, tinnitus, nausea, hearing loss plus myalgias and neuralgias of neck; worse with tension and anxiety
Cogan's syndrome	Generalized vasculitis	Usually follows vaccination, antibiotics, or URI; symptom complex of (1) vestibuloauditory abnormalities (vertigo, tinnitus, hearing loss, ear pain; possible nausea, vomiting, ataxia), (2) interstitial keratitis (photophobia, lacrimation, keratitis, decreased vision), (3) absence of syphilis Patients die in acute phase or follow indolent chronic course

glomus jugulare, or a vascular lesion in the temporal bone may result in extension of disease before appropriate work-up and treatment.

Ear Trauma

Ear trauma that is likely to present to the urgent care setting includes the categories of minor auricle lacerations, auricle hematomas, minor lacerations of the external auditory canal, burns and frostbite of the auricle, traumatic TM perforations, ossicular chain disruption, and labyrinthine fistula. Special consideration is given to blast trauma and barotrauma as mechanisms of injury.

Table 10. Central Causes of Vertigo *(Columns continued)*

Examination	Treatment	Follow-up and Precautions
Normal ear examination, frequently focal neurologic findings; other signs of vascular disease; signs may resolve (transient ischemic attack) or persist (cerebral infarct)	Neurologic consultation for hospitalization and work-up (CT, MRI, possible cerebral angiogram)	With neurologist or primary care physician
Supraclavicular fossa bruit, unequal upper extremity blood pressure or pulses; symptoms elicited by arm exercise	Surgery; prompt vascular consultation needed	With surgeon or primary care physician
Normal ear examination, possible scattered neurologic findings; look for visual deficit	Symptomatic	Referral to neurologist for definitive diagnosis Probable lumbar puncture, CT/MRI
May be normal	Neurology consult for work-up if first seizure; nature of lesion may be determined by CT/MRI, electroencephalography or lumbar puncture Possibly antiepileptics	With neurologist or primary care physician
Normal ear examination, focal neurologic abnormalities	Prompt ENT/neurosurgery consultation for audiometric and vestibular tests, radiographs, CT/MRI	With ENT and/or neurosurgery
Vesicular rash involving TM, auditory canal	Analgesics, antivertiginous drugs; consult ENT for opinion about antiviral agents and corticosteroids	ENT follow-up in 3–5 days
Evidence of neck injury or disease, cervical tension, normal ear examination, focal neurologic	Heat, massage, exercise, soft cervical collar, muscle relaxants, analgesics	ENT follow-up for confirmation of diagnosis; then primary care
Normal ear examination, abnormal eye examination; may have evidence of vasculitis in heart, gastrointestinal tract, spleen; may have focal neurologic findings	Medicine consultation; probably hospitalization for steroids with or without immunosuppressants; treat vertiginous symptoms with antihistamines, sedation	Must be distinguished from multiple sclerosis, cerebellopontine angle

Auricle Laceration

Differential Diagnosis. The examiner should determine whether the laceration is new or more that a few hours old, whether it is actually a cut or potentially a human or other animal bite, whether cartilage has been lost or crushed, and whether skin loss has occurred. Simple, clean, recent lacerations of the auricle may be well managed by the urgent care physician; more complicated injuries of the auricle require plastic surgery or ENT consultation because the cosmetic preservation of delicate cartilaginous structures is of the utmost concern. The need for tetanus and rabies prophylaxis should be determined.

Table 11. Causes of Tinnitus

Conductive Lesions	Sensorineural Lesions
External ear	**Cochlea**
EAC obstruction secondary to external otitis	Paget's disease
Furuncles	Otosclerosis
Cerumen impaction	Perilymph fistula or infection
Foreign body	Ménière's disease
Osteophytes	Organ of Corti lesions secondary to ototoxicity, atrophy, noise,
Middle ear	allergies, edema, viropathy, vascular lesions
TM perforations or adhesive fibrosis	**Cranial nerve VIII**
Middle ear fluid (e.g., pus, blood, effusion)	Nerve VIII tumors, inflammation, vascular anomalies
Ossicular chain disruption or immobility	Tumors
Spasms of TM muscles	Vascular anomalies of cerebellopontine angle
Vascular anomalies of jugular bulb or carotid artery	
Tumors	

Management. Simple lacerations not involving the cartilage may be closed in standard fashion with nonabsorbable, simple, interrupted sutures. If the cartilage is cut, the cartilage and perichondrial layer should be approximated with fine absorbable sutures before skin closure. Meticulous cleansing and sterile technique are important to minimize the risk of potentially deforming cartilage infection. Anesthesia of all but the concha and external canal can be achieved by infiltration about the base of the pinna with 1% lidocaine without epinephrine; the concha and external canal must be anesthetized by direct infiltration if they are involved. Antibiotics are recommended in contaminated cases. A pressure dressing may be necessary to prevent accumulation of a hematoma (see below).

Pitfalls in Practice. Failure to recognize an animal or human bite as the mechanism of laceration may result in inappropriate closure or inadequate antibiotic prophylaxis. Failure to refer more complicated lacerations for repair may result in less than optimal cosmetic repair.

Auricle Hematoma

Differential Diagnosis. A hematoma of the auricle is due to extravasation of blood between the perichondrium and the cartilage; usually as a result of blunt trauma. Swelling may obliterate the contours of the pinna. If allowed to form a firm, organized clot, blood can cause permanent thickening (cauliflower ear).[8]

Management. Small, acute hematomas may be aspirated with a large-bore needle under strict aseptic conditions after administration of local anesthesia (without epinephrine). The needle must not penetrate the cartilage. Large or subacute hematomas should be incised with a small scalpel under sterile conditions. A $1/4$-inch incision parallel to the margin of the helix at the most dependent part of the hematoma allows aspiration of the hematoma with a small suction catheter. If the blood clot is too well organized to pass through the catheter, the incision may need to be enlarged to allow removal with a small forceps. To prevent hematoma or seroma accumulation after repair or drainage of the pinna, a pressure dressing should be applied. Pieces of cotton or gauze moistened with povidone-iodine solution or petroleum jelly are placed behind the ear for support and into the recesses of the auricle. The ear is then generously covered with fluffed gauze and the head firmly encircled with gauze and an elastic bandage. The pressure dressing should be left in place for 2 days, then removed for wound inspection and replaced for 3–4 days. Reaccumulation of clot necessitates repeat aspiration or incision. Consultation should be sought for complex clots.

Pitfalls in Practice. Failure to evacuate a hematoma and to apply an effective pressure dressing may lead to marked cosmetic deformity of the auricle.

External Auditory Canal Laceration

Differential Diagnosis. Fairly mild direct trauma to the external auditory canal may result in laceration; frequently it results from children putting objects into their ears or adults attempting to clean the ear canals. The TM should be adequately visualized for evidence of perforation in all such injuries. If necessary, the canal may be suctioned to facilitate visualization, but irrigation must be avoided until the integrity of the TM has been ensured. Blunt trauma to the head that results in bleeding from the ear or a canal laceration must raise the suspicion of middle ear damage or temporal bone fracture, either of which necessitates complete otologic and neurologic evaluation.

Management. Small canal laceration may be managed by simple cleansing and 3–5 days of a prophylactic antibiotic-steroid preparation such as Cortisporin otic suspension. A wound check in 2–3 days is recommended. Active bleeding from a small canal laceration can be controlled by direct pressure with a cotton-tipped swab. Tetanus immunization should be administered, if indicated. Large lacerations and inability to visualize the TM when injury is suspected are indications for prompt otolaryngologic referral.

Pitfalls in Practice. Failure to appreciate the possibility of middle ear damage with penetrating injury to the EAC and failure to suspect temporal bone fracture when canal laceration accompanies a history of blunt head trauma may result in delay in appropriate diagnosis and treatment.

Auricle Burns and Frostbite

Chapter 8 describes the differential diagnosis and management of burns and frostbite injuries to the external ear.

Traumatic Tympanic Membrane Perforation

Differential Diagnosis. Traumatic TM perforation is the most common serious ear injury. Causes are easily identified by the history and include direct injury from flying objects such as slag and sticks; self-inflicted injury with cotton-tipped applicators, pencils, bobby pins, and paper clips; concussive injury from an explosion or a blow to the ear that suddenly compresses the air in the EAC; sudden changes in atmospheric pressure; lightning injury; and tears from temporal bone fracture. Any of these mechanisms may produce injuries ranging from tiny tears to extensive TM damage. Likewise, any mechanism may be associated with disruption of the ossicular chain or damage to the labyrinth or facial nerve. Any patient with significant head trauma, suspected temporal bone fracture, or lightning injury generally needs more complete evaluation than can be accomplished in the urgent care setting.

The EAC and TM should be examined carefully to identify the type and extent of perforation. A picture of the perforation drawn in the medical record is helpful in describing the injury. Blood and debris may be removed by suction, but the canal should not be irrigated when perforation is suspected. Facial nerve function, hearing status, and vestibular function should be assessed.

Management. Most perforations less than 2 mm heal spontaneously; perforations occupying less than one-fourth of the TM area may require simple patching; larger perforations are likely to require tympanoplasty. Initial care is directed to cleansing the canal of debris (avoiding irrigation) and preventing contamination of the middle ear by instructing the patient not to put anything in the ear and by placing the patient on water precautions (described above). Systemic antibiotics are recommended by some physicians.[8] The patient with an isolated TM perforation should be reexamined periodically until the TM is healed. Immediate otolaryngologic consultation should be sought when associated injuries are detected or suspected.

Pitfalls in Practice. Failure to detect an associated middle or inner ear injury is the most probable pitfall in managing traumatic TM ruptures.

Blast Injury

Differential Diagnosis. Sudden build-up of pressure from an explosion or blow to the ear can cause injury. TM perforation and middle ear damage such as disruption of the ossicular chain are common. Inner ear damage is possible, however, and must be considered even when no visual evidence of injury is present. Ossicular disruption results in marked conductive hearing loss. Tinnitus may accompany the blast exposure without significant injury, but vertigo is rare and must alert the physician to the possibility of perilymph fistula.[9,10] (See Table 6 for characteristics and treatment.)

Management. If middle ear or labyrinth damage is suspected, immediate otolaryngologic consultation is indicated.

Pitfalls in Practice. Failure to look for evidence of middle ear or labyrinth damage despite a normal EAC and TM can result in unnecessary morbidity.

Barotrauma

Differential Diagnosis. Barotrauma is a special category of otologic trauma caused by changes in ambient pressure over a relatively short time, as in airplane travel and scuba diving. Because of the popularity of these activities, barotrauma is fairly common. Barotrauma may affect the EAC, middle ear, or inner ear. Careful history taking and otologic examination generally delineate the nature of the injury. Specific injuries, their presentation, and recommendations for treatment are detailed in Table 12.

Management. Appropriate management entails specific treatment for the injury noted, as described in Table 12, and avoidance of further exposure to changes in atmospheric pressure until the problem is resolved.

Pitfalls in Practice. Failure to recognize changes in atmospheric pressure as mechanism of injury and failure to appreciate the possibility of inner ear damage from this mechanism constitute two potential pitfalls. In addition, the diver complaining of tinnitus, vertigo, and sensorineural hearing loss must bring to mind the possibility of inner ear decompression sickness (DCS). When the condition is suspected, a diving physician should be consulted (e.g., through the Divers Alert Network, 919-684-8111) because Hyperbaric treatment for DCS may be indicated.

Table 12. Barotrauma of the Ear

Etiology	Mechanism	Presentation	Findings	Treatment and Precautions
EAC baro-trauma	Obstruction of EAC (cerumen, plug, hood) causes negative pressure in EAC, producing edema, hemorrhage, blebs on canal or TM	History of pressure change; painful ear	Tender to palpation; blebs, hemorrhage, edema	Not serious; analgesics, follow-up as needed, avoid reexposure
Middle ear barotrauma	Eustacian tube dysfunction results in negative middle ear pressure relative to environment; causes TM retraction, vascular enlargement, middle ear effusion or bleeding; may rupture TM	History of pressure exposure, often preexisting URI; pain, ear fullness, conductive hearing loss	TM retracted, middle ear fluid or blood possible perforation	Decongestants; antibiotics if also infected, avoid pressure exposure until ear looks and feels normal; follow-up ear examination in 1–2 weeks
Inner ear barotrauma	Failure to equalize middle ear pressure or sudden change in middle ear pressure may damage cochlea or disrupt round or oval window, causing perilymph fistula	History of pressure change; sensorineural hearing loss, ear fullness, vertigo, tinnitus, nystagmus, nausea, vomiting, ataxia	Evidence of middle ear barotrauma on TM examination	If fistula suspected, immediate ENT consultation; hospitalization, bed rest

Foreign Bodies in the External Auditory Canal

Foreign bodies are most commonly found in the EACs of children, but patients of any age may present when symptoms of pain, irritation, or decreased hearing call attention to the foreign body.

Differential Diagnosis. The history and examination generally reveal the nature of the foreign body. Vegetable foreign bodies (e.g., peas or peanuts) tend to swell, macerate, and cause marked local inflammation. Live insects can be extremely aggravating. Objects external to the isthmus of the canal are most amenable to removal; those medial to the isthmus and appearing to fill the isthmus are difficult to remove without anesthesia. General anesthesia is recommended in the uncooperative child.

Management. Regardless of the type of foreign body in the EAC, removal is usually easiest on the first attempt. Ear injury from foreign bodies generally occurs during removal rather than during placement, and careful consideration of the technique to be used, availability of the proper equipment, and proper positioning and immobilization of the patient should precede any attempt at removal. If an attempt at removal appears to be ill advised or is unsuccessful, ENT consultation should be obtained within 24 hours. Specific management options include instrument removal, suction, and irrigation.

Instrumentation. Grasping the object with forceps under direct vision is likely to be successful with irregular objects or macerated vegetable matter but is likely to push a round, smooth, or hard object deeper into the canal. A hook or dull ring curette passed along the canal wall distal to such an object may be used to gain purchase from behind and to tease it forward. Insects may first be drowned with water, lidocaine, or mineral oil and then removed with forceps. Care must be taken in using instruments to avoid damaging the TM or the delicate canal. Because the posterosuperior aspect of the meatal wall is the least sensitive, instruments are best placed along this surface.

Suction. Pus, liquid, macerated material, and small beads may sometimes be removed by suction with the use of a small, angulated metal suction tip.

Irrigation. Irrigation should not be performed in patients with suspected TM perforation because of the risk of contamination of the middle ear. If the TM is intact, irrigation of the canal may help to remove the foreign body. The irrigation fluid should be at body temperature to avoid unpleasant caloric stimulation of the labyrinth. Water and saline are acceptable; addition of sodium bicarbonate or hydrogen peroxide may be helpful for removing cerumen. Successful irrigation depends on fluid passing by the foreign body and causing an extrusive force from behind it. It follows that a totally occluding foreign body cannot be removed by this technique but instead becomes jettisoned more deeply into the canal. Impacted cerumen can be gently teased from the superior meatal wall with a blunt instrument to facilitate successful removal by irrigation. The irrigating stream should be directed against the meatal wall and not against the TM because rupture can occur. The meatus should be inspected periodically during the procedure and inspected and gently dried at the completion of irrigation.

Pitfalls in Practice. The most common pitfall in managing EAC foreign bodies is failing to organize needed equipment and to secure the cooperation of the patient before initiating attempts at removal. Attempts to remove a foreign body without suitable equipment or with the patient protesting hinder the success of the procedure and raise the risk of mechanical damage to the ear during the process. Failure to appreciate the possibility of TM perforation by the history and the nature of the foreign body is another pitfall because it can lead to an unwise choice of irrigation as a method of removal, thus contaminating the middle ear. Once it has been decided that the foreign body is to be removed in the urgent care center, only the simplest and gentlest of maneuvers should be used; subsequent vigorous procedures are unlikely to be successful and only increase the risk of complications.

References

1. Canafax DM, Giebink GS: Antimicrobial treatment of acute otitis media. Ann Otol Rhinol Laryngol 103:11–14, 1994.
2. Gliklich RE, Eavey RD, Iannuzzi RA, Camacho AE: A contemporary analysis of acute mastoiditis. Arch Otolaryngol Head Neck Surg 122:135–139, 1996.
3. Olshaker JS: Vertigo. In Rosen P, Barkin R, et al (eds): Emergency Medicine: Concepts and Clinical Practice, 4th ed. St. Louis, Mosby, 1998, pp 2165–2173.
4. Greenberg DA, Aminoff MJ, Simon RP: Disorders of equilibrium. In Greenberg DA, Aminoff MJ, Simon RP (eds): Clinical Neurology. Norwalk, CT, Appleton & Lange, 1993, pp 92–120.
5. Dix MR, Hallpick LS: The Pathology, symptomology, and diagnosis of certain common disorders of the vestibular system. Proc R Soc Med 45:341–354, 1952.
6. Epley JM: Particle Repositioning for benign paroxysmal positional vertigo. Otolaryngol Clin North Am 29:323–331, 1996.
7. Seligmann H, Podoshin L, Ben-David J, et al: Drug induced tinnitus and other hearing disorders. Drug Safety 14(3):198–212, 1996.
8. Shulman JB: Traumatic diseases of the ear and temporal bone. In Goodhill V (ed): Ear Diseases, Deafness, and Dizziness. Hagerstown, MD, Harper & Row; 1979, pp 504–516.
9. Goodhill V: Tinnitus. In Goodhill V (ed): Ear Diseases, Deafness, and Dizziness. Hagerstown, MD, Harper & Row, 1979, pp 731–738.
10. Mawson SR, Ludman H: Diseases of the Ear. Chicago, Edward Arnold, 1979, pp 469–472.

Chapter 12

Urgencies of the Nose and Paranasal Sinuses

Laura Schrag, MD
Robert Rusnak, MD

Sinusitis

The sinuses of the skull are closed air spaces drained by ostia and lined with pseudo-stratified ciliated columnar epithelium studded with mucin-producing goblet cells. Bacterial or viral infection of these spaces produces sinusitis. Although septal deformities, polyps, foreign bodies, mass lesions, allergies, dental disease, trauma, or systemic disorders may potentiate or be associated with sinusitis, most cases occur after viral upper respiratory tract infections (URIs). The urgent care physician must correctly separate patients who require specific treatment for sinusitis from patients who require only symptomatic or supportive treatment for a URI or no treatment at all.

The presenting signs and symptoms of sinusitis depend on the sinus or sinuses involved, the presence or absence of complications, and the patient's age. Most physicians rely on a constellation of signs and symptoms to diagnose acute sinusitis in children. The common course of sinusitis is the persistence of a URI for more than 7–10 days without improvement, a fever > 101° F, facial swelling and discomfort associated with purulent nasal secretions, and cough worse when the child first goes to bed. Some authors suggest using major and minor criteria to aid in the diagnosis of sinusitis in children (Table 1). The presence of two major or of one major plus two or more minor criteria for more than 7 days signifies acute sinusitis.[1,2]

Table 1. Diagnostic Criteria for Sinusitis in Children

Major Criteria	Minor Criteria	
Nasal discharge	Periorbital edema	Sore throat
Purulent pharyngeal discharge	Headache	Foul breath
Cough	Facial pain	Increased wheeze
	Tooth pain	Fever
	Earache	

In diagnosing sinusitis in adults, the signs and symptoms become more focal. Most patients with true sinusitis complain of facial pain, nasal congestion, and mucous purulence associated with headache or high temperatures. No diagnostic criteria have been set to diagnose sinusitis in adults; instead, clinical judgment is used to make the diagnosis of sinusitis; on occasion, a few ancillary tests are performed to confirm the diagnosis.

Normal sinuses do not contain bacteria. During health, the sinuses are protected from infection by the quality of normal mucus, ciliary action, and patent ostia. Infection occurs when normal mechanisms are disrupted. Viral infections produce ciliastasis and edema of the nasal mucosa. Because epithelial mucus production continues, mucus accumulates in a closed space with subsequent secondary bacterial infection. Infected mucopus results in further ciliastasis and inflammatory changes in the sinus ostia when it is discharged into the nasal cavity, thus perpetuating the cycle of sinus infection.

Acute sinusitis involves changes lasting days to weeks, and chronic sinusitis involves changes lasting months to years. Chronic maxillary sinusitis may exist alone, but chronic ethmoid or frontal sinusitis is usually associated with maxillary sinus infection.

Maxillary Sinusitis

History and Physical Examination. Maxillary sinusitis is the most frequent type of sinusitis. Typical maxillary sinus pain extends from the inner canthus of the eye to the molars or even the ears.[3] The signs and symptoms of maxillary sinusitis are listed in Table 2.

Table 2. Sinusitis Syndromes *(Columns continue on facing page)*

Involved Sinus	Presentation	Examination	Epidemiology
Maxillary	Onset: acute, days to weeks; chronic, years. Signs and symptoms: facial pain (worse on bending over), altered facial sensation, purulent nasal discharge, headache, fever, tooth pain, severe URI symptoms.	Elevated temperature, purulent nasal discharge, facial tenderness, facial pain on percussion over sinus, or molar teeth.	Occurrence: after viral URI, especially in presence of predisposing factors. Organisms involved: *Streptococcus pneumoniae*, *S. pyogenes*, *Hemophilus influenzae*, *Branhamella catarrhalis*, anaerobes (usually chronic).
Ethmoid	Onset: gradual, acute pain with abrupt obstruction of ostia. Signs and symptoms: facial pain, eyelid edema, periorbital cellulitis, pansinusitis, headache around eyes.	Elevated temperature, purulent nasal discharge, periorbital cellulitis, orbital cellulitis; tenderness, swelling over ethmoid sinus; tenderness over all sinuses (pansinusitis).	Occurrence: after viral URI; if isolated, consider cancer, mucoceles, pyomucoceles. Organisms involved: *Streptococcus pneumoniae*, β-hemolytic streptococci, *Hemophilus influenzae*, *Staphylococcus aureus*, *Klebsiella pneumoniae*.
Frontal	Onset: gradual. Signs and symptoms: facial pain, frontal headache, frontal swelling, erythema; frontal tenderness; pansinus involvement.	Elevated temperature, purulent nasal discharge, tenderness, swelling over frontal sinus (Potts' puffy tumor); tenderness over all sinuses (pansinusitis).	Occurrence: after viral URI; in setting of closed head trauma, skull fracture, barotrauma. Organisms involved: acute infections, *Streptococcus pneumoniae*, *H. influenzae*, anaerobes; chronic infections, *Staphylococcus aureus*, anaerobes.
Sphenoid	Onset: gradual. Signs and symptoms: pansinus involvement, nasal discharge, headache (bitemporal, parietal, periorbital, frontal), pain (vertex of head, retro-orbital, occipital, mastoid regions), pain and paresthesias in V1, V2 distribution of trigeminal nerve.	Elevated temperature, purulent nasal discharge, tenderness over all sinuses (pansinusitis); cranial nerve IV, V, VI dysfunction.	Occurrence: after viral URI; in setting of barotrauma, recent head trauma, skull fracture. Organisms involved: same as in frontal frontal sinusitis.

Sinus infections in children most often are associated with cough (constant, dry, possibly night-time); nasal discharge that may be thick, thin, clear, mucoid, or purulent; and foul breath. Intermittent, painless morning periorbital swelling also may be present. Older children complain of facial pain and headache. These symptoms in children and adults often occur in the setting of a cold that is prolonged or more severe than usually experienced by the patient. In adults, the initially clear nasal discharge becomes yellow, brown, or green. In children, nasal discharge and cough persist longer than the usual 5–7-day course of viral URIs. Even when symptoms last longer than usual for viral syndromes, there is almost always a history of improvement over time. The persistence of URI symptoms for more than 10 days or symptoms that do not improve suggest sinusitis.

Diagnostic Aids. Antral puncture is the most accurate tool for diagnosing acute maxillary sinusitis and provides specific bacteriologic information. This procedure is rarely done in the outpatient setting without specialty consultation. The bacteriology of maxillary sinusitis has been well studied in adults and children (see Table 2). Nasal or

Table 2. Sinusitis Syndromes (Columns continued)

Diagnosis	Treatment	Follow-up Issues
Water's view: opacity in maxillary sinus, air-fluid level, mucosal thickening > 8 mm adults, > 5 mm children. Transillumination: unilateral opacity. CT scan is the gold standard.	Adults: amoxicillin-clavulanic acid (500/125 mg 3 times/day or 875/125 mg 2 times/day × 10 days), cefuroxime (250 mg 2 times/day × 10 days). Children: amoxicillin (40 mg/kg/day in 3 divided doses for 2 weeks). Penicillin-allergic patients: trimethoprim-sulfamethoxazole (Bactrim; BID), cefaclor, erythromycin (Pediazole), azithromycin. If *H. influenzae* resistance is present in the community: chloramphenicol, 2.5–25 mg/kg 4 times/day for 14 days. If *S. pneumoniae* with high resistance level, consider levofloxacin, 500 mg. Hospitalize if severe symptoms or pain. If no response to outpatient therapy in 3–5 days, change to second drug.	Follow-up: acute infections, 34 wk; chronic infections, 6 wk Estimated disability: acute infections, 1 wk; chronic infections, variable
Caldwell's view: opacification of ethmoid sinus, elevated white blood cell count. CT scan with air fluid.	Adults and children: outpatient treatment for only mildest cases; treat as maxillary sinusitis. Hospitalize if severe symptoms, pain, any eye involvement (decreased visual acuity, proptosis, ophthalmoplegia), any orbital involvement (orbital, periorbital, cellulitis), and toxic-appearing condition.	Follow-up: acute infections, 3 wk or sooner if symptoms worsen; chronic infections, determined
Towne's view, lateral skull; Water's view: opacification of frontal sinus. Transillumination: absent, reduced. CT scan definitive.	Adults and children: outpatient treatment for only mildest cases; treat as maxillary sinusitis. Hospitalize all other cases.	Follow-up: all outpatients within 24 hr; acute infections 3 wk after therapy starts; chronic infections, per ENT. Estimated disability: 1 wk with complete recovery if treated.
Routine sinus views: parasinusitis. CT defines infection, delineates spread of infection.	Adults and children: outpatient treatment only for patients in nontoxic condition who are able to comply; treat as maxillary sinusitis. Hospitalize all other cases.	Follow-up: all outpatients within 24 hr; acute infections 3 wk after therapy starts; chronic infections, per ENT. Estimated disability: 1 wk with complete recovery if treated.

oropharyngeal cultures do not correlate with organisms obtained by sinus aspiration and are of no value in the diagnosis of sinusitis.

Transillumination of the maxillary sinus may assist in the diagnosis. This procedure is done in a completely darkened examination room. The physician places a lighted penlight into the patient's mouth. The patient closes his or her lips around the light, and the physician notes differences in illumination between the two sides of the face. Evans and colleagues found that an opaque sinus correlates strongly with purulent sinus infection as determined by sinus puncture.[4] Other studies, however, have found transillumination to be unreliable in the diagnosis of maxillary sinusitis.[5] Transillumination is often not possible in the urgent care setting because examination rooms are usually not dark enough to permit accurate interpretation of the results.

Ultrasonography also has been used to diagnose maxillary sinusitis; however, it is neither sensitive nor specific enough when compared with sinus x-rays to be used as a substitute for radiographic studies in the diagnosis of sinus disease.[3] Ultrasonography may have a place in the evaluation of pregnant patients with rhinitis who do not wish to have radiation exposure. In this setting, it is important to recognize its inherent limitations.[3]

Radiologic examination of the sinuses is designed to give information that complements the clinical findings. Computed tomography (CT) has replaced standard radiography as the modality of choice in the evaluation of the paranasal sinuses and adjacent structures.[6] The maxillary sinus appears to be the "best" sinus studies by conventional radiography. As a screening exam for a children with chronic respiratory complaints, especially when costs and radiation exposure are considered, a Water's view remains an acceptable diagnostic procedure.[3]

Management. Most clinicians recommend antibiotic treatment for sinusitis (see Table 2). Therapy is recommended for 10–14 days. Concurrent adjunct therapy should include steam or moist heat to the face several times each day, humidifying the patient's environment (especially at night), nasal cleaning with physiologic saline, and use of topical nasal decongestants for no more than 3–5 days to enhance sinus drainage. Most clinicians avoid using systemic antihistamines because of their drying effect on the nasal mucosa; the associated increased viscosity of nasal secretions hinders rather than helps sinus drainage.

Pitfalls in Practice. Complications of maxillary sinusitis are rare. Hospitalization should be considered for patients who have extreme symptoms or severe pain or who do not respond to outpatient treatment in 3–5 days. In such patients, a specialist should perform sinus puncture for drainage and culture, and other surgical procedures, such as a nasoantral window, should be considered to ensure adequate sinus drainage. CT of the sinuses is associated with a high false-positive rate because a high proportion of individuals with viral URI have fluid and mucosal thickening in their sinuses.

Ethmoiditis

Isolated bacterial infection of the ethmoid sinus is rare. The final common pathway, as in all sinus infections, is obstruction of the sinus ostia. Cancer, mucoceles, and pyomucoceles are considered in the differential diagnosis as causes of isolated ethmoiditis. Ethmoiditis usually has few symptoms and is recognized only when patients develop complications, which are most common in children and young adults. Most cases of ethmoiditis occur as a component of pansinusitis.

History and Physical Examination. Tenderness and swelling are usually present over the region of the ethmoid sinuses. Fever is common. Ethmoid sinus disease localizes pain over the bridge of the nose and behind the eyes, and pain may increase with eye movement.[3] Most patients present with signs of edema or cellulitis of the eyelids or periorbital tissues without orbital involvement. Orbital cellulitis, which is characterized by tenderness of the globe, ophthalmoplegia, chemosis, and erythema and edema of the lids may occasionally be present. Other complications are listed in Table 3.

Table 3. Complications of Sinusitis

Type of Sinusitis	Potential Complications
Maxillary	Sepsis, abscess formation, bony destruction, osteomyelitis, development of pansinusitis (with orbital complication)
Ethmoid	Subperiosteal abscess formation, orbital abscess formation with or without proptosis, meningitis, epidural abscess formation, cavernous sinus thrombosis
Frontal	Orbital extension (inflammatory edema, orbital cellulitis, subperiosteal abscess), meningitis, cerebral abscess formation, cavernous sinus thrombosis
Sphenoid	Orbital cellulitis, cranial nerve palsies, blindness, subdural abscess, meningitis, hypopituitarism, cavernous sinus thrombosis

Diagnostic Aids. On radiographic evaluation, Caldwell's view may show opacification of the ethmoid sinuses. CT scan is the modality of choice to look at the ethmoid sinuses.[6]

Management. Outpatient medical treatment for ethmoiditis is the same as that recommended for maxillary sinusitis; however, outpatient treatment of ethmoiditis should be attempted only in mild cases without orbital involvement. Outpatient antibiotic therapy should be continued for 3 weeks in children younger than 12 years and for 10–14 days in adults. Because of the high complication rate, patients who present with more than mild illness should be hospitalized and treated with high-dose intravenous antibiotics with early otolaryngologic consultation. Urgent otolaryngologic consultation and possible surgery are necessary for patients who present with ophthalmoplegia, proptosis, or decreased visual acuity.

Pitfalls in Practice. Failure to recognize the seriousness of symptoms (especially ophthalmologic) results in increased morbidity. Failure to ensure follow-up or to obtain immediate consultation in patients with signs or symptoms of orbital cellulitis or central nervous system involvement also results in poor outcomes and potential mortality.

Frontal Sinusitis

History and Physical Examination. The signs and symptoms of frontal sinusitis are presented in Table 2. Frontal sinus pain typically radiates from the forehead to the temple and occasionally to the occiput.[3] Other sinuses may be involved. The classic appearance is Pott's puffy tumor, which is a swollen, tender, erythematous mass over the frontal sinus.[7] Predisposing factors are similar to those for maxillary sinusitis; occasionally the patient has a history of barotrauma, recent head injury, or skull fracture.

On physical examination, patients may have fever and purulent nasal discharge. All sinuses should be examined to detect the presence of pansinusitis. Complications of frontal sinusitis are listed in Table 3.

Diagnostic Aids. Transillumination of the frontal sinus is done by placing a bright light under the medial border of the supraorbital ridge and evaluating the symmetry of the light transmittance over the frontal bone. One study has shown that transillumination is useful in the diagnosis of sinusitis if light transmission is absent or reduced. Towne's view, a lateral skull x-ray, and Water's view show the frontal sinuses, and may be useful in establishing the diagnosis. A CT scan may identify any degree of extension of infection.

Management. Outpatient treatment of frontal sinusitis should be attempted only after consultation with an otolaryngologist. Treatment of acute frontal sinusitis often requires hospitalization, intravenous antibiotics, and adjunct measures, including topical nasal decongestants and analgesics. Indications for surgery are progressive proptosis, decreasing visual acuity, localized pus, and orbital involvement with failure to respond to medical management after 24–48 hours.

Pitfalls in Practice. Significant morbidity and mortality can result from unrecognized frontal sinusitis. Mortality from meningitis, abscess formation, and cavernous sinus thromboses has been reported. Osteomyelitis of the frontal bone can be missed because of antibiotic masking or lack of suspicion. Computed tomography (CT) is invaluable in detecting complications of frontal sinusitis.

Sphenoid Sinusitis

Sphenoid sinusitis is frequently misdiagnosed on initial evaluation and may not be suspected until the appearance of one or more potentially fatal complications. The incidence of sphenoid sinusitis is low compared with other types of sinusitis.

History and Physical Examination. The signs and symptoms of sphenoid sinusitis are presented in Table 2. Sphenoid sinusitis may present as pansinusitis after a URI or as an isolated entity. Predisposing factors include barotrauma (e.g., swimming or diving in infected water), recent URI, and skull fracture. The area over each sinus should be examined to detect the presence of pansinusitis. Sphenoid sinusitis produces pain localized to the vertex of the head or the retro-orbital, occipital, or even the mastoid region. Unexplained tenderness over the cranial vertex or mastoid region also may be due to sphenoid sinusitis. Pain and paresthesias in the V1, V2, and V3 distribution of the trigeminal nerve may be noted. Nasal discharge is a common feature of sphenoid sinusitis but may not be present if the sinus openings have become obstructed by swollen mucosa. Fever frequently is detected in patients with acute sphenoid sinusitis but may be absent in patients with chronic disease.

Diagnostic Aids. Radiographic examination is mandatory in any patient suspected of having acute sphenoid sinusitis. Routine sinus x-rays were not satisfactory for the diagnosis in one series of case reports, however, and even linear sagittal tomography may not provide adequate information.[7] Therefore, most clinicians recommend obtaining a CT scan in cases of suspected sphenoid sinusitis.[6] This study also helps define spread of infection to the brain or cavernous sinus.

Management. Outpatient treatment may be tried in selected reliable patients who appear nontoxic, have no evidence of complications, are certain to follow up, and can comply with a regimen of oral antibiotics, intranasal decongestants, steam, and local heat. Outpatient treatment should not be attempted without first consulting an otolaryngologist with a follow-up visit in 24 hours to allow re-examination for signs and symptoms

of clinical worsening or the presence of complications. The complications of sphenoid sinusitis are listed in Table 3. Many authorities continue to recommend inpatient treatment with high-dose intravenous antibiotics, intranasal decongestants, local heat, steam,
and analgesics.

Pitfalls in Practice. The walls of the sphenoid sinus can be extremely thin. Sometimes
bone is absent, so that adjacent structures, which include the internal carotid artery,
optic nerve, and cavernous sinus (which contains cranial nerves V, VI, and IV) are separated from the sinus cavity only by a thin mucosal barrier. Therefore, spread of infection
is frequent if treatment is delayed or ineffective. Recognition of complications requires a
careful examination of the cranial nerves. Immediate referral is mandatory if cranial
nerve signs and symptoms are present.

Sphenoid sinusitis is a frequent cause of cavernous sinus thrombosis in adults. Clinical
features of cavernous sinus thrombosis include the sudden onset of photophobia,
headache, chemosis, ophthalmoplegia, proptosis, blindness, and sensory changes in the
V1 or V2 distribution of the trigeminal nerve. Signs and symptoms are reported to begin
unilaterally but can be bilateral. With pus in a closed vascular space, bacteremia can
occur together with fever and systemic infection.

Epistaxis

With the exception of menstrual bleeding, epistaxis is the most common form of spontaneous bleeding.[8] There are two types of epistaxis: the more easily controllable anterior
epistaxis, in which nasal bleeding originates from the anterior part of the nasal septum,
and the more severe posterior epistaxis, which can produce significant morbidity and,
rarely, mortality. Approximately 80–90% of nosebleeds are anteriorly located.[8] A unilateral nosebleed is almost always anterior, but in patients older than 40 years of age, up to
28% of nosebleeds may originate posteriorly. Most anterior epistaxis originates in
Kiesselbach's area, which is an anastomosing of the sphenopalatine artery, greater pala-
tine, and labial vessels. This area is easily visible on examination of the nasal septum.

Differential Diagnosis. Some of the many causes of nasal bleeding are listed in Table 4.
Most nasal bleeding is caused by mechanical factors that dry the nasal mucosa and lead
to cracking and bleeding. Local factors such as injury or inflammation also can cause
epistaxis. People who experience chronic crusting of the nose, such as those with atrophic rhinitis or nasal septal perforations, bleed profusely when the crusts are removed.
Arteriosclerosis involving nasal vessels, such as those on the septum and posterior end of
the inferior turbinate, can cause increased vessel fragility and rupture, especially in elder
patients with associated hypertension. Leukemia, hemophilia, and von Willebrand's disease

Table 4. Primary Causes of Epistaxis

Mechanical causes leading to muscosal dryness	Local factors
Overheated indoor air	Minor trauma (nose picking)
Lowering of atmospheric pressure or humidity	Inflammation secondary to upper respiratory infection or allergies
Interruption of laminal air flow due to septal irregularities	Vigorous noseblowing, sneezing
	Exposure to noxious agent (cocaine)
	Topical steroid nasal sprays

rarely present solely as epistaxis. Once bleeding has started, coagulopathies such as those associated with vitamin C and K deficiencies and alcoholism may make bleeding difficult to control. Despite a long list of possible etiologies for nasal bleeding, many nosebleeds have an indeterminate cause.

Management. Most patients can manage a bleeding episode without physician intervention. When bleeding is uncontrollable, persistent, or recurrent, however, patients seek evaluation. Thus, physicians see the most difficult, self-selected cases. Because nasal bleeding can be life-threatening, the goal of urgent care treatment must be to stop the bleeding while evaluation proceeds.

When a patient presents with epistaxis, the history taking of the current complaint should be brief and pertinent. It should determine that nasal bleeding is in fact present, not hemoptysis or hematemesis. The medical history should center on similar past episodes, medications, illnesses, allergies, polyps, nasal operations and habits. A family history of nasal bleeding or a bleeding disorder should be sought. A brief review of systems should establish nose breathing or mouth breathing to determine whether nasal obstruction is due to intrinsic or extrinsic causes. Orthostatic vital signs should be obtained, if possible.

The initial step in management of epistaxis is to have the patient pinch the nostrils together for 10 minutes. An ice pack applied to the neck or face helps during this phase of treatment by inducing reflex vasoconstriction of the nasal vessels. This technique is sound telephone advice, if a patient calls for instructions about the out-of-facility treatment of a nosebleed. During self-applied pressure, the vital signs can be determined and both patient and physician can prepare for examination. Both physician and patient should be draped in sheets or gowns; the physician should wear glasses and surgical gloves. The necessary instruments are a head light, nasal speculum, bayonet forceps, and suction catheters.

In preparing the nose for examination, the patient is asked to blow the nose lightly to remove clots, and any residual blood is gently suctioned from the nasal chamber with a suction catheter. Large clots are removed with the aid of a nasal speculum and bayonet forceps, and the bleeding nostril is packed with cotton pledgets soaked in an anesthetic solution. Cocaine (5–10%) is an excellent anesthetic (maximal dose, 200 mg). Benzocaine (Hurricaine, 20%) also can be used and is preferred to Cetacaine (14% benzocaine, 2% tetracaine). In patients younger than 2 years or in elderly patients with marked hypertension, 4% lidocaine with epinephrine (1:100,000) is used. The ideal situation is to insert cotton pledgets rolled onto cocaine applicators and soaked in 4% cocaine solution, placing one under each turbinate and one against the nasal septum. The nasal ala are compressed for 10 minutes. The pledgets are then removed, and residual blood is suctioned away.[8]

If a bleeding site is visible, a silver nitrate stick is applied for 20–30 seconds; excessive silver nitrate is removed with a cotton applicator to prevent spread of the chemical to the normal mucosa. Electric cautery also can be done if a prominent vessel (usually at the mucocutaneous junction on the nasal septum) is involved. Cautery is done with multiple light touches; heavy pressure is not necessary and can cause perforation of the mucosa. Cautery requires excellent nasal anesthesia and a dry field. Blind stabbing into a hemorrhaging site should never be done.

If the bleeding is now controlled, the patient should be observed for 15–30 minutes before discharge to ensure that the bleeding does not recur. During this time, further history taking and physical examination can be done. Neosporin or petroleum jelly is then applied to the bleeding site, and the patient is instructed to apply the same ointment to the nasal vestibule 3 times a day for 7–10 days. The patient also should be instructed to treat the bleeding site as a cut that should be handled carefully. As with any cut, a scab or crust forms when the bleeding stops; if the scab is removed prematurely, bleeding can recur. The patient also should be instructed not to scratch the nose; if a sneeze is inevitable, it should be done through the mouth. The patient should rest at home and drink plenty of fluids; aspirin and nonsteroidal anti-inflammatory drugs are to be avoided, if possible. The orthostatic blood pressure should be checked before discharge. If a significant change occurs, complete blood count, prothrombin time, partial thromboplastin time, and platelet count should be assessed and intravenous hydration begun; if symptoms are severe, hospitalization should be considered.

Most bleeding can be controlled with either pressure or cautery (chemical or electrical). When a bleeding site cannot be identified and blood continues to pool in the throat or to run out the nose, the bleeding originates either from an area of the nose that was not apparent on examination or from a true posterior site. If a bleeding point cannot be identified, a suction catheter can be advanced slowly along the floor of the nose until blood enters the suction tubing. This maneuver indicates the approximate distance of the bleeding site from the nares. An anterior nasal pack is then used to attempt to stop the bleeding.

The classic nasal pack is petroleum jelly gauze (¼ inch by 72 inches) impregnated with antibiotic ointment. Anterior nasal packing requires excellent nasal anesthesia and meticulous attention to the details of packing. Packing applied so that it bunches in the anterior portion of the nose promotes rather than controls hemorrhage by acting as a wick. Instead, the gauze should be passed with a bayonet forceps along the nasal floor to the posterior tip of the inferior turbinate. Successive folds should be placed from anterior to posterior in a ribbon candy–like arrangement, wedging the packing inferiorly and superiorly. To ensure that the packing does not prolapse into the nasopharynx or hang down into the oropharynx, both the starting end and the finishing end are extended outward through the anterior nares. Packing should be as tight as possible to achieve hemostasis, but excessive pressure, which can cause septal ulceration and necrosis, should be avoided. An average nose properly packed should accommodate approximately 72 inches of packing. Daily follow-up is mandatory for patients with anterior nasal packing, which is usually left in place for 24–48 hours.

An alternative to anterior nasal packing is an anterior nasal balloon. Among the advantages of the nasal balloon are simplicity of use and easy reversibility.[9] There are various nasal balloons from which to choose. An example is the Epistat nasal catheter, which is a dual-cuff silicone catheter with a central airway and two independently inflatable balloons. The balloon is inserted along the nasal floor to the junction of the three ports of the device, and the anterior port of the device is inflated. If oozing or bleeding continues, the posterior balloon is then inflated. Once the bleeding stops, the balloon is deflated, coated with antibiotic ointment, and reinflated with saline.[10] When nasal balloons are used to control posterior bleeding, overinflation must be avoided; inflation should be sufficient to control posterior bleeding but not enough to cause obvious bulging of the soft palate.

Compressed sponges (Merocel, Mystic, CT) are easy alternatives to gauze packing. The advantages of Merocel packs are that they can be inserted quickly and easily with little experience. The Merocel should be placed on the floor of the nose in a horizontal plane. If the sponge does not adequately expand with blood, saline or lidocaine with 1% epinephrine can be dripped onto the sponge. A recent study showed that the Merocel was successful at controlling epistaxis in up to 90% of patients.[11] The Merocel packing should be left in place for 3–5 days. After gauze packing or Merocel placement, oral antibiotics should be considered.[11] The patient should follow up with his or her primary physician; if the bleeding is recurrent, referral to an ear, nose, and throat specialist is appropriate.

In some circumstances, patients may require bilateral anterior nasal packing to provide tamponade of the bleeding site. The septum is easily displaced, and often bleeding continues, unless the septum is buttressed on the contralateral side with an additional anterior pack. Patients who require bilateral nasal packing may require hospitalization to observe for the development of potential complications (see below). Elderly patients and patients who have significant medical illness may require oxygen if bilateral nasal packing produces hypoxia. Required pain medications may further depress ventilation.[10]

Posterior bleeding can occasionally be controlled with anterior nasal packs. Failure to control bleeding with anterior packs necessitates a posterior pack and usually mandates admission to the hospital. When a posterior pack is necessary, an intravenous line should be placed and blood should be obtained for complete blood count, prothrombin time, partial thromboplastin time, and platelet count. Posterior bleeding not controlled in this manner may require posterior balloon tamponade. This procedure is best done in an emergency department.

Local complications of anterior nasal packing are otitis media and purulent sinusitis. When a nasal balloon catheter is used, the incidence of local complications increases when bilateral tamponade is required, the duration of cuff inflation is more than 24 hours, or the posterior cuff is inflated and produces eustachian tube obstruction.[9] Oral antibiotics should be considered in patients with nasal packing to avoid the risk of sinusitis secondary to blocked sinus ostia. Decongestants to the unaffected nostril and analgesics to control local pain and headache are also important. When patients are sent home, they should be instructed to apply ice to the nose to reduce oozing (if present), to use a humidifier, to reduce oral dehydration from mouth breathing, and to keep the lips moist with a petroleum-based ointment.

Pitfalls in Practice. Substantial hazards are associated with the use of nasal packing to control nasal bleeding. Most severe nosebleeds occur in the fifth to eighth decades of life, when associated medical disease often complicates all forms of therapy.

A specific nasovagal reflex has been demonstrated in dogs.[12] Stimulation of canine nasal mucous membranes produces prolonged bradycardia, reduction of cardiac output, decrease in blood pressure, and apnea. This reflex could be abolished with topical nasal anesthesia. If this reflex is also present in humans, inadequate nasal anesthesia before nasal packing may cause similar events.

Topical anesthetics and vasoconstrictors have toxic properties. A 200-mg dose of cocaine (2 ml of a 10% solution) is safe in healthy adults. A smaller amount should be used in elderly, and/or hypertensive patients; 4% viscous lidocaine with epinephrine (1:100,000) may be safer.

Local complications associated with posterior nasal packing include laceration of the soft palate and damage to the nostrils by anchoring packs over buttresses to secure the packs. A posterior nasal pack may become dislodged and aspirated with fatal results. Posterior nasal packing with a balloon catheter has been reported to cause acute compressive optic neuropathy that was reversed on removal of the catheter.[13]

Nasally packed patients may become hypoxic. Numerous cases of unexpected death have been reported in patients with posterior epistaxis treated with anterior and posterior nasal packs and sedation. Aspiration of blood and exaggeration of pulmonary dysfunction in the elderly are the primary causes of such hypoxia, especially when compounded by acute blood loss. A bulky posterior pack that overfills the nasopharynx and depresses the soft palate can create relative upper airway obstruction, especially during sleep, and lead to hypoventilation.[14] Supplemental oxygen is recommended to improve hypoxemia but may remove the respiratory drive in patients with chronic carbon dioxide retention, who are dependent on hypoxic drive to maintain ventilation. Serial measurements of oxygen saturation, therefore, are prudent in patients with posterior nasal packing.

Sinusitis results from occlusion of sinus ostia by nasal packing and blood accumulation. Otitis media with effusion and even hemotympanum has been reported. Toxic shock syndrome, secondary to nasal packing, was first reported in 1982 by Thomas and coworkers.[15] Considering the numerous possible infectious complications of nasal packing, antistaphylococcal antibiotics are often used for the entire duration of packing.

All patients with nasal hemorrhage requiring nasal packing should have a thorough examination of the nose and nasopharynx after removal of the pack to detect anatomic abnormalities, tumors, and complications of packing.

Nasal Foreign Bodies

Children and occasionally adults may insert foreign bodies into the nasal passages or the external ear canals during play or exploratory activities. The type of foreign body is limited only by the kinds of small objects in the environment; therefore, during medical management it is imperative to remind caregivers of the danger to prevent subsequent occurrences.

Differential Diagnosis. Patients usually seek medical care after attempting to remove the foreign body at home, thus selecting the most difficult cases for the physician. Acute complaints include pain, foreign body sensation, witnessed event, recurrent "colds," persistent unexplained unilateral nasal discharge, and recurrent sinus infection (most often maxillary sinusitis). In children, a nasal foreign body should be considered with a history of persistent rhinitis, halitosis, or otitis media.

Detection is usually made after careful physical examination of the nasal passages. Vasoconstrictors, commonly 0.5% or 0.25% Neo-Synephrine, injected with a tuberculin syringe through an appropriately sized nasal speculum, are often necessary to complete a careful examination. In cases of a suspected intranasal foreign body not visualized on physical examination or recurrent sinus infection, a Water's view and lateral nasopharyngeal radiograph may be helpful.

The only true emergency occurs when button batteries are inserted into the nasal passages. They can injure mucosal surfaces by several mechanisms. Burns can result from electrolyte leakage or the production of alkali if external currents are generated when the battery is in contact with moist mucosal surfaces. Pressure necrosis and mercury toxicity from leaky mercury button batteries also can occur. Mucosal injury from button batteries can occur in as little as 4 hours.[16]

Management. Once found, a foreign body requires expeditious removal. Bright illumination with a head mirror or head light, nasal specula, and bayonet forceps are invaluable for attempting to remove foreign bodies from the nasal passages. Placing the patient in an upright position decreases the chance of aspiration of the foreign body and the risk of blood flowing posteriorly into the pharynx. Local anesthetics and vasoconstrictors aid visualization, enable patients to cooperate without struggling, and minimize bleeding if the nasal mucous membranes are inadvertently abraded during removal attempts. For infants, 4% viscous lidocaine is recommended; for toddlers older than 2 years and young children, it is safe to use 4% cocaine solution. Cocaine (maximum dose, 200 mg) is also recommended for adults; cocaine solution with epinephrine (1:100,000) also may be useful. Occasionally sedation and anesthesia are required for the safe removal of a nasal foreign body. Anteriorly lodged foreign bodies usually can be visualized and, if their edges permit, grasped with a forceps, bayonet, wire loop, or angled hook. With smooth-edged foreign bodies, a suction catheter may be useful.

Deep foreign bodies that cannot be reached by other means may be removed by using balloon catheters. An appropriately sized Fogarty catheter (2F, 4F, or 6F) is advanced into the nasal passage beyond the point of the visualized foreign body. The balloon is then inflated with water or saline and the catheter withdrawn, thus pushing the foreign body outward through the anterior nare.

Air pressure has been used to blow objects out of nares. This technique is especially useful in children. The patient lies supine, and the uninvolved nostril is occluded. Air is then briskly introduced into the mouth and pushes the foreign body from the unoccluded nostril. Air can be introduced by mouth-to-mouth ventilation or gentle use of a bag-valve mask.[17] Parents can perform this maneuver on their children, thus reducing the child's anxiety.

Pitfalls in Practice. After appropriate anesthesia and sedation, foreign body removal is usually possible. In cases in which the foreign body is inaccessible or becomes so during removal attempts, specialty consultation should be obtained. If removal attempts result in complications, appropriate urgent referral is needed. In addition, inserted button batteries that are not immediately removed demand urgent specialty consultation and removal.

Failure to diagnose and remove a nasal foreign body can result in recurrent sinusitis or persistent nasal discharge. Tetanus in an unimmunized child has been reported after insertion of a nasal foreign body[18]; thus, it is important to inquire about the tetanus immunization status of patients with nasal foreign bodies and to provide primary immunizations or booster shots as required.

Nasal Injuries

Most injuries to the nose result from motor vehicle accidents, falls, assaults, or play. Patients frequently complain of pain, bleeding, and a new deformity of the nasal contours.

Soft tissue swelling and edema can obscure subtle changes in the external contour of the nose during the first examination. Deviation of the medial nasal septum may be seen when the nose is examined with a nasal speculum; crepitus may be noted on palpation of the nose. Detection of crepitus or mobility of skeletal parts on palpation of the nasal septum is usually diagnostic of fracture.

Management. All patients with nasal trauma should undergo a speculum examination for septal hematoma, which most often appears as a purplish (occasionally fluctuant) symmetric bulge of the medial nasal septum. Septal hematomas are treated emergently by aspiration with an 18-gauge needle attached to a 12-ml syringe after adequate nasal anesthesia.[17]

All patients suspected of having a nasal fracture should be referred to an otolaryngologist within 5 days for re-examination and treatment because most fractures that are seen early can be treated by closed techniques. Fractures seen more than 2 weeks after injury usually require treatment with more extensive open procedures. In patients with septal hematoma aspirated in the urgent care center, an anterior pack should be placed on the aspirated side, and the patient should be reexamined in 24 hours to ascertain that the hematoma has not reaccumulated.

Radiographs of the nasal bones are often not helpful during the initial visit because normal divisions between adjacent pieces of cartilage may be mistaken for fracture. Radiographs add nothing to the diagnosis when an obvious deformity is present and are obtained most often for medicolegal purposes. Most patients with fractures report a change in the contour of the nose. If the clinician has a high index of suspicion that the nose may not be solely involved, CT scan gives better assessment of the extent of fractures. CT scans also show associated sinus wall fractures. For the first 2 days after injury, ice packs to the area and slight elevation of the head, whenever possible, decrease the nasal swelling.

Pitfalls in Practice. Unrecognized septal hematomas usually become infected and are complicated by septal abscesses, destruction of septal cartilage with medial septal perforations, "saddle nose" deformations, or occluded airway. The cartilage of the nasal septum does not have direct vascular supply and receives nutrients from the surrounding perichondrial tissues. If the blood accumulates, the septum loses its nutrient supply and the stagnant blood may get infected. With blood or pus accumulation cartilage necrosis may occur.

References

1. Shapiro GG, Rachelevsky GS: Introduction and definition of sinusitis. J Allergy Clin Immunol 90:417–418, 1992.
2. Gungor A, Corey JP: Pediatric sinusitis: A literature review with emphasis on the role of allergy. Otolaryng Head Neck Surg 116:4–15, 1994.
3. Incaudo GA, Wooding LG: Diagnosis and treatment of acute and subacute sinusitis in children and adults. Clin Rev Allergy Immunol 16:157–204, 1998.
4. Evans FO Jr, Sydnor JB, Moore WE, et al: Sinusitis of the maxillary antrum. N Engl J Med 293:735–739, 1975.
5. Spector SL, Lotan A, English G, et al: Comparison between transillumination and the roentgenogram in diagnosing paranasal sinus disease. J Allergy Clin Immunol 67:22–26, 1981.
6. Zinreich S: Imaging of inflammatory sinus disease. Otolaryngol Clin North Am 26: 535, 1993.
7. Ramsey PG, Wegmu EA: Complications of bacterial infection of the ears, paranasal sinuses and oropharynx in adults, Emerg Med Clin North Am 3:15–152, 1985.

8. Emanuel JM: Epistaxis. Otolaryngology Head Neck Surgery, 3rd ed. St. Louis, Mosby, 1998.
9. Elwang S, Kamel T, Mekhamer A: Pneumatic nasal catheters: Advantages and drawbacks. J Laryngol Otol 100:641–647, 1986.
10. Cook PR, Renner G, Williams F: A comparison of nasal balloon and posterior gauze packs for posterior epistaxis. Ear Nose Throat J 64:79–82, 1985.
11. Pringle MB, Beasley P, Brightwell AP: The use of Merocel nasal packs in the treatment of epistaxis. J Laryngol Otol 110:543–546, 1996.
12. Angell-lames IE: Nasal reflexes. Proc R Soc Med 62:1287–1293, 1969.
13. Sadowsky AK, Leavensworth N, Wirtschafter ID: Compressive optic neuropathy induced by intranasal balloon catheter [letter]. Am J Opthalmol 99:487–489, 1985.
14. Fairbanks DNF: Complications of nasal packing. Otolaryngol Head Neck Surg 94:412–415, 1986.
15. Thomas SW, Baird IM, Frazier RD: Toxic shock syndrome following submucous resection and rhinoplasty. JAMA 247:2402–2403, 1982.
16. Capo IM, Lucente FE: Alkaline battery foreign bodies of the ear and nose. Arch Otolaryngol Head Neck Surg 112:562–563, 1986.
17. Manthey DE, Harrison BF: Otolaryngologic procedures. In Roberts JR, Hedges JR (eds): Clinical Procedures in Emergency Medicine, 3rd ed. Philadelphia, W.B. Saunders, 1998, pp 1120–1149.
18. Sarniak AP, Venkat G: Cephalic tetanus as a compilation of a nasal foreign body. Am J Dis Child 135:571–572, 1981.

Chapter 13

Urgencies of the Oropharynx

Susan Krieg, MD
Karen Kuo, MD

Pharyngitis

The diagnostic category of pharyngitis includes tonsillitis, tonsillopharyngitis, and nasopharyngitis. Regardless of the extent of pharyngeal involvement, pharyngitis is defined as an inflammatory illness of the pharynx accompanied by sore throat. Sore throat is a common complaint that is caused by multiple agents (Table 1). In many patients, however, no specific cause of pharyngitis can be defined.

Table 1. Common Causes of Pharyngitis

Infectious		Noninfectious	
Nonviral:	Group A β-hemolytic *Streptococcus pyogenes*	Mechanical:	Trauma (thermal injuries, abrasions)
	Neisseria gonorrhoeae		Foreign bodies in pharynx
	Corynebacterium diphtheriae		Chemical exposure (inhalations or
	Mixed anaerobic infection (fusobacterium,		ingestions of irritants)
	spirochetes)		Dehydration
	Hemophilus influenzae		Mouth breathing
	Mycoplasma pneumoniae		Sinus drainage
	Treponema pallidum		Drug reactions
	Candida sp.		Chemotherapy
	Cryptococcus sp.	Systemic:	Glossopharyngeal neuralgia
	Histoplasma sp.		Subacute thyroiditis
	Toxoplasma sp.		Systemic lupus erythematosus
	Chlamydia trachomatis		Carotidynia
Viral:	Rhinovirus		Cricoarytenoid arthritis
	Coronavirus		Leukemia
	Adenovirus		Multiple myeloma
	Herpes simplex		Hodgkin's disease
	Epstein-Barr		Pharyngeal, laryngeal cancer
	Cytomegalovirus		Other cancers
	Coxsackie A, B		Immunodepressed states
	Rubeola		
	Rubella		
	Influenza viruses		

In the urgent care setting, management of patients with pharyngitis involves determination of the need for antibiotics, emergent referral, or hospitalization. Timely follow-up is important. It is necessary, therefore, to determine the most probable cause of the pharyngitis and to arrive at a treatment plan. Causes, characteristics, diagnostic aids, and therapy for bacterial, viral, and miscellaneous causes of pharyngitis are presented in Tables 2, 3,

Table 2. Bacterial Syndromes of the Oropharynx *(Columns continue on facing page)*

Syndrome	Presentation	Examination	Epidemiology
Streptococcal pharyngitis (Group A β–hemolytic)	Onset: gradual, 2–3 days Age: children, young adults rare in children under age of 2 yr Complaints: sore throat, dysphagia, fever, chills, headache, abdominal pain, vomiting Peak incidence: Jan. to May Duration: untreated, 1–6 wk; treated, 24–48 hr	Elevated temperature, scarlatiniform rash, tender cervical adenopathy, beefy red pharynx, swollen tonsils pharynx, swollen tonsils, white patchy exudate on tonsils, and pharyngeal walls, palatal petechiae, lack of cough	Air-borne spread of oro-pharyngeal discharge Incubation: 1–3 days Communicability: not infectious hours after starting antibiotics
Gonococcal pharyngitis (*Neisseria gonorrhoeae*)	Onset: 1–2 days after exposure Age: all age groups Complaints: sore throat, mouth sores, rectal sores, genital complaints, fever, malaise Duration: untreated weeks to months; treated, 3–5 days	Red oropharynx, pharyngeal exudate, pharyngeal ulcers	Oral-genital route of spread Incubation: 1–2 days Communicability: until treated for genital gonococci, but low infectivity Frequent concomitant chlamydial infection
Epiglottitis (*Hemophilus influenzae*)	Onset: Abrupt, often after mild respiratory illness Age: unimmunized children 2–7 yr old; adults, 20–40 yr old Complaints: severe sore throat, dysphagia, brassy cough, muffled voice or aphonia, fever, respiratory distress, drooling Duration: untreated, rapid progression to airway obstruction, respiratory arrest.	Elevated temperature, pulse, respiratory rate; inspiratory and possibly expiratory stridor; nasal flaring; intercostal retractions; diminished breath sounds; erythematous pharynx; pooled secretions; minimal adenopathy or neck edema; altered mental status; epiglottitis red, swollen (do not attempt to visualize unless airway equipment and management skills available)	Airborne spread of oral and nasal discharge Incubation: 2–4 days Communicability: until treated
Diphtheria (*Coryne-bacterium diphtheriae*)	Onset: insidious Age: unimmunized children 5–15 yr old; unimmunized adults Complaints: sore throat, respiratory symptoms, dysphagia, malaise, headaches, fever, chills, nausea. Duration: untreated, rapid progression to coma, death within 7 days; treated, 3-7 days.	Elevated temperature (to 104° F), tender cervical adenopathy, neck edema, erythematous pharynx; thick, gray, adherent pseudomembrane on tonsils, pharynx, uvula, palate	Airborne spread of oro-pharyngeal secretions Incubation: 2–6 days Communicability: 1–2 days after start of therapy (until bacilli can no longer be isolated), 2–4 wk preceding therapy
Trench mouth, Vincent's angina (mixed anaerobic infection)	Onset: abrupt Age: 15–35 yr, immunosuppressed patients, poor oral hygiene, smokers Complaints: sore throat, mouth sores, metallic taste in mouth, foul breath, bleeding gingiva. Duration: untreated, becomes chronic, or spontaneous resolution in weeks; treated, 2–7 days.	Low-grade temperature elevation, tender cervical adenopathy; interdental papillae; painful hyperemic bleeding gingiva, erythematous oropharynx and tonsils; necrotic ulcers on gingiva, tonsils pharyngeal walls	Spread by direct contact with ulcerative material Incubation: not determined Communicability: during ulcerative stage if direct oral contact

Table 2. *(Columns continued)*

Diagnosis	Treatment	Follow-Up Issues
Rapid strep screening, throat culture, evidence of scarlatiniform rash, clinical suspicion	Antibiotics: adults, penicillin G benzathine (1.2 million U IM), procaine/benzathine penicillin (1.2 million U IM) or penicillin VK (500 mg PO bid for 10 days) or erythromycin (500 mg PO bid for 10 days) Children: penicillin G benzathine (600,000 U IM if < 30 kg body weight), procaine/benzathine penicillin (300/900,000 U IM for children up to 64 kg, causes significantly less pain and tenderness at injection site), penicillin VK (250 mg PO bid for 10 days) or erythromycin (40 mg/kg/day in 4 divided doses PO for 10 days) Hospitalize if patient is unable to swallow fluids, is significantly dehydrated, or if potential complications exist.	Follow-up in 2–3 weeks; rapid strep or culture for symptomatic family contacts, prophylaxis for asymptomatic family contacts with history of rheumatic fever Estimated disability: complete recovery in 5–6 days with treatment. Children may return to school or day care 1 day after antibiotic administration.
Positive growth on Thayer-Martin agar False positives in oropharynx from other *Neisseria* strains which are normal flora Culture of oropharynx, cervix or penis and rectum can increase yield.	Antibiotics: adults, children more than 50 kg body weight: ceftriaxone (125 mg IM) plus either azithromycin (1 g PO once) or doxycycline (100 mg PO bid for 7 days); alternative: ciprofloxacin (500 mg PO single dose) plus either azithromycin (1 g PO once) or doxycycline (100 mg PO bid for 7 days) Children: ceftriaxone (125 mg IM) or sulfamethoxazole-trimethoprim plus azithromycin (20 mg/kg PO single dose)	Follow-up in 7 days after completion of therapy; suspect child abuse in diagnosed children; prophylaxis for contacts is advised. Estimated disability: minimal distress before and during treatment, complete recovery after treatment Potential complication: disseminated disease.
Enlarged epiglottis seen on lateral neck soft tissue x-ray "thumb" sign, positive throat and blood cultures, elevated white blood cell count, left shift, hypoxemia	Support: never leave patient unattended; allow patient to assume most comfortable position; give high-flow humidified oxygen if tolerated. For sick-appearing patients, immediate transport to a facility with airway skills (including surgical airways) given high risk of airway obstruction. Transport: by ambulance with medical personnel skilled in airway management with airway equipment and bag-valve mask available.	Follow-up per primary care physician Prophylaxis for contacts in households with children (other than index case) younger than 4 yr of age, day care centers if two cases occur within 60 days; rifampin (20 mg/kg qid for 4 days, maximum 600 mg per day) Estimated disability: complete recovery in 3–7 days with treatment
Positive growth on Loeffler's medium, PCR testing, methylene blue stain of pseudomembranes, fluorescent labeling with diphtheria antitoxin; gram-positive pleomorphic bacilli	Support: IV fluids, hydration, airway support if needed Transport to intensive care unit, isolation with cardiac monitor. Antitoxin: 20–40,000 U IM, or if severe, 40–80,000 U, half given IV. Then antibiotics: erythromycin 40 mg/kg/day PO for 14 days; or procaine penicillin G (600,000 U IM bid for 14 days)	Follow-up per primary physician; prophylaxis for contacts: if previously immunized, tetanus-diphtheria toxoid booster plus penicillin G procaine (600,000 U IM single dose) or erythromycin (children 40/mg/kg/day in 4 divided doses for 10 days); if unimmunized, 3000 U antitoxin IM immediately or start tetanus-diphtheria toxoid series. Daily evaluation important. Estimated disability: 2–3 wk after discharge with bed rest. Potential complications: hematogenous spread; delayed neurologic, cardiac or pulmonary problems; complete airway obstruction from pseudomembrane.
Clinical examination only (mixed bacterial culture growth and Gram stain)	Refer to dentist for local debridement Antibiotics: adults: penicillin VK (250 mg PO qid for 7 days), metronidazole (250 mg PO tid for 7 days), penicillin G procaine (600,000 U IM bid for 7 days) Support 3% peroxide mouth wash, analgesics	Follow-up after antibiotic course complete. recovery in 5–7 days with treatment. Estimated disability: complete recovery in 5–7 days with treatment Potential complications: septicemia, jugular venous thrombosis, lung abscess if aspiration occurs

Table 3. Viral Syndromes of the Oropharynx *(Columns continue on facing page)*

Syndrome	Presentation	Examination	Epidemiology
Infectious mononucleosis (Epstein-Barr virus)	Onset: gradual Age: adolescents, young adults Complaints: sore throat, headache, fever, rash, malaise, anorexia Duration: < 4 wk	Low-grade temperature elevation, rubella-like rash, splenomegaly, hepatomegaly, occasionally jaundice, eyelid edema, petechiae on soft palate, tonsillar enlargement; thick white tonsillar exudate	Airborne or direct spread of oropharyngeal discharge Incubation: 2–7 wk Communicability: undetermined
Viral pharyngitis (rhinovirus, coronavirus, adenovirus, influenza virus)	Onset: gradual Age: all ages Complaints: sore throat, cough, rhinorrhea, hoarseness, malaise, headache, abdominal pain	Low-grade temperature elevation, cervical adenopathy, tonsillar exudate (adenovirus), conjunctival inflammation (adenovirus), coryza, normal oropharynx	Airborne spread of oropharyngeal discharge Incubation: 48 hr Communicability: several days.
Croup (parainfluenza, RSV, adenovirus, measles)	Onset: gradual, 1–2 days Age: 3 mo to 5 yr Complaints: sore throat, hoarseness, fever, barking cough, respiratory distress; worse at night Duration: 3–4 days	Low-grade temperature elevation, tachypnea, respiratory distress, stridor, expiratory rhonchi; barking, seal-like cough; normal oropharynx	Airborne spread of oropharyngeal secretions Incubation: 1–4 days Communicability: undetermined.
Herpangina (coxsackie A)	Onset: acute Age: children younger than 6 yr Most common in months of June to October Complaints: sore throat, dysphagia, headaches, abdominal pain, anorexia Duration: 1–4 days	Temperature elevation, erythematous oropharynx; occasional parotitis; exanthem (hand, foot and mouth disease); vesicular lesions in clusters throughout oropharynx; scattered, shallow gray ulcers surrounded by red halos	Airborne or direct spread of oropharyngeal discharge Incubation: 1–4 days Communicability: while symptomatic
Herpetic stomatitis (herpes simplex, varicella-zoster)	Onset: precipitous Age: 1–3 yr, 20–40 yr Complaints: sore throat, mouth sores, in recurrent cases patients frequently experience a prodrome of tingling or burning Duration: 7–10 days	Temperature elevation; red, swollen gingiva; erythematous oropharynx; painful, vesicular and/or ulcerative lesions throughout the oropharynx; cervical adenopathy; lesions secondary to herpes zoster will not cross the midline	Airborne or direct spread of oral secretions Incubation: 1–3 days Communicability: undetermined

and 4. Many infectious agents can cause tonsillar or pharyngeal exudates, and the characteristics of these exudates can aid in the diagnosis (Table 5). Oral and pharyngeal lesions can present as part of the pharyngitis or as the primary cause of oral or pharyngeal pain. Table 6 lists various differentiating characteristics of oropharyngeal lesions.

In the evaluation of patients with a sore throat, important historical points include onset and progression of symptoms, associated or additional symptoms, exposure to irritants or toxins (inhaled or ingested); exposure to other symptomatic individuals, smoking history, past medical history, and current medications.

Physical examination should include the ears, nose, oropharynx, neck, chest, heart, and abdomen. Vital signs, general appearance, and state of hydration are also important in determining treatment and disposition.

Table 3. *(Columns continued)*

Diagnosis	Treatment	Follow-Up Issues
Positive monospot test, heterophile titer, lymphocytosis (> 50% lymphs), with presence of atypical lymphocytes	Support: bed rest acutely; saline gargles, antipyretics, fluids; restrict activity if splenomegaly Medications: steroids occasionally used in cases where airway is compromised. Hospitalize if airway compromised, significant dehydration.	Estimated disability: 2–4 wk, although fatigue may last 3–4 months, with complete recovery. Potential acute complications: airway obstruction, splenic rupture, and bacterial superinfection with group A strep.
Viral isolation, antibody titers	Support: bed rest acutely: saline gargles, topical anesthetics, antipyretics, and fluids.	Estimated disability: 3–4 days with complete recovery. Potential complication: bacterial superinfection.
Viral isolation, antibody titers, "steeple" sign on postero-anterior soft tissue neck x-ray (narrowed column of air in trachea appearing in form of steeple in subglottic area)	Support: bed rest, fluids, humidified oxygen Medication: epinephrine for moderate to severe symptoms (0.5 ml/kg of 1:1000 solution diluted 1:8 with water, delivered by aerosol over 15 min; patients tend to return to baseline in 2 hr), dexamethasone (0.6 mg/kg IM, PO or IV, single dose). Hospitalize if patients are unreliable, if declining level of consciousness, if condition appears to be toxic, if severe respiratory distress.	Estimated disability: 3–4 days with complete recovery Potential acute complications: extension of airway edema, airway obstruction
Viral isolation, antibody titers	Support: bed rest, fluids, antipyretics, analgesics, topical anesthetic agents (i.e., "magic mouthwash": lidocaine, diphenhydramine, aluminum hydroxide).	Estimated disability: 5–7 days with complete recovery Potential complications: dehydration
Viral isolation, antibody titers	Oral antivirals have been shown to reduce severity and duration of symptoms if begun during prodromal phase. Adults: acyclovir (400 mg PO tid for 5 days), famciclovir (250 mg PO tid for 5 days), valacyclovir (1000 mg PO bid for 5 days) Support: topical anesthetic agents, normal saline agents, oral analgesics.	Estimated disability: 5–7 days with complete recovery Many who experience primary outbreak will have recurrent outbreaks, usually with less severe symptoms Potential complications: dehydration

Streptococcal Pharyngitis

Group A beta-hemolytic streptococcus (GABHS) is thought to be the most common cause of bacterial pharyngitis in both adults and children. The prevalence of GABHS ranges from 15% to 30% in children with signs and symptoms of pharyngitis. It is rarely encountered in children younger than 2 years. Streptococcal pharyngitis is most common from January to May but may occur at other times as well. The classic characteristics of streptococcal pharyngitis are sore throat; pain with swallowing; beefy red pharynx; swollen erythematous tonsils; thick, white, and patchy exudate on tonsils or pharyngeal walls; fever; and tender cervical adenopathy. Other possible findings include nausea, vomiting, headache, red swollen uvula, petechiae on the soft palate, and a scarlatiniform

Table 4. Miscellaneous Syndromes of the Oropharynx *(Columns continue on facing page)*

Syndrome	Presentation	Examination	Epidemiology
Mycoplasma pneumoniae	Onset: gradual Age: school age children and young adults Complaints: sore throat, earache, persistent cough, headache, fever Duration: untreated, 2–6 wk; treated, 1–3 wk	Low-grade temperature elevation, congested tympanic membranes, bullous and hemorrhagic myringitis, erythematous oropharynx, mild tonsillar swelling; wheezing, rales, rhonchi	Airborne spread of respiratory secretions, direct contact Incubation: 1–2 wk Communicability: weeks, low infectivity
Oral thrush (*Candida albicans*)	Onset: gradual Age: infants, immunosuppressed adults Complaints: mild dysphagia, mild sore throat Duration: untreated, 5–10 days; treated, 3–7 days.	White, cheesy patches of exudate over shallow, bleeding ulcers scattered throughout oropharynx	Airborne spread of spores Incubation: 2–3 days Communicability: undetermined, but low infectivity
Canker sore (aphthous ulcers)	Onset: precipitous with burning or tingling prodrome Age: all ages Complaint: recurrent mouth sores Duration: 7–14 days	Small, shallow, painful vesicles with membranous base surrounded by red halo	Airborne or direct spread from oropharyngeal secretions Incubation: undetermined Communicability: undetermined
Chlamydia trachomatis	Onset: gradual Age: children, young adults Complaints: mild sore throat, upper respiratory symptoms Duration: untreated, 1–3 wk; treated, 7–10 days	Erythematous oropharynx, mild tonsillar swelling; conjunctivitis or genital symptoms	Orogenital spread or from conjunctive drainage into oropharynx

rash. Clinical findings that point away from GABHS and toward viral etiology include absence of fever and presence of cough, coryza, and diarrhea.[2]

In the 1980s, acute rheumatic fever (ARF) and suppurative complications of streptococcal pharyngitis re-emerged in North America. The reasons are unclear but may involve more virulent serotypes of the bacteria, as well as host factors.[3] For this reason, accurate diagnosis and treatment of GABHS may be even more important than previously thought.

Diagnostic Aids. Rapid streptococcal testing has emerged at the diagnostic forefront in recent years. A multitude of rapid screens can indicate the presence of group A streptococci in minutes. The sensitivity and specificity of these tests, however, are widely variable. Overall, latex agglutination tests have a median sensitivity of around 80% and specificity of 96%. Enzyme-linked immunosorbent assays (ELISAs) demonstrate a median sensitivity of 78% and specificity of 97%. Optical immune assay, a newer form of rapid test, may be more sensitive, with a median test sensitivity of about 91% and specificity of 95%.[4] Although these tests are helpful in the early definition of the disease, diagnosis still requires correlation of test results with the clinical picture. These screens identify streptococcal antigen in the pharynx but do not differentiate between infected patients and asymptomatic carriers. A positive streptococcal screen in the presence of clinical symptoms strongly suggests the diagnosis.

Table 4. *(Columns continued)*

Diagnosis	Treatment	Follow-Up Issues
Elevated cold agglutinin titer for patients older than 12 yr PCR	Antibiotics: adults, erythromycin (500 mg PO qid for 10 days) or tetracycline (250 mg PO qid for 10 days); children, erythromycin (40 mg./kg/day in 4 divided doses for 7–10 days); clarithromycin and azithromycin also effective. Support: bed rest, humidity, fluids, analgesics, antipyretics	Estimated disability: complete recovery in 7–10 days. Consider isolating immuno-compromised contacts
Potassium hydroxide wet prep, positive Gram stain for yeast, hyphae	Medications: adults, nystatin suspension (5 ml qid, swish and swallow) or nystatin tablets (1 tablet PO qid). Children, nystatin suspension (5ml qid, painted on or swish and swallow); infants, nystatin suspension (1 ml qid); oral fluconazole may also be used. Hospitalize if significant dehydration, immuno-compromised patient.	Estimated disability: until no eating and drinking problems. Consider isolating immunosuppressed contacts. Potential complications: systemic dissemination
Clinical exam	Medications: topical anesthetics (tincture of benzoin, viscous lidocaine); adults, tetracycline suspension (250 mg qid for 7 days, usefulness unclear); steroids in severe cases	Estimated disability: complete healing, but disease recurs
PCR, ELISA-type assay, culture isolation, antibody titers	Antibiotics: adults, erythromycin (500 mg PO qid for 10 days), doxycycline (100 mg PO bid for 10 days); children, erythromycin (40 mg/kg/day in 4 divided doses PO for 10 days): azithromycin and clarithromycin also acceptable	Suspect child abuse in pediatric cases. Estimated disability: complete recovery in 2–3 days after treatment. Prophylaxis for contacts advised

Throat culture is considered the gold standard for the diagnosis of GABHS. The sensitivity of culture is approximately 90–95%.[1] As with the rapid tests, false-positive tests can occur in asymptomatic carriers; the estimated false-positive rate is 10–50%.[4] False-negative cultures probably reflect inaccuracy in culturing techniques or sample collection. The posterior pharyngeal wall or tonsils need to be vigorously swabbed to obtain an adequate sample for culture.

Table 5. Oropharyngeal Exudates

Agent	Appearance	Location
Group A β-hemolytic streptococci	Thick, purulent, patchy, white-yellow	Tonsils, pharynx, uvula (unusual)
Neisseria gonorrhoeae	Diffuse over ulcerative lesions	Tonsils, pharynx
Corynebacterium diphtheriae	Gray, adherent, thick pseudomembrane	Tonsils, pharynx, nares, uvula
Mixed anaerobes	Gray, adherent over swollen ulcerative regions regions	Tonsils, pharynx, gingiva
Adenovirus	Patchy, thick, white	Tonsils, pharynx
Epstein-Barr virus	Thick, white	Tonsils, pharynx
Candida albicans (oral thrush)	White, cheesy, plaquelike over swollen, bleeding ulcerations with inflamed bases	Palate, uvula, pharynx, tongue, buccal mucosa, gingiva

Table 6. Oropharyngeal Lesions

Agent or Syndrome	Appearance	Location
Group A β-hemolytic streptococci	Petechiae	Palate
Neisseria gonorrhoeae	Small, yellow, irregular ulcers	Oropharynx (diffuse)
Mixed anaerobes	Solitary to multiple, punched-out, necrotic ulcers covered with gray exudate.	Tonsils, gingival, pharyngeal walls
Epstein-Barr virus	Petechiae	Palate
Rubeola	Small, white vesicles with erythematous margins (Koplick's spots)	Buccal mucosa
Herpes simplex	Multiple, 2–3 mm, shallow, yellow, painful, punctate vessels that ulcerate; gray membrane over ulcers	Oropharynx (diffuse); preferentially on mucosa attached to periosteum
Aphthous ulcers (canker sores)	Few, 2–10 mm, shallow painful vesicles with white membranous base and well-circumscribed margin surrounded by red halo	Anterior mouth; preferentially on mucosa not attached to periosteum
Treponema pallidum	Primary: erosive, painful chancre appearing 3 wk after infection, covered by gray membrane	Lips, tongue, tonsils
	Secondary: multiple, painless, gray-white plaques over ulcerative lesion	Tongue, gingival, buccal mucosa
	Tertiary: gumma (hard nodular, painless mass)	Oropharynx (diffuse)
Mycobacterium tuberculosis	Solitary erosive granuloma	Oropharynx
Coxsackie A (herpangina)	Multiple, 1–2 mm, painful vesicles in clusters that form gray ulcers surrounded by red halo	Soft palate, uvula, tongue, tonsils
Pemphigus vulgaris	Large, painful, nonconfluent bullae filled with clear fluid	Oropharynx, lips
Oropharyngeal cancers	Painful, nonhealing ulcers	Oropharynx

Management (Fig. 1). The primary purpose of treating GABHS is the prevention of acute rheumatic fever. Antibiotic therapy also helps prevent suppurative complications, such as peritonsillar or retropharyngeal abscess, otitis media, sinusitis, cervical adenitis, necrotizing fasciitis, malignant scarlet fever, bacteremia, and streptococcal toxic shock syndrome. Furthermore, treatment speeds clinical recovery and reduces infectivity, helping the patient return to school or work more quickly. Antibiotic treatment has not been shown to prevent post-streptococcal glomerulonephritis.

Evidence-based studies have devoted considerable attention to the cost-effectiveness of GABHS management strategies. These studies take into account not only the cost of testing and treatment, but also the cost of treating acute rheumatic fever, suppurative complications, and penicillin reactions. The best management strategy depends on the available diagnostic tests, the symptom profile, patient reliability, and the ability to establish follow-up.

A well-validated strategy, found to be cost-effective in urban emergency departments, is to perform a rapid streptococcal test on all patients with pharyngitis. Treat patients with positive rapid streptococcal tests, and send cultures on all those with negative screen.[2,5] The American Heart Association and the Infectious Diseases Society of America currently recommend that a culture be obtained on all negative rapid streptococcal tests.[6]

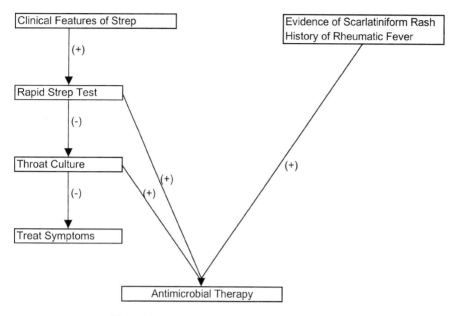

Figure 1.   Management strategies for pharyngitis.

The higher sensitivity of the newer rapid streptococcal tests has created debate over whether backup culture is truly necessary.[7,8] Because sensitivities of both rapid streptococcal tests and cultures may vary significantly from lab to lab,[8] the sensitivities of the tests in the local lab should be taken into account in deciding which tests to employ.

Empiric treatment of GABHS is appropriate in certain cases. Patients who present with a sore throat and scarlatiniform rash do not need further testing. The rash is virtually diagnostic of GABHS.[9] Some clinicians advocate empiric treatment based on a constellation of symptoms or scoring system. Commonly cited are the Centor criteria: fever, pharyngeal exudate, anterior cervical lymphadenopathy, and absence of cough. Three of the four findings confer a high probability of GABHS.[6] Positive predictive values of such systems range from 39% to 59%.[4] Some authors believe that this approach leads to an unacceptably high risk of penicillin reactions.[5]

Certain people in close contact with an infected patient may need antibiotic prophylaxis. Examples include patients with rheumatic heart disease or recent ARF. The duration of prophylaxis depends on many factors that are best determined and followed by the patient's primary care physician.

Penicillin is the mainstay of treatment of GABHS. Despite years of use, penicillin-resistance has apparently not become an issue with GABHS infection.[10] Treatment options include intramuscular injection of benzathine penicillin G or CR bicillin, and oral penicillin V. Erythromycin is recommended for patients who are allergic to penicillin. Other options include amoxicillin, clindamycin, azithromycin, and first-generation cephalosporins.[6] For dosing recommendations, see Table 2. Antibiotic therapy needs to be initiated within 9 days of symptom onset to reduce effectively the incidence of ARF.

Pitfalls in Practice. Complete or partial obstruction of the upper airway because of swollen tonsils or soft tissues can occur in patients with pharyngitis and requires emergent airway intervention. Patients with an impeding obstruction should not be left alone during their evaluation and should not be allowed to leave the urgent care facility to go to the hospital alone; they need rapid transport in the company of a health professional who is skilled in airway management (i.e., ACLS-level transport).

Serious complications of streptococcal pharyngitis and other oropharyngeal infections that require consultation or hospitalization are listed in Table 7 (next page). Substantial morbidity and possible mortality can occur if these rare complications of pharyngitis are not recognized and treated.

The persistence of symptoms beyond 7 days of treatment is usually due to lack of medical compliance. Changing from penicillin to another antibiotic is not effective. For such patients who were initially treated with oral antibiotics, intramuscular injections should be considered. If compliance is not an issue, failure to improve should bring the original diagnosis into question.

Recurrent streptococcal pharyngitis (more than two episodes within a few months) is rare. Patients who repeatedly test positive may be streptococcal carriers who suffer from episodes of viral pharyngitis. Such patients should be referred for further evaluation of the cause of the pharyngitis and immune status.

Gonococcal Pharyngitis

Differential Diagnosis. Pharyngitis caused by *Neisseria gonorrhoeae* is usually asymptomatic, but on rare occasions it can cause severe exudative pharyngitis and oral lesions (see Tables 2 and 5). It is not an uncommon cause of pharyngitis in patients with genital infections who engage in orogenital sexual practices.

Diagnostic Aids. *N. gonorrhoeae* can be isolated from the oropharynx, but often the culture is overgrown or confused by other species of *Neisseria* that are normal flora in the oral cavity. Patients with pharyngitis and a positive culture for *N. gonorrhoeae* from a nonpharyngeal source should be questioned about the possibility of orogenital spread of the organism.

Management. Gonococcal pharyngitis is a self-limited disease that usually resolves spontaneously in several weeks without treatment. Treatment can reduce the time course of the infection and reduces the severity of symptoms. Treatment options include ceftriaxone and ciprofloxacin. See Table 2 for dosing recommendations.

Pitfalls in Practice. Gonococcal pharyngitis is almost always due to orogenital contact. It is recommended, therefore, that patients and their sexual partners undergo genital cultures for *N. gonorrhoeae*. If a child presents with gonococcal pharyngitis, sexual abuse must be suspected.

Mycoplasmal Pharyngitis

Mycoplasma pneumoniae causes pharyngitis in school-aged children and young adults. The most common symptom is a mild sore throat. The infection may progress to the lower airway, causing tracheobronchitis, pneumonia, and persistent cough.

Table 7. Complications of Oropharyngeal Infections

Complication	Presentation	Examination	Management
Peritonsillar abscess	Onset: insidious after 3–4 days of untreated or unresponsive sore throat Complaints: unilaterally worse sore throat, dysphagia, ipsilateral otalgia, trismus	Elevated temperature, coarse, raspy, or muffled voice, anterior cervical adenopathy (can be unilateral), asymmetric tonsillar enlargement, soft palate distortion and fluctuance, drooling, pooled secretions	Airway support if needed, consultation with ear, nose, and throat (ENT) specialist for incision and drainage (inpatient or outpatient) Complications: airway obstruction, continued extension, dehydration
Retropharyngeal abscess	Onset: insidious after dental disease, pharyngeal trauma, oropharyngeal infection Complaints: sore throat, dysphagia, neck pain	Elevated temperature, noisy breathing, possible stridor, muffled voice, erythematous bulging of posterior pharyngeal wall, anterior neck swelling, cervical adenopathy	Lateral soft tissue neck x-ray (increase in prevertebral soft tissue space to 1.5–2.0 times normal), airway support if needed, admission to intensive care unit after ENT drainage under general anesthesia; do not leave patient unattended Complications: airway obstruction, aspiration.
Parapharyngeal infection	Onset: insidious after oropharyngeal or dental infections Complaints: unilateral neck pain, sore throat, otalgia, trismus	Elevated temperature, swelling along mandible, unilateral cervical adenopathy, unilateral medial displacement of lateral pharyngeal wall	Lateral soft tissue neck x-ray (nonspecific prevertebral tissue swelling), airway management, ENT admission to intensive care unit; do not leave patient unattended Complications: airway obstruction, septic thrombophlebitis, carotid sheath erosion
Submandibular cellulitis (Ludwig's angina)	Onset: insidious after dental extractions, lacerations of floor of mouth or tongue Complaints: pain in floor of mouth and neck, sore throat, dysphagia, trismus, fever, respiratory distress.	Elevated temperature, drooling pooled secretions, brawny anterior neck edema; tender, edematous, erythematous, indurated submandibular and sublingual spaces; tongue elevated from floor of mouth	Lateral soft tissue neck x-ray (submandibular tissue swelling), airway management, ENT admission to intensive care unit; do not leave patient unattended Complications: generalized sepsis, airway obstruction
Epiglottitis		See Table 2	
Acute rheumatic fever	Onset: 14–18 days after untreated streptococcal infection Complaints: fever, migratory polyarthritis, precordial pain, rash, abdominal pain	Elevated temperature; painless,hard, subcutaneous nodules on bony prominences; heart murmur; friction rub; tachycardia; erythema marginatum (flat red lesions with clear centers)	Hospitalize if carditis, chorea, other symptoms of generalized toxicity. Medications (outpatient): penicillin G benzathine (1.2×10^6 U intramuscularly) or penicillin G procaine (0.6×10^6 U intramuscularly every day for 10 days), aspirin for symptomatic relief: steroids occasionally given for carditis (prednisone, 60–120 mg in four divided doses every day)
Poststreptococcal glomerulonephritis	Onset: 10 days after streptococcal infection Complaints: edema in dependent portions of body, dark or bloody urine, decreased urinary output	Edema, occasionally hypertension, occasionally encephalopathy, proteinuria, hematuria, red cell casts, electrolyte abnormalities	Support: bed rest, fluid restriction; consider diuretics; medical therapy if severe hypertension Medications: penicillin if streptococcal infection not yet treated

Diagnostic Aids. The most accurate way to diagnose mycoplasma infection is polymerase chain reaction (PCR) testing. Mycoplasmal infection also evokes a positive cold agglutinin reaction. This simple test is rapid and can be performed easily in the urgent care setting. A high cold agglutinin titer (≥ 1/64) is a good diagnostic marker in patients over the age of 12, provided that the patient has evidence of lower respiratory tract infection.[11] False-positive reactions frequently occur with adenovirus or Epstein-Barr virus infections; positive results, therefore, must be interpreted in light of the clinical picture.

Management. Mycoplasmal pharyngitis is a benign disease with a self-limited but prolonged course of 2–6 weeks without treatment. Treatment can reduce the symptoms by 1–2 weeks and therefore is of clinical benefit. Erythromycin is effective in treatment, as are clarithromycin and azithromycin. Tetracycline also may be used but is not recommended in children. See Table 4 for specific recommendations.

Because of its prolonged incubation period and because shedding of the organism occurs for a prolonged period even after treatment, household contacts often develop mycoplasmal infection. No recommendations about antibiotic prophylaxis have been advanced, but immunocompromised contacts should be isolated, if possible, and evaluated frequently if symptoms develop.

Pitfalls in Practice. The diagnosis of mycoplasmal pharyngitis is infrequent because culturing for the mycoplasma organisms is not standard. This diagnosis should be considered in patients with persistent sore throats in the absence of streptococcal or mononucleosis infection.

Chlamydial Pharyngitis

Chlamydia trachomatis is less well studied as an etiologic agent of pharyngitis. Symptoms are mild and nonspecific unless accompanied by other signs of chlamydial infection, such as conjunctivitis or genital symptoms.

Diagnostic Aids. Throat cultures for chlamydial organisms are not routinely done. Serologic testing of acute- and convalescent-phase serum demonstrates elevated antibody titers if chlamydial infection has occurred, but this test is frequently unavailable. A positive cervical or urethral culture for chlamydial organisms in a patient who also complains of sore throat should prompt questioning about the possibility of orogenital spread of this organism.

Management. Chlamydial pharyngitis is a benign disease with a self-limited course of 1–3 weeks. Erythromycin is effective in treatment. Tetracycline is also effective but is not recommended for children (see Table 4).

The route of transmission of chlamydial infection may be drainage from the eye to the lacrimal duct and oropharynx or orogenital spread. If the orogenital route is suspected, genital cultures or PCR samples should be obtained from patients and their intimate contacts. Patients with positive PCR or cultures should be treated. If conjunctivitis is present and thought to be the source of the organism, care must be exercised to avoid contamination of contacts from eye drainage.

Both mycoplasmal and chlamydial infections are responsive to erythromycin but not to penicillin. Therefore, if a patient has been started on penicillin empirically for presumed streptococcal pharyngitis but has not responded, a reasonable next choice for antibiotic therapy is erythromycin.

Pitfalls in Practice. Chlamydial pharyngitis is not routinely diagnosed because chlamydial throat cultures are infrequently obtained. If cultures are obtained and are positive for chlamydial organisms, urogenital spread may have occurred; in children, sexual abuse must be considered.

Viral Pharyngitis

Most cases of pharyngitis are due to viral causes, which are self-limited. Viral syndromes of the oropharynx are described in Table 3.

Diagnostic Aids. Viral cultures rarely provide useful information in the urgent care setting and require special culturing techniques. Viral titers are costly to measure and often are not detected until several days after infection. The monospot test for the presence of infectious mononucleosis may be useful. Positive responses can sometimes be delayed for up to 4 weeks and can remain positive for 4 weeks. A rising heterophile titer can help diagnose infectious mononucleosis but is not readily available in the urgent care setting.

Management. Treatment for viral pharyngitis consists of supportive care, adequate hydration and analgesia. In certain cases, such as herpes stomatitis, antiviral medications may be helpful (see Table 4). In general, antihistamines, decongestants, and antiseptic mouth washes do not shorten the duration of symptoms and may cause unpleasant side effects, especially in children. Symptomatic relief can be obtained from salt water gargles and topical anesthetic sprays, lozenges, or viscous lidocaine. Nonsteroidal anti-inflammatory drugs and acetaminophen also may aid in pain control and maintaining fluid hydration in patients who are otherwise unable to drink. Anesthetics should not be used when sore throat is secondary to trauma or when handling secretions may be a problem because such therapy may mask delayed complications or compromise protective physiologic reflexes.

Pitfalls in Practice. Regional adenopathy is characteristic of several viral and bacterial causes of pharyngitis, most notably infectious mononucleosis and streptococcal pharyngitis. Typically, lymphadenopathy due to streptococcal infection resolves within 1 month of the infection, and adenopathy due to mononucleosis resolves within 2 months of infection. If adenopathy has persisted beyond these periods, other causes must be considered, such as lymphoma, leukemia, granulomatous diseases, or autoimmune diseases. Patients with persistent symptoms need referral to a specialist for further evaluation.

Hoarseness

Laryngitis is inflammation of the larynx that presents with the complaint of hoarseness. Usually this disease is due to a viral infection and is associated with an upper respiratory tract infection. The symptom of hoarseness also may be a primary or a chronic complaint and is frequently seen in patients with a history of smoking, irritant inhalation, and voice abuse. Hoarseness may mean complete loss of the voice or vocal roughness. Hoarseness is the term used by most people to describe a change in normal voice quality. The goal of urgent care management of the patient presenting with hoarseness is to differentiate serious life-threatening disease from less serious disease.

Differential Diagnosis. The differential diagnosis of hoarseness is described in Table 8. Hoarseness that has persisted in an adult for more than 6 weeks should raise suspicion of cancer, especially in a smoker.[12] Important historical information that may help define pathology includes the duration of the symptoms, voice use, associated symptoms, exposure history, smoking and alcohol use, medical history, medication history, and allergies. Presbylaryngeus, the most common cause of hoarseness in elders, is due to the loss of muscle tone of the laryngeal complex with increasing age.

Management. In most cases, acute voice changes are part of a syndrome of upper respiratory tract infection and resolve spontaneously as the disease runs its course. Some acute causes of hoarseness, such as laryngeal foreign body, allergic reaction, or trauma, are suggested by the history. Patients should be advised of good vocal hygiene, including adequate hydration, and avoidance of caffeine and alcohol because of the diuretic effect.

When hoarseness has persisted 7–10 days longer than symptoms of upper respiratory tract infection or is of more than 2–3 weeks' duration, visualization of the patient's larynx is essential. This is best done at the time of the initial examination by indirect laryngoscopy. Indirect laryngoscopy with a head light and warmed laryngeal mirror is a time-honored method and provides an excellent view of the area. Fiberoptic scans are excellent adjuncts to the examination but may not be readily available in the urgent care center. For the gagging patient, premedication with 10 mg of diazepam orally and an analgesic throat spray (Cetacaine, Xylocaine 1% spray) may facilitate examination. For patients with uncontrollable gag reflexes, cords that cannot be visualized, indirect laryngoscopy revealing abnormal vocal cord structure or movement, or unexplained hoarseness of more than 2–3 weeks' duration, referral to an otolaryngologist should be made for further evaluation. Any patient with hoarseness and concurrent dyspnea requires emergent evaluation for causes of patient upper airway obstruction.

Pitfalls in Practice. Failure to include cord visualization in the initial assessment of a patient presenting with persistent hoarseness with the absence of associated symptoms of upper respiratory tract infection may delay the diagnosis of potentially life-threatening pathology. Because delayed complications may develop after laryngeal trauma, patients with histories suggesting trauma (even those with a normal initial examination) need close follow-up or inpatient observation.

Dysphagia or Lump in the Throat

Dysphagia is defined as the subjective sensation of difficulty in swallowing. Frequently the patient describes the sensation of a "lump in the throat," which may be associated with dysphagia or a completely separate concern.

The patient who cannot swallow needs careful evaluation because this sign may indicate serious pathology. Diagnosis is often difficult to make in the urgent care setting because most necessary diagnostic studies are not readily available (e.g., barium swallow, cineradiography, esophagoscopy).

The goals of urgent care management of patients who complain of dysphagia are to rule out the presence of a foreign body, to make appropriate and timely referral for patients who may have serious pathology, and to evaluate and offer therapy to patients whose symptoms are probably due to self-limited medical illness.

Table 8. Causes of Hoarseness

Cause	Agent	Signs and Symptoms	Therapy	Follow Up Issues
Acute infectious laryngitiis	Viral, occasionally bacterial	Onset: gradual Age: all ages Complaints: upper respiratory symptoms, dry cough, mild sore throat, hoarseness Duration: 1–7 days Voice quality: whisper Indirect laryngoscopy (IDL): red, edematous, mobile cords; pooled, thick yellow mucus	Support: voice rest for 3–4 days, steam inhalation (humidity), analgesics, cough suppressants, warm sialogogues	Repeat exam if patient is not better in 7–10 days
Acute allergic laryngitis (angioedema)	Drug reaction, allergic reaction	Onset: sudden, rapidly progressive Age: all ages Complaints: allergic or anaphylactic symptoms, hoarseness, and occasionally severe respiratory distress Duration: until antigen is removed and treatment is started Voice quality: spastic IDL: red, edematous, mobile cords; edematous soft tissues See text	Support: airway intervention if needed Medications: treat for allergic reaction Adults, aqueous epinephrine (0.3–0.5 ml or 1:1,000 solution intramuscularly) or diphenhydramine (Benadryl) (25–60 mg IV or intramuscularly) Children, epinephrine (0.01 ml/kg, up to 0.5ml of 1:1,000 solution) or Benadryl (12.5–25 mg IV or intramuscularly)	Potential acute complications: airway obstruction, recurrence if continued exposure to allergen
Laryngeal trauma	Blunt direct anterior neck trauma, strangulation	Onset: sudden Age: all ages Complaints: Hoarseness, dysphagia, pain, and variable degrees of respiratory distress Voice: rough; aphonia IDL: abnormal structure, abnormal mobility of cords, hemorrhage or edema of surrounding soft tissues Neck: occasional subcutaneous emphysema	Support: never leave patient unattended if in any respiratory distress; support airway if needed. Neck x-ray may show free air or abnormal air column Hospitalize all patients with significant complaints for observation of delayed complications	Potential acute complications: tracheal tear, rupture, complete airway obstruction, laryngeal disruption
Reflux laryngitis	Gastropharyngeal or laryngo-pharyngeal reflux	Onset: variable Age: adults, elders Complaints: chronic hoarseness, chronic cough, and throat irritation with frequent throat clearing Voice: rough IDL: inflammatory changes of posterior pharynx, mucosa between arytenoids may be erythematous and thickened	Treat like gastroesophageal reflux: avoiding meals or snacks within 2 hours of bedtime, avoiding spicy foods, elevation of head of bed, H_2 blocker	Follow up with GI
Laryngeal nodule or polyp	Voice abuse, mucous cysts, granulation tissue, and papillomas	Onset: gradual Age: all ages Complaint: persistent hoarseness Voice: breathy, deep IDL: Abnormal cord structure with normal mobility and color	Support: voice rest Medications: consider steroids for professional singers	ENT consultation for possible excision if no improvement with voice rest

(Cont'd on next page)

Table 8. Causes of Hoarseness *(Continued)*

Cause	Agent	Signs and Symptoms	Therapy	Follow Up Issues
Chronic nonspecific laryngitis	Smoking, dust inhalation, voice abuse, mouth breathing	Onset: gradual Age: all ages Complaint: persistent hoarseness Voice: rough IDL: hyperemic, hyperplastic cords with normal mobility	Support: reduce irritant exposure, warm sialogogues, cough suppressants, humidity, voice rest	ENT consultation for routinely repeated examinations
Laryngeal cancer	Predisposition in smokers	Onset: gradual Age: adults, men more often than women Complaints: hoarseness, progressive dysphagia Duration: > 6 weeks Voice quality: harsh IDL: abnormally thickened cords or obvious lesion, abnormal cord movement	ENT consultation Hospitalize if airway compromised Smokers should be told to quit	ENT consultation for biopsy and excision
Lung cancer	Compression of recurrent laryngeal nerve; predisposition in smokers	Onset: gradual Age: adults Complaints: hoarseness, weight loss, hemoptysis, and dyspnea Duration: > 6 weeks Voice quality: harsh IDL: normal cord structure, abnormal unilateral cord movement or paralysis	Chest x-ray may reveal pathology	Medical consultation for further evaluation and supportive therapy
Systemic disease	Arthritis, hypothyroidism, diabetes, gastroesophageal reflux, systemic lupus erythematosus	Onset: gradual Age: usually adults Complaints: variable Duration: variable Voice: variable IDL: normal or thickened cords, abnormal morbidity	Treat primary disease	ENT consultation for repeated examinations

Differential Diagnosis. Important historical points in the evaluation of dysphonia include onset, duration, presence of pain, degree of disability incurred because of the discomfort, history of exposure to inhaled chemical irritants, history of caustic ingestions, history of peptic ulcer disease, history of irradiation of the neck or chest, gastrointestinal complaints, or neurologic complaints. Physical examination requires careful examination of the oropharynx, head, neck, and chest. The differential diagnosis for dysphagia is described in part in Table 9.

Dysphagia is best approached by considering swallowing as two separate processes: the oropharyngeal phase and the esophageal phase. The pharyngeal phase, also known as transfer dysphagia, moves food from the mouth into the esophagus. Eighty-percent of oropharyngeal dysphagia is caused by neuromuscular disease.[13] Complaints include inability to initiate swallowing, fear of eating, coughing during swallowing, aspiration, nasal speech, and gagging. Medical history is often remarkable for secondary pneumonia, bronchitis, or asthma.

The esophageal phase, also known as transport dysphagia, moves food from the esophagus into the stomach. Eighty-five percent of esophageal dysphagia is due to obstructive disease. In this phase swallowing is initiated well, but there are complaints of food sticking

Table 9. Causes of Dysphagia

Oropharyngeal lesions		Esophageal lesions
Neuromuscular disorders	Structural abnormalities	Mechanical narrowing
Cerebrovascular accident	Zenker's diverticulum	Carcinoma
Polymyositis, dermatomyositis	Tracheostomy	Esophageal ring (Schatzki's ring) or web
Multiple sclerosis	Carcinoma	Expanding esophageal diverticula
Amyotrophic lateral sclerosis		Strictures
Parkinson's disease	Collagen vascular disorders	Osteophytes
Poliomyelitis	Scleroderma	Vascular anomalies* (dysphagia lusoria)
Pseudobulbar or bulbar palsy		Aortic aneurysm
	Inflammatory disorders	Goiter
Myopathies of metabolic and	Pharyngitis	Foreign bodies
endocrine disorders	Tonsillitis	
Myxedema	Diphtheria	Motility disorders
Thyrotoxicosis	Mass lesions/abscesses	Achalasia
Alcoholism		Symptomatic diffuse esophageal
Diabetic neuropathy	Other	spasm (SDES)
Amyloidosis	Foreign body ingestion	
Lead poisoning	Mouth breathing	Other
Magnesium deficiency	Dehydration	Hiatal hernia
Hypercalcemia		Reflux esophagitis

* Dysphagia lusoria: when anomalous blood vessel is present, usually the right subclavian artery, which crosses behind the esophagus, is involved.

or hanging up, generally within 10–15 seconds of ingestion. Correlation of pain and site of pathology are not accurate because of referred pain. "Heartburn" is a frequent complaint and may suggest gastroesophageal reflux with transient spasm and/or esophagitis.[13] Figure 2 illustrates an approach to the evaluation of dysphagia.

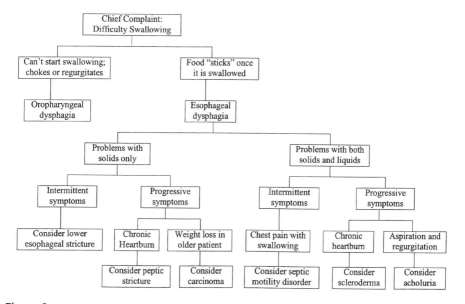

Figure 2. Approach to the patient with dysphagia. (Adapted from Young HS: Esophageal disorders. In Dale DC, Federman DD (eds): Scientific American Medicine. New York, Scientific American, 1999, pp 3–5, with permission.)

Management. Occasionally patients in whom mass lesions cause dysphagia present with compression of the trachea as well as the esophagus and can have impending respiratory compromise. Such patients may need emergent consultation and hospitalization. Dysphagia due to systemic disease is a serious and usually long-standing symptom. Evaluation with appropriate consultation should be arranged. If dysphagia is due to strictures secondary to a caustic ingestion or long-standing esophagitis, dilation is the appropriate therapy, and consultation should be arranged. Dysphagia is commonly associated with hiatal hernia and reflux esophagitis. In such cases, a trial of antacids may be of symptomatic benefit. In general, dysphagia due to tonsillitis or pharyngitis is short-lived. The history and physical examination suggest this diagnosis. Functional dysphagia, which is described as a feeling of throat tightness or fullness, may be independent of pathologic dysphagia.[13]

Pitfalls in Practice. It is often difficult to give much credence to the well-nourished, well-hydrated patient who claims that he or she cannot swallow. It is a serious error to minimize such symptoms and to fail to make appropriate referral for further evaluation. High-risk patients for serious pathology are those with long-standing, progressive symptoms or a history of heavy smoking. All patients with the complaint of dysphagia, even if the cause is evident, need appropriate follow-up care planned before discharge from the urgent care center.

Because most causes of dysphagia are due to potentially dangerous pathology, the diagnosis of globus hystericus is one of exclusion that is made only after thorough evaluation. Reasonable organic causes should be considered first. If the patient is complaining of heartburn or related types of chest discomfort, consider cardiac disease. An electrocardiogram should be obtained to rule out unsuspected myocardial infarction.

Caustic Ingestions

Caustic ingestions are usually accidental in children and intentional in adults. Acid ingestions produce a coagulative necrosis in exposed tissue, which limits damage to relatively superficial tissue layers of the oropharynx and esophagus. Acids can cause significant damage to the mucosal lining of the stomach. Alkali ingestions produce a liquefying necrosis and penetrate tissues deeply by direct extension. Alkali ingestion can cause significant immediate and long-term dysfunction of the oropharynx and esophagus. Many different corrosive agents have been reported to be responsible for chemical injuries, but readily available household alkali compounds are the most frequently ingested corrosives.[14] Bleaches have a neutral pH and are considered esophageal irritants.

Differential Diagnosis. The degree of damage due to a caustic ingestion depends on the type, concentration, form (e.g., a liquid reaches the esophagus more easily than a solid), and quantity of the injested substance as well as the presence of food in the stomach, gastroesophageal reflux, gastrointestinal transient time, and duration of contact. Patients who recently have ingested a caustic substance present with a sore mouth, dysphagia, and nausea. Frequently they have an elevated temperature and have vomited spontaneously. Fifty percent of patients with two or more of the signs and symptoms of vomiting, drooling, and stridor have serious esophageal damage. The presence of oropharyngeal burns does not necessarily identify patients with serious esophageal injury.[14]

If the material is held in the mouth, oral burns may occur. If a liquid form of caustic substance has been ingested, the oropharynx may appear to be completely normal; therefore, the absence of oral injuries cannot accurately predict the presence or absence of esophageal injuries. Table 10 lists some signs and symptoms of caustic ingestion.

Table 10. Signs and Symptoms of Caustic Ingestion

Pharyngeal or laryngeal	Esophageal	Gastric
Odynophagia	Dysphagia	Epigastric pain or tenderness
Mucosal erythema, ulceration	Odynophagia	Vomiting
Drooling	Chest or back pain	Hematemesis
Tongue edema		
Stridor		
Hoarseness		

Management. Patients with significant oral mucosal burns, tongue edema, hoarseness, stridor, and dyspnea should be observed carefully for airway obstruction. Laryngeal edema is frequently seen in the first 24 hours in association with severe caustic burns of the esophagus. Fiberoptic laryngoscopy in the awake patient, if available, can be valuable to assess hypopharyngeal damage and risk of airway compromise. No attempts to induce vomiting should be made because emesis is associated with reinjury of the mucosa and increased chances of aspiration. Gastric acidity may neutralize ingested alkali. Attempts to dilute the injected caustic with water or other liquids is of little value and may produce additional vomiting or retching that aggravates the situation. If oral lesions are present, the mouth should be irrigated with large amounts of water to dilute and wash out the caustic substance.

Patients who present with a history of caustic ingestion need hospital admission with direct visualization of the esophagus (esophogoscopy) after 2 or 3 days to determine the degree of injury. Such patients should receive nothing by mouth and should be maintained on intravenous fluids. Early consultation with a poison control center may be helpful.

Pitfalls in Practice. The complications of caustic ingestions are associated with serious morbidity and are often lethal. Therefore, if caustic ingestion is suspected, a conservative approach to management should be taken. Because many complications of a caustic ingestion do not occur immediately, a patient may initially appear to be perfectly normal. Severe symptoms may not develop until hours to days later. The maximal extent of esophageal burns in caustic ingestions may not manifest until up to 12 hours after ingestion. All patients with a history of caustic ingestion need consultation and hospital admission and should not be discharged from the urgent care facility until such arrangements have been made.

Foreign Bodies in the Respiratory Tract

Ingestion of foreign objects is common in children and occasionally occurs in adults. Ingested foreign objects usually are swallowed. If not swallowed, most are expelled by reflex coughing. Those that are not expelled can lodge in the respiratory tract and cause acute or delayed problems.

Differential Diagnosis. History and Physical Examination. The history of foreign body ingestion and subsequent aspiration is often unobtainable or forgotten. The presentation depends on the size of the object or food bolus, the site at which it is lodged, and the degree of obstruction. A foreign object lodged in the oropharynx is often visible on examination. Small objects lodged in the larynx produce localized discomfort or more serious symptoms, such as dyspnea, hoarseness, gagging, or reflex coughing. Sharp objects can damage surrounding mucosa, and resultant edema may cause airway obstruction. A patient who has aspirated an object into the trachea or bronchi may present with a symptom-free period of minutes to weeks after the initial choking episode. Pulmonary symptoms, such as wheezing, dyspnea, cough, hemoptysis, and even fever and sepsis, may then develop. Bronchial obstruction can result in unilateral decreased air movement, atelectasis, localized wheezing, or emphysema beyond the obstruction. If the bronchial obstruction is incomplete, the pulmonary examination may be normal.

Diagnostic Aids. Lateral soft-tissue neck x-rays help locate radiopaque laryngeal foreign bodies. If the object appears to be anterior, it is probably in the larynx; if it appears to be posterior, it is probably lodged in the esophagus or the hypopharynx. Chest x-rays may be useful in locating tracheal or bronchial foreign bodies by identifying the object itself or by revealing complications of obstruction such as air trapping or lobar collapse. Acute pulmonary lesions, especially in young children, should raise the suspicion of aspirated foreign bodies.

Management. Foreign bodies lodged in the oropharynx, at the base of the tongue, or in the lateral pharyngeal walls can be removed with a curved forceps if they are clearly visible.

Patients with suspected laryngeal foreign bodies should not be left unattended, and neck x-rays should be obtained only if the patient is in no distress. If a foreign body is present, direct laryngoscopy or endoscopy is needed to remove it. Until removal is achieved, the patient should be kept calm and comfortable, with the head, chest, and shoulders slightly dependent. A laryngeal foreign body has the potential to obstruct the airway completely. All medical personnel should be trained in basic life support and prepared to intervene if the airway is suddenly obstructed. A surgical airway may be necessary if attempts to relieve the obstruction fail. Patients with laryngeal foreign bodies should be transported to a hospital by ambulance. They should not be allowed to leave the urgent care facility on their own. Bronchoscopy under general anesthesia is generally used to remove bronchial or tracheal foreign bodies.

Pitfalls in Practice. Most foreign bodies lodged in the respiratory tract cause substantial morbidity and mortality if not removed. Attempts to remove a visible object with the fingers may force the object farther toward the larynx or induce a gag reflex that may dislodge it. Slapping a patient on the back to relieve a partial obstruction may dislodge a foreign body, or produce a complete obstruction. Turning an infant upside-down to retrieve an aspirated foreign object may dislodge it from the trachea or bronchus, only to have it lodge on the inferior side of the larynx and cause total obstruction. Using positive pressure to support ventilation may forcibly lodge an aspirated foreign body farther down the respiratory tract. This approach may convert a partial airway obstruction to a complete airway obstruction. In the face of complete obstruction, however, positive pressure may force the foreign body down the mainstem bronchus, allowing ventilation of the other lung until bronchoscopy can be arranged to remove the foreign body. If a patient is not able to ventilate adequately, one must use whatever means are available to provide adequate ventilation. If the obstruction is partial and if the patient ventilates adequately, the foreign body should be removed as quickly as possible in the operating room with the best equipment and specialists available.

Salivary Gland Disorders

Acute inflammation of the salivary glands can be caused by acute parotitis, acute bacterial sialadenitis, or sialolithiasis. Acute parotitis is most commonly caused by mumps and other viruses although many drugs and systemic diseases can cause enlargement of the parotid glands on a chronic basis. Acute sialadenitis is most often due to a bacterial infection that spreads in a retrograde fashion from the oral cavity and is seen primarily in debilitated, dehydrated adults coupled with poor oral hygiene. Salivary duct stones can obstruct the salivary duct partially or completely, resulting in a swollen, painful gland.

Differential Diagnosis. Acute parotitis may be caused by mumps or other viral infections, such as influenza, enterovirus, cytomegalovirus, and HIV. Symptoms may begin with fever and malaise and progress to pain and stiffness with chewing, and/or swelling of the parotid gland. The diagnosis of mumps can be made solely on clinical grounds. It may be difficult to differentiate viral and suppurative parotitis.

Salivary duct obstruction due to salivary stones presents with sudden, painful swelling of a salivary gland, most commonly the submandibular gland, that worsens after eating and eases within a few hours. The second most common location for obstruction is in the parotid gland. Episodes may occur intermittently over years. Often the stone can be palpated or visualized on x-ray. Gout is known to cause salivary gland calculi composed of uric acid. Otherwise most calculi are largely calcium phosphate with small amounts of magnesium, ammonium, and carbonate. Despite their similar chemical makeup, 90% of submandibular calculi are radiopaque, whereas 90% of parotid calculi are radiolucent. The submandibular duct is believed to be more susceptible to calculus formation because its saliva is more alkaline and has a higher concentration of calcium and phosphate coupled with a higher mucus content.[15] If the duct is only partially occluded, saliva can be observed flowing from the duct. If an infection occurs behind the obstruction, the patient may be febrile.

Patients with sialadenitis due to bacterial causes present with local pain and swelling, fevers, chills, and generalized sepsis. The gland feels firm and is tender. Sometimes pus can be expressed from the salivary duct. Facial edema and paralysis can occur. An obstruction due to a stone is frequently associated with infection. Bilateral obstruction occurs in a minority of cases.

Management. Salivary duct stones occasionally can be milked out of the duct. If this approach is unsuccessful, patients should be started on analgesics and antibiotics. Vigorous probing can initiate an inflammatory episode. Referral to an ear, nose, and throat specialist or oral surgeon should be made because surgical excision of the stone may be necessary.

In bacterial sialadenitis the usual causative organisms include *Staphylococcus aureus*, *Streptococcus pneumoniae*, *Escherichia coli*, and *Haemophilus influenzae*. Initial treatment includes adequate hydration to ensure salivary flow, improved oral hygiene, repeated massage of the gland, and sialogogues (such as lemon drops). If purulent saliva can be seen at the duct orifice, especially with massage of the gland, the saliva should undergo Gram stain, and culture for both aerobes and anaerobes.[15] Empiric therapy with a penicillinase-resistant antistaphylococcal antibiotic should be started while culture results are awaited. Acute bacterial sialadenitis is a serious life-threatening disease, and diagnosed patients require hospital admission for hydration and intravenous antibiotics.

Antibiotic management of parotitis and sialoadenitis, if needed, consists of dicloxacillin, 500 mg orally 4 times/day, or cephadrine, 500 mg 4 times/day; amoxicillin/clavulanate or ampicillin/sulbactam for a 7–10 day course, covering for *S. aureus* and anaerobes.

Treatment for acute viral parotitis is symptomatic. Analgesics, sialogogues, and application of warm or cold compresses to the parotid area may be helpful.

Pitfalls in Practice. Overmanipulation of a salivary duct stone during attempts to remove it can result in significant swelling and may delay surgical excision.

References

1. Tsevat J, et al: Management of sore throats in children: A cost-effectiveness analysis. Arch Pediatr Adolesc Med 153:681–688, 1999.
2. Bisno AL, Gerber MA, Gwaltney JM, et al: Diagnosis and management of group A streptococcal pharyngitis: A practice guideline. Clin Infect Dis 25:574–583, 1997.
3. Kaplan EL: Recent epidemiology of group A streptococcal infection in North America and abroad: An overview. Pediatrics 97(Suppl):954–959, 1996.
4. Stewart M, et al: Evaluation of the patient with sore throat, earache, and sinusitis: An evidence based approach. Emerg Med Clin North Am 17:153–184, 1999.
5. Lieu TA, Fleisher GR, Schwartz JS: Cost-effectiveness of rapid latex agglutination testing and throat culture for streptococcal pharyngitis. Pediatrics 85:246–256, 1990.
6. Dajani AS, et al: Treatment of acute streptococcal pharyngitis and prevention of rheumatic fever: A statement for health professionals. Pediatrics 97:758–764, 1995.
7. Webb KH: Does culture confirmation of high-sensitivity rapid strep test make sense? A medical decision analysis. Pediatrics 101:209–300, 1998.
8. Gerber MA, Tanz RR, Kabat W, et al: Optical immunoassay test for group A β-hemolytic streptococcal pharyngitis. JAMA 277:899–903, 1997.
9. Lowe R, Hedges JR: Early treatment of streptococcal pharyngitis. Ann Emerg Med 13:440–448, 1984.
10. Wilde JA: Antibiotic resistance and the problems of antibiotic overuse. Emerg Med Rep 6(5):45–56, 2001.
11. Cimolai N: *Mycoplasma pneumoniae* respiratory infection. Pediatr Rev 19:327-332, 1998.
12. Wilson WR: Approach to the patient with hoarseness. In Gorroll AH (ed): Primary Care Medicine, 3rd ed. Philadelphia, Lippincott-Raven, 1995, pp 999–1001.
13. Young HS: Esophageal disorders. In Dale DC, Federman DD (eds): Scientific American Medicine. New York, Scientific American, 1999, pp 3–5.
14. Brown JD, Thompson JN: Caustic ingestion. In Cummings CW, Fredrickson JM, Harker LA, et al (eds): Otolaryngology Head and Neck Surgery, 3rd ed. St. Louis, Mosby, 1998, pp 366–375.
15. Rice DH: Salivary gland disorders. Med Clin North Am 83:197–206, 1999.

Chapter 14

Dental Urgencies

Jill L. Benson, MD

General Approach to Dental Problems

Dental injury, infection, and odontogenic pain are frequent complaints in the urgent care setting. Because the source of the problem is sometimes difficult to localize, patients with dental problems frequently present to a medical setting instead of to a dentist. Although most problems of the oral cavity do not require emergent dental care, a few require aggressive immediate therapy to avoid serious and possibly life-threatening complications of dental disease. The urgent care physician must be able to recognize and begin treatment of true dental emergencies as well as provide temporary care and symptomatic relief to patients with less serious dental problems.

The use of dental terminology allows accurate description and documentation of physical examination and facilitates dental consultation and subsequent reevaluation. Some commonly used terms are listed in Table 1.

Table 1. Dental Terminology

Term	Definition
Alveolus	Tooth socket
Apex	Tip of the root
Buccal	Adjacent or pertaining to the intraoral surface of the cheek
Cementum	Substance that coats that root surfaces
Dentin	Substance beneath the enamel (supports the enamel)
Gingivae	Gum tissue
Incisal surface	Biting surface of the canines
Labial surface	Incisor and canine surface toward the lips
Lingual surface	Tooth surface toward the tongue
Mucobuccal fold	Sulcus between the gums and cheeks
Occlusal surface	Biting surface of the premolars and molars
Odontalgia	Toothache
Periodontal ligament	Fiber supporting the tooth in the alveolus with attachments to the cementum
Pulp	Center area of the tooth comprising nerves and blood vessels

The evaluation of patients with problems of the oral cavity and teeth requires an understanding of dental development and anatomy. The sequence of dental eruption and tooth numbering are illustrated in Figure 1. There are 20 primary and 32 permanent teeth. Primary dentition is normally lost and replaced with permanent teeth between the ages of 6 and 12 years; permanent second molars erupt at ages 11–13 years, and third molars erupt at ages 17–21 years.[1] It is important to ascertain the status of the patient's dentition because the therapy of certain dental problems depends on whether the involved tooth is primary or permanent.

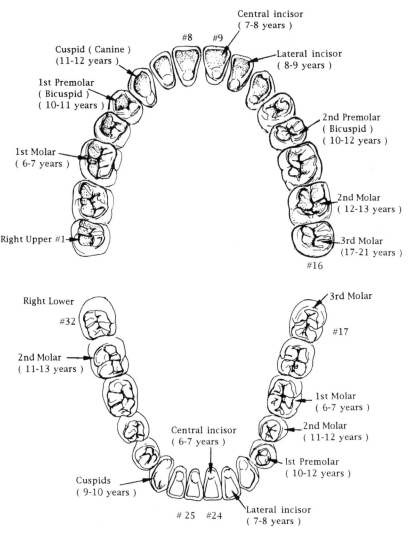

Figure 1. Tooth numbering and age of eruption of permanent teeth.

Patients with problems of the oral cavity and teeth should be asked about the circumstances that led to their presentation and whether any recent dental manipulation was performed. Further necessary history includes whether they have been systemically ill, have had recent trauma or any major medical illnesses, take any medications, or have any allergies. Knowing how the problem has interfered with the patient's normal activity, ability to eat and drink, or any recent changes in a chronic dental problem may aid in the diagnosis and direct subsequent management. The natural history of a disease that has progressed may suggest the diagnosis. Knowing factors that aggravate dental pain (e.g., hot or cold substances, lying in a prone position, or opening the mouth) can help differentiate between various possible causes of the presenting dental problem.

Physical examination includes determination of the vital signs, evaluation of the face and neck, assessment for cervical and submental adenopathy, and evaluation of the hard and soft palate, salivary glands and ducts, tonsils, tongue, floor of the mouth gingiva, and teeth. A more detailed general physical examination may be indicated if the patient has a significant medical history or vague complaints.

Dentoalveolar Trauma

Dentoalveolar trauma can produce a wide spectrum of injuries to the teeth and surrounding structures. Dental trauma may be isolated or occur in association with other significant injury that must be managed first. Trauma involving the teeth and surrounding structures is commonly seen in adults after motor vehicle accidents. Children frequently sustain dental trauma in falls. The anterior teeth are the most frequently involved structures. Significant bleeding from the site of injury may obscure the extent and exact location of the damage.

Tooth Fractures

Differential Diagnosis. The anatomy of a tooth and its surrounding structures is illustrated in Figure 2. Fractures of the teeth can present with pain or be totally asymptomatic. The type of fracture and subsequent management depend on the extent of disruption of the layers of the tooth.

Table 2 lists the characteristics and management of tooth fractures. Crown infraction is an incomplete fracture of the crown of the tooth and is usually asymptomatic. On examination, a crack or defect of the crown may be found. If the fracture involves the enamel only, it is termed an Ellis 1 fracture, and a defect in the enamel may be seen. The patient may complain of pain due to rubbing of the sharp edge of the tooth against oral tissue surfaces but will not experience thermal sensitivity. An Ellis 2 fracture involves the enamel and dentin. Exposed dentin is ivory-yellow and microporous so that bacteria can track down into the pulp. Subsequent pulp necrosis occurs in up to 10% of cases, but if treatment is delayed beyond 24 hours the risk of necrosis increases. The surrounding soft tissue should be inspected for embedded chips of tooth. Fractures that expose the pulp (Ellis 3) are true dental emergencies because the likelihood of pulp contamination and subsequent infection is high. These fractures result from significant oral trauma and can be associated with concomitant alveolar bone fracture or gingival lacerations. Pulp exposure can be determined if the tooth is wiped clean and then observed for the development of a pink blush or drop of blood at the site of injury. Physical examination should include palpation of the bony structure to assess for defects and careful inspection of soft tissues to detect embedded pieces of broken teeth. Radiographs of the area (mandibular or maxillary) are useful to detect fractures or embedded foreign material not found on physical examination.

Management. The management of dental fractures is described in Table 2. A crown infraction requires no urgent treatment. When the fracture involves the enamel only, the

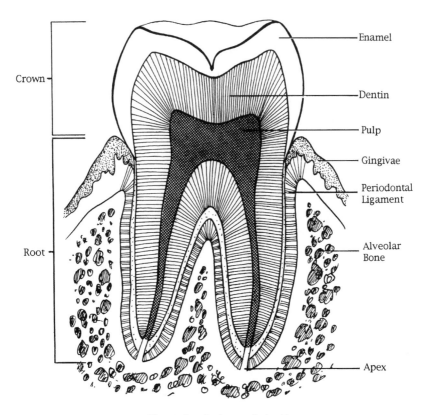

Figure 2. Anatomy of a tooth.

Table 2. Tooth Fractures

Fracture	Description	Examination	Management	Comments
Crown infarction	Incomplete fracture of enamel without loss of tooth tooth substance	Painless, no thermal sensitivity; may appear as crack or line in tooth surface	No urgent therapy required; general dental referral	Pulp necrosis uncommon
Uncomplicated crown fracture (Ellis 1 and 2)	Fracture of enamel (Ellis 1) or enamel and dentin (Ellis 2) without pulp involvement	Irregular, sharp tooth margin; painful if dentin involved; thermal sensitivity if dentin involved	Ellis 1: Smooth out sharp edges, general dental referral. Ellis 2: Calcium hydroxide paste (Dycal) or cotton soaked in eugenol (oil of cloves) and zinc oxide, analgesics, soft diet; general dental referral as soon as possible	Pulp necrosis in about 10% of Ellis 2 fractures; risk increases if treatment delayed more than 24 hours
Complicated crown fracture (Ellis 3)	Fracture involving enamel, dentin, pulp	Capillary bleeding or blush noted if surface is cleaned and dried;	Immediate general dental referral or calcium hydroxide paste or eugenol-soaked cotton and zinc oxide, repair of gingival laceration (4-0 or 5-0 Vicryl, simple closure), analgesia, soft diet	Pulp necrosis common

sharp irregular edge resulting from the trauma can be smoothed with an emory board. If the dentin is exposed, a calcium hydroxide paste (Dycal) should be applied to cover the defect and then covered with an enamel-bonded plastic.[2] If this approach is not possible, a cotton pledget soaked in eugenol (oil of cloves) will reduce the pain as dental consultation is obtained. The patient should be instructed to follow a soft diet to avoid disrupting the covering, and analgesics should be prescribed. Complicated fractures exposing the pulp (Ellis 3) should be seen immediately by a specialist. If dentistry is not immediately available, the exposed pulp should be covered with calcium hydroxide paste. Any gingival lacerations should be sutured, and analgesia should be given.

Pitfalls in Practice. Although dental trauma may be isolated, other traumatic injuries should be sought with special attention to the head and neck. Failure to diagnose an Ellis 3 fracture may result in delay in definitive dental therapy and the subsequent development of pulp necrosis with possible infection or tooth loss.

Periodontal Injuries

Differential Diagnosis. Table 3 describes common periodontal injuries. A tooth concussion that results from minor trauma may result in injury to the periodontal ligament. The tooth may be loose only when palpated, but no displacement is noted on visual

Table 3. Periodontal Injuries

Injury	Description	Examination	Management	Comments
Tooth concussion	Minor damage to periodontal ligaments	No displacement, or mild tooth loosening; may be sensitive to percussion	No urgent treatment required; general dental referral	
Tooth subluxation	Significant damage to periodontal supporting structure with loosening but no displacement	Tooth not displaced, moves with manipulation; gingival sulcus blood; tooth sensitive to percussion	With minor mobility: soft diet for 1–2 weeks, general dental referral. With gross mobility: immediate general dental referral, immobilize tooth with temporary splint	
Tooth luxation, intrusive	Displacement of tooth into alveolar bone with associated bony fracture	Tooth shortening, ginigival bleeding or laceration; tooth firm to palpation (impacted)	Immediate general dental referral. For primary dentition, wait. For permanent dentition: extraction, possible realignment with immobilization	Consider with suspected avulsion
Tooth luxation, extrusive	Partial tooth displacement out of socket	Tooth lengthening, gingival bleeding	Immediate general dental referral. For primary dentition: wait. For permanent dentition: realign and immobilize	Pulp necrosis common
Tooth avulsion	Complete tooth displacement out of socket	Tooth missing from socket, gingival bleeding	For primary dentition: do not replace. For permanent dentition: rinse tooth with water, store in milk or normal saline, attempt to replace; immediate general dental referral for immobilization; consider tetanus prophylaxis antibiotics	Replacement within 2 hr is optimal for tooth survival

inspection. Tooth luxation can be **intrusive**, in which case the tooth is impacted downward into the bone, or **extrusive**, in which case the tooth is partially out of its socket. Associated intraoral trauma should be sought. An avulsed tooth is completely displaced from its socket. It is essential to determine the location of the avulsed tooth, especially in elderly and very young patients, because aspiration or impaction in soft tissue may have occurred at the time of the trauma. A complete intrusive luxation can present as a missing tooth and must be considered during evaluation.

Management. The management of periodontal injuries is described in Table 3. If a tooth is partially avulsed, it is sometimes possible to reposition the tooth with light pressure of the fingers and to splint it to adjacent teeth.[3] If a patient contacts the urgent care center with a history of recent avulsion of a permanent tooth, he or she should be instructed to rinse gently (not to scrub) the tooth and socket with warm water, and then to reimplant the tooth immediately. This approach provides a physiologic environment until the patient arrives at the urgent care center for further assessment and tooth stabilization. If the patient is unable to reimplant the tooth, it should be stored under the patient's tongue or in the buccal fold to bathe it in saliva until the patient arrives at the urgent care center.[2] If the tooth is to be transported outside the mouth (as with a young child or elderly patient with increased risk of aspiration), it should be placed in milk, which is protein-rich and has physiologic osmolarity,[4] or, ideally, Hank's solution. Alternatively, the tooth can be transported in a liquid medium such as normal saline if the other options are not available.

Once the patient arrives, the tooth and socket are cleaned and the tooth replaced into the socket. Emergent dental consultation should be obtained. Reimplantation with immobilization is done if the supporting structures are still intact. Antibiotics (penicillin or erythromycin) are recommended in cases of tooth avulsion.[2] If the patient's tetanus immunization is not current, tetanus toxoid should be given. The success of reimplantation of an avulsed tooth depends on the vitality of the periodontal ligament. The best result is obtained if reimplantation is done within 30 minutes of avulsion. If reimplantation is delayed by more than 2 hours, clots formed in the socket and retraction of the periodontal tissue decrease the likelihood of success.[2] The patient should be placed on a liquid diet for several days; then a soft diet may be continued for the next 2 weeks.

Pitfalls in Practice. Tooth chips from fractures that become embedded in the soft tissue of the oral cavity act as foreign bodies and must be removed to reduce the risk of infection. Patients with trauma to the teeth must be assessed for other injury, especially to the bony structures of the mouth.

Primary teeth that are avulsed should not be reimplanted. Reimplanted primary teeth will fuse to the alveolar bone, and the reimplantation site will not grow at the same rate as the rest of the face. Reimplanted primary teeth also may interfere with the eruption of the permanent dentition.[2] Either scenario may result in a cosmetic deformity. Children may be referred to their dentist for management.

Lacerations of Oral Tissues

Differential Diagnosis. Lacerations of the oral tissue can involve the gingiva, lip, and tongue and may be through-and-through to the cheek. Frequently these injuries result from accidental biting of the tissue or direct trauma to the area. Physical examination should assess the function of underlying structures in the vicinity of the laceration (facial nerve, salivary ducts, and so forth) as well as determine the extent of the obvious injury.

Management. Basic wound care, as described in Chapter 8, should be followed in oral tissue lacerations, including anesthesia, irrigation, debridement, and tetanus immunization, if necessary. Antibiotics to cover oral flora are usually recommended. Penicillin VK (500 mg or 40 mg/kg orally 4 times/day for 7 days) or Bicillin CR (1.2 million U IM) plus aqueous penicillin G (1 million U IM) are usually given. In penicillin-allergic individuals, erythromycin is an acceptable alternative.

Table 4 describes the management of specific oral tissue lacerations. In general, intraoral lacerations of the buccal mucosa and the tongue that are not through-and-through, are not bleeding, and are small (< 1 cm) with little risk of trapping food can be left open.[5] Through-and through lacerations to the cheek should be repaired in layers; a water-tight closure is important. Repair of lip lacerations that involve the vermillion border requires careful approximation of the edges of the lip to achieve a cosmetically acceptable result.

Table 4. Oral Tissue Lacerations

Site	Surgical Repair	Comments
Gingivae	Simple closure, 4-0 Vicryl	Check for underlying bony defects
Through-and-through cheek	Simple water-tight mucosa closure, 3-0 Vicryl or silk; skin closure, 5-0 or 6-0 monofilament Nylon	Rule out facial nerve or Stenson's duct involvement; take skin suture out in 4–5 days
Lip	Simple closure of external lip surface, 4-0 monofilament nylon; mucosal closure, 4-0 Vicryl or silk; skin closure, 5-0 or 6-0 monofilament nylon	Approximate vermillion border first; take skin suture out in 4–5 days
Tongue	Simple closure of involved muscles, 3-0 or 4-0 Vicryl or chromic suture; simple closure of mucosa, 4-0 Vicryl	Hemostasis essential

Pitfalls in Practice. Lacerations that have the potential to trap foreign material, such as food, require surgical repair. All oral tissue lacerations should be digitally explored to ensure that there are no bony defects or embedded materials, such as food or tooth fragments, within the laceration.

Complications of Dental Procedures

Pain after Tooth Extraction

Differential Diagnosis. Pain occurring immediately after a tooth extraction is common and easily treated with analgesics. If pain occurs 2–3 days after tooth extraction, alveolar osteitis (dry socket) has probably developed. This condition occurs as a postextraction syndrome most often associated with extraction of the third molars.[6] The pain is caused by the loss of a blood clot that formed at the extraction site and incomplete healing of the alveolar bone with subsequent bacterial contamination.[4] The patient presents with intense local pain due to irritation of the exposed nerve tissue at the extraction site. A foul mouth odor usually is associated with this condition, but frank pus from the exposed socket is not seen.

Management. Patients with complaints of pain immediately (up to 24 hours) after tooth extraction should be given oral analgesia (Tylenol with codeine every 4 hours as needed). If alveolar osteitis is present, the socket should be gently irrigated with warm water to clear debris. Packing with iodoform gauze soaked in eugenol provides pain relief; packing should be changed daily. A local nerve block may also be use for pain relief. Oral analgesia should be prescribed, and the patient should be started on an antibiotic (penicillin VK or erythromycin, 500 mg orally 4 times/day for 10 days).[2] The patient should arrange daily follow-up with a dentist for dressing changes and definitive care.

Pitfalls in Practice. Although the complaint of dental pain is used by some patients to obtain drugs, pain after tooth extraction is common and real. Patients with this complaint and a recent history of a procedure should be treated for pain. Pain that persists beyond 24 hours is a sign of a possible serious complication (such as alveolar osteitis) and requires dental referral. It is essential to avoid any additional trauma to the socket during irrigation or inspection; this is associated with increased risk of osteomyelitis.[2]

Postextraction Bleeding

Differential Diagnosis. Postextraction bleeding can present a few hours after a dental procedure, most often just about the time when the vasoconstrictive action of the local anesthetics used for the procedure wears off. The bleeding is usually not profuse, and with gargling or irrigation the site is easy to visualize.

Management. If the site is oozing, it usually stops bleeding after the application of direct pressure. Firm pressure should be applied over the site with sterile gauze. The patient can apply this pressure by biting down for approximately 20 minutes on a gauze pad placed over the site. This protocol may be repeated after a local infiltration of lidocaine with epinephrine. If the bleeding continues or is moderately brisk, the socket should be suctioned to remove any clots and to allow visualization of the bleeding site. If the site cannot be visualized, iodoform gauze packing should be used to tamponade the bleeding site. If an obvious site of bleeding is seen, a suture may be placed with 3-0 Vicryl or chromic suture across the site. Hemostatic aids (Surgicel or Gelfoam) may be useful in stopping the bleeding or slowing it to facilitate placement of a suture. Silver nitrate sticks and other topical hemostatic are rarely useful in a moist field.[3] If the bleeding continues after these measures have been tried, the dentist who performed the procedure should be consulted. If the bleeding is stopped, the patient should be instructed to avoid rinsing, gargling, spitting, using a straw, smoking, or any activity that could disrupt the newly formed blood clot. Follow-up should be arranged with the patient's dentist.

Pitfalls in Practice. Spontaneous gingival bleeding (not associated with extraction or trauma) suggests gingival disease or blood dyscrasias. Such patients should be carefully assessed for other bleeding, other symptoms, and hemodynamic stability and then emergently referred for additional evaluation.

Pain after Root Canal

Differential Diagnosis. Pain after root canal can result from the trauma of the procedure itself or from gas build-up in the sealed canal. Swelling of the tissues may cause the tooth to be slightly raised and cause pain during chewing. This pain may be intense with a paucity of associated physical findings.

Management. Palliative therapy includes systemic and local anesthetics. True relief of the pain may not be achieved with palliative therapy, and the cause of the pain may not be discerned on physical examination. Therefore, consultation with the patient's dentist or endodontist is advised.

Pitfalls in Practice. Persistent or increasing pain after root canal or other endodontic procedures must be assessed for infection of the soft tissue or underlying bone.

Subcutaneous Emphysema

Differential Diagnosis. Subcutaneous emphysema may result from an endodontic procedure or cavity preparation if forced air is used in cleaning or preparing the site for the procedure. The accumulation of air is noted a few hours after the procedure and may last as long as 1 week.[7] Air may be forced through tissue planes of the face and neck, and marked swelling may occur with associated crepitus.

Management. Although subcutaneous emphysema after a dental procedure may be alarming to the patient, it is usually benign. The patient should be reassured that it is not uncommon after certain procedures and that the air will resorb completely in about 7–10 days. Analgesics should be prescribed if pain is associated with the emphysema. Broad-spectrum antibiotics (e.g. cephalosporins) are recommended along with daily follow-up with the patient's dentist or endodontist.[7]

Pitfalls in Practice. It is essential to differentiate subcutaneous emphysema due to forced air used in dental procedures from the subcutaneous emphysema that results from an anaerobic soft tissue infection after dental manipulation. Microorganisms can be carried from the oral cavity into deep tissues during dental procedures when pressurized air is used (e.g., for cleaning tooth surfaces). A subsequent possible complication that should not be overlooked is infection of tissues of the oral cavity and the face.

Loss of a Crown or Filling

Differential Diagnosis. Patients who have lost a crown or filling may present with no symptoms or may have intense local pain at the site. Examination should determine the previous location of the restoration as well as where it is now (i.e., lost, swallowed, or aspirated).

Management. A cotton pledget soaked in eugenol or a mixture of zinc oxide and eugenol should be placed over the exposed area. Irritants to the exposed dentin and pulp should be avoided. Dental consultation for replacement of the restoration should be done as soon as possible.

Pitfalls in Practice. Locating the lost restoration is important, especially in elderly and very young patients, who are prone to aspiration. If aspiration is suspected, a chest x-ray or soft tissue lateral neck x-rays may be useful in determining whether or not the restoration is in the airway or lungs.

Odontogenic Pain

Odontogenic pain is a frequent complaint in primary practice and prompts visits to urgent care centers at all hours of the night and day. Patients are certain about the presence of pain but sometimes have difficulty localizing it within the oral cavity. Additionally, many nondental diseases can produce pain that is referred to the oral cavity. Many systemic diseases have oral manifestations. The goals of urgent care evaluation are to differentiate these possibilities, to determine the presence of potentially serious diseases or complications, and to treat symptomatically less serious problems until definitive dental treatment can be arranged.

Differential Diagnosis. Patients with primary odontogenic disorders of pain complain of pain of variable intensity that usually starts within the oral cavity. Frequently, the patient can pinpoint a single tooth as the source of the pain, but occasionally the pain radiates to other structures in the oral cavity as well as to structures of the face, head, and neck, making localization of the disease process difficult. Knowing the onset, duration, and periodicity of pain may help in determining its cause. Many dental diseases are affected by hot or cold exposure, the presence of chemical irritants such as acids or chocolate, or physical or mechanical stimulants such as air movement, chewing, or physical manipulation of the involved tooth. Response of pain to prior self-medication should be noted.

To determine whether the pain is originating from an oral source, visual inspection of the oral cavity is performed to detect tooth fractures, loose restorations, caries, abnormal coloration, abrasions of the enamel, and exposure of the dentin or pulp. The gingiva should be evaluated for erythema, swelling, lesions, or exudates. Percussion of the tooth suspected to be the source of the pain can be accomplished with a tongue blade or an instrument handle; the tooth and surrounding tissues should be palpated for loose findings, foreign bodies embedded in soft tissue (usually food particles), or soft tissue fluctuance. Swollen, tender lymph nodes should be noted as well as the presence of a fever or other abnormal vital signs. In patients who appear to be ill or have complicated past medical histories, a more general and comprehensive history and physical examination should be performed.

Table 5 lists the characteristics of several odontogenic causes of pain. Dental caries is one of the most common diseases in humans[6] and, with its complications, probably causes most cases of acute odontogenic pain. Most odontogenic diseases can be diagnosed on the basis of history and physical examination alone, and most require dental procedures for ultimate cure. Laboratory studies in the urgent care center, therefore, are not usually useful or necessary.

Management. The management of common causes of odontogenic pain is listed in Table 5. In general, management includes ruling out complications of these diseases, determining whether or not antibiotics are indicated and delivering symptomatic treatment.

Table 5. Characteristics and Management of Some Causes of Odontogenic Pain

Cause	Presentation	Physical Examination	Management	Comments
Hypersensitive dentin	Due to acquired loss of dentin from any cause; pain is sharp, brief, worse with thermal or physical stimulation	Tooth appears to be normal, or small areas denuded of enamel are visible	No specific urgent management, eugenol on cotton may be helpful; general referral	

(Cont'd on next page)

Table 5. Characteristics and Management of Some Causes of Odontogenic Pain *(Continued)*

Cause	Presentation	Physical Examination	Management	Comments
Caries: without pulpitis	Intermittent dull pain, increased sensitivity to chemical and thermal stimulation	Poor dentition, yellow or brown area on enamel	Local analgesia with block or topical agents, systemic analgesia, general dental referral	Caries around previous restorations are hard to detect on examination
Caries: with pulpitis	Continuous spontaneous, severe pain, worsened by thermal stimulation; may worsen when patient lies down	Patient uncomfortable; pulp exposed; pain on tooth percussion; possible ill appearance	Same as above plus penicillin VK (500 mg 4 times/day for 7 days)	Pain may radiate to other areas of oral cavity and face
Tooth eruption	Primary teeth erupt at approximately 6–7 months; associated fretfulness, diarrhea, low-grade fever (< 100°F) Third molars erupt at age 17–25 years	Pale, taut, stretched mucous membrane over site; surrounding tissues red, tender, and swollen	Local analgesia with topical agents; ensure adequate hydration	Pain is short lived, temperature does not rise above 100°F; children frequently have concurrent symptoms of upper respiratory tract infection that increase their irritability[5]
Periapical abscess	Throbbing, severe, persistent pain; not affected by thermal changes; worse with physical manipulation	Tender, loose tooth; lymphadenopathy, trismus, facial swelling, fever, malaise, pain on tooth percussion; tooth may extrude slightly from socket; tooth decay usually obvious	Analgesia with local blocks, systemic agents; penicillin VK (500 mg 4 times/day for 7 days); refer for incision and drainage of abscess or extraction of tooth	Serious infectious complications are possible if not adequately treated
Pericoronitis	Due to debris trapped in tissue crevices around erupting third molars; tissue further injured by impaction against other teeth; seen at ages 17–25 years	Gingival inflammation near erupting tooth, local pain on contact, tissue edema, erythema, dysphagia, trismus, possible fever, systemic signs	Remove trapped debris with saline rinses, peroxide irrigation; if infected, give penicillin VK (500 mg 4 times/day for 7 days); refer for removal of third molar	Must consider peritonsillar abscess in differential diagnosis; pain can be referred to ear, throat, floor of mouth
Periodontal abscess	Due to food debris trapped between gum and tooth; gnawing, continuous pain, not thermally sensitive	Local swelling at or near gumline, purulent drainage; overlying tissue erythematous; tooth loosened; lymphadenopathy, fever	Local and systemic analgesia. Incision and drainage of abscess; give penicillin VK (500 mg 4 times/day for 7 days); refer for follow-up	Serious infectious complications are possible if not adequately drained
Gingivitis	Acute onset of rapidly progressing pain in gingivae; due to plaque formation in interdental papillae	Gingivae inflamed, bleeding, tender	Irrigate, debride; general dental referral for plaque removal	Condition improves rapidly with improved oral hygiene
Acute necrotizing ulcerative gingivitis	Sudden onset; gnawing, diffuse pain in gums; metallic taste in mouth; usually due to *Fusiformis* organisms or spirochetes, poor oral hygiene	Foul breath, systemic illness, increased salivation; gingivae swollen, ulcerated, spontaneously bleeds; lymphadenopathy, gray pseudomembranes can form on gums	Extensive debridement of pseudomembranes; irrigate with hydrogen peroxide, warm saline; systemic, topical analgesia; if patient dehydrated or ill, hospitalize for IV fluids, antibiotics (tetracycline, penicillin VK, erythromycin)	No evidence to date that this is communicable; predisposes to other periodontal diseases

Pain relief can be achieved by topical application of anesthetic agents such as viscous lidocaine or eugenol solutions and is particularly useful in the treatment of some local gingival and tooth disorders. Cotton pledgets soaked in the solution and applied to the involved area deliver prompt pain relief.

Dental blocks are simple procedures that can deliver immediate relief to patients with odontalgia from pulpitis, periapical abscess, and some periodontal abscesses. Dental blocks are also extremely useful in repairing oral lacerations or in pain management of dentoalveolar trauma. The choice of block depends on the area to be anesthetized. Examples of common anesthetic agents include 2% lidocaine (Xylocaine), 2% mepivacaine (Carbocaine), and 0.5% bupivacaine (Marcaine); they should be delivered with a 25-gauge needle.[8] The allergic history of the patient should be elicited before any agent is used. As with the delivery of all anesthetic agents, the syringe should be aspirated before the agent is injected. Useful local nerve blocks are described in Table 6, and Figure 3 illustrates the application of the inferior alveolar nerve block. The correct choice of block results in anesthesia to most areas of concern. The duration of anesthesia depends on the agent. The average duration of action of bupivacaine 0.5% with epinephrine ranges from 40 minutes for maxillary infiltration to 4 hours for an inferior alveolar block in the pulpal tissues, and the duration of action is longer in the soft tissues. Lidocaine 2% with epinephrine lasts an average of 60–85 minutes in the pulpal tissues.[9]

Table 6. Dental Nerve Blocks

Block	Landmarks	Anesthetized Area
Inferior alveolar nerve	Palpate coronoid notch of ascending ramus; injection site is between coronoid notch and pterygomandibular raphe (see Fig. 3). Advance needle 1.5–2.0 cm, and aspirate before injection	Mandibular teeth, bone, and gingivae
Anterior superior alveolar nerve	Identify cuspid tooth, and deposit 1–2 ml of anesthetic at bone near apex	Central and lateral incisor and cuspid; associated gingivae, alveolus; upper lip
Maxillary/mandibular supraperiosteal infiltration	Deposit 1–2 ml of anesthetic at apex of involved tooth	Individual tooth; associated gingivae, alveolus
Palatine nerve	Nasopalatine nerve blocked with a few tenths of a milliliter of anesthetic deposited behind incisors on the hard palate; greater palatine nerve blocked with a few tenths of a milliliter of anesthetic deposited at level of second molar, 1 cm from margin of gingivae, at junction of soft and hard palates	Upper incisors, canines, bicuspids with nasopalatine nerve; upper teeth, side of nose, upper lip, lower eyelid, maxillary sinus with greater palatine nerve

Patients who have odontalgia may require systemic analgesia for continued pain relief after local or dental blocks have worn off. Nonsteroidal anti-inflammatory drugs (NSAIDs) are frequently sufficient. If the pathology is severe or if NSAIDs were previously tried and were not effective, a narcotic agent such as codeine may be necessary. Patients with an identifiable and reasonable cause of pain should never be denied adequate analgesia. Occasionally drug abusers use dental pain as an excuse for seeking oral pain medications. If this scenario is suspected, a local block alone or followed with NSAIDs should be tried; the use of narcotics for such patients is discouraged.

In cases of odontalgia in which infection is a possibility or is already established and detectable on clinical examination, antibiotics should be prescribed as suggested in Table 5.

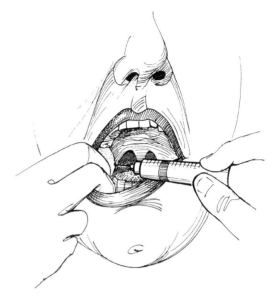

Figure 3.   Inferior alveolar nerve block.

Broad-spectrum coverage of oral flora can be obtained with penicillin. If the patient is penicillin allergic, erythromycin (500 mg 4 times/day) or tetracycline (500 mg 4 times/day in nonpregnant adults) are alternatives.

Patients who are evaluated in the urgent care setting for odontalgia from any cause require dental referral for continued evaluation and definitive care. Complications of dental infections from any source include spread to adjacent structures with the possibility of deep space infections of the head and neck. Hematogenous spread through bacteremia is also possible and may seed infection at distant sites, including lesions of heart valves. Endocarditis is also a possibility for high-risk patients undergoing routine dental procedures, and prophylaxis is recommended (Table 7).[10] Patients who present with complications of dental disease may require emergent dental evaluation and hospitalization for intravenous antibiotics.

Pitfalls in Practice.   The sources of pain in the oral cavity are not always the dentoalveolar structures. Table 8 lists etiologies of pain that can be referred to the mouth. Pain is usually referred through dermatomes on the ipsilateral side of the true source. These entities must be considered when the source of dental pain is not obvious from the history and physical examination. Some of these diseases, such as angina, are extremely dangerous, and delay in diagnosis may result in significant morbidity and possibly mortality.

Dental manifestations of systemic disease are not uncommon, and failure to recognize them can prolong the course of dental involvement and perhaps delay adequate therapy of the underlying disease process. Table 9 describes the dental presentation of some systemic diseases.

The spread of dental infections may cause infections of the head and neck. Complications include facial and periorbital cellulitis, maxillary sinusitis, meningitis, deep space infections, osteomyelitis, cavernous sinus thrombosis, and bacterial endocarditis.

Table 7. Antibiotic Prophylaxis for Prevention of Endocarditis in High-Risk Patients Undergoing Dental Procedures

	Moderate Risk Patients*	High-Risk Patients†
Non–penicillin-allergic	Adults: amoxicillin 2 gm orally 1 hour before procedure, follow with 1.5 gm 6 hours after first dose	Adults: ampicillin, 2.0 gm plus gentamicin, 1.5 mg/kg IM or IV, 30 minutes before procedure; follow with oral amoxicillin 1 gm oral or ampicillin, 1 gm IM/IV 6 hours after first dose of antibiotics
	Children (< 30 kg body weight): penicillin V, 1 gm orally 1 hour before procedure, follow with 500 mg 6 hours	Children (< 30 kg body weight): ampicillin, 50 mg/kg IM or IV, 30 minutes before procedure; follow with ampicillin, 25 mg/kg IM/IV, or amoxicillin, 25 mg/kg orally IM/IV, or amoxicillin, 25 mg/kg 6 hours after first dose of antibiotics
Penicillin-allergic	Adults: clindamycin 600 mg 1 hr before procedure then 300 mg 6 hours after first dose	Adults: vancomycin, 1 gm IV over 60 minutes; start 60 minutes before procedure, no repeated dose necessary
	Children: clindamycin 20 mg/kg orally 1 hour before procedure, follow with 10 mg/kg 6 hours after first dose	Children (< 30 kg body weight): vancomycin, 20 mg/kg IV over 60 minutes; start 60 minutes before procedure

* Past history of bacterial endocarditis, congenital cardiac malformations.
† Prosthetic heart valves, known valvular heart disease, cyanotic heart disease.

Table 8. Some Causes of Pain Referred to the Teeth

Maxillary sinusitis or carcinoma	Bell's palsy
Salivary gland infection or stone	Trigeminal neuralgia
Temporomandibular joint syndrome or arthritis	Glossopharyngeal neuralgia
Masseter muscle spasm	Vascular headaches
Pharyngitis	Rheumatic disorders (giant cell arteritis, polymyalgia rheumatica)
Peritonsillar abscess	Angina or myocardial ischemia
Otitis media or externa	

Table 9. Oral Manifestations of Some Systemic Diseases

Disease	Oral Manifestation
Diabetes mellitus	Hemorrhagic gingivitis, periodontitis, periodontal abscesses
Erythema multiforme	Vesicular lesions, usually on lips, buccal mucosa, tongue; breakdown to erosions and ulcerations covered with gray pseudomembranes
Pemphigus	Vesicular lesions, usually collapsed or ulcered, next to normal-looking tissue
Angioedema	Swollen oropharyngeal soft tissue, often associated with generalized urticaria, itching
Systemic lupus erythematosus	Ulcerated, necrotic intraoral lesions
Leukemia	Hemorrhagic gingivitis with occasional ulcers on tongue or buccal mucosa
Immunocompromise	Gingivitis, gingival ulcerations, oral candidiasis
Drug-induced allergic reaction	Diffuse or patchy inflammation with occasional maculopapular lesions on oral mucosa

Because many of these infectious complications are life-threatening, failure to recognize and treat them emergently can result in significant morbidity and mortality.

References

1. Nelson LP, Shusterman S: Dental emergencies. In Fleisher G, Ludwig S (eds): Textbook of Pediatric Emergency Medicine. Baltimore, William & Wilkins, 1993, pp 1403–1409.

2. Amsterdam JT: Dental disorders. In Rosen P, Barkin RM, et al (eds): Emergency Medicine: Concepts and Clinical Practice, 4th ed. St. Louis, Mosby, 1998, pp 2680–2697.
3. Kelly JP: Dental emergencies. In Kravis TC, Warner CG, Jacobs LM (eds): Emergency Medicine: A Comprehensive Review. New York, Raven Press, 1993, pp 1331–1337.
4. Medford HM: Dental trauma and infection. In Callaham M (ed): Current Practice of Emergency Medicine. Philadelphia, B.C. Dekker, 1991, pp 170–172.
5. Beaudreau RW: Oral and dental emergencies. In Tintinalli JE, Kelen GD, Stapczynski JS (eds): Emergency Medicine: A Comprehensive Study Guide. New York, McGraw-Hill, 2000, pp 1539–1556.
6. MacLeod DK: Common problems of the teeth and oral cavity. In Barker LR, Burton JR, Zieve PD (eds): Principles of Ambulatory Medicine. Baltimore, Williams & Wilkins, 1994, pp 1479–1492.
7. Dembo JB: Diagnosis and management of oral surgical complications. In Falace DA: Emergency Dental Care. Baltimore, Williams & Wilkins, 1995, pp 227–253.
8. Jastak JT, et al: Anesthetic equipment. In Jastak JT, Yagiela JA, Donaldson D (eds): Local Anesthesia of the Oral Cavity. Philadelphia, W.B. Saunders, 1995, pp 147–170.
9. Jastak JT, et al: Clinical preparation and drug selection. In Jastak JT, Yagiela JA, Donaldson D (eds): Local Anesthesia of the Oral Cavity. Philadelphia, W.B. Saunders, 1995, pp 87–126.
10. Lynch MA: Diseases of the cardiovascular system. In Lynch MA, Brightman VJ, Greenberg MS (eds): Burket's Oral Medicine. Philadelphia, J.B. Lippincott, 1994, pp 449–473.

Chapter 15

Common Gynecologic Problems in Urgent Care

Christine A. Kletti, MD
Steve Sterner, MD

Women with gynecologic problems frequently present to urgent care settings for evaluation of symptoms. Presentations range in severity from a minor vaginal discharge to a life-threatening hemorrhage from an ectopic pregnancy. The most important distinction to be made early in the evaluation is whether the woman is pregnant. Currently available urine pregnancy tests are highly sensitive and should be obtained as part of the evaluation of most women of reproductive age presenting with gynecologic or lower abdominal complaints. (Management of problems related to pregnancy is discussed in Chapter 16.) The physician also must consider the implications for the patient's sexual partner(s) when formulating a treatment plan.

The success of diagnosing gynecologic problems is highly dependent on the quality of the history and physical examination. Even when both are performed well, diagnostic accuracy is not high. The urgent care physician should not feel uncomfortable discharging the patient with a presumptive diagnosis after imminently dangerous conditions have been ruled out. The goal of urgent care physicians is to identify and stabilize patients with life-threatening problems, to begin evaluation and treatment of patients with less serious problems, and to arrange appropriate referral or follow-up care.

Vaginal Discharge

Vaginal discharge is both a symptom and a physical finding. Most healthy women report some amount of vaginal discharge that they consider normal. Typically a woman presents for evaluation of discharge because it has somehow changed. The physician's responsibility is to determine what the patient believes is abnormal about the current vaginal discharge. Inflammation of the vagina, cervix, uterus or fallopian tubes can cause an abnormal discharge. Usually this inflammation is due to an infectious agent, but other causes such as a foreign body should be considered. Some organisms cause an inflammation that is limited to the vaginal epithelium, whereas others cause cervicitis. Cervicitis is more concerning because it has the potential to ascend to the uterus and fallopian tubes.

Differential Diagnosis. Vulvovaginal candidiasis is usually caused by an overgrowth of *Candida albicans*, which typically is not considered a sexually transmitted infection. Immunocompromised patients, diabetics, patients recently treated with broad-spectrum antibiotics, and healthy women with no discernable risk factors are susceptible to vulvovaginal candidiasis. Patients generally complain of a white vaginal discharge and vaginal pruritus, but they may also present with dysuria, vulvar or vaginal soreness, or dyspareunia.

Trichomonas vaginalis is a flagellated protozoan that is typically spread by sexual contact. Women with a trichomonal infection often describe a foul smelling, yellow-green discharge and vulvovaginal discomfort. They also may complain of dysuria, dyspareunia, and mild low abdominal discomfort. Most men with *T. vaginalis* are asymptomatic.[1]

Bacterial vaginosis is the most commonly accepted term for the syndrome once called gardnerella vaginosis. Bacterial vaginosis occurs when aerobic *Lactobacillus* sp., which are part of the normal vaginal flora, are replaced by high concentrations of anaerobes and *Gardnerella vaginalis*.[2] Bacterial vaginosis is not believed to be a sexually transmitted disease, but it rarely affects women who have never been sexually active.

Neisseria gonorrhoeae and *Chlamydia trachomatis* are the most common agents responsible for cervicitis. Approximately one million new cases of gonorrhea are diagnosed in the U.S. each year. *C. trachomatis* has surpassed *N. gonorrhoeae* as the most common sexually transmitted bacterial infection.[3] *N. gonorrhoeae* is a gram-negative diplococcus. whereas *C. trachomatis* is an obligate intracellular organism. The spectrum of disease caused by these organisms ranges from urethritis or cervicitis to a fulminant pelvic infection. *N. gonorrhoeae* also can cause a systemic infection that includes arthritis and skin lesions. Chlamydial infections are often asymptomatic. One study of patients evaluated in the emergency department setting showed that 79% of women with *C. trachomatis* and 27% of women with *N. gonorrhoeae* infections were underrecognized and undertreated, suggesting that the symptoms often are subtle.[4] *C. trachomatis* infection of the fallopian tubes is considered a leading cause of female infertility.

History and Physical Examination. A thorough history of the patient presenting with an abnormal vaginal discharge includes the date of her last menstrual period, the characteristics of the discharge, associated vulvovaginal or urinary symptoms, and the course of the symptoms. It also should determined whether the patient is experiencing fever, chills, vomiting, or abdominal pain, which may suggest an infection involving the uterus and fallopian tubes. Abdominal pain is not usually a symptom of simple vaginitis. The clinician should elicit a careful sexual history including the number of partners in the past year, use of prophylaxis against pregnancy and sexually transmitted diseases. Finally, the patient should be questioned about her medical history and medication use. It is important to know whether the patient is immunocompromised or diabetic or recently took antibiotics.

The physical examination should include temperature measurements. The clinician should perform a careful evaluation of the abdomen and inguinal region in addition to the pelvic examination. The pelvic examination begins with careful inspection of the external genitalia. A generalized inflammation of this region is characteristic of a candidal infection. The vagina is examined for signs of infection and abnormal vaginal discharge. A sample of the discharge should be obtained by swabbing the vaginal fornices. The sample can be suspended in normal saline and applied to a microscope slide at a later time. The physician should search for a foreign body or neoplasm, which can also cause an abnormal vaginal discharge. Next, the cervix is examined for inflammation, lesions, and discharge. Specimen collection for *C. trachomatis* and *N. gonorrhoeae* is performed by inserting a cotton swab into the cervical os. Generally the swab must be rotated and left in the os for 15–30 seconds to allow adequate specimen collection. The next step involves the bimanual exam. During this examination the physician palpates for cervical motion tenderness, uterine or adnexal tenderness, and uterine or adnexal enlargement. Such findings suggest a process involving the upper genital tract. A rectal examination should be performed on patients also complaining of abdominal pain. Finally, the skin should be carefully inspected for lesions suggestive of syphilis or systemic gonorrhea.

Diagnostic Aids. The most important test for evaluating the patient with a gynecologic compliant is the human chorionic gonadotropin (hCG) urine test. A positive test changes both the differential diagnosis and the treatment options. Currently available hCG urine tests are greater than 99% sensitive and specific. The urine pregnancy tests can be positive as early as 6 days after conception.

A wet preparation is made by suspending a sample of vaginal discharge in normal saline and applying it to two microscope slides. Potassium hydroxide 10% should be added to one slide to enhance the fishy odor of bacterial vaginosis and define the pseudohyphae of candidal organisms. Swimming, flagellated organisms are diagnostic for *T. vaginalis*. Clue cells, which are vaginal epithelial cells with multiple, small, oval bacilli studding their surfaces, are suggestive of the diagnosis of bacterial vaginosis. The level of skill of the microscopist, the time and effort spent in examining the slide, and the quality of the sample influence the sensitivity of the test. The absence of clue cells does not exclude the diagnosis of bacterial vaginosis. Classically, three of the four following criteria should be met to make the diagnosis of bacterial vaginosis: (1) vaginal pH > 4.5; (2) presence of thin, homogenous vaginal discharge; (3) fishy odor after placement of KOH on wet mount; and (4) presence of clue cells on wet mount.[5]

Other methods of detecting *N. gonorrhoeae* and *C. trachomatis* include culture, Giemsa or Gram stain, fluorescent antibody stain, enzyme-linked immunosorbent assay (ELISA), and nucleic acid detection techniques. Culture is still considered the gold standard for diagnosing gonorrhea, but it requires careful handling of the specimen, and at least 48 hours is required for the return of the diagnosis. The accuracy depends greatly on how appropriately the specimen was handled. Amplified DNA tests seem to have the most favorable profile of the nucleic acid detection techniques with sensitivities of 97% and specificities of 98% for detecting *N. gonorrhoeae*.[6] In the case of *C. trachomatis*, amplified DNA tests are actually more sensitive than culture. They identify 25–35% more positive results. In addition, the amplified DNA tests have been shown to be 99.8% specific for *C. trachomatis*.[7] Another advantage of an amplified DNA test is that the results are often available within a few hours. Some nucleic acid tests also allow use of first morning urine specimens. It is important for the urgent care clinician to know which method is used in his or her facility and to understand its sensitivity and specificity profile.

The physician also should consider syphilis serology for patients at high risk for sexually transmitted diseases. HIV testing may be indicated, but it is controversial in the urgent care setting. The appropriateness of HIV testing and the ability to provide adequate follow-up and counseling for patients found to be HIV-positive should be discussed with urgent care administrators. A written policy about this issue is useful in case subsequent questions arise.

Management. Management of the patient with a vaginal discharge is described in Table 1. Before prescribing a treatment plan, the physician must be clear about the patient's pregnancy status. When a patient states that a sexual partner was recently diagnosed with a STD, the clinician might consider presumptively treating for that disease. Routine tests for gonorrhea and chlamydial infection may be done for documentation. After performing a careful history and physical examination and collecting the appropriate specimens, a diagnosis may be evident. If vaginitis appears to be likely, yet the wet preparation is negative, consider other diagnoses. The patient may have a normal vaginal discharge, allergic vaginitis, or mechanical or chemical irritation. Allergic vaginitis can be caused by exposure to feminine hygiene products, condoms, and spermicidal creams.

Table 1. Vaginal Discharge: Diagnosis and Treatment

Diagnosis	Physical Findings	Laboratory Findings	Treatment
Candida albicans infection	White discharge, mucosal inflammation no cervical inflammation	Wet preparation— spores and hyphae	Intravaginal agents: (multiple acceptable options including clotrimazole 1% cream 5 gm or 100 mg vaginal tablets once/day for 7 days; miconazole 2% cream 5 gm once/day for 7 days or 200 mg vaginal suppository once/day for 3 days; nystatin 1000,000 unit vaginal tablet, once/day for 14 days Oral agents: fluconazole 150 mg, 1 tablet single dose[19]
Trichomonas vaginalis infection	Yellow or green discharge, possible mucosal inflammation, no cervical inflammation	Wet preparation— flagellated trichomonads	Metronidazole, 2 gm orally as single dose or 500 mg orally 2 times/day for 7 days (not safe in pregnancy; substitute clotrimazole 100 mg vaginally once/day for 7 days)
Bacterial vaginosis	Thin, homogenous discharge	Wet preparation—clue cells, pH > 4.5, fishy odor with KOH	Metronidazole, 500 mg orally twice/day for 7 days; clindamycin cream 2%, 5 gm intravaginally at bedtime for 7 days; metronidazole gel 0.75%, 5 gm intravaginally twice/day for 5 days[8]
Chlamydia trachomatis infection	Cervical inflammation, cervical discharge, may be minimal	Gram stain, fluorescent antibody, DNA amplification	Azithromycin, 1 gm orally in a single dose; doxycycline, 100 mg orally twice/day for 7 days[20]; ofloxacin, 300 mg orally twice/day for 7 days[8] In pregnancy: erythromycin base, 500 mg orally 4 times /day for 7 days; amoxicillin, 500 mg orally 3 times/day for 7 days[8]
Neisseria gonorrhoeae infection	Cervical inflammation, cervical discharge	Gram stain, positive culture, fluorescent antibody, DNA amplification	Cefixime, 400 mg orally in single dose; ceftriaxone, 125 mg IM in a single dose; ciprofloxacin, 500 mg orally in a single dose; ofloxacin, 400 mg orally in a single dose[8] In pregnancy: If cephalosporin not tolerated, spectinomycin, 2 gm orally as a single dose[8]
Pelvic inflammatory disease	Lower abdominal, cervical motion, and adnexal tenderness, possible cervical discharge, fever	Positive *N. gonorrhoeae* or *C. trachomatis* test, elevated ESR, CRP or WBC	Outpatient: ofloxacin, 400 mg orally twice/day for 14 days, *plus* metronidazole, 500 mg orally twice/day for 14 days, or ceftriaxone, 250 mg IM single dose, *plus* doxycycline orally twice/day for 14 days[8] Inpatient: cefotetan, 2 gm IV every 12 hr, or cefoxitin, 2 gm IV every 6 hr, *plus* doxycycline, 100 mg IV/oral every 12 hr or clindamycin 900 mg IV every 8 hr *plus* gentamicin load (2 mg/kg) followed by maintenance (1.5 mg/kg) every 8 hr[8]

In a patient who appears to have cervicitis, *N. gonorrhoeae* and *C. trachomatis* are the most likely causes. At this point the physician should estimate the likelihood of infection and how reliable the patient will be to make a follow-up appointment if treatment is necessary. Often laboratory confirmation is not available for 1–3 days. Patients with cervicitis on examination may have a subclinical upper genital tract infection. If treatment is delayed, the patient may develop pelvic inflammatory disease (PID). A delay also increases the risk of transmission to other people. Outpatient notification and follow-up are often unreliable, resulting in delay of treatment for days to weeks, if it is ever sought.[4] If the patient is going to be treated presumptively for a STD, the treatment should be carefully explained to her. She should then be treated for both gonorrhea and chlamydia. In addition, it is important to discuss testing for HIV in patients at risk for STDs.

The urgent care physician also has a responsibility to the sexual partners of the patient. The patient should be counseled to notify all sexual partners for the 60 days before the onset of symptoms, if an STD is documented. If the patient had no sexual partner during this interval, she should notify her most recent sexual partner. The partners should be evaluated, tested, and treated as appropriate. The patient should be advised to refrain from sexual intercourse for 7 days after completion of the antibiotic therapy. If symptoms persist, the patient should continue abstinence and be reevaluated by her physician.[8]

Patients who are treated with one of the recommended regimens for *N. gonorrhoeae* and *C. trachomatis* generally do not need to return for reevaluation and cultures (i.e., a test of cure). If symptoms persist, the patient should be reevaluated. Patients with persistent symptoms who were previously diagnosed with gonorrhea should be evaluated and recultured at this time so that antibiotic susceptibility also can be tested. It is generally of no use to repeat DNA tests for *C. trachomatis* less than 3 weeks after completion of drug therapy.[8]

Pitfalls in Practice. If evidence of cervicitis is present, the patient may develop PID while waiting for laboratory confirmation before treatment for chlamydial infection or gonorrhea. Such patients should be treated at the first visit. Bacterial vaginosis may be accompanied by little or no discernible discharge, but patients report improvement in other symptoms after treatment. Finally, it is the responsibility of the physician to discuss the importance of safe sexual practices and the risk of exposure to HIV in patients diagnosed with an STD. Failure to do so places the patient at risk of reinfection and increases the odds of further transmission of the disease.

Genital Lesions

Genital Ulcers

Genital ulcers are typically caused by infectious organisms that are transmitted sexually. The vast majority of genital ulcers in the United States are caused by herpes simplex virus 2 (HSV-2), but syphilis and other uncommon organisms cause genital ulcers as well. Because these organisms tend to be difficult to culture, a diagnosis is difficult to make. Perhaps the most useful finding differentiating genital ulcers is whether they are painful.

Differential Diagnosis. HSV-2 causes **genital herpes** and is transmitted through sexual contact. Initial lesions appear on the external genitalia and in the vagina as small, painful, grouped vesicles on an erythematous base that break down to form painful ulcers. The virus invades the sensory nerves in the affected area and after days becomes dormant in the nerve ganglion. Some patients have only one episode, but most have recurrent episodes at variable intervals. The primary infection is usually the worst. The lesions may last for days to weeks. The patient may develop inguinal adenopathy, dysuria, and a low-grade fever. It has long been known that people are contagious when lesions are present, but now it is believed that the virus can also be shed during asymptomatic periods. Approximately 21% of the U.S. population is seropositive for HSV-2. Most people are unaware of the infection.[9]

Syphilis is caused by *Treponema pallidum*, a spirochete that is transmitted by sexual contact when lesions are present. Initially it causes one or more chancres that usually ulcerate. These lesions tend to be painless and located in the genital area or any other area of contact. If untreated, they disappear spontaneously over 2–6 weeks. The chancres are usually associated with adenopathy that is characteristically tender. During this time the infection becomes systemic, manifesting again at about 6 weeks as secondary syphilis, with maculopapular skin lesions and lymphadenopathy. These lesions can mimic almost any kind of rash and often appear in unusual locations, such as on the palmar surfaces of the hands and the plantar surfaces of the feet. If untreated, these lesions resolve and the organism slowly invades the central nervous and cardiovascular system.[10]

Lymphogranuloma venereum is caused by a serotype of *Chlamydia trachomatis* and tends to cause painless genital ulcers with inguinal lymphadenopathy. The lesions look much like a syphilitic chancre or a single herpetic vesicle. The adenopathy usually occurs 2–6 weeks after the lesion. It is most commonly unilateral. The inguinal ligament may cause a groove in the adenopathy, leading to the term *groove sign*. The groove sign is reported in only 20% of infected women.[10] Most believe that lymphogranuloma venereum is transmitted sexually. It is uncommon in most of the United States.

Chancroid is a sexually transmitted disease caused by *Hemophilus ducreyi*. It is characterized by painful genital ulcers and tender inguinal lymphadenopathy. Chancroid is relatively rare, but it is endemic in some areas of the United States. It often occurs as outbreaks. Chancroid is a cofactor for HIV transmission. Large ulcers may require more than 2 weeks to heal.[8]

Granuloma inguinale is caused by *Calymmatobacteriuim granulomatis*. It, too, is rare in the United States. Granuloma inguinale is characterized by painless ulcers without inguinal adenopathy. The lesions are beefy and vascular. They can be quite disfiguring and are at risk for secondary infection.[10]

Other Genital Lesions

Condylomata acuminata (genital warts) is transmitted both sexually and nonsexually. Genital warts are caused by certain strains of the human papillomavirus (HPV). The strains most likely to cause genital warts are oncogenic and are associated with cervical cancer. The lesions range in appearance from papules to cauliflower-like masses. The incubation period can range from weeks to year. Patients may complain of vaginal discomfort or dyspareunia.[11]

Lichen sclerosus is a chronic atrophic skin disease characterized by well-demarcated white plaques of the vulva and perineum. It can cause pruritus, discomfort, dysuria, and dyspareunia. It is most common in postmenopausal women but can occur in all age groups.

Bartholin's cysts and abscesses are relatively common gynecologic problems. The Bartholin's glands are small glands located in the labia minora at the 4 and 8 o'clock positions in relation to the introitus. A Bartholin's cyst results when the gland becomes obstructed and dilates. Most are asymptomatic, but if they become large enough, they may cause local discomfort. Bartholin's gland abscesses are typically quite painful. They develop quickly over a few days. Many different bacteria typical of vaginal flora have been isolated from cultures obtained from these abscesses.

History and Physical Examination. Characteristics and management of genital ulcers are listed in Table 2. Multiple painful vesicles are almost certainly due to herpes. Painless ulcers are highly suggestive of syphilis, but the diagnosis of genital ulcers by physical examination alone is often inaccurate.

Diagnostic Aids. Patients presenting for evaluation of genital ulcers should generally be evaluated for HSV and syphilis. A physician can obtain a specimen for diagnosing herpes simplex by scraping the base of an open ulcer or by puncturing a vesicle. This fluid can be sent for culture, polymerase chain reaction (PCR), and Tzank smear. Blood samples can also be obtained to test for HSV-2 antibodies. All patients with a genital ulcer should be screened by a syphilis serology test such as the Venereal Disease Research Laboratory (VDRL) test or rapid plasma reagin (RPR) test, both of which have high sensitivity but low specificity. A positive VDRL or RPR does not necessarily diagnose syphilis because there are many false positives. If VDRL is positive, a fluorescent treponemal antibody test also should be performed, which is a highly specific test and is considered diagnostic for syphilis. Culturing the other organisms mentioned above is difficult and rarely attempted.

Management. The patient with multiple painful genital ulcers almost certainly has herpes. If the physician desires confirmation, a herpes culture can be performed. If it is a first episode for the patient and if the visit to the urgent care center is within 6 days of onset of the lesions, a course of acyclovir (Zovirax) will shorten the duration of the episode by up to 5 days (see Table 1). If it is a subsequent episode, therapy is not as effective. If acyclovir is begun within 2 days of onset of recurrent symptoms, it will shorten the episode by 1 day on average. Patients with severe lesions may be unable to void and require catheterization for a few days. This, together with difficulty in controlling severe pain, occasionally requires hospitalization.

The patient with primary syphilis should be treated with penicillin G benzathine (see Table 2) and followed for repeat serology in 3 months. The patient with primary syphilis should be referred to her primary physician for careful follow-up. The patient with secondary syphilis also should be treated and referred. The fluorescent antibody test, once positive, remains positive for life. RPR and VDRL titers should decline after treatment, and the titers usually return to normal within 1 year. If they do not, the patient may have had a treatment failure and needs further evaluation, including a test for HIV. Any patient with a genital ulcer should be evaluated again in 5–7 days. If no symptomatic improvement or signs of healing are noted, the original diagnosis should be questioned.

Table 2. Genital Ulcers: Diagnosis and Treatment

Disease	Physical Findings		Treatment
	Painful Ulcer	Inguinal Adenopathy	
Herpes	+	+	First episode: acyclovir, 400 mg orally 3 times/day or 200 mg orally 5 times/day for 7–10 days; famcyclovir, 250 mg orally 3 times /day for 7–10 days; or valacyclovir 1 gm orally twice/day for 7–10 days Recurrent episodes: acyclovir, 400 mg orally 3 times/day, 200 mg orally 5 times/day, or 800 mg orally twice/day for 5 days; famcyclovir, 125 mg orally twice/day for 5 days; valacyclovir, 500 mg orally twice/day for 5 days Suppressive therapy: acyclovir, 400 mg orally twice/day; famcyclovir, 250 mg orally twice/day; valacyclovir, 250 mg orally twice/day, 500 mg orally once/day, or 1,000 mg orally once/day Inpatient/severe disease: acyclovir, 5–10 mg/kg IV every 8 hr[8]
Syphilis	–	±	Primary/secondary: benzathine penicillin G, 2.4 million units IM in a single dose Penicillin allergic: doxycycline, 100 mg orally twice/day, or tetracycline, 500 mg orally 4 times/day for 2 wk[8]
Chancroid	+	+	Azithromycin, 1 gm orally in a single dose; ceftriaxone, 250 mg IM in a single dose; ciprofloxacin, 500 mg orally twice/day for 3 days; erythromycin base, 500 mg orally 4 times/day for 7 days[8]
Lymphogranuloma venereum	–	+	Doxycycline, 100 mg orally twice/day for 21 days, or erythromycin base, 500 mg orally 4 times/day for 21 days[8]
Granuloma inguinale	–	–	Trimethoprim-sulfamethoxazole DS, 1 tablet orally twice/day, or doxycycline, 100 mg orally twice a day for at least 3 wk Alternatives: ciprofloxacin, 750 mg orally twice/day for at least 3 wk[8]
Carcinoma	–	+	Refer for biopsy to diagnose.

Table 2 describes the recommended treatment regimens for chancroid, granuloma inguinale, and lymphogranuloma venereum. There are many different options for the treatment of genital warts, including cytotoxic agents (e.g., podophyllin), surgical procedures, liquid nitrogen, and interferons. Patients should be referred to their primary care physician or a dermatologist for therapy. Multiple treatments are usually required for resolution of lesions.[11,12]

The initial treatment of lichen sclerosus is topical corticosteroids. Bartholin's cysts can be managed conservatively if they are not causing the patient much discomfort. Warm sitz baths may encourage the spontaneous rupture of the cyst. For patients with large, uncomfortable cysts or abscesses, definitive treatment is indicated.

Definitive treatment involves incision and drainage with placement of a Word catheter, marsupialization, or application of silver nitrate. Description of this treatment is beyond the scope of this text.[12,13] Patients should be treated for concurrent vaginal or cervical infections, if present, because the same organisms may have contributed to the formation of the Bartholin Gland abscess.

Pitfalls in Practice. Because the diagnosis of genital ulcers by physical examination is inaccurate, it is important to test for syphilis, especially if one plans to treat for an alternative diagnosis. Any genital ulcer should be followed after therapy until its resolution. Lesions that are not responding appropriately to therapy should be biopsied for malignancy and reevaluated for alternative infectious causes. Carcinoma is an unusual cause of genital ulcers in young women but should be considered seriously in elderly patients. The physician must stress the importance of follow-up to ensure the resolution of the lesion with the chosen treatment. Patients should be carefully warned about the sexually transmitted nature of the lesion to avoid further transmission.

Lower Abdominal Pain

Differential Diagnosis. The first step in limiting the differential diagnosis in the evaluation of abdominal pain is to determine whether the patient is pregnant. Evaluation of abdominal pain in pregnant patients is discussed in Chapter 16. In nonpregnant patients, the next step in evaluation is to determine whether the abdominal pain originates in the reproductive organs. Often this goal can be accomplished by the physical examination. The differential diagnosis of lower abdominal pain in young female patients is listed in Table 3.

Table 3. Differential Diagnosis of Lower Abdominal Pain

Nonpregnant	Pregnant
PID	Ectopic pregnancy
Endometriosis	Spontaneous abortion
Ovarian cyst rupture, torsion, hemorrhage	Corpus luteum cyst
Acute appendicitis	Acute appendicitis
Abdominal pain of unclear etiology	Abdominal pain of unclear etiology

History and Physical Examination. As always, the history of women with abdominal pain should include the time and course of onset of the pain. Pain that begins suddenly, in a matter of seconds or minutes, should lead the physician to suspect the rupture (cyst or ectopic pregnancy) or torsion of a structure (ovary or ovarian cyst). Pain of a more gradual onset, over hours to days, is more suggestive of an inflammatory process. It is useful to know if the patient has had this type of pain before. Is the pain associated with menstrual cycles? Does it occur in a cyclic pattern? The physician should also ask about the quality of the pain. Is the pain constant or colicky? What has the patient tried to relieve the symptoms? Abnormalities in the menstrual history may be helpful as well, particularly a missed menstrual period. However, this history does not obviate the need for an objective urine pregnancy test. The physician should inquire about the presence of any vaginal discharge, which tends to indicate an infectious cause for the pain, such as PID.

Physical examination should begin with an assessment of vital signs, including temperature, respiratory rate, and pulse and blood pressure, both supine and standing. The presence of fever is strongly associated with infection. An orthostatic rise in pulse and a fall in blood pressure are associated with hypovolemia due to dehydration or hemorrhage. The chest and abdomen should be carefully examined, with special concern for localizing tenderness and signs of peritoneal inflammation. The pelvic examination is particularly important. The cervix is examined for discharge, and a swab for *C. trachomatis* and *N. gonorrhoeae* should be obtained. The uterus should be palpated for abnormal size and tenderness. The adnexal areas should be palpated for masses or tenderness. In most patients, one can distinguish pelvic tenderness from general abdominal tenderness. Pelvic tenderness increases the probability of a gynecologic cause of the pain. The most difficult patients to assess are those with poorly localized peritoneal inflammation who have general abdominal tenderness as well as pelvic tenderness. Many such patients have serious pathology of either abdominal or pelvic origin and need further evaluation, including laparoscopy or laparotomy if necessary. It is also important to perform a rectal examination, which adds another dimension to the bimanual examination.

Diagnostic Aids. Few diagnostic aids are helpful in the evaluation of abdominal pain. A urinalysis should be performed to detect signs of a urinary tract infection. White blood cell count, ESR, and C-reactive protein are nonspecific indicators of inflammation. If they are elevated, the physician may be more concerned about an infectious cause of the pain, but no more sure of the diagnosis. The importance of the urine pregnancy test has been discussed. Pelvic ultrasonography may help in the diagnosis of patients with a pelvic mass, ovarian cyst, ovarian torsion and tubo-ovarian abscess. Magnetic resonance imaging and CT scanning are also adjuncts in the evaluation of low abdominal pain.

Specific Causes of Lower Abdominal Pain

Pelvic Inflammatory Disease

Pelvic inflammatory disease (PID) is an infection of the upper genital tract and may include endometritis, salpingitis, tubo-ovarian abscess, and pelvic peritonitis. PID is commonly caused by a sexually transmitted organism that ascends the genital tract. Most PID is caused by *C. trachomatis* or *N. gonorrhoeae*, but polymicrobial disease, including *Escherichia coli*, *H. influenzae*, and anaerobes, has also been identified. It is suggested that an estimated 1 million women in the U.S. suffer from an episode of PID every year.[14] Until further studies are performed, clinicians need to accept the fact that the clinical diagnosis of PID is relatively inaccurate.

The spectrum of clinical presentation is broad, ranging from women who are essentially asymptomatic to those with fever and severe abdominal pain. Patients may even develop localized or generalized peritonitis secondary to purulent drainage from the fallopian tubes into the peritoneal cavity. Many criteria have been offered for the diagnosis of PID, but laparoscopy is considered the gold standard. The minimal requirements for making the diagnosis of PID include lower abdominal pain, cervical motion tenderness, and adnexal tenderness. The specificity increases if the patient has a temperature > 101° F and elevated ESR or C-reactive protein, an abnormal vaginal discharge, or a laboratory test confirming *N. gonorrhoeae* or *C. trachomatis*. Finally, a definitive diagnosis can be made with endometrial biopsy, ultrasonography, or laparoscopy.[8]

The long-term sequelae of PID include infertility, chronic pelvic pain, and ectopic pregnancy. Because the real concern for increased morbidity if the infection is not treated early, it may be in the patient's best interest to make a presumptive diagnosis of PID and to treat with antibiotics before the diagnosis is completely clear.

Management. Women with severe abdominal pain, significant fever, or complicating factors should be hospitalized. Complicating factors may include a previous failure of outpatient therapy, poor likelihood of compliance with antibiotic regimen, or possibility of an alternative diagnosis, which may require surgery. Advantages of hospitalization include certain medication compliance, use of intravenous antibiotics, and the opportunity for frequent reevaluation of the patient. If the patient is not improving, it is likely that either the wrong antibiotics are being used or the wrong diagnosis has been made. Most women with PID can be treated as outpatients but should be reevaluated at 24- to 48-hour intervals until they are clearly improving. The recommended treatment regimens are listed in Table 1.

Ovarian Cysts

Ovarian cysts—whether functional, endometriotic, benign, or malignant—can cause pelvic pain in a number of ways. Pain of sudden onset is more likely to be caused by rupture, hemorrhage, or torsion related to the cyst, whereas gradual, mild chronic pain may result simply from the enlarging cyst. When a follicular cyst ruptures to release an egg, a small amount of fluid may leak. Some women experience midcycle discomfort with this process, which is known as *mittelschmerz*. The pain rarely lasts more than 2 days and is usually associated with a benign pelvic and abdominal examination. Rupture of larger cysts can cause more impressive symptoms and physical examination findings when the fluid irritates the peritoneum. It is also possible to have hemorrhage from an ovarian cyst. Such patients can become unstable and require emergent laparotomy. Finally, ovarian cysts or tumors can cause acute pelvic pain by torsion. This, too, is a surgical emergency, requiring immediate diagnosis and laparotomy.

Management. In general, patients with severe pain or signs of peritoneal inflammation should be further evaluated in the hospital environment. Pelvic ultrasonography can be helpful in diagnosing ovarian cysts, evaluating for free fluid in the pelvis, and detecting ovarian blood flow abnormalities suggestive of torsion.[10,15]

Endometriosis

The true incidence of endometriosis is unknown because many women with endometriosis never seek medical care. The abdominal pain associated with endometriosis is caused by islands of endometrial tissue in the peritoneal cavity, which break down and bleed during the menstrual cycle. The blood and dead tissue collect in the peritoneal cavity, causing pain and possibly focal peritoneal inflammation and tenderness. Patients with endometriosis may complain of dysmenorrhea, pelvic pain, or dyspareunia. They may also give a history of infertility.

Management. Treatment of endometriosis is controversial and beyond the scope of this text. The difficult task is making the diagnosis. History of chronic dysmenorrhea is suggestive, but only laparoscopic diagnosis is definitive. Patients diagnosed with endometriosis need to discuss the many treatment options, including various hormonal and surgical therapies.[15,16]

Acute Appendicitis

Although acute appendicitis accounts for only a small fraction of women with abdominal pain, it must be seriously considered in any woman with localized right lower abdominal pain that is not clearly localized to the right adnexal area on pelvic examination. It is not unusual to diagnose PID on laparotomy or laparoscopy when appendicitis was initially suspected. Likewise, in the patient with PID whose pain worsens and localizes to the right lower quadrant, appendicitis is a distinct possibility.

Management. Acute appendicitis is managed by surgical appendectomy.

Abdominal Pain of Unclear Etiology

Not much is written about abdominal pain of unclear etiology, probably because most physicians dislike vague diagnoses. Clearly, many if not most patients with acute abdominal pain improve, no matter what therapy is prescribed or whether a definitive diagnosis is made. Many young women who fit into this category, however, receive a diagnosis of and treatment for PID.

Pitfalls in Practice. The diagnosis of the cause of abdominal pain must be considered presumptive unless confirmed by direct surgical visualization. The patient should be reexamined at frequent intervals until she is clearly improving. Because of the associated morbidity, the physician may consider presumptively treating for PID if the diagnosis is likely.

Vaginal Bleeding

Typically the patient with abnormal vaginal bleeding is experiencing an increase in volume or a change in the timing or duration of the bleeding. The bleeding may be a bothersome spotting or a life-threatening hemorrhage. Patients with significant hemorrhage usually should be transferred immediately to a hospital emergency department. If possible, IV access should be obtained before transfer. Again, it is most important to identify the pregnant patient early, because pregnancy drastically changes the differential diagnosis (see Chapter 16). If the patient is not pregnant, the next most important factor is her age. Young women tend to bleed abnormally because of hormonal reasons, and older women tend to bleed because of anatomic abnormalities. The urgent care physician can initially evaluate such women but should refer them to a specialist for further care.

Differential Diagnosis. The most common cause of abnormal bleeding in young, postmenarchal, premenopausal women is anovulatory cycles. During a normal menstrual cycle, estrogen stimulates endometrial proliferation. Progesterone plays a role in ovulation and also stabilizes the endometrium and prepares it for implantation. Withdrawal of progesterone finishes the cycle by causing endometrial shedding. In the typical anovulatory cycle, estrogen causes endometrial proliferation, but for some reason ovulation does not occur. As a result, the estrogen continues to stimulate endometrial proliferation. Without progesterone the endometrium grows so large that the estrogen levels can no longer support it, and bleeding begins. To start the cycle again, progesterone is needed to mature the endometrium. Withdrawal of this progesterone then causes the endometrium to slough in an organized manner. Although such hormonal imbalances are the most common cause of abnormal vaginal bleeding in young women, they should be considered a diagnosis of exclusion. When all other causes have been eliminated, the diagnosis of dysfunctional uterine bleeding can be made.

Other endocrine imbalances can cause abnormal vaginal bleeding in woman of any age group. Hyperthyroidism and hypothyroidism are examples of such imbalances. Disorders of the coagulation system, such as von Willebrand's disease, can cause abnormal bleeding in any system, including the reproductive system. It is important to include a medication history in the evaluation of patients with abnormal vaginal bleeding. A history of Depo-Provera use or oral contraceptive pill noncompliance may alter a previously normal menstrual cycle. To complete the differential diagnosis the physician should include the possibility of fibroids, endometriosis, trauma, infection, and neoplasm.[17]

In older women, tumors are a common cause of abnormal vaginal bleeding. Vaginal bleeding after menopause should be considered tumor until proved otherwise.

History and Physical Examination. The history should determine whether the problem is acute or chronic, whether the patient has any underlying medical problems, and whether she is taking any medications. The physician should try to quantify the amount of bleeding. The frequency with which the patient needs to change her tampon or pad is an indication of the amount of bleeding. The clinician also should ask questions to help determine whether the patient is experiencing hypovolemia or anemia. The physician may be able to elicit information suggesting an underlying endocrine imbalance or coagulopathy.

The physical examination should include vital signs to evaluate for evidence of hypovolemia. Evidence of endocrine imbalance or bleeding from other organ systems also should be sought. A thorough genital and pelvic examination should be performed. A few patients have bleeding lesions of the vulva, vagina, or cervix. Such lesions may be benign or malignant and require further evaluation. Most bleeding comes from the cervical os. Bimanual examination of the uterus and adnexa may reveal a mass as the cause of the bleeding, but probably the examination will be normal.

Diagnostic Aids. A hemoglobin or hematocrit measurement is helpful if bleeding has been substantial. Clotting studies should be ordered with any suspicion of clotting disorder. Levels of thyroid hormones can be measured if hypothyroidism is suspected. Endometrial biopsy is the most useful tool for evaluating abnormal vaginal bleeding; it accurately identifies the stage in the endometrial cycle. In an anovulatory cycle, a proliferative endometrium is observed.

Management. The urgent care physician probably will not be able to make a definitive diagnosis of abnormal vaginal bleeding. All patients need to be referred for continued management and evaluation. If the patient is experiencing no ill effects of the bleeding, it is acceptable to observe and have her follow up with a primary care physician. If the bleeding is bothersome or causing symptoms, the clinician may consider presumptive treatment for dysfunctional uterine bleeding, assuming no other cause has been discovered. A common regimen is medroxyprogesterone (10 mg/day orally for 10 days).[18] This regimen is acceptable in a young, nonsexually active woman. In sexually active women who are not interested in pregnancy, combination oral contraceptive pills are a good option. The patient can take 3 or 4 tablets/day until the bleeding stops and then continue with the regular dose of 1 tablet/day. Patients who are bleeding so heavily as to cause hemodynamic changes should be transferred to an emergency department with IV access in place.

Pitfalls in Practice. It is an error to believe that treating the patient with vaginal bleeding on the initial visit will resolve the problem. Patients with abnormal vaginal bleeding should be followed by a physician who is willing to continue the work-up until a diagnosis is established. It is the responsibility of the urgent care physician to make an appropriate referral to a gynecologist as part of the patient's disposition.

References

1. Heine P, McGregor JA: Trichomonas vaginalis: A reemerging pathogen. Clin Obstet Gynecol 36:137–144, 1993.

2. Biswas MK: Bacterial vaginosis. Clin Obstet Gynecol 36:166–175, 1993.
3. Peter G (ed): 1997 Red Book: Report of the Committee on Infectious Diseases, 24th ed. Elk Grove Village, IL, American Academy of Pediatrics, 1997.
4. Yealy DM, Greene TJ, Hobbs GD: Underrecognition of cervical Neisseria gonorrhoeae and *Chlamydia trachomatis* infections in the emergency department. Acad Emerg Med 4:962–967, 1997.
5. Amsel R, Totten PA, Speigel CA, et al: Nonspecific vaginitis. Am J Med 74:14–22, 1983.
6. Jephcott AE: Microbiological diagnosis of gonorrhoea. Genitourin Med 73:245–52, 1997.
7. Schachter J: DFA, EIA, PCR, LCR and other technologies: What tests should be used for diagnosis of *Chlamydia* infections? Immunol Invest 26:157–161, 1997.
8. Centers for Disease Control and Prevention: 1998 Guidelines for treatment of sexually transmitted diseases. MMWR 47(no. RR-1), 1998.
9. Fleming DT, McQuillan GM, Johnson RE, et al: Herpes simplex virus type 2 in the United States, 1976–1994. N Engl J Med 337:1105–1111, 1997.
10. Elgart ML: Sexually Transmitted diseases of the vulva. Dermatol Clin 10:387–403, 1992.
11. Von Krogh G, Gross G: Anogenital warts. Clin Dermatol 15:355–368, 1997.
12. Gross G, Von Krogh G: Therapy of anogenital HPV-induced lesions. Clin Dermatol 15:547–570, 1997.
13. Hill DA, Lense JJ: Office management of Bartholin gland cysts and abscesses. Am Fam Phys 57:1611–1616, 1998.
14. Rolfs RT, Galaaid EI, Zaidi AA: Pelvic inflammatory disease: Trends in hospitalization and office visits, 1997 through 1988. Am J Obstet Gynecol 166(3):983–990, 1992.
15. Tepper R, Zalel Y, Goldberger S, et al: Diagnostic value of transvaginal color Doppler flow in ovarian torsion. Eur J Obstet Gynecol Reproduct Biol 68:115–118, 1996.
16. Kettel LM, Hummel WP: Endometriosis. Obstet Gynecol Clin 24:361–373, 1997.
17. Brenner PF: Differential diagnosis of abnormal uterine bleeding. Am J Obstet Gynecol 175:766–769, 1996.
18. Chuong CJ, Brenner PF: Management of abnormal uterine bleeding. Am J Obstet Gynecol 175:787–792, 1996.
19. Sobel JD, et al: Single dose fluconazole compared with conventional clotrimazole topical therapy of *Candida* vaginitis. Am J Obstet Gynecol 172:1263–1268, 1995.
20. Thorpe EM, et al: Chlamydial cervicitis and urethritis: Single dose treatment compared with doxycycline for seven days in community based practices. Genitourin Med 72:93–97, 1996.

Chapter 16

Management of Pregnant Patients in Urgent Care

Carrie Tibbles, MD
Steve Sterner, MD

This chapter reviews the common medical problems that may present during pregnancy to an urgent care (UC) facility. Certain basic principles are important to keep in mind when caring for pregnant women.

1. Suspect pregnancy in all women of reproductive age, regardless of the chief complaint. Many women present to UC early in the pregnancy and do not know that they are pregnant. The practitioner must have a high degree of suspicion for pregnancy in such patients. Pregnancy may be related to the chief complaint, such as morning nausea or, in the worst case, abdominal pain from an ectopic pregnancy. The final diagnosis may be unrelated to the pregnancy, but prescription medications or radiologic studies may have potential adverse effects on a developing fetus. A careful menstrual history and routine use of pregnancy tests should avoid these types of errors.

2. Pregnant patients present with two types of medical problems: those related to the pregnancy and those that are independent of pregnancy. Most medical problems are treated alike in pregnant and nonpregnant patients. However, pregnancy can have a significant influence on both the diagnosis and treatment of medical problems. Pregnancy also places a woman at higher risk for certain conditions, such as pyelonephritis or deep vein thrombosis. Do not automatically attribute a symptom such as abdominal pain or nausea to the pregnancy without first considering other possible causes.

3. Clarify the patient's delivery date as much as possible. The specific trimester of a pregnancy, to a large extent, predicts the type of problems that occur. In the initial trimesters, nausea, abdominal pain, and vaginal bleeding are common. A large variety of obstetrical problems are seen in the third trimester.

Problems of the First Trimester

Ectopic Pregnancy

Differential Diagnosis. Ectopic pregnancy, defined as any pregnancy occurring outside the uterine cavity, complicates 16 in every 1000 pregnancies. Although the incidence of ectopic pregnancy has been steadily rising, the associated morbidity and mortality rates have steadily declined secondary to improved detection and treatment. However, it is estimated that 50% of all ectopic pregnancies are still missed at the first encounter with a physician. In most cases, the cause of the ectopic pregnancy is mechanical interference with the migration of the ovum to the uterus because of disease or scarring in the fallopian tube. Risk factors for ectopic pregnancy include prior pelvic inflammatory disease, tubal ligation or surgeries, and in vitro fertilization. Some ectopic pregnancies abort or resorb spontaneously with no treatment. In other ectopic pregnancies, the gestational sac ruptures resulting in bleeding into the peritoneal cavity. Consequently, the clinical presentation of an ectopic pregnancy varies from asymptomatic to hypovolemic shock. Most ectopic pregnancies present before 8 weeks' gestation.

History and Physical Examination. Abdominal pain is the most common presenting complaint, followed closely by amennorhea. The pain is typically sharp, stabbing, and unilateral, but presentation varies. Abnormal vaginal bleeding occurs in up to 80% of cases. A large amount of vaginal bleeding is more suggestive of a complicated interuterine pregnancy. Approximately 20% of patients have a low-grade fever. Physical exam findings are notoriously inaccurate in the diagnosis of ectopic pregnancy. Abdominal or adnexal tenderness is common. An adnexal mass may be palpated. The uterus is normal in size in 70% of patients. Hypotension and peritoneal signs may be present if a rupture has occurred. The differential diagnosis of ectopic pregnancy is presented in Table 1.[2]

Table 1. Differential Diagnosis of Ectopic Pregnancy

Normal intrauterine pregnancy	Threatened or complete abortion
Salpingitis	Ovarian torsion
Appendicitis	Ovarian cyst rupture
Gastroenteritis	Endometriosis

Adapted from Marcet V: Ectopic pregnancy. In Pearlman M, Tintinalli J (eds): Emergency Care of the Woman. New York, McGraw-Hill, 1998, pp 21–28.

Diagnostic Aids. Urine beta human chorionic gonadotropin (β-HCG) immunoassays are sensitive to 20–50 mIU/ml and are used to initially make the diagnosis of pregnancy. Few, if any, ectopic pregnancies are missed using this screening tool. If the urine pregnancy test is positive, a quantitative serum β-HCG level should be ordered; it is used in conjunction with ultrasonography to make the diagnosis of ectopic pregnancy. At a serum level of 1000–1500 mIU/ml, an intrauterine fetus should be visible by transvaginal ultrasound; the discriminatory level is institutionally variable. A fetus is visible at 6000 mIU/ml if transabdominal ultrasonography is used. An ectopic pregnancy is very likely when no intrauterine pregnancy (IUP) is seen and the serum β-HCG is higher than these cutoff values. β-HCG levels predictably double every two days in a normal intrauterine pregnancy. Serial measurement of HCG levels can be used in the stable patient, if the measured HCG level is below the cutoff values and no IUP is seen on ultrasonography.

Management. Once the diagnosis of ectopic pregnancy is made, treatment should begin immediately. Laparoscopy may be performed for confirmation of the diagnosis, and many ectopic pregnancies can be excised through the laparoscope. Surgical management has traditionally been the standard of care, but many patients are now treated medically with methotrexate. This decision rests with the obstetrical consultant and should not be made by the urgent care practitioner.

Pitfalls in Practice. Consider the possibility of ectopic pregnancy in all women of reproductive age with abdominal pain or vaginal bleeding. Remember that physical exam findings are unreliable in the diagnosis of ectopic pregnancy.

Spontaneous Abortion

Differential Diagnosis. Spontaneous abortion is loss of pregnancy before 20 weeks or loss of a fetus weighing < 500 grams (World Health Organization). To evaluate accurately uterine bleeding in early pregnancy, it is helpful to review the following definitions.[3]

Threatened abortion: uterine bleeding in the first 20 weeks without passage of tissue or cervical dilation.

Inevitable abortion: gestation < 20 weeks, with bleeding and cervical dilation but no passage of fetal tissue.

Complete abortion: passage of all fetal tissue before 20 weeks of gestation, accompanied by closure of the cervix.

Incomplete abortion: passage of only part of the products of conception.

Missed abortion: fetal death at < 20 weeks without passage of any fetal tissue.

Septic abortion: any stage of abortion accompanied by intrauterine infection.[2]

History and Physical Examination. The rate and amount of bleeding should be determined. Vital signs and orthostatic changes should be carefully evaluated. Abdominal examination should reveal little or no tenderness.

Pelvic examination typically reveals blood in the vagina; clots also may be present. Clots usually indicate more rapid bleeding because blood remaining in the uterus for a long period is defibrinated. The uterus is usually somewhat increased in size. If a complete abortion has already occurred and if all the products of conception have been expelled, the uterus is normal or slightly increased in size. If some or all of the products of conception remain in the uterus, it is enlarged up to 12- to 14-weeks' size. The cervix should be examined. Usually the bleeding comes from the cervical os, but occasionally a lesion on the cervix may bleed. Such bleeding can be controlled with local cautery. If the cervix seems to be closed on fingertip examination, it should be considered to be closed. Instruments must not be forced through the cervical os. If the cervix is dilated, tissue also may be seen protruding from the os. Because abortion is inevitable at this stage, it is best to grasp the tissue with a ring forceps and extract it gently. Tissue that is extracted or spontaneously expelled should be examined to determine whether it represents a complete gestational sac with placenta and fetal pole.

Diagnostic Aids. Measurement of hemoglobin level may be helpful in patients with significant bleeding over a period of time. Measurements of serum HCG levels over a period of days help to determine whether the HCG level is increasing (as it should with a viable fetus) or decreasing (as it does if the fetus is dead). The serum HCG level falls with a half-life of 0.63 day for the first 2 days and of 3.85 days thereafter. The urine pregnancy test almost always is negative within 2 weeks after abortion. Ultrasonography has now become standard for evaluation of threatened abortion. The following are basic guidelines:

1. At a HCG level > 6000, a gestational sac should be visualized on abdominal ultrasound. At HCG > 1500, a gestational sac should be visible on transvaginal ultrasound.

2. A yolk sac is usually seen at 36 days, with cardiac activity noted at 41–47 days from the LMP.

3. At 8 weeks, the gestational sac (generally 25 mm) and embryo (14 mm) should be seen.

Management. In threatened abortions, no evidence suggests that reduction in activity or medical treatment can affect pregnancy outcome. Patients should be given instructions to return if bleeding increases or if they pass tissue. Sensitivity to the patient's feelings are important aspects of management, and she should be reassured that the problem is not her fault. An incomplete abortion is best managed by evacuating the uterus with vacuum curettage. This technique allows the uterus to contract without impediment from intrauterine tissue, thereby improving hemostasis. Vacuum curettage is easily done on an outpatient basis with intravenous analgesia, but the support services of a hospital must be available. The patient is observed for 2–3 hours in case of continued bleeding; if bleeding has lessened or stopped, she may then be discharged home and treated with ergonovine (0.2 mg orally 3 times daily for 2 days). The management of complete abortion is somewhat controversial, because it is sometimes difficult to determine whether the abortion was actually complete. If the tissue passed appears to be an intact gestational sac with complete placenta and fetal pole and if bleeding is minimal, the diagnosis of complete abortion can be made provisionally. If an incomplete abortion is suspected, especially if bleeding is heavy, vacuum curettage is an option. Any patient with complete or incomplete abortion who is Rh-negative should be treated with Rh immunoglobulin.

Pitfalls in Practice. A woman presenting at 8–10 weeks' gestation with vaginal bleeding and abdominal pain may be assumed to have a threatened abortion because of the time of gestation, but an ectopic fetus may be implanted at or near the end of the fallopian tube, where it can grow longer than other ectopic pregnancies before the patient becomes symptomatic.

Abdominal Pain in Early Pregnancy

Differential Diagnosis and Physical Examination. The diagnosis and management of a pregnant patient with abdominal pain often are challenging for the health care provider. Abdominal pain is quite common in early pregnancy and frequently self-limited; however, a large number of potentially serious causes, both gynecologic and nongynecologic must be considered[3] (Table 2).

Table 2. Differential Diagnosis of Acute Abdomen In Early Pregnancy

Corpus luteal cyst	Adnexal torsion/masses
Ectopic/spontaneous abortion	Degenerating leiomyomata
Pelvic inflammatory disease/tubo-ovarian abscess	Gastroesophageal reflux disease/reflux
Pyelonephritis	Cholecystitis
Appendicitis	Bowel obstruction

During early pregnancy, a physiologic corpus luteal cyst develops and secretes hormones necessary to maintain the pregnancy. Sometimes this cyst fills with fluid that may leak or suddenly rupture into the peritoneal cavity. Pelvic ultrasound may assist in the diagnosis. A uterine leiomyoma may increase in size secondary to hormonal stimulation during pregnancy, or it may undergo hemorrhagic infarction, resulting in pain, fever, and possibly uterine contractions. Ultrasound and a known history of a myoma are useful for this diagnosis. Treatment consists of analgesics; surgical intervention is rarely required. Obstetric consultation is recommended. The nongynecologic causes of abdominal pain, such as appendicitis and cholecystitis, are discussed in a later section; the diagnosis of these conditions is more challenging in later pregnancy. In general, these conditions are treated the same as in nonpregnant patients, and significant morbidity is associated with delay in diagnosis and treatment.

Management. The specific treatment depends on the diagnosis. If the patient has abdominal pain that does not appear to represent a serious process, identifying a definitive cause may be impossible. The physician, however, must ensure that the patient is followed closely, usually within 24 hours, and that the patient is improving.

Nausea and Vomiting in Pregnancy

Differential Diagnosis. Nausea and vomiting, particularly in the morning, are extremely common in pregnancy, affecting 50–90% of all pregnant women.[4] In most women, symptoms are limited to the first trimester, but they can persist throughout pregnancy. **Hyperemesis gravidarum** is a prolonged course of nausea and vomiting associated with weight loss, dehydration, ketone formation, and electrolyte disturbances.[4] The cause of nausea and vomiting in pregnancy is still unknown.

History and Physical Examination. The history should include duration and type of symptoms, and ability to tolerate any liquids or food. It is also important to investigate other causes of nausea and vomiting unrelated to pregnancy, especially in patients with abdominal pain. Assess the patient carefully for signs of dehydration.

Diagnostic Aids. Lab tests include urinalysis to assess for ketones. In severe and intractable vomiting, serum electrolyte levels may be required. In hyperemesis gravidarum, an ultrasound may be helpful to rule out multiple gestations or molar pregnancy. If the history or physical exam suggests a nonobstetric cause of the vomiting, other diagnostic tests may be ordered as needed.

Management. In straightforward cases, counseling about the nature of nausea and vomiting in pregnancy and rehydration is usually sufficient. If the patient is dehydrated or has ketonuria, IV hydration with D5 normal saline or D5 lactated Ringer's solution is recommended. Some patients require antiemetics acutely or for maintenance therapy (Table 3). In hyperemesis gravidarum, in addition to aggressive rehydration and antiemetics, the patient may require admission if weight loss is > 10%, the cause of vomiting is unclear, electrolyte disturbances are present, or the patient has severe persistent vomiting despite no oral intake.[4]

Table 3. Antiemetics for Nausea and Vomiting in Pregnancy

	PO	Rectal	IV
Acute			
Prochlorperazine (Compazine)	10 mg every 6–8 hr	25 mg every 12 hr	10 mg/2 min 40 mg/24 hr
Promethazine (Phenergan)	25 mg every 4 hr	25 mg every 4 hr	25–50mg IV push 50 mg/500 ml over 2 hours
Maintenance			
Doxylamine with pyridoxine	25 mg at bedtime 25 mg every 8 hr		
Trimethobenzamide (Tigan)	250 mg every 6–8 hr	200 mg every 6–8 hr	200 mg IM

Pitfalls in Practice. Consider other causes of nausea and vomiting before attributing symptoms to pregnancy. Caution patients who are discharged home on phenothiazines about the possibility of dystonic reactions. Patients should be instructed to return for re-evaluation if symptoms worsen or if signs of orthostatic hypovolemia appear.

Problems of the Second and Third Trimester

Spontaneous Abortion and Vaginal Bleeding

Differential Diagnosis and Physical Examination. Spontaneous abortion during the second trimester is a grave situation, because bleeding tends to be profuse. The patient with second trimester bleeding should not be considered to be aborting but should be evaluated for other causes. For example, placenta previa and placental abruption can present with bleeding in the second trimester. A pelvic examination may exacerbate bleeding and usually should not be performed before an ultrasonographic examination of the placenta.

Management. Any patient with heavy vaginal bleeding should have intravenous (IV) access before transport or further evaluation. Blood transfusion may be required. Management should be in a hospital because patients may continue to bleed significantly after vacuum curettage.

Pitfalls in Practice. Placenta previa should be considered and ruled out before a pelvic exam in second- and third-trimester bleeds. Failure to secure IV access and transport a patient with heavy bleeding to an ED can result in significant maternal morbidity and possible mortality.

Placenta Previa

Differential Diagnosis. Normally the placenta implants high on the uterine wall away from the cervical opening. In placenta previa, the placenta implants partially at a lower site or completely covers the cervical opening. The incidence of placenta previa is roughly 1/200 term births.[1] History of placenta previa, multiparity, previous cesarean section, and prior abortion with curettage increase the risk of placenta previa. Marginal separation of the placenta away from the lower uterine segment results in bleeding. Classically, the patient presents with painless, sudden vaginal bleeding, either spontaneously or provoked by intercourse, activity, or vaginal exam. Abdominal pain may be present.

Management. A pelvic exam may precipitate severe hemorrhage, and ultrasound localization of the placenta is crucial before the pelvic exam. An ultrasound earlier in the pregnancy can confirm the location of the placenta. Initial management involves assessment of the patient's hemodynamic status and volume resuscitation, as needed, with blood sent for type and cross-match. Consultation with an obstetrician is appropriate for all cases of second- or third-trimester bleeding, and hospitalization is usually required. Life-threatening hemorrhage is an indication for urgent caesarean section.

Pitfalls in Practice. Curiosity tends to compel the physician to perform a quick pelvic exam to determine the site of the bleeding. This approach should not be done. It is best to start an IV line and transport the patient to the hospital for an ultrasound and subsequent management as quickly as possible.

Placental Abruption

Differential Diagnosis. Placental abruption is defined as premature separation of the placenta from its uterine implantation site after 20 weeks' gestation. Abruption is associated with maternal hypertension and other conditions, such as diabetes and renal disease, that predispose to vascular compromise. Blunt abdominal trauma and acceleration/deceleration injuries also may result in an abruption. Multiparity, cigarettes, advanced maternal age, and cocaine use also are associated.[5] In severe abruption, the patient presents with sudden severe abdominal/back pain and fetal demise. Hemodynamic instability and coagulopathy, including disseminated intravascular coagulation are sequalae. Mild-to-moderate abruptions are more difficult to diagnose. Patients may present with pain and superimposed uterine contractions. Vaginal bleeding is common but may be absent if the abruption occurred away from the cervix (concealed abruption).

Management. Detection of abruption by ultrasound is difficult, but ultrasound is used to rule out placenta previa in pregnant patients with bleeding. Laboratory tests to detect subclinical coagulopathy include a low platelet count, prolonged prothrombin time and partial thromboplastin time, elevated D-dimer, and low serum fibrinogen. A Kleihauer-Betke test is useful to identify fetal cells in the maternal circulation. Management centers on the expedient delivery of the fetus if necessary. Begin fetal monitoring early, as fetal demise may occur quickly. Maternal volume resuscitation or blood transfusion may be required. Method and timing of delivery depend on the amount of hemodynamic instability and the status of the fetus. Immediate consult with an obstetrician and rapid transfer to an appropriate facility are warranted.

Pitfalls in Practice. A high index of suspicion for placental abruption should be maintained in pregnant patients with vaginal bleeding, because smaller abruptions have a variable and often subtle presentation. Ultrasound should not be relied on to diagnose placental abruption. IV access should be obtained as quickly as possible, because hemorrhage may be brisk.

Premature Labor

Differential Diagnosis. Any woman presenting with abdominal pain during the third trimester may be in premature labor. It may take several hours of observation or monitoring to determine if labor is commencing. Common symptoms of premature labor include menstrual-like cramps, low dull backache, pelvic pressure, increasing vaginal discharge or spotting, or frequent painful uterine contractions. Risk factors for premature labor include infection, cervical incompetence, multiple gestation, and drug use (cocaine, amphetamines). Initial evaluation includes a careful obstetrical history, including estimated date of confinement and past preterm deliveries as well as evaluation for predisposing factors, such as infection. Physical exam includes estimating fetal lie, fundal height, the presence of rupture of membranes, and assessment of the degree of cervical dilation and effacement. Placenta previa should be ruled out in any pregnant patient with vaginal bleeding before a pelvic exam. A new assay for the presence of fetal fibronectin shows promise in predicting preterm labor but may have a long turnaround time and is not available in all areas.[6]

Management. Typically the best place to monitor and observe the patient is a labor and delivery unit equipped with fetal monitoring equipment. Management of preterm labor includes bedrest, hydration, and tocolysis typically with beta-sympathometics or magnesium. Glucocorticoids are given before 34 weeks' gestation to promote fetal lung maturity.

Pitfalls in Practice. Even experienced clinicians encounter difficulty in determining whether or not labor is commencing. Only observation over time is an accurate means of making the diagnosis. In most circumstances, this should be done in a labor and delivery unit.

Premature Rupture of Membranes

Differential Diagnosis and Physical Examination. Premature rupture of membranes (PROM) is defined as rupture of the membranes more than 1 hour before the onset of labor. Before 37 weeks' gestation PROM is termed preterm premature rupture of membranes. Patients with PROM are at increased risk for fetal and maternal infection as well as cord prolapse. Patients report a watery discharge that may be sudden or a slow leak. Sterile speculum exam should be performed. Diagnosis is confirmed by visualizing the pooling of fluid in the vagina, determining its pH, and a Fern test. Amniotic fluid has pH approximately 7.4, whereas vaginal secretions are typically acidic. The fluid should be examined closely for meconium. Amniotic fluid has a fern-like appearance under the microscope after it has dried on a glass slide.

Management. Women with PROM require admission to a labor and delivery unit. If the woman is at term, delivery should be within 24 hours to decrease the risk of amnionitis. Penicillin or clindamycin (in penicillin-allergic patients) should be started empirically if rupture has been greater than 18 hours or if the patient has a fever.

Pitfalls in Practice. Women with rupture of membranes may be unable to discern the source of the fluid and complain instead of urinary incontinence or vaginal discharge. Unless a high index of suspicion is maintained, this history may mislead the clinician. In documented rupture of membranes serial digital exams should be avoided because they increase the risk of chorioamnionitis.

Preeclampsia and Pregnancy-Induced Hypertension

Differential Diagnosis. Preeclampsia is defined as increased blood pressure (> 140/90 mmHg) accompanied by proteinuria (> 300mg/24 hrs) and edema, usually occurring in the last 20 weeks of gestation.[7] Chronic hypertension, renal disease, nulliparity, advanced maternal age, and African-American race are among the risk factors predisposing to preeclampsia. In **severe preeclampsia** the blood pressure is often markedly elevated (160–180/> 110 mmHg), and the patient also may complain of severe headache, visual disturbances, marked edema, and epigastric or right upper quadrant pain. The physical exam may be remarkable for hyperreflexia and clonus, and generalized edema, particularly of the hands and face. A particularly severe variant of preeclampsia is known as HELLP syndrome, which is characterized by **h**emolysis, **e**levated **l**iver enzymes and **l**ow **p**latelets. Recognition and prompt treatment of preeclampsia are important to prevent the development of eclampsia or seizures.

Management. The laboratory evaluation for preeclampsia includes complete blood count (CBC) with smear, liver function tests, blood urea nitrogen, creatinine, urinalysis, and 24-urine collection for protein; creatinine clearance also should be started. Most women should be admitted for initial evaluation and treatment. Timing of delivery depends on the severity of the symptoms and the gestational age of the fetus. Severe hypertension (i.e., diastolic pressure > 110 mmHg) should be treated pharmacologically. Methyldopa, hydralazine, and labetolol have been used as first-line agents.[8] In severe preeclampsia, seizure prophylaxis with magnesium sulfate, 6 gm IV over 15 minutes followed by 2 gm/hr maintenance drip, should be started. A target therapeutic level of 4–7 mg/dl is desirable, and the patient should be monitored for magnesium toxicity, manifested by loss of deep tendon reflexes and respiratory depression.

Pitfalls in Practice. Routine vital signs and urinalysis in pregnant women are key to early diagnosis of preeclampsia. Preeclampsia should be considered in all hypertensive pregnant women, regardless of the presenting medical complaint.

Abdominal Pain in Advanced Pregnancy

Differential Diagnosis. The differential diagnosis of abdominal pain in later trimesters is listed in Table 4.[3]

Table 4. Differential Diagnosis of Abdominal Pain in Late Pregnancy

Labor	Placental abruption
Severe preeclampsia	Uterine rupture/dehiscence
Acute fatty liver	Appendicitis
Cholecystitis	Peptic ulcer disease/gastroesophageal reflux disease
Acute pancreatitis	Bowel obstruction

The most common cause of abdominal pain in late pregnancy is the onset of labor. Characterized by intermittent contractions of the uterus and dilation and effacement of the cervix, onset of labor is generally straightforward to diagnosis. However, uterine irritability can be associated with other causes of abdominal pain, such as pyelonephritis or appendicitis.[3] A digital vaginal exam should be done to assess for dilation and effacement, however, it should be avoided if the patient complains of vaginal bleeding (possible placenta previa), or preterm leakage of amniotic fluid. Other conditions of abdominal pain already have been discussed. Acute fatty liver of pregnancy is a rare complication, occurring in 1/10,000 pregnancies, usually in the third trimester.[3] Clinical findings include epigastric pain, malaise, nausea, vomiting, jaundice, proteinuria, hypertension, and edema. Hypoglycemia is used to distinguish this entity from severe preeclampsia. Diagnosis requires a complete history, physical exam, and laboratory profile. It is associated with a high mortality rate. Consultation with an obstetrician and possibly with a GI specialist is recommended.

Appendicitis. Appendicitis occurs at the same rate in pregnant as in nonpregnant patients. Incidence is evenly divided among trimesters.[3] Physiologic and anatomic changes of pregnancy make the diagnosis challenging. The classic physical findings of localized tenderness with peritoneal inflammation may not be present until late in the course of the disease, because the expanding uterus tends to push the appendix upward and posteriorly away from the parietal peritoneum (Fig. 1). In pregnancy, appendicitis may be associated with right upper quadrant pain. Leukocytosis can be helpful in making the diagnosis. Bryant's sign (pain that does not move to the left when the patient is turned to

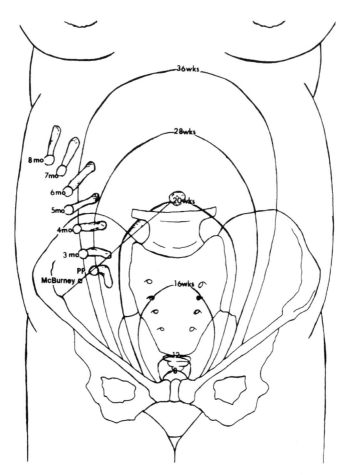

Figure 1.   Changes in location and direction of appendix during pregnancy in relationship to McBurney's point and height of fundus at various weeks of gestation. (From Ratcliffe SD, Baxley EG, Byrd JE, Sakornbut EL: Family Practice Obstetrics, 2nd ed. Philadelphia, Hanley and Belfus, 2001, with permission.)

the left decubitus position) may be associated with acute appendicitis.[3] Surgical appendectomy is the accepted treatment; both the surgery and anesthesia are generally well tolerated by the mother and fetus.

Gallbladder Disease.   Gallstones are common in pregnant women, and asymptomatic women generally do not require therapy. However, acute cholecystitis requires prompt recognition and treatment. Presentation is similar to that in nonpregnant women, and ultrasonography is the diagnostic modality of choice. Medical management consists of IV hydration, analgesia, and cessation of oral intake. Surgery is considered for women who do not respond to initial conservative therapy or if complications are suspected.

Pitfalls in Practice.   White blood cell count is normally elevated in pregnancy but should not be dismissed in the evaluation of abdominal pain. Labor may present atypically and should be considered in all patients in the third trimester who present with abdominal pain. Significant morbidity and mortality are associated with delay in the treatment of appendicitis in pregnancy.

Urinary Tract Infection and Pyelonephritis

Differential Diagnosis and Physical Examination. Urinary tract infections are common bacterial infections in pregnancy. Pregnant women are at more risk of developing upper urinary tract infections because pregnancy results in urinary tract dilation as well as increased urine stasis. *E. coli* is the most common pathogen. Asymptomatic bacteriuria may be detected on routine culture. Cystitis typically presents with dysuria, frequent urination, and urgency. The patient may or may not have a fever, and physical exam is typically remarkable for suprapubic tenderness. Pyelonephritis presents with fever and chills, flank or low back pain, and abdominal pain. Anorexia, nausea, or vomiting are also associated. Costovertebral angle tenderness is frequently elicited on physical exam.

Management. Urinalysis and urine culture should be obtained. Blood culture may be obtained in suspected urosepsis. Asymptomatic bacteriuria and cystitis are treated as outpatients using a wide variety of antibiotic regimens. Most pregnant women with acute pyelonephritis require admission and treatment with hydration and IV antibiotics. Ampicillin, a cephalosporin, or an extended-spectrum penicillin are appropriate empiric antibiotics.

Pitfalls in Practice. Asymptomatic bacteriuria should be treated in pregnancy because one-fourth of patients develop a symptomatic infection. In a woman not responding to typical antibiotic regimens, urinary tract obstruction or resistant organisms should be suspected.

Pulmonary Embolism and Deep Vein Thrombosis

Differential Diagnosis. Venous thromboembolism is five times more likely to occur in a pregnant woman than in nonpregnant women of the same age and complicates 1 in every 1000–2000 pregnancies.[9] Pregnancy, in addition to being a hypercoagulable state, also is associated with increased venous capacitance resulting in venous stasis. An enlarging uterus often compresses pelvic vessels, increasing venous stasis in the lower extremities. Signs and symptoms accompanying deep vein thrombosis are variable but include leg pain, tenderness, and swelling. Although less common, a palpable cord, engorged superficial veins, redness, or edema may be present. Homan's sign (pain in calf on dorsiflexion of the foot) is present in fewer than one-third of patients with deep vein thrombosis.[9] The diagnosis of pulmonary embolism (PE) is a continued challenge. Given the previously mentioned risk factors, the possibility of a pulmonary embolism should be considered in a pregnant woman with acute dyspnea and/or chest pain. Cough or hemoptysis also may be present. Elevated respiratory rate, tachycardia, and pulmonary rales or crackles are common physical exam findings.

Diagnostic Aids. Electrocardiogram, chest x-ray, and arterial blood gases may support the diagnosis of pulmonary embolism. As in nonpregnant patients, a ventilation/perfusion scan, followed by a pulmonary angiogram if needed, is used to make the diagnosis of pulmonary embolism. Spiral CT is used with increasing frequency to diagnose pulmonary embolism. Compression ultrasonography, impedance plethysmography, or duplex Doppler scanning are the initial screening tests for deep vein thrombosis (DVT). Venography or serial noninvasive tests (day 2 and day 7) should be used if initial test is negative, but the clinical suspicion of DVT is high.

Management. Pregnant patients with documented DVT or suspicion for PE should be hospitalized for anticoagulation and supportive care. Hypoxia must be aggressively treated. Heparin is considered the safest anticoagulant in pregnancy because it does not cross the placenta.[9] After documented venous thromboembolism, the patient requires chronic anticoagulation for the remainder of the pregnancy. Typically subcutaneous heparin is used, because warfarin is associated with adverse effects on fetal development and readily crosses the placenta.

Pitfalls in Practice. Early diagnosis and treatment of PE and DVT improve patient outcome, and a high index of suspicion is warranted in pregnant women.

Problems of the Postpartum Period

Acute Endometritis

Differential Diagnosis. Abdominal pain during the postpartum period should be evaluated as usual, with the exception that endometritis should be prominent in the differential diagnosis. After delivery of the infant, the uterine cavity fills with blood as the endometrial lining is sloughed, making it susceptible to bacterial infection. Most cases of endometritis are polymicrobial (anaerobes and aerobes), and arise from ascending infection from organisms in the normal indigenous vaginal flora. Established risk factors include operative delivery, prolonged ruptured membranes, prolonged labor, and repeated vaginal exams in labor. Of note, enterococcus is commonly isolated from patients who receive cephalosporin prophylaxis in labor.[10]

History and Physical Examination. The hallmarks are lower abdominal pain and fever, which may be rapid or develop slowly; foul-smelling, purulent vaginal discharge may be present. Uterine tenderness may involve the fundus or only the lower uterine segment.

Diagnostic Aids. A cervical culture for gonnorrhea and chlamydial infection is recommended. The white blood cell count is typically elevated. Urinalysis should be obtained because urinary tract infection is in the differential diagnosis. Endometrial cultures are generally not clinically useful, but blood cultures and endometrial cultures may be helpful in a patient not responding to conventional therapy.

Management. The large majority of patients should be admitted for broad-spectrum intravenous antibiotics. Compliant patients who are not toxic may be given a trial of outpatient antibiotics if they are followed carefully. See Table 5 for commonly used regimens.[11]

Table 5. Antibiotics Frequently Used in Endometritis

Cefoxitin	1–2 g IV every 6 hr
Cefotetan	1–2 g IV every 12 hr
Ampicillin-sulbactam	1.5–3 g IV every 6 hr
Piperacillin-tazobactam	3.375 g IV every 6 hr
Ticarcillin-clavulanic acid	3.1 g IV every 6 hr
Clindamycin and gentamicin	Clindamycin, 900 mg IV every 8 hr Gentamicin, 2.0 mg/kg bolus followed by 1.5–1.7 mg/kg every 8 hr

Adapted from Maccato M: Postpartum infections. In Pearlman M, Tintinalli J (eds): Emergency Care of the Woman. New York, McGraw-Hill, 1998, pp 149–154.

Pitfalls in Practice. Women treated as outpatients require close follow-up to ensure that they are improving. If not, they should be hospitalized for treatment with broad-spectrum intravenous antibiotics.

Acute Mastitis

Differential Diagnosis. Acute mastitis presents as a swollen, tender breast in the post-partum period. Acute mastitis complicates breast feeding in 1–10% of postpartum women.[10] Some cases are infectious, with staphylococcal organisms predominating. Other cases do not seem to be infectious but instead are attributed to milk congestion.

History and Physical Examination. The history is one of breast tenderness and swelling over a period of hours to days. The patient may have a fever. On examination, the breast is swollen and tender and is often warm and erythematous. Abscesses occur, and areas of fluctuance should be sought. The presence of an abscess can be confirmed by needle aspiration or ultrasound, if desired, before drainage.

Management. Unless the exam reveals a benign condition, mastitis should be attrib-uted to infection with staphylococcal organisms. A penicillinase-resistant penicillin, such as dicloxacillin or a first-generation cephalosporin, should be used for 7–10 days. Frequent breast emptying, either by nursing or pumping, also has been shown to be helpful. Many women cease breast feeding on the side of the infection, although it is not mandatory to do so. If breast feeding is discontinued, the breast should be mechanically emptied on the affected side, while the infant continues to nurse on the other side, until the infection resolves. If an abscess is present, it should be drained. Patients require close follow-up.

Pitfalls in Practice. Patients should be examined closely for abscess formation, partic-ularly if the infection does not appear to respond to antibiotics. If an abscess is present, antibiotic therapy will be of limited success; definitive management is drainage of the abscess.

Postpartum Vaginal Bleeding

Differential Diagnosis. Most significant postpartum bleeding occurs in the immediate postpartum period. Normally, women pass small amounts of brownish blood with an oc-casional spotting of red for several weeks after delivery. Occasionally, a woman begins to bleed heavily some time after delivery. Delayed hemorrhage is believed to result from either subinvolution of the uterus or retained placental fragments. A clotting disor-der also should be considered.

History and Physical Examination. The rate and amount of bleeding should be de-termined. Pulse and blood pressure with orthostatic positioning should be evaluated for any sign of hypovolemia. During a pelvic examination, the rate of bleeding can be esti-mated. Oozing from the cervical os indicates brisk bleeding. The uterus should be pal-pated. In uterine atony, the uterus is enlarged, and the fundus feels boggy.

Diagnostic Aid. Low hemoglobin indicates significant chronic blood loss, but a normal level does not exclude significant acute blood loss. Clotting studies are usually normal but may reveal a coagulopathy. Ultrasound has been suggested as a method for visualizing the presence of retained placental tissue, but sensitivity and specificity are currently undefined.

Management. An IV line should be placed as soon as it is determined that significant bleeding is occurring. The patient requires uterine currettage if heavy bleeding occurs because she is at risk for hypovolemia or anemia. The procedure usually should be done in a hospital, but it may be done on an outpatient basis, depending on the severity of the bleeding and the response to treatment.

Pitfalls in Practice. A large-bore IV (16-gauge or larger) should be started, because patients can be very hypovolemic and progress to profound shock. Most patients will require hospitalization. If significant bleeding cannot be controlled with curettage, emergency surgery may be indicated.

Trauma During Pregnancy

Differential Diagnosis. Trauma during pregnancy severe enough to harm the fetus is usually not managed in an urgent care facility. However, serious fetal injury and placental abruption after minor injuries have been reported. Such circumstances include minor falls and motor vehicle accidents in which the mother received no significant injuries.

History and Physical Examination. Any history or sign of vaginal bleeding or abdominal pain after blunt trauma is worrisome. Fetal heart rate should be assessed (normal range: 120–160 beats/min). Injuries to pregnant and nonpregnant patients generally should be evaluated in the same manner.

Diagnostic Aids. Radiographic studies with appropriate shielding of the fetus should be performed as needed. Studies should be done for clear medical indications only. Ultrasonography of the fetus and placenta may be helpful. Fetal monitoring for a period of time is indicated if there is concern that significant abdominal trauma has occurred. The first indication of injury is often reflected by fetal distress on continuous monitoring.

Management. Any pregnant patient with vaginal bleeding or abdominal pain after blunt trauma should be hospitalized for fetal monitoring. Hospitalization may be advised even in the absence of these indications if significant trauma, such as a motor vehicle accident, has occurred. If trauma occurs in the first trimester, unfortunately nothing can be done to alter fetal outcome. Management of other injuries to the mother should not be affected by pregnancy.

Pitfalls in Practice. Fetal injury and placental abruption have been reported after minor trauma. If any doubt exists about the seriousness of abdominal trauma, the patient should be hospitalized for fetal monitoring. A large number of pregnant women experience domestic violence, sometimes beginning or escalating in pregnancy. Any nonvehicular trauma in pregnancy requires careful screening for domestic violence. Suspicious injuries include bruises to head and neck, or breasts and abdomen, or bruises in various stages of healing. Suspicion also should be heightened if the severity and pattern of the injury is inconsistent with the patient's explanation of how the injury occurred. In addition to treatment of the acute injuries, the health care provider should be familiar with the resources in his facility and community to aid victims of domestic violence (i.e., advocates, shelters). The national Domestic Violence Hotline is 1-800-799-SAFE.

Emergency Childbirth

Differential Diagnosis. The urgent care center is not the ideal environment for delivering babies; nevertheless, women in active labor occasionally present and must receive care. In the free-standing urgent care facility, the patient must be assessed and treatment individualized depending on the time and distance to the nearest hospital. If delivery is imminent or if transport time will be long, it may be best to deliver the infant before transport.

Any pregnant woman presenting with active labor or abdominal pains needs a quick examination to estimate the time until delivery. If the infant's head is not crowning, a quick digital pelvic exam should be done to determine the degree of cervical dilation. Vital signs should be assessed, including fetal heart rate.

Management. If the infant's head is crowning, delivery probably will occur in the next few minutes, allowing no time for transport. If the cervix is completely dilated, delivery also will be soon, unless the head is high in the pelvis. A multiparous woman also may deliver quickly, even if the cervix is not yet completely dilated. If there is time, transport should be initiated immediately, and a medical professional experienced in vaginal delivery should accompany the patient. If delivery in the urgent care center is elected, a few basic principles are helpful.

Vertex Presentation

1. Have a delivery pack available (sterile gloves, sterile towels, 10% povidone-iodine solution, suction bulb aspirator, two sterile umbilical cord clamps, sterile scissors).

2. Support the perineum with one hand while controlling delivery of the head with the other.

3. Once the head is delivered, immediately suction the nose and mouth clear before the infant starts breathing.

4. Check to make sure that the umbilical cord is not wrapped around the neck. If a nuchal cord is present, attempt to slide it over the infant's head. If it will not slide over the head, quickly place two clamps on it and cut it between them (Figure 2).

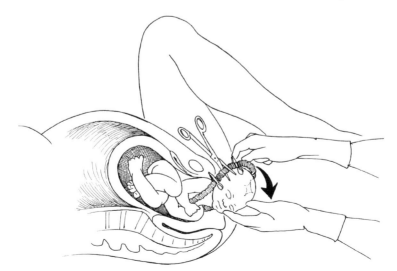

Figure 2.   Delivery of infant with nuchal cord. (From Tintinalli J, Pearlman M (eds): Emergency Care of the Woman. New York, McGraw-Hill, 1998, with permission.)

5. Downward traction on the head allows delivery of the anterior shoulder; gentle upward traction will then allow delivery of the rest of the infant.

6. Support the infant with the head down, and suction the mouth and nose one more time.

7. Dry the infant and keep it warm.

8. If the infant does not begin to breathe, a few mouth-to-mouth ventilations are usually adequate for resuscitation. If unsuccessful, begin cardiopulmonary resuscitation according to ACLS guidelines.

9. Gently massage the mother's uterus to stimulate contractions.

10. If the placenta does not deliver within 15 minutes, begin transport to the hospital.

Breech Delivery

1. If the buttocks or both feet present initially, it is probably best to attempt delivery before transport. If delivery is not progressing quickly, transport the patient.

2. If the buttocks present initially, the feet will usually deliver spontaneously, but the physician may assist by inserting the fingers and gently pulling the feet out.

3. Once the feet are out, the infant's body is usually delivered quickly while the head is left inside. This is potentially dangerous because the infant's oxygenation is still coming through the cord, which may be obstructed by pressure from the infant's head.

4. Deliver the head as quickly as possible by sliding the middle finger of one hand into the infant's mouth and pulling gently down to slide the head under the mother's pubis (Figure 3).

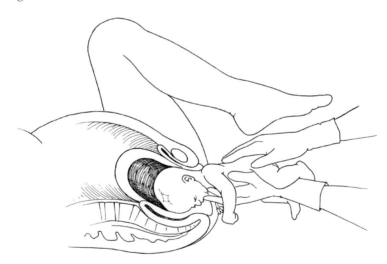

Figure 3. Delivery of the head in a breech presentation. (From Tintinalli J, Pearlman M (eds): Emergency Care of the Woman. New York, McGraw-Hill, 1998, with permission.)

5. If the head cannot be delivered, the mother must be immediately transported to a delivery room, where forceps can assist. Meanwhile, attempt to hold the vaginal wall away from the infant's nose and mouth so that it can breathe.

6. Once the infant is delivered, proceed as for a normal delivery.

Pitfalls in Practice. An unusual complication of vaginal deliveries is prolapse of the umbilical cord before delivery of the infant. This is usually associated with abnormal presentations (breech) and lack of engagement of the presenting part. The infant's oxygenation may be cut off by pressure on the cord. The treatment is rapid delivery, usually by caesarean section. To decompress the cord, the patient is placed in the knee-chest position to allow gravity to assist in decompressing the cord. The physician then gently pushes up on the presenting part with the fingers of one hand to decompress the cord further (Figure 4). Do not attempt to replace the cord into the cervix; it cannot be done. Shoulder dystocia is the inability to deliver the shoulders of the infant after the head is delivered. This complication is more common in infants of diabetic mothers. Suprapubic pressure and the McRobert's manuever may assist in the delivery of the anterior shoulder. A delivery may be complicated by uterine atony and postpartum hemorrhage. Bimanual compression of the uterus can help control the bleeding (Figure 5). Pitocin and ergotamines are also used in postpartum hemorrhage to stimulate contraction of the uterus, which will decrease the amount of bleeding.

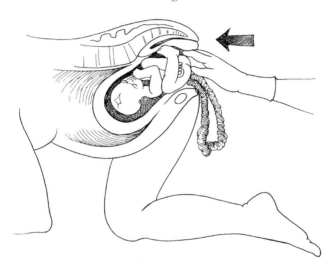

Figure 4.   Prolapse of the umbilical cord. Keep pressure off the cord. (From Tintinalli J, Pearlman M (eds): Emergency Care of the Woman. New York, McGraw-Hill, 1998, with permission.)

Drugs in Pregnancy

The fetal effects of most drugs given during pregnancy are poorly understood. Some drugs are known to be harmful to a fetus, and many drugs are believed to be generally safe. The Food and Drug Administration uses the following labeling classification system for drug use in pregnancy.

Category A: Controlled studies in women fail to demonstrate a risk to the fetus in the first trimester, and the possibility of fetal harm appears remote.

Category B: Animal data do not indicate a risk to the fetus. There are no controlled human studies, or animal studies show an adverse effect on the fetus, but well-controlled studies in pregnant women have failed to demonstrate a risk to the fetus.

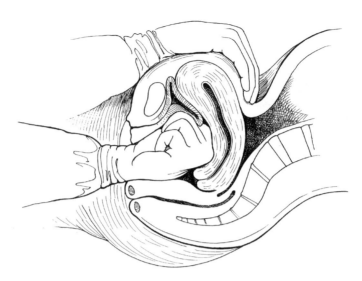

Figure 5. Bimanual compression of uterus for hemorrhage due to uterine atony. (From Tintinalli J, Pearlman M (eds): Emergency Care of the Woman. New York, McGraw-Hill, 1998, with permission.)

Category C: Studies have shown the drug to have animal teratogenic or embryocidal effects, but no controlled studies in women are available or no studies are available in either animals or women.

Category D: Positive evidence of human fetal risk exists, but benefits in certain situations (e.g., life-threatening situations or serious diseases for which safer drugs cannot be used or are ineffective) may make the use of the drug acceptable despite its risks.

Category X: Studies in animals or humans have demonstrated fetal abnormalities, or evidence demonstrates fetal risk based on human experience, or both, and the risk clearly outweighs any possible benefit.

Drugs prescribed for the pregnant patient should be given only for clear indications. The pregnant patient should also be warned of the potential effects of the medication to her infant, even (or especially) if those effects are unknown. In addition, the possibility of pregnancy should always be considered before prescribing medications to women of childbearing age. An excellent reference for current thought on the use of specific drugs in the pregnant patient is *Drugs in Pregnancy and Lactation.*[11] Table 6 lists some common medications that are contraindicated in pregnancy and their adverse effects on the fetus.

Table 6. Commonly Used Medications Contraindicated in Pregnancy

Drug	Effect
Angiotensin-converting enzyme inhibitors	Renal failure, oligohydramnios
Aminoglycosides	Ototoxicity
Androgenic steroids	Masculinize female fetus
Anticonvulsants	Dysmorphic syndrome, anomalies
Antithyroid agents	Fetal goiter

(Cont'd on next page)

Table 6. Commonly Used Medications Contraindicated in Pregnancy *(Continued)*

Drug	Effect
Aspirin	Bleeding antepartum, postpartum
Cytotoxic agents	Multiple anomalies
Isotretinoin	Hydrocephalus, deafness, anomalies
Lithium	Congenital heart disease (Epstein's)
Methotrexate	Anomalies
Nonsteroidal antiinflammatories (prolonged use after 32 weeks)	Oligohydramnios, constriction of fetal ductus arteriosus
Tetracycline (after first trimester)	Discoloration of decidous teeth; inhibits bone growth
Thalidomide	Phocomelia
Warfarin	Embryopathy

Adapted from Niebyl J: Drug use in pregnancy and lactation. In Pearlman M, Tintinalli J (eds): Emergency Care of the Woman. New York, McGraw-Hill, 1998.

References

 1. Mallett V: Ectopic pregnancy. In Pearlman M, Tintinalli J (eds): Emergency Care of the Woman. New York, McGraw-Hill, 1998, pp 21–28.
 2. Yashar C: Bleeding in the first 20 weeks of pregnancy. In Pearlman M, Tintinalli J (eds): Emergency Care of the Woman. New York, McGraw-Hill, 1998, pp 29–35.
 3. Bloom S, Gilstrap L: Abdominal pain in pregnancy. In Pearlman M, Tintinalli J (eds): Emergency Care of the Woman. New York, McGraw-Hill, 1998, pp 229–237.
 4. van de Ven CJM: Nausea and vomiting in early pregnancy. In Pearlman M, Tintinalli J (eds): Emergency Care of the Woman. New York, McGraw-Hill, 1998, pp 49–56.
 5. VanDekerhove K, Johnson T: Bleeding in the second half of pregnancy: Maternal and fetal assessment. In Pearlman M, Tintinalli J (eds): Emergency Care of the Woman. New York, McGraw-Hill, 1998, pp 77–97.
 6. Iman JD, Casal D, McGregor JA, et al: Fetal fibronectin improves the accuracy of diagnosis of preterm labor. Am J Obstet Gynecol 173:141, 1995.
 7. National High Blood Pressure Education Program Working Group: Report on high blood pressure in pregnancy. Am J Obstet Gynecol 163:1689, 1990.
 8. American College of Obstetricians and Gynecologists: Hypertension in Pregnancy. ACOG Technical Bulletin 219. Washington, DC, ACOG, 1996.
 9. Toglia M: Management of venous thromboembolism during pregnancy. In Pearlman M, Tintinalli J (eds): Emergency Care of the Woman. New York, McGraw-Hill 1998, pp 183–189.
10. Maccato M: Postpartum infections. In Pearlman M, Tintinalli J (eds): Emergency Care of the Woman. New York, McGraw-Hill, 1998, pp 149–154.
11. Briggs GG, Freeman RK, Yaffe SJ: Drugs in Pregnancy and Lactation, 4th ed. Baltimore, Williams & Wilkins, 1994.

Chapter 17

Dermatologic Disorders

Howard J. Haines, MD
Louis Ling, MD

Skin conditions prompt 10–15% of all visits to primary care physicians.[1] Rashes, although often alarming and readily apparent to the patient, are rarely life-threatening. Some skin conditions, however, can represent life-threatening disease or signs of systemic illness. The goals of the urgent care evaluation are to differentiate serious skin disease from mild skin disease, to institute appropriate therapy and comfort measures for mild skin disease, and to make appropriate and timely referral to a dermatologist, if necessary.

The temptation with skin disorders is to look only at the obvious rash and to ignore important clues in the history and physical examination that may suggest the diagnosis. Clues from the history include duration and course of the symptoms, previously affected body parts, effects of sunlight, and other modifying factors. Medication and drug use are important points as well. Many patients have already tried a topical or systemic medication, which may have modified the skin's appearance or even caused a hypersensitivity reaction. The patient's general health should be assessed, looking for underlying systemic diseases that can predispose the patient to certain skin conditions and other systemic symptoms that suggest the diagnosis. An exposure history, including occupational, recreational, and travel factors, may be helpful in diagnosis.

Physical examination includes visual inspection of the entire skin surface and palpation of affected areas and associated lymph nodes. A small, hand-held magnifying glass is useful for close inspection of skin lesions. Oral mucosa, scalp, hair, and nails should be evaluated. Other symptoms should be further assessed to determine the possibility of underlying disease.

Although the vast majority of conditions can be treated by a nondermatologist, occasionally specialty consultation is necessary. A basic understanding of descriptive terms for skin lesions facilitates accurate and precise documentation and communication with dermatologists. Key definitions are given in Table 1 and Figure 1; illustrations are provided in Figures 1 and 2.

Common Acute Rashes

Differential Diagnosis. There are many types of rashes, and most are chronic or recurrent with periodic exacerbations. A new rash of acute onset is of great concern to most patients, particularly to parents of young children. The first task of the physician is to categorize the overall appearance of the rash.

Table 1. Descriptive Terms for Skin Lesions

Term	Definition
Macule	Flat, circumscribed area of skin color change; diameter less than 1 cm.
Papule	Solid elevation of the skin; diameter less than 0.5 cm.
Plaque	Flat-topped papule larger than 0.5 cm in diameter.
Wheal	Erythematous, pruritic papule or plaque caused by acute accumulation of serum into the dermis.
Vesicle	Elevation of skin smaller than 1 cm in diameter caused by accumulation of clear fluid just under or within the epidermis.
Bulla	Fluid-filled elevation of skin larger than 0.5 cm caused by accumulation of clear fluid just under or within the epidermis.
Pustule	Pus-filled skin lesion.
Scales	Flakes of dried epidermis.
Crust	Honey-colored, dried exudate.
Ulcer	Localized, circumscribed area of destruction of the epidermis and superficial dermis.
Petechia	Nonblanching, bright red or purple skin lesion smaller than 1 cm in diameter caused by an extravasation of blood into the skin.
Purpura	Nonblanching, purple-hued skin lesion caused by extravasation of blood into the skin.

Most vesicular or bullous rashes (Table 2) are easily differentiated from nonvesicular rashes. Other causes of an acute vesicular eruption include acute contact dermatitis, trauma, sunburn, occasional drug reactions, and diabetes mellitus. Vesicles that are fragile may have broken and present to the examiner as small craters or erosions but should still be considered in the differential diagnosis of a vesicular rash. A helpful diagnostic sign for toxic epidermal necrolysis and pemphigus vulgaris is the Nikolsky sign; if light fingertip pressure is applied to the affected area, the epidermis rubs off.

Papulosquamous diseases are characterized by sharply demarcated, scaling, red lesions without crusting or erosions. This class includes the whole spectrum of psoriatic diseases as well as fungal infections and several unknown etiological disorders.

Eczematous diseases usually present with pruritus, excoriation, and lichenification or thickening of the skin. Acutely, the disease may look vesicular with oozing and weeping of clear, straw-colored fluid.

Management. Tables 2, 3, and 4 describe the management for various rashes. Most often, management is directed toward patient comfort while the rash spontaneously resolves, but some specific treatments may be appropriate to start in the urgent care setting.

Pitfalls in Practice. Although most skin diseases are not medically serious, a common pitfall in the evaluation of skin rashes is the failure to recognize and treat anaphylaxis in a patient presenting with urticaria or to diagnose a life-threatening cause of a bullous disease. Always consider secondary syphilis in the differential of a new rash. If the rash is suggestive of a systemic disease, failure to refer the patient for additional medical evaluation may delay the diagnosis. Patients with toxic epidermal necrolysis may benefit from referral to an experienced burn center.

PRIMARY LESION	DEFINITION	MORPHOLOGY	EXAMPLES
Macule	Flat, circumscribed skin discoloration that lacks surface elevation or depression		Café au lait Vitiligo Freckle Junctional nevi Ink tattoo
Papule	Elevated, solid lesion <0.5 cm in diameter		Acrochordon (skin tag) Basal cell carcinoma Molluscum contagiosum Intradermal nevi Lichen planus
Plaque	Elevated, solid "confluence of papules" (>0.5 cm in diameter) that lacks a deep component		Bowen's disease Mycosis fungoides Psoriasis Eczema Tinea corporis
Patch	Flat, circumscribed skin discoloration; a very large macule		Nevus flammeus Vitiligo
Nodule	Elevated, solid lesion >0.5 cm in diameter; a larger, deeper papule		Rheumatoid nodule Tendon xanthoma Erythema nodosum Lipoma Metastatic carcinoma
Wheal	Firm, edematous plaque that is evanescent and pruritic; a hive		Urticaria Dermographism Urticaria pigmentosa
Vesicle	Papule that contains clear fluid; a blister		Herpes simplex Herpes zoster Dyshidrotic eczema Contact dermatitis
Bulla	Localized fluid collection > 0.5 cm in diameter; a large vesicle		Pemphigus vulgaris Bullous pemphigoid Bullous impetigo

Figure 1. Primary skin lesions. (From Corvette DM: Morphology of primary and secondary skin lesions. In Fitzpatrick JE, Aeling JL (eds): Dermatology Secrets. Philadelphia, Hanley & Belfus, 1996, pp 8–14, with permission.) *(Continues on next page)*

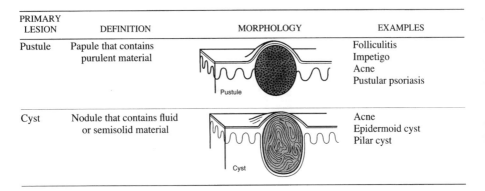

PRIMARY LESION	DEFINITION	MORPHOLOGY	EXAMPLES
Pustule	Papule that contains purulent material		Folliculitis Impetigo Acne Pustular psoriasis
Cyst	Nodule that contains fluid or semisolid material		Acne Epidermoid cyst Pilar cyst

Figure 1. Primary skin lesions (Continued).

Environmental Skin Disorders

Differential Diagnosis. The diagnosis of environmental traumatic skin disorders is easily made on the basis of historical information about exposure to the traumatic condition and characteristic clinical examination. Acute rashes caused or exacerbated by trauma or irritation are summarized in Table 5. If occupational exposure to a caustic or corrosive agent is suspected, refer to the Material Safety Data Sheet (MSDS) regarding the agent for specific identification and treatment guidelines.

Management. The management of environmental skin disorders is included in Table 5. Patients with burns that are large or involve the hands, feet, perineum, and face should be considered for referral and admission.[1] Burns and frostbite injury covering small surface areas do not require topical antibiotics. Even minor repeated trauma when the skin is already damaged causes a great deal of pain and further injury and must be avoided.

Pitfalls in Practice. Prophylactic use of systemic antibiotics is not indicated in the treatment of minor burns. Close follow-up is necessary for all second-degree or greater burns and frostbite. Tetanus prophylaxis is always indicated if the patient's immunization status is unknown or it is more than 5 years since the patient's last booster. Remove the offending agent (i.e., toxins, cold, sunlight, allergens) by appropriate washing, protective garments, and sunscreens. Failure to do so may allow continued skin damage.

Pediatric Skin Conditions:

Differential Diagnosis. Childhood viral exanthems are usually self-limited conditions but are quite concerning to parents. Rash is often preceded by febrile illness. Examination of the mouth should be included in the assessment to look for mucosal involvement (enanthems) such as erosions, Koplik spots, and vesicles.[2,3] Table 6 presents descriptions and management recommendations for many pediatric rashes. Rubella and rubeola are uncommon in developed countries but have been reported in unimmunized immigrants. Beware of toxic-appearing children with rashes: meningococcemia, Kawasaki disease, and toxic shock syndrome are life-threatening conditions associated with a rash and require immediate referral to an emergency department. Diaper rash is dermatitis of a particular anatomic

SECONDARY LESION	DEFINITION	MORPHOLOGY
Crust	A collection of cellular debris, dried serum, and blood; a scab Antecedent primary lesion is usually a vesicle, bulla, or pustule	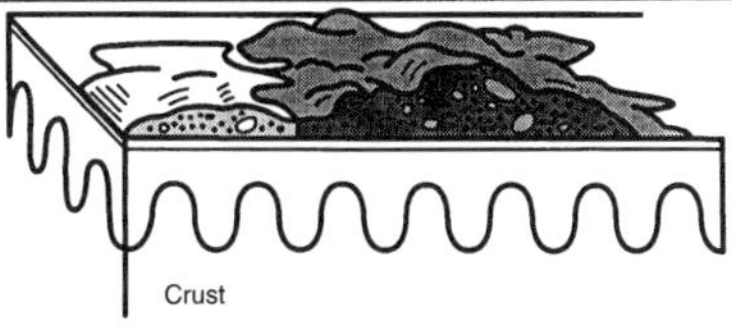
Erosion	A partial focal loss of epidermis; heals without scarring	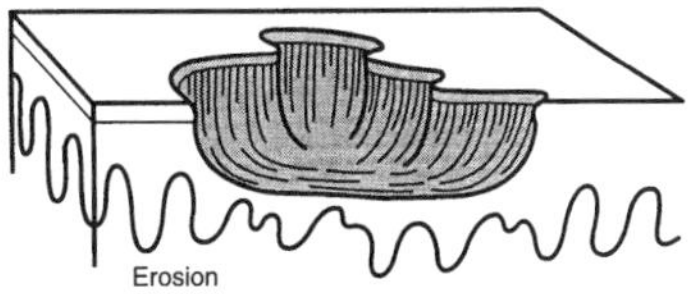
Ulcer	A full-thickness, focal loss of epidermis and dermis; heals with scarring	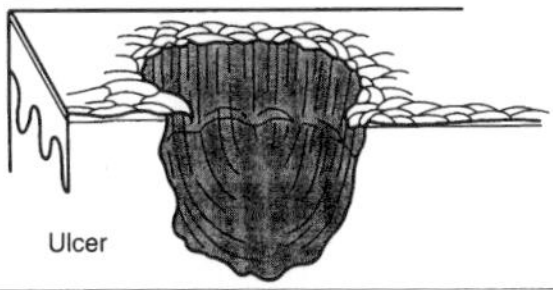
Fissure	Vertical loss of epidermis and dermis with sharply defined walls; crack in skin	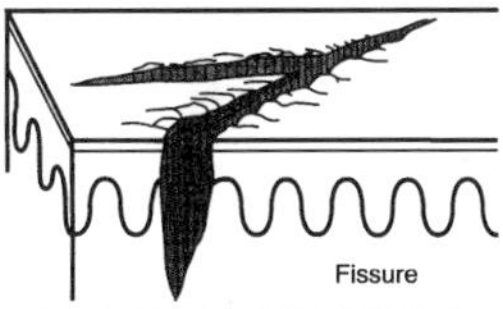
Excoriation	Linear erosion induced by scratching	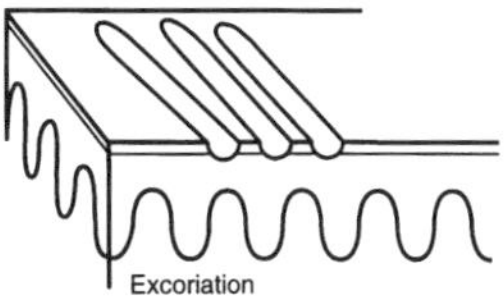
Scar	A collection of new connective tissue; may be hypertrophic or atrophic Scar implies dermoepidermal damage	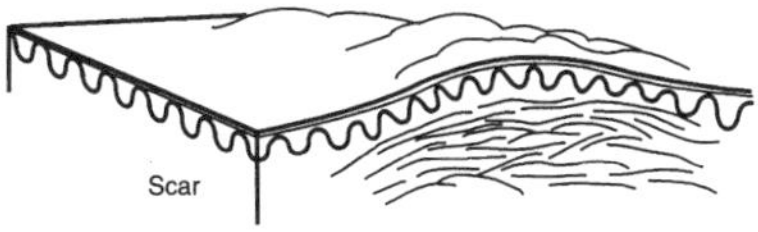
Scale	Thick stratum corneum that results from hyperproliferation or increased cohesion of keratinocytes	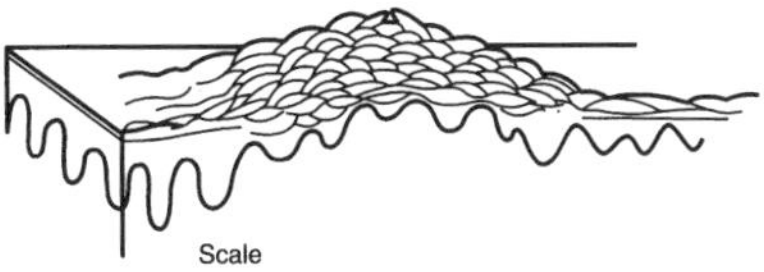

Figure 2.   Primary skin lesions. (From Corvette DM: Morphology of primary and secondary skin lesions. In Fitzpatrick JE, Aeling JL (eds): Dermatology Secrets. Philadelphia, Hanley & Belfus, 1996, pp 8–14, with permission.)

area. The diagnosis of diaper rash does not define the cause. More than one condition may be responsible for the rash at any one time. Table 7 describes various diaper rashes.

Management.   Most pediatric rashes are benign, self-limited diseases requiring only symptomatic treatment. Specific treatment and management are described in Tables 6 and 7.

Table 2. Vesicular and Bullous Diseases

Rash	Etiology	History	Exam	Management
Herpes simplex virus (HSV)	Direct contact with lesions Type 1, oral; Type 2, genital Reactivation from latent viral DNA in sensory nerve roots	Incubation: 3–14 days after exposure of broken skin Duration: 1–3 wk	Painful, burning group of vesicles on erythematous base Erosions, crusting later	Acyclovir 200 mg orally 5 times/day, antipruretics, penciclovir ointment for cold sores OB/GYN referral if pregnant
Varicella/ chicken pox	Viral infection with varicella zoster virus	Incubation period: 13–17 days One week prodrome with fever, malaise Communicable 5 days before to 5 days after vesicles	Initially maculopapular, then vesicles and crusting Occur in crops, start on trunk May get secondarily infected with staphylococci	Antivirals not routinely used, but may shorten duration if started < 24 hr from onset of rash Acyclovir 20 mg/kg orally 4 times/day for 5 days Treat if > 12 yr old No aspirin use Antihistamines for itching
Varicella/ zoster	Reactivation from previous infection	Pain, paresthesias in dermatome prior to vesicular rash Immunosuppression or stress reactivation	Grouped vesicles on red base in derma-tomal pattern Stops at midline; rash at tip of nose means ophthalmic nerve involvement	Analgesics, sedation, acy-clovir 800 mg orally 5 times/day for 7–10 days Prednisone taper 30 mg 2 times/day for 7 days, 7.5 mg 2 times/day for 7 days Admit for IV antiviral and VZIG treatment in immunosuppressed Ophthalmology consult if tip of nose is involved
Pemphigus vulgaris	Autoimmune disease in 40–60 year old group May be genetic com-ponent vs. reaction to drugs	Bullae start in oral mucosa; then gen-eralize to other areas over weeks Nonpruritic	Fragile blisters, ero-sions with crusting No erythema Positive Nikolsky's sign = sloughing of epi-dermis with slight pressure blister	Admission for high-dose steroids and fluid management High risk of secondary infections and dehydration
Bullous pemphigoid	Possible autoimmune with antibodies against dermal-epidermal junction	Chronic, persistent blisters that may be pruritic Usually benign/self-limited course	Subepidermal blisters, negative Nikolsky's sign Starts on extremities, spreads to trunk and scalp	Dermatology referral, steroids (topical vs. systemic) Consider admission for differentiation from pemphigus vulgaris, in ex-tensive disease and elders
Bullous impetigo	Bacterial infection, usually *Staphylococcus aureus* or group A beta-hemolytic streptococci	Minor trauma, fissures around mouth, face, intertriginous zones.	Easily ruptured blisters, erosions with honey colored crust Usually afebrile	Soak/scrub to remove blisters and crust First-generation cephalo-sporins (Duricef, 500 mg orally 2 times/day for 7 days)
Staphylococcal scalded skin syndrome	Group 2 *Staphylococcus aureus* with epiderm-olytic toxins	Initial infections of naso-pharynx, conjunctiva, ears	Febrile infants with - widespread blistering, peeling in sheets	Admission for hydration, sedation, skin care and antistaph antibiotics

(Cont'd on next page)

Table 2. Vesicular and Bullous Diseases *(Continued)*

Rash	Etiology	History	Exam	Management
Staphylococcal scalded-skin syndrome *(cont'd.)*		Tender skin, then wrinkling and bullae formation	Neck and groin first, then body Mucous membranes spared	Rapid course with usual complete healing in 5–7 days.
Erythema multiforme (EM) minor	Vascular hypersensitivity reaction caused by exposure to medications or infectious agents	Recent or current HSV, EBV, or bacterial infection Recent new culprit medication	Targetoid lesions with concentric rings, central clearing and flattened papules Usually first appear on hands and feet	Elimination of allergen by antiviral treatment if suspected or stop offending medications PM antipruritic and sedation with antihistamines Oral steroids helpful early in course: prednisone 40–60 mg/day for 7 days in adults (1–2 mg/kg/day in children)
Toxic epidermal necrolysis, Stevens-Johnson syndrome, erythema multiforme major	Autoimmune/hypersensitivity reaction: 90% association with drugs Occasionally herpes infection.	Systemic illness, recent culprit on medication list: sulfa drug, penicillins, barbiturates, phenytoin, NSAIDs	Lesions as with EM minor, followed by widespread blistering, exfoliation, positive Nikolsky's sign Oral mucosal involvement	Refer for admission; stop drug, IV fluids, and high-dose steroids Antiviral treatment for herpes if suspected

EBV = Epstein-Barr virus.

Pitfalls in Practice. Consider the diagnosis of measles in nonimmunized children or adults presenting with a rash. Toxic-appearing children with a rash and with altered level of consciousness need immediate referral to an emergency department; meningitis must be considered in the differential diagnosis.

Bacterial Skin Infections

Differential Diagnosis. Recognition and initiation of proper treatment of bacterial skin infections prevent progression and complications of the disease. Table 8 describes differentiating characteristics of common bacterial skin infections.

Management. Hospitalization should be considered for immunocompromised hosts; patients with cellulitis of the face, perineum, or orbit; patients with fever or lymphangitis; patients who cannot care for themselves; and patients with crepitus (suggesting anaerobic involvement).[1] Although most patients who do not have systemic signs can be managed as outpatients, close follow-up is essential, with wound checks at 2 days. Marking the borders of erythema with a pen can assist in following the progress of the infection. Management techniques are summarized in Table 8.

Pitfalls in Practice. Good hygiene must be followed to prevent spread of impetigo. Furuncles of the face may be drained with needle aspiration to avoid scarring and damage to the facial nerve; supplemental antibiotics should be given. Deep cutaneous abscesses (i.e., pilonidal or perirectal) should be opened, explored, and drained with wick placement. This approach may not be appropriate for the urgent care setting; patients should be referred to a nearby emergency department. Systemic antibiotics are not necessary for simple abscesses.

Table 3. Papulosquamous Diseases

Rash	Etiology	History	Exam	Management
Psoriasis Common Guttate Pustular Erythro- dermic	2% of population Familial predisposition Unknown etiology	Chronic and recurrent; onset in 20s–30s Guttate during streptococcal infection with small papules	Epidermal proliferation Thickened plaques with silvery scale on extensor surfaces Nail pitting	Topical high-potency steroids in emergency department Dermatology referral for further treatment options Admission for generalized pustular disease with fever Erythrodermic with confluent plaques; often hospitalization to distinguish from other entities
Pityriasis rosea	Common, probable viral etiology	Pruritic; herald patch initially, then generalized rash	Large annular scaling, maculopapular patch Pink plaques along skin lines in Christmas tree pattern on trunk and proximal extremities	Self-limited, resolves in 6–8 wk Oral diphenhydramine, topical low-potency steroids Consider VDRL for syphilis
Lichen planus	Unknown etiology	5 Ps: polygonal, plaques, papules, purplish, pruritic	Wickham's striae: fine white crisscrossing lines often revealed after alcohol wiping Wrist flexures and lower legs; mucous membranes/genitalia	Mid-potency steroids with derm follow-up for non-mucosal Oral gel steroids and oral steroids for severe oral lesions
Miliaria	Occlusion of sweat into tissue	Early childhood in hot, humid conditions Chronic with acute exacerbations	Tiny, diffuse papules in areas of perspiration	Ventilate, cool skin
Seborrheic dermatitis	Inflammatory condition from scale build-up	Chronic-debilitated, unable to shampoo Cradle cap in neonates	Salmon-colored greasy scale; eyelids, eyebrows, skin folds, scalp May cause diaper rash	Scrubbing off scale Antiseborrheic shampoos with tar, zinc pyrithione in adults Mineral oil brushing for cradle cap Low potency topical steroid cream to facial areas
Tinea Corporis Versicolor	Fungal infection acquired from soil, animals or humans	Starts as papule that evolves into annular erythema- tous patch with peripheral scale	Ring-like lesions with central clearing and peripheral fine scale Versicolor may show up as hypo- or hyper- pigmented areas with scaling	Topical antifungals for corporis: ketoconazole or terbinafine Oral griseofulvin 500 mg twice daily (20 mg/kg) for pustular or bullous tinea Selenium sulfide shampoo, 50% propylene glycol in water, or oral single dose ketoconazole for versicolor
Urticaria	Immune response/ allergic reaction to various stimuli	Pruritic lesions appear and disappear in minutes to hours Exposure to allergen (food, soaps, insect bites, stress, temperature)	Red, thickened, edematous epidermis Anxious, itching, uncomfortable patients Look for signs of anaphylaxis: respiratory difficulty, hypotension, edema, airway compromise	Severe: SQ epinephrine (0.3 ml of 1:1000), repeat every 20 min for 3 times if needed; diphenhydramine, 50 mg IM; consider cimetidine, 300 mg IM, and systemic steroids Careful airway evaluation and management if necessary Monitor for recurrence for 2–4 hr Moderate: antihistamines, observation; identify and remove stimuli if known Consider oral steroids at discharge for 5 days Consider Epi autoinjector for severe reactions

VDRL = Venereal Disease Research Laboratory test.

Table 4. Eczematous Diseases

Rash	Etiology	History	Exam	Management
Atopic dermatitis	Chronic allergic disease with family history	Long personal and family history of allergic diseases like asthma, hayfever Chronic course with acute exacerbations	Neck, wrists, antecubital and popliteal areas with pruritic, erythematous and often excoriated, lichenified plaques May show papular, vesicular, crusting lesions in acute phase	Avoid/remove irritants: wool, solvents, harsh soaps, temp extremes Bathing in lukewarm water with mild soaps Topical moisturizers after washing Topical steroids of potency dependent on sites and severity of disease Break itch-scratch cycle with antihistamines, gloves, trimming nails
Allergic/ contact dermatitis	Immune response in skin after previous sensitization, usually to *Rhus* species (poison ivy, oak, sumac) Also with nickel-containing jewelry	Recent exposure to plants or fumes from burning plants Clearing brush, camping, pulling weeds Rapid onset of rash	Small blisters, papules in characteristic linear patterns in exposed areas Excoriations from rubbing and scratching common	Remove stimuli, wash skin to remove *Rhus* oils and remove and wash exposed clothing Remove belt buckles, earrings or chains that may be culprits Topical steroids depending on area of body affected Antihistamines for sedation and breaking itch-scratch cycle Ten-day to 2-week tapering course of oral prednisone (40 mg/day) for extensive cases
Stasis dermatitis	Inflammation of skin from chronic edema, fissuring and secondary excoriations	Chronic diseases with LE edema: CHF, DM, cellulitis	Chronic edema, hyperpigmentation, thickened skin Erythematous plaques with fissuring, erosions and ulceration	Control of underlying disease process/ edema Compression stockings, Unna boots, elastic wraps as appropriate Mid-potency steroid ointment such as triamcinolone 0.1% twice daily Control of secondary infection and itching with antibiotic and antihistamines
Scabies	Infestation with mites Inflammation/ eczema from mite and feces Not related to hygiene	Insidious onset of pruritus with excoriations History of close contact with infected persons	Erythematous, scaling rash with oral papules/burrows Volar wrist creases, finger webs, skin folds May be on face and scalp in infants Rarely above the neck in adults	Treatment from head to toe with 5% permethrin cream, left on 8–12 hr, then washed off Sexual and close personal contacts should be treated simultaneously Clothing, towels, and linens used in last 24 hr should be washed in hot water Antihistamines for pruritus. May continue to itch up to 2 weeks from dead mites and feces under skin; lindane no longer recommended due to neurotoxic potential

LE = lower extremity, CHF = congestive heart failure, DM = diabetes mellitus.

Hair and Scalp Disorders

Differential Diagnosis. Loss of hair can be extremely distressful to the patient, and it may be difficult to identify the underlying cause. Diffuse alopecia frequently has systemic causes such as drugs (e.g., contraceptives, warfarin, heparin, allopurinol, beta blockers, amphetamines, iodine, thiouracil, trimethadione), pregnancy, surgery, severe weight loss, severe illness, thyroid disease, or iron deficiency. Fever can cause hair to stop growing and to shed prematurely within 3 months. Identifying the pattern of hair loss and the

Table 5. Environmental Skin Disorders

Disorder	Etiology	History	Exam	Management
Sunburn	Direct irritation from sunlight/UV	Longer than normal outdoor activity at peak times (10 AM–2 PM) Only in sunexposed areas of skin	Diffuse, tender erythema with demarcation at clothing edges Edema and blistering in severe cases	Remove from exposure Cold compresses, aspirin or other NSAIDs, low-potency steroid creams with or without .25% menthol added
Photosensitivity reaction	Reaction to light source with concomitant medication use: tetracycline, sulfa drugs, phenothiazines, sulfonylureas, and griseofulvin	Immediate onset of burning, erythema and vesiculation in severe cases	Like severe sunburn to exposed skin	Remove offending agent, treat as above for severe sunburn Protective clothing/sunblock if medications need to be continued
Burns	Direct contact with heat source causes tissue damage	Exposure to source or steam Immediate onset of pain, erythema, blistering	First degree: erythema, edema, pain Second degree: blistering, weeping, pain Third degree: painless, leathery, white surface	Tetanus prophylaxis if needed Cold water compresses/immersion, pain control; debride ruptured blisters and devitalized tissue; silvadene or bacitracin, sterile nonstick dressing Refer/admit for > 10% body surface area, second or third degree burns to hands, feet, face or genitals
Frostbite	Necrosis/damage to tissue by direct cold exposure	Pain, parasthesias, hypesthesias in exposed areas Toes, fingers, nose and ears most often affected Later bullae and necrosis of tissue	May be initially painless, mottled or blanched Pain, erythema, bullae with rewarming Later necrosis, gangrene, desquamation and secondary infection	Rewarming in lukewarm water; debride ruptured blisters; topical antibiotic and bulky dressing Refer/admit for severe cases, secondary infection, and inability to protect from reexposure
Insect bites	Inflammation/irritation to substance left behind by insect	Exposure to insects, outdoors/ camping Exposed areas on extremities, face	Varies with species Mosquito bites show erythematous, papular areas that become excoriated with scratching Spider bites may have central necrotic areas that develop late and become infected	Removal from insect-infested areas, antihistamines for pruritus, topical mid-potency steroids for eczematous reactions Refer for questionable cases of necrosis or severe secondarily infected lesions Antistaph antibiotic for minor cellulitis at bite site Ask about foreign travel or exotic animal exposure

degree of inflammation/scalp involvement is an easy method of approaching the diagnosis of these disorders[2,3] (Table 9).

Management. The management of these disorders is summarized in Table 9.

Pitfalls in Practice. Failure to treat aggressively the underlying cause of inflammation or to identify a correctable cause of diffuse alopecia results in continued hair loss. Secondary syphilis should be considered in patchy hair loss with other systemic signs

Table 6. Pediatric Exanthems

Rash	Etiology	History	Exam	Management
Roseola	Human herpesvirus 6 infection (6 mo–3 yr)	High fever spikes PM for 2–4 days, usually resolve prior to rash	Red/pink non-scaling maculopapular rash on head and trunk	Symptomatic treatment with acetaminophen, fluids for fever Resolves in 2 days
Erythema infectiosum/ fifth disease	Human parvovirus B19 infection (5–15 yr old)	Mild fever, URI Symptoms followed by red "slapped-cheek" facial rash Later characteristic body rash	Erythematous, non-scaling cheek rash Pink, lacy, reticular rash on extremities and buttocks Well child otherwise	No treatment other than reassurance Rash may wax and wane up to 3 weeks Noninfectious after rash develops
Rubella/ German measles	Rubella virus infection Rare now in developed world with MMR vaccinations Preschool age; usually in spring	Incubation 12–15 days Fever, sore throat, malaise prodrome 1–5 days Rash starts on face and moves to trunk, then extremities	Pink, non-scaling macules, which coalesce into generalized eruption	Symptomatic treatment only Rash resolves in 2–4 days in same pattern as development Congenital rubella with birth defects/blueberry muffin spots in neonates
Rubeola/ measles	Rubeola virus infection Rare in developed world with MMR vaccinations Preschool age or non-vaccinated winter/ spring prevalence	Ten-day incubation period, then 3 day prodrome of URI symptoms with fever, cough, coryza, and malaise Rash starts first in mouth then hairline, face then trunk	Koplick spots in mouth: whitish spots on buccal mucosa Pink, confluent macular rash on face, neck spreading to trunk and extremities	Supportive treatment only Rash lasts about 7 days
Scarlet fever/ scarlatina	Bacterial infection with group A beta hemolytic streptococci Rash is related to bacterial toxins Typically 2–10 years old *Staphylococcus aureus* can cause similar disease	Fever, pharyngitis, abdominal pain, vomiting are common Bright red oral mucosa with "white straw-berry"-coated tongue Truncal rash follows with skin fold predilection	"Sandpapery" feel of rash and linear petechiae on flexion skin folds Rash will fade followed by desquamation	Rapid streptococcal screen/ culture, ASO titer Oral or parenteral penicillin, erythromycin or cephalo-sporins for 10 days Supportive care with fluids, rest and acetaminophen
Lyme disease/ erythema migrans	Infection with *Borrelia burgdorferi* from tick bite	Rash develops 2–4 weeks after tick bite Associated flu-like symptoms of fever, sore throat, headache, and vomiting are common	Starts as red macule at bite site, which enlarges into annular, nonscaling plaque with central clearing Lymphadenopathy and arthralgias common	Diagnosis on clinic basis as serology is unreliable Pregnant women or children < 8 yr: amoxicillin, 10 mg/kg orally 3 times/day, cefurox-ime or clarithromycin in penicillin-allergic, doxycy-cline 100 mg orally 2 times/day in adults
Kawasaki disease	Unclear etiology with speculation of hyper-immune response to viral, bacterial, chemical or other stimulus Children < 9 yr old	Prolonged fever with: conjunctivitis, rash, edema, and erythema of extremities, LAD, otopharyngeal changes	Strawberry tongue, erythematous rash especially in diaper area that desquamates late	Rapid referral for treatment and further evaluation IVIG and oral aspirin are effective Coronary arterial aneurysms in 20% if untreated

LAD = lymphadenopathy, URI = upper respiratory infection, IVIG = intravenous immunoglobulin.

Table 7. Diaper Rashes

Rash	Etiology	Exam	Management
Occlusion dermatitis	Trapped moisture, friction, infrequent diaper changing	Redness, maceration in intertriginous areas; inguinal, genital folds, inner thighs	Mild soaps, allow to dry after changing, zinc oxide creams
Seborrheic dermatitis	Unknown	Salmon-colored rash with greasy scales Not only in creases; may involve face, scalp and posterior auricular areas	Physically remove scale with mineral oil rubbing Hydrocortisone 1% cream twice daily only
Candidal dermatitis	Superficial skin infection with *Candida albicans* May be concurrent with both of the above	Intense, erythematous, confluent rash with sharp borders and satellite lesions of pustular character Whitish plaques in mouth (thrush) may be present	Clotrimazole 1% or nystatin cream to rash twice daily Oral nystatin for thrush 4 times/day

(e.g., rash, lymphadenopathy, mucous membrane patches). Some systemic illnesses present with changes in hair pattern, growth, or texture; patients with these complaints require further evaluation.

Pruritus

Differential Diagnosis. Pruritus is a common complaint that is often frustrating to patient and physician alike. Several common causes are listed in Table 10. Patients with known or apparent systemic diseases, such as renal or hepatic failure, may have pruritus

Table 8. Bacterial Skin Infections

Rash	Etiology	History	Exam	Management
Impetigo	Superficial infection with staphylococci or streptococci Associated with poor hygiene	Rapid developing, pruritic lesions accompanied by crusting and erosions Afebrile	Lesions on face and extremities with fissuring	Removal of crust, good hygiene, oral first-generation cephalosporins
Erysipelas	Superficial streptococcal infection of broken skin, usually on face	Sudden onset of facial redness in ill-appearing patients	Sharply demarcated, edematous red plaques on face	Prompt referral for admission, intravenous antibiotics and pain control
Cellulitis	Infection of dermis and subcutaneous tissues by skin flora	Painful, red, swollen area of skin near break in skin	Associated with fever, elevated WBC, and local lymphadenopathy Poorly demarcated areas of rash	Elevation of affected side with intravenous vs. oral anti-staphylococcal antibiotics Consider admission if severe or follow-up and compliance in question
Cutaneous abscesses	Localized staphylococcal infections of hair follicles lead to abscesses of various sites and sizes	History of similar lesions in past Diabetics are more susceptible	Red, painful, indurated lump on neck, back, axilla, or groin Afebrile	Incision and drainage, warm packs and pain control More extensive treatment and referral in DM or immunosuppression

Table 9. Hair and Scalp Disorders

Disorder	Etiology	History	Exam	Management
Alopecia areata	Probably autoimmune, may be related to thyroid disease	Waxing and waning course of patchy hair loss and regrowth New hair is finer and lighter than original with tapered tips	Well demarcated patches of hair loss with normal scalp Hair easily detaches with intact roots (club hairs) Wide range of severity from small patch to "alopecia totalis"	Stimulation of regrowth with topical steroids (0.1% triamcinolone cream) Intralesional steroid injections effective for small areas Early referral to dermatologist
Trichotillo-mania	Hair loss secondary to chronic pulling and twisting	Psychological stress, anxiety disorders common; patchy hair loss in fixed areas	Hair broken off close to scalp Normal scalp with normal roots, not easily detached	Patient education, anti-pruritic with sedative properties if PM itching is problem Close follow-up with primary physician for possible psychological evaluation
Traction alopecia	Hair loss from chronic tension due to tightly braided hair left braided for long periods	African-American children and women with hair loss mani-fested as receding hairline in frontal and parietal areas	Normal scalp with fringe of short, unbraidable hairs at margins of hair loss Actual permanent loss of hair follicles	Loose or no braiding in children No good nonsurgical treatments available
Tinea capitis	Fungal infection with scalp inflammation	Well-demarcated plaques with hair loss, scale and crusting	Inflamed scalp with pustules, induration and drainage possible	Oral antifungals required for resolution Griseofulvin 20 mg/kg/day for 2 months or until scalp inflammation resolved Oral fluconazole, terbinafine also effective
Discoid lupus erythe-matosus	Autoimmune to skin elements	Chronic, complete, permanent, hair loss with inflammatory scalp lesions with central crust	Red, crusted plaques of complete hair loss; central depigmentation with peripheral hyperpigmentation	High-potency topical steroids: fluocinonide 0.05% cream twice daily Referral to dermatologist for evaluation of SLE and further treatment with hydroxychloroquine
Acne keloid/ bacterial cellulitis of the scalp	Foreign body reaction to ingrown hairs from shaving with or with or without bacterial infection	Inflammation, purulent discharge from scalp in occipital area	Hair loss with pustules, discharge Consider pediculosis if signs of lice/eggs on hair shafts	Gentle shampooing, anti-staphylococcal antibiotic or erythromycin for 7 days Stop shaving scalp Treat lice if present with permethrin 1%

SLE = systemic lupus erythematosus.

from build-up of toxic substances. Screening lab samples should be drawn, if possible, for liver function and blood urea nitrogen. Complete blood count can help define poly-cythemia and anemia of chronic disease.[1] The most common cause of pruritus in elder patients is xerosis or dry skin, especially in winter and low-humidity conditions.

Management. Detect and treat systemic disease as needed. Referral for further evalua-tion usually is required. Showers with mild soaps are less drying to the skin than baths. Lubricating creams such as Eucerin or Aquaphor after showers may be helpful. Oral an-tihistamines are helpful for pruritus, provide sedation, and may be useful at night when

Table 10. Causes of Pruritus

Type	Etiology	History	Exam	Management
Systemic	Numerous toxic, metabolic substances Consider: hepatic or renal dysfunction, blood dyscrasias (polycythemia, lymphoma), endocrine (diabetes, hypo- or hyperthyroid), pregnancy and hypercalcemia	Variable, depends on disease process and onset	Consistent with underlying disease Look for edema, hepatomegaly, lymphadenopathy, bruising	Screening labs for systemic disease: CBC with differential, electrolytes including calcium, BUN, UA, TSH
Xerosis	Excessive dry skin with decreased lipid content from low humidity, bathing/usually worse in winter	Seasonal waxing and waning of symptoms Absence of other diseases	Dry, scaly skin with linear excoriations	Short showers instead of bathing limited to once daily Lubricating creams after bathing (Eucerin) Humidification of environment and night-time antihistamines
Irritants	Contact with irritant such as fiberglass, wool causes mechanical irritation	Exposure to irritant	Normal skin with excoriations	Remove irritant, observe for contact dermatitis
Psychogenic	Compulsive behavior with or without formication	Anxious, insistent patient with numerous office visits; may report seeing bugs or worms	Normal exam except excoriations No bugs, worms, or eggs present	Treat as for dry skin with lubricants, antihistamines, limited bathing Psychological referral for behavior modification

symptoms are more bothersome. Doxepin and amitriptyline are tricyclic antidepressants that have significant antihistaminic and sedative effects. They may be helpful in extreme cases of night-time itching.

Pitfalls in Practice. If no cause of pruritus is found, placebo therapy should not be used; the effectiveness is often short-lived, and when symptoms return the patient is convinced that real disease is present. If pruritus is suspected as a symptom of systemic disease, failure to ensure timely follow-up can delay diagnosis of a potentially serious medical illness.

Drug Use in Dermatologic Disorders

Topical medications for use on the skin are formulated in various vehicles. The choice of vehicle depends on a variety of factors, including disease process, degree of inflammation, area of the body affected, and patient profile. If not indicated by the prescribing physician, the default vehicle is usually cream.[1] See Table 11 for applications of the various vehicles.

Steroids are a mainstay in treatment of skin disorders, both systemic and topical. The appropriate potency and vehicle can be critical in proper treatment of disease processes and limiting of side effects. Table 12 shows the various topical steroid preparations classified by potency. Because there is no real advantage of one preparation over another within groups, the clinician's repertoire needs to include only one type from each group. Generally, hydrocortisone 1% as low-potency, triamcinolone 0.1% as mid-potency, and

Table 11. Common Vehicles in Dermatology

Vehicle	Contents	Advantages	Disadvantages	Common Uses
Ointment	Petroleum jelly/ medicines	Occlusive, a little goes a long way; lubricating; fewer additives	Greasy feel, messy Can cause maceration in moist areas (skin folds)	Fissured, inflamed, dry skin areas
Cream	Oil in water/ medicines and preservatives	Easily absorbed without greasy feel Cosmetically pleasing	Less moisturizing, more needed for given area Increased risk of allergic reactions to preservatives	Intact skin, skin folds, cosmetically obvious areas and maintenance therapy
Lotion	Water/alcohol and medicines	Nongreasy, cooling feeling from evaporation, no maceration	Drying agent, irritating to broken or inflamed skin Allergic potential	Hairy areas, scalp, for large surface area coverage Damp areas such as web spaces

Table 12. Potencies of Common Steroid Preparations

Potency	Generic Name	Concentration	Preparation	Brand Name
Ultra	Clobetasol	0.05%	Ointment	Temovate
	Betamethasone	0.05%	Ointment, gel, lotion	Diprolene
	Diflorasone	0.05%	Ointment	Psorcon
	Halobetasol	0.05%		Ultravate
High	Amcinonide	0.1%	Ointment	Cyclocort
	Betamethasone	0.05%	Cream	Diprolene AF
	Desoximetasone	0.05%; 0.025%	Gel; cream, ointment	Topicort
	Diflorasone	0.05%	Cream	Psorcon
	Fluocinonide	0.05%	Cream	Lidex
	Halcinonide	0.1%	Cream	Halog
	Mometasone	0.1%	Ointment	Elocon
Middle	Desoximetasone	0.05%	Cream	Topicort LP
	Fluocinolone	0.025%	Ointment	Synalar
	Hydrocortisone	0.2%	Ointment	Westcort
	Mometasone	0.1%	Cream	Elocon
	Triamcinolone	0.1%	Ointment, cream	Aristocort, Kenalog
Mild	Alclometasone	0.05%	Ointment, cream	Aclovate
	Desonide	0.05%	Cream	Tridesilon, DesOwen
	Fluocinolone	0.01%	Cream, lotion	Synalar
Low	Hydrocortisone	0.5, 1, 2%	Cream	Hytone

fluocinonide 0.05% as high-potency are acceptable for use in an urgent care setting and are available in generic formulations in most pharmacies. Ultra-potent formulations should be used with caution and reserved for cases with good follow-up plans. Clobetasol 0.05% and betamethasone 0.05% are common choices in this group.

References

1. Edwards L: Dermatology in Emergency Care. New York, Churchill Livingstone, 1997.
2. Fitzpatrick TB, et al: Color Atlas and Synopsis of Clinical Dermatology, 3rd ed. New York, McGraw-Hill, 1997.
3. Habif TP: Clinical Dermatology: A Color Guide to Diagnosis and Therapy, 3rd ed. St. Louis, Mosby, 1996.

Chapter 18

Special Problems in Pediatrics

Marc Martel, MD
Cara Ellman Black, MD
Michelle H. Biros, MS, MD

Fevers in Infants and Children

Fever is a common complaint of children presenting to the urgent care facility. Most children have benign causes of febrile illness, but some have serious pathology that may cause morbidity and even mortality, if left untreated. The clinician must determine which children with a fever are seriously ill and which are not. We use many factors to help determine the child's wellness—age, history, clinical exam, laboratory studies, radiographic measures, and parent's reliability. Often, the symptoms and signs of infection are vague or nonspecific. Although a daunting task at times, following a systematic approach can make the evaluation of the febrile child much easier.

History and Physical Examination

Fever is defined as a temperature $\geq 38.0°C$ (100.4°F). For infants 0–90 days, a temperature of $< 36.0°C$ (96.8°F) may signify serious infections or sepsis.[1] In small children, rectal temperatures are more accurate than tympanic, oral, or axillary measures. A history of an elevated temperature provided by a reliable parent should never be ignored. Tactile temperatures by parents have been shown to be accurate approximately 75% of the time.[2]

The management of a febrile child with an identified infectious source is usually straightforward, and based on the cause of the fever, general health of the child, adequacy of parental involvement, and available pediatric follow-up. This discussion concentrates on children who present with a fever for which no obvious infectious source can be identified by history and physical examination. Without an obvious source, the search for the cause of fever depends on the age of the child. Younger children pose greater challenges. Their clinical exam can be unreliable in detecting the source of the fever as well as in determining the severity of the illness.

Important historical considerations in febrile infants include birth history, infectious exposures, immunization status, recent travel or immigration, current activity and attitude, appetite, presence of vomiting or diarrhea, respiratory patterns, rashes, and parents' assessment of hydration status (i.e., wet diapers, making tears). Recent diphtheria-pertussis-tetanus (DPT) vaccinations can cause fever 12–24 hours later, which persist for 24–48 hours.[1]

Examination. Many studies have evaluated the height of fever as a predictor of serious bacterial illness (SBI). Although it appears that higher fevers suggest an increased likelihood of SBI, some infants with lower temperatures have SBI, and others with higher fevers have minor illness.[1]

The examination of the febrile infant may be nonspecific or misleading. For instance, meningitic signs are often absent in infants less than 3 months old with meningitis.[3] The work-up therefore often relies on diagnostic testing.

Diagnostic Evaluation. The diagnostic evaluation of the febrile infant without a source can be time-consuming and frustrating, since obtaining samples (i.e., blood, urine) for analysis is often difficult. The usefulness and interpretations of each diagnostic screen, therefore, must be fully understood if they are to provide direction in the evaluation and management of the febrile infant.

Complete Blood Count with Differential/Blood Cultures. The risk of bacteremia appears to increase with increasing temperatures. Therefore, with fevers ≥ 39.0°C (102.2°F) a complete blood count (CBC) is helpful. An abnormal CBC has limited sensitivity or specificity to predict SBI in febrile infants, but a normal CBC is somewhat reassuring.[4] The absolute band count is most predictive. For a white blood cell count > 15,000/mm³, the relative risk of bacteria is fivefold higher. In this situation, blood cultures should be sent and antibiotics given. Ceftriaxone (50 mg/kg IM) is often the empiric choice. Follow-up in 12 hours is recommended for re-evaluation and review of the pending blood cultures. Common organisms of positive blood cultures are *S. pneumoniae*, *H. influenzae* type b, and *Neisseria meningitides*.

Urinalysis and Urine Culture. Catheter specimens are recommended for more accurate results. Urinalysis (UA) is recommended for all males ≤ 6 months of age (older for uncircumcised males) and females ≤ 24 months of age. A normal dipstick UA usually rules out UTIs.[1] If the UA results are positive, a culture should be sent, and the child should have follow-up arranged for further testing regarding the etiology of the UTI.

Chest Radiographs. The likelihood of pneumonia, as diagnosed by chest x-ray findings, is low in febrile children with no pulmonary symptoms or signs.[5] Reasons to obtain a chest x-ray include a cough, asymmetric lung exam/rales or rhonchi, diminished oxygen saturation, tachypnea, temperature ≥ 40.0°C or white blood cell count > 15,000/mm³.

Cerebrospinal Fluid Analysis. Cerebral spinal fluid (CSF) analysis must take into account the age-dependent normal values for white blood cells (WBC). In general, the CSF WBC count and Gram stain are the most predictive tests for meningitis that are readily available. The predictive value of this combination has not been validated, however.[1]

General Age-Dependent Approach to Fever Without a Source

1. Fever without a source in infants less than 28 days of age

Patients should be admitted to the hospital with consideration given to a complete sepsis work-up. Cefotaxime, 50 mg/kg IV, and ampicillin, 100 mg/kg IV, are considered for empiric treatment before the results of cultures are obtained. This regimen protects against the most common bacterial agents in this age group, including Group B streptococci, *E. coli*, and *Listeria* sp. Ceftriaxone is not recommended in children < 8 weeks of age because of its effects on biliary sludging.

2. Fever in infants 28–90 days of age

The work-up of infants 28–90 days old can be separated into two categories: **low-risk** and **high-risk infants**. The criteria for low-risk febrile infants include previously healthy condition, no focal bacterial infection on exam (except otitis media), nontoxic clinical appearance, and negative laboratory screening (WBC between 5,000 and 15,000/mm^3, with < 1500 bands/mm^3; normal urinalysis, normal stool sample if diarrhea present, and negative chest x-ray).[6]

Outpatient management of **low-risk infants** can be considered as an alternative to hospitalization. Parents must be deemed reliable, and close follow-up must be guaranteed. However, before low-risk febrile infants can be discharged home, a CSF specimen should be obtained and a dose of IM antibiotics should be given. Since lumbar punctures (LPs) may be beyond the scope of diagnostic evaluation available in most urgent care settings, patients in this category should be transferred to an emergency department (ED) for further evaluation and treatment. **High-risk infants** should be transferred emergently to an ED for further evaluation and admission.

3. Fever without a source in children 3–36 months of age

This group can be separated into two categories: **toxic-appearing and non–toxic-appearing**. On clinical exam, "toxicity" is determined by the quality of cry, reaction to parent stimulation, wakefulness, color, hydration, interaction, and meningeal signs.[6] Toxicity should be re-evaluated after antipyretics have been given, and toxic-appearing children need transfer to an ED for further evaluation. Admission should be arranged. A CSF specimen should be obtained as soon as possible. However, antibiotics should not be withheld if an LP cannot be obtained. If concerns of meningitis are present, antibiotics should be given promptly. The recommended treatment is ceftriaxone, 100 mg/kg IV.

After appropriate diagnostic evaluation, **non–toxic-appearing febrile children** 3–36 months of age can be managed as outpatients as long as parents are reliable and close follow-up can be ensured.

Pitfalls in Practice. Failure to adequately work up the infant with a fever or minimization of parental history of symptoms has the potential to result in substantial morbidity and mortality, especially in the presence of a nonfocal examination. All young children with fever need expedient evaluation. If urgent care facilities are not equipped to meet the special needs of such children, they should be promptly referred and transferred for immediate diagnostic work-up and management.

Acute Otitis Media

One of the most common infections of childhood is acute otitis media (AOM). Although the diagnosis is often straightforward, the treatment of this pathology has become controversial. Several issues are at the center of the current clinical debate, including the antibiotic of choice for first and recurrent AOM, duration of treatment, necessity of treating mild cases, and whether AOM alone can explain an extremely high fever in a toxic-appearing child.

Acute otitis media arises from eustachian tube dysfunction and colonization of the middle ear with pathogenic bacteria. The most common pathogens are *Streptococcus pneumoniae*, *Haemophilus influenzae*, and *Moraxella catarrhalis*. Viruses are also frequent causative agents. Often the patient has had a preceding upper respiratory infection. Other risk factors for the occurrence of AOM include day care attendance and second hand cigarette smoke.[7]

Examination. The diagnosis of AOM is established by history and clinical exam. Patients usually complain of ear pain, which may begin suddenly. Fever also may be present, along with diminished hearing, ear pulling in infants, irritability, vomiting, vertigo, and ear drainage.

On examination, the tympanic membrane may appear erythematous, bulging, dull, immobile to insufflation, or scarred from previous infectious episodes. Tympanocentesis with culture of the middle ear fluid is the gold standard for definitive identification of the offending organism.[7]

Management. The management of AOM has been a source of controversy for several years. A recent meta-analysis describes a spontaneous cure rate for AOM of up to 81%,[8] suggesting that many cases are viral or bacterial with low virulence.[7] Some authorities, therefore, choose to watch a child for clinical progression and begin treatment if fever and symptoms persist for more than 24–72 hours.[9] Most studies have not followed patients over the long term for complications related to AOM, and a recent increase in the incidence of mastoiditis has been described in Germany, thought to be due to inadequate or absent treatment of AOM.[7] The differentiation of bacterial from viral causes cannot be done on the basis of the clinical exam. In most developed countries, AOM is treated with antibiotics.

Figure 1 presents a risk stratification for the treatment of AOM in children more than 6 months of age. Since tympanocentesis is rarely done, treatment is empiric and aimed at the most likely organism. The mainstay of antibiotic treatment has been amoxicillin. Recently, because inconsistent antimicrobial activity has been demonstrated, alternative agents and/or dosing has been recommended (Table 1; Figure 1).

Table 1. Antibiotics for AOM in Children

First-line antibiotics	
Amoxicillin	80–90 mg/kg, 2 or 3 daily doses for 10 days
Amoxicillin-clavulanate	80/20 mg/kg/day × 10 days
Azithromycin	10 mg/kg/day × 1; 5 mg/kg days 2–5
Cefuroxime	30 mg/kg/day × 10 days
Ceftriaxone	50mg.kg/day IM × 1–3 days
Second-line antibiotics	
Trimethoprim-sulfamethoxazole	8/40 mg/kg/day × 10 days
Clarithromycin	15 mg/kg/day × 10 days
Cefpodoxime	10 mg/kg/day × 10 days

Pitfalls in Practice. When the ear appears normal but the patient presents with ear pain, referred pain from other head and neck sources must be considered. Especially common are dental abscesses, temporomandibular joint syndrome, and sinus infections.[7] It is easy to attribute a fever in an infant or toddler to AOM; other sources also should be considered and ruled out.

Febrile Seizures

Childhood seizures may be due to an idiopathic seizure disorder, infection, metabolic abnormality, toxic disorder, structural lesion, or other cause. Many are simple febrile seizures for which no other underlying cause can be identified. Risk factors for a febrile seizure and recurrent febrile seizures are presented in Table 2. The principal objective of

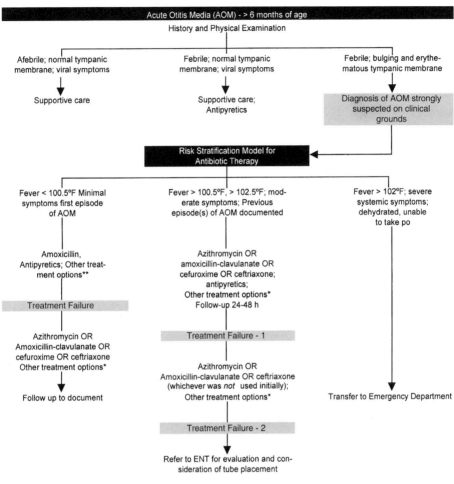

Figure 1. Risk stratification for the treatment of AOM in children more than 6 months of age. (Adapted from Bosker G: Acute Otitis Media (AOM) Year 2000. Update: A rational and evidence based analysis of current controversies in antibiotic therapy and drug selection. Emerg Med Rep 21(7): 75–80, 2000.)

Table 2. Risk Factors for Febrile Seizures

Initial Febrile Seizure	Recurrent Febrile Seizures
Family history of febrile seizure	Young age
Neonatal hospital discharge ≥ 28 days	Family history of febrile seizure
Delayed development	Short duration of fever before initial seizure
Child care attendance	Relatively low fever before onset of seizure
Hyponatremia	Family history of seizure disorder
Significant degree of fever	

the UC physician is to differentiate the simple febrile seizure without an underlying cause from a febrile seizure with an underlying cause. The characteristics of simple and complex febrile seizures are listed in Table 3.

Table 3. Simple vs. Complex Seizures

Simple Febrile Seizures	Complex Febrile Seizures
Ages 6 months to 5 years	Younger than 6 months
Duration 15 minutes or less	Prolonged seizure > 15 minutes
Nonfocal (generalized)	Focal
Single seizure	Recurrent seizures
Normal neurologic examination	Abnormal neurologic examination
Brief postical period	Underlying etiology present

Differential Diagnosis. The most important components of the evaluation are a careful history and a complete physical examination. Laboratory studies should be performed as directed by the history and physical examination. The most frequently helpful tests to explain the seizure are electrolyte measurements (hyponatremia) and lumbar puncture (meningitis). Other studies, as in the evaluation of the febrile child, may be indicated.

Management. A child older than 15 months of age with characteristics of a simple febrile seizure and a known febrile source and who appears to be entirely well after observation may be discharged with early follow-up by a primary care physician. Younger children are more difficult to assess and generally should be referred directly to an emergency department (ED). Any child with characteristics of a complex seizure should be transferred to an ED for further evaluation.

Simple seizures do not require treatment other than aggressive fever control. Evidence suggests that recurrence rates are lower when continuous phenobarbital is administered. However, most practitioners believe that the adverse consequences of this measure outweigh the advantages. Intermittent phenobarbital administration with febrile illness is not effective.[10] The decision to initiate anticonvulsant prophylaxis in high-risk situations or after multiple simple febrile seizures should be left to the primary care physician.

Pitfalls in Practice. Simple febrile seizure is a diagnosis of exclusion. A specific cause must be presumed to be present until shown to be absent on the basis of the evaluation outlined above.

Pediatric Pulmonary Disorders

Asthma

Asthma is a disease of intermittent symptoms caused by hyperactive airways and reversible airway obstruction. Asthma can be extrinsic (immunologically mediated) or intrinsic (no identifiable cause).

Examination. Expiratory wheezing and a prolonged expiratory phase are usually noted. However, with insufficient air movement, expiratory wheezing may not be appreciated. Other symptoms include dyspnea, coughing, and retractions/accessory muscle use.

Diagnostic Aids. Peak flows and pulse oximetry are helpful diagnostic tests in the initial evaluation. Chest radiographs should be considered for patients with hypoxia, fever, asymmetric lung exam, or no improvement after multiple nebulizer treatments.

Management. Initial treatment includes bronchial smooth muscle relaxants such as albuterol and atrovent nebulizers. Oral prednisone, 1–2 mg/kg, is also recommended. If the child does not improve after 3 nebulizers, transfer to an ED for further evaluation and possible admission to the hospital.

Bronchiolitis

Bronchiolitis is a common disease of the lower respiratory tract. Peak incidence occurs between 6 and 8 months of age, although it can affect children within the first 24 months of life. Causative agents include respiratory syncytial virus (RSV; most common), parainfluenza virus 3, adenovirus, *Mycoplasma* sp. and *H. influenzae*.

Examination. Clinical presentation includes serous nasal discharge, sneezing, and mild fever. With worsening symptoms, expiratory wheezing, cough, intercostal retractions, tachypnea, nasal flaring, cyanosis, and rales may be noted.

Diagnostic Aids. If checked, the CBC is usually normal. Oxygen saturation may be normal or low. Nasal washing can be obtained to verify for RSV. A chest radiograph may reveal hyperinflation and scattered areas of consolidation and perihilar haziness.

Management. Therapy is supportive (oxygen, IV fluids if the child is dehydrated). Antibiotics are not indicated unless a secondary bacterial infection is present. Bronchodilators (albuterol) often relieve acute symptoms. The patient's disposition depends on the clinical appearance and age of the child. The most concerning period during the illness is at 48–72 hours, often the onset of a cough. Infants with moderate-to-severe wheezing and dyspnea (especially early on in the illness) should be observed for worsening symptoms. Infants with mild symptoms and reliable parents can be managed at home with close follow-up.

Croup (Laryngotracheobronchitis)

Croup is a self-limited, benign viral illness caused by influenzae, adenovirus, and parainfluenza. It usually affects children less than 7 years old and occurs more often in colder months of the year.

Examination. The clinical course usually begins with upper respiratory infection symptoms and may progress to a "seal-like" cough that is worse at night. Disease progression usually occurs over a 7-day period. The "seal-like" or barking cough increases when the patient is agitated and is caused by edema in the subglottic region of the trachea. Often the patient is afebrile. With worsening disease, stridor with expiratory wheezing may be noted at rest, and respiratory efforts become labored. Typically this pattern occurs in younger infants.

Diagnostic Aids. The diagnosis is made by history and clinical exam. Pulse oximetry may be helpful. Obtaining a CBC is not necessary, but if obtained, it usually shows lymphocytosis. A posterior-anterior chest radiograph may demonstrate a narrowed tracheal air column (steeple sign).

Management. Management depends on the child's level of comfort at rest. If no stridor is present at rest, the child can be discharged home with symptomatic treatment.

Steam or cool air usually alleviates the seal-like cough. Children with stridor at rest should be treated with nebulized racemic epinephrine (2.25% solution diluted 1:5 or 1:8 with water and given 4 ml nebulized over 15 minutes). If the stridor improves, a minimum of 2 hours of continued observation is recommended before discharge home. Rebound stridor usually occurs within 2 hours after the racemic epinephrine nebulization is given. A single dose of 0.6–1.0 mg/kg of dexamethasone IM is recommended. If the child does not improve after this regimen or if the parents are unreliable, the child should be admitted to the hospital.

Epiglottitis

Epiglottitis is not as prevalent as in the past, probably due to the decline of *H. influenzae*. However, epiglottitis occasionally occurs among both pediatric and adult patients. Given the life-threatening nature of the disease, knowledge about proper management is vital.

Etiology. Epiglottitis usually occurs in children 3–7 years old, although it can occur outside this range. The most common causative agent is *Haemophilus influenzae*, although *S. pneumoniae*, *S. aureus*, viruses, or allergic reactions can be the culprit.

Examination. Clinical exam is the key to the diagnosis. Always suspect epiglottitis in a toxic, drooling child without a cough. Older children may present in the sitting position with their head extended.

Diagnostic Aids. A lateral cervical x-ray shows the "thumb-print sign" (a swollen epiglottis) along with obliteration of the vallecula.

Management. If epiglottitis is suspected, the child should not be left unattended. Ambulance transfer to the nearest ED should be arranged immediately. While awaiting transfer, the child should not be aggravated. High flow oxygen should be administered unless it aggravates the child. Avoid IVs until the airway is secure. It is preferable to intubate the child in an operating room under a controlled setting.

Peritonsillar Abscess

A peritonsillar abscess can occur when acute bacterial tonsillitis progresses to form a pocket of purulent material in the pharyngeal pillar. Serious complications can occur, such as airway compromise and extension into the mediastinum.

Examination. The examination reveals a fever, muffled voice, difficulty swallowing, drooling, difficulty opening the mouth, foul smelling breath, and a unilaterally enlarged and edematous tonsil with a deviation of the uvula to the contralateral side.

Management. If a peritonsillar abscess if suspected, transfer to an ED, where the abscess can be incised and drained (I&D), is recommended. Often abscesses can be drained in the ED. If the patient is toxic and concerns about the airway remain, the patient should be admitted.

Pneumonia

Pneumonia is an infection of the pulmonary parenchyma. Predisposing risk factors include diabetes, sickle cell disease, asplenia, and chemotherapy.

Examination. The exam may be nonspecific (i.e., minimal fever, normal lung exam) or may reveal a fever, cough, tachypnea, ausculatory findings, purulent sputum, or retractions. The patient may be toxic-appearing or non–toxic-appearing.

Diagnostic Aids. Diagnostic evaluation should include pulse oximetry. Young children without lung disease normally have oxygen saturations of 99–100%: If they are lower, a chest x-ray should be obtained.

Management. Antibiotic therapy should be directed at the most likely bacterial cause. Causative agents of pneumonia are age-dependent, and include the following:

> Neonates: Group B Streptococci, *E. coli*, *H. influenzae*, *S. pneumoniae*
> 1–4 mos: *Chlamydia trachomatis, S pneumoniae, H. influenzae*
> 4 mos to 5 yrs: Viruses, *S. pneumoniae, H. influenzae*
> Older children: *Mycoplasma* sp., viruses, *S. pneumoniae*

Admission to the hospital is recommended if the child is toxic-appearing, dyspneic, or hypoxic (pulse oximeter < 95%); if the parents appear unreliable; or if close follow-up cannot be ensured.

Pitfalls in Practice. Infants and young children frequently have nonspecific or difficult pulmonary examinations. Often the history may be quite vague, and the clues to the diagnosis of a pulmonary disorder may be subtle. A high index of suspicion must be maintained and a careful history obtained if pulmonary pathology is a possible cause of the presenting complaint. Children with hypoxia may appear relatively well, despite a worrisome history. Oxygen saturation measurement is an important adjunct to the investigation and should be performed whenever a suspicion of pulmonary pathology exists.

Pediatric Gastrointestinal Disorders

Acute Infectious Diarrhea

Diarrhea is a common pediatric complaint encountered in the UC setting. Diarrhea accounts for approximately 11% of hospital admissions of children less than 5 years old and between 300 and 400 deaths per year, typically in the first year of life.[11] Children are at increased risk for complications associated with diarrheal illnesses because of volume loss and electrolyte abnormalities due to their size, developing immune system, and dependence on adults for hydration.

Osmotic diarrhea is a colonic response to increased amounts of osmoticly active substances in the gut lumen. This results in the movement of fluid and electrolytes into the colon and hence increased volumes of hypertonic fluid. Diagnosis is assisted if diarrhea slows with decreased oral intake, the pH of stools is less than 5, and reducing substances are found in the stool.

Secretory diarrhea is due to enterotoxins causing an increase in cyclic adenosine monophosphate (cAMP) in the luminal endothelial cell with resulting chloride secretion. Offending agents include *Salmonella, Shigella, Vibrio cholerae, E. coli,* and *C. difficile* species. Noninfectious causes are rare. Diagnosis is suggested by a history of no change of the stooling pattern with altered oral intake, a stool pH greater than 6, and no reducing substances in the stool. Organisms responsible for secretory diarrhea typically attach to endothelial cells. This results in cell damage with bleeding and mucous production and the potential for access to the systemic circulation.

Acid–base abnormalities are commonly found in patients with diarrhea, often in conjunction with significant volume alterations. Typically metabolic acidosis with variable respiratory compensation is found. The acidosis is due to primary loss of bicarbonate and chloride in the stool, but contributions from lactic acid, ketones, and salicylates may also occur. Maximum respiratory compensation may occur within hours of the onset of diarrheal illness. Correction is based on replacement of intravascular fluid losses rather than bicarbonate replenishment.

Etiology. Viruses are implicated in most cases of pediatric diarrhea. Infectious diarrhea in the pediatric population is associated most often with poor hygienic practices. Table 4 describes the clinical presentation and treatment of selected causes of pediatric acute infectious diarrhea.

Table 4. Pediatric Diarrhea

Agent	Presentation	Treatment	Comments
Rotavirus	F, V, D, URI	Rehydration	Diagnosis: antigen in stool
Adenovirus	F, V, D	Symptomatic	
Norwalk agent	F, V, D	Symptomatic	
Hepatitis A (HAV)	F, V, A, M	Symptomatic	Household contact: offer prophylaxis*
Shigella	F, D, Y	TMP-SMX (5 mg/kg PO BID × 7–10 days)	Peak 6 mos–10 yrs
Salmonella	F, N, D	Symptomatic	Recurrence risk[†]
Campylobacter[‡]	F, D, Y, P	Symptomatic, erythromycin may shorten course	Diagnosis by darkfield microscopy
Yersinia	V, D, P(Ma)		Symptoms may last > 14 days
C. difficile	F, D, C	Vancomycin (40 mg/kg/24 hr)	Most common after antibiotics
S. aureus	V, D, C	Symptomatic	Preformed enterotoxin, rapid onset and resolution of symptoms

F = febrile illness, V = vomiting, D = diarrhea, A = anorexia, M = malaise, Y = dysentery, C = cramps, P = pseudoappendicitis, Ma = pseudoappendicitis secondary to mesenteric adenitis, URI = upper respiratory infection symptoms.
* HAV immunoglobulin prophylaxis should be offered to household contacts.
† Treatment with amoxicillin or ampicillin is associated with reoccurrence of symptoms.
‡ *C. jejuni* and *E. coli* most common.

Diagnosis. Examination of fluid and electrolyte status is essential. Decreased intake in conjunction with vomiting and diarrhea requires careful correction of volume, electrolytes, and acid–base disturbances. Quantification of lost volume is generally difficult. Questions involving the number of diapers changed or deviation from normal bowel habits may assist parents in providing a more accurate history. Details should be obtained about the course, duration, and severity of symptoms. Constitutional symptoms as well as a history of associated pain, hematemesis, hematochezia, or melena is relevant. Travel history may be useful.

Physical examination should be directed at fluid status. Vitals sign are critical, but it is important to recognize the physiologic compensating abilities of the pediatric population. Significant hypovolemia may exist before considerable alterations in vital signs are apparent. Mucous membranes, capillary refill, skin elasticity, and urine output may provide useful information.

Stool examination on an outpatient basis is generally not indicated. In this setting, studies for fecal leukocytes and occult blood may be used to differentiate acute gastroenteritis and dysentery. When a pathogen invades the endothelium, the risk of systemic invasion exists, and is demonstrated by the presence of leukocytes and blood in the stool. Typically fecal leukocytes are present with infections caused by *Shigella, Salmonella, Campylobacter, Yersinia enterocolitica*, invasive *E. coli*, and *Vibrio parahaemolyticus*. Liver function tests may be used as an adjunct to delineate hepatic involvement. Urinalysis may provide information on renal function, hydration status, and infection. CBC, blood cultures, and extensive stool studies or cultures may be indicated in severe disease or immunocompromised patients.

Management. The use of IV rehydration acutely in diarrheal illness has become commonplace because of the role that fluid and electrolyte abnormalities play in this setting. In some cases, oral management may be used in diarrhea associated with volume depletion. Oral rehydration therapy is most appropriate in the UC setting. It has been shown to be safe and effective in the pediatric population with acute gastroenteritis and volume depletion.[12] Oral rehydration may be a lengthy process and may not be appropriate for all settings. If significant dehydration is evident, transfer of care to a tertiary care facility may be warranted. A simple algorithm for the management and treatment of acute gastroenteritis is shown in Figure 2.

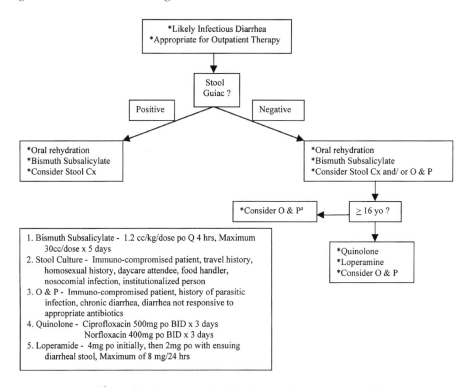

Figure 2.   Management and treatment of acute gastroenteritis.

Pitfalls in Practice. Serious sequelae may result from prolonged and extensive volume depletion. Aggressive management should be initiated early and referral made when necessary.

Constipation

The presenting complaint of constipation is common in the pediatric population. Constipation is defined by a combination of three factors: (1) stool consistency, (2) stool frequency, and (3) physical examination. Alteration in the patient's norm for stool consistency and frequency, in conjunction with the physical exam finding of a large fecal mass in the rectum, confirms the diagnosis of constipation. The patient's age and etiology of constipation make the clinical presentation highly variable.

Diagnosis. A detailed history and physical examination generally reveal the diagnosis of constipation. Flat and upright radiographs may be helpful. In all age groups evaluation for decreased oral intake, anal fissures, systemic illness, and an acute surgical problem as the inciting reason for constipation is required.

Management. If no specific etiology is discovered, symptomatic treatment may be initiated. Increased oral hydration and a gentle laxative is an appropriate treatment option for the UC physician. Increased dietary fiber should be suggested for prevention.

Pitfalls in Practice. Constipation is a common and generally benign problem. It is important to not dismiss a more serious presenting complaint as constipation.

The Acute Abdomen

The diagnosis of the acute abdomen continues to be a challenge for primary physicians and is particularly difficult in children. A consistent approach to evaluation is the key to diagnosis, including a thorough history, associated symptoms, physical examination, and ancillary testing. Surgical consultation should be considered early, particularly in the UC setting, where transportation delays may be encountered. It is important to recognize that both surgical and medical conditions produce an acute abdomen, and early distinction between the two is essential.

Important historical features include characteristics of the pain and location (with changes), radiation, intensity, and exaggerating and alleviating factors. Relationship to meals, anorexia, nausea, and vomiting may also be useful. Diarrhea is not usually associated with peritoneal involvement.

Examination of the pediatric patient with abdominal pain may be difficult. Time, reassurance, patience, and observation are useful adjuncts to gentle palpation. Rectal examination is essential including occult blood studies.

Diagnosis. Laboratory and radiographic exams may include CBC, electrolytes (with associated volume loss history), flat and upright abdomen films, and an upright chest radiograph. Extended testing may add liver function tests, serum amylase and lipase, abdominal ultrasound or computed tomography, or barium (or air contrast) enema.

Common causes of abdominal pain in all age groups of the pediatric population include acute gastroenteritis, appendicitis, Meckel's diverticulum, intestinal obstruction (various etiologies), and trauma. The causes of abdominal pain in the infant age group are extended to include intussusception, volvulus, necrotizing enterocolitis, and colic. The adolescent years involve diagnoses including peptic ulcer disease, cholecystitis, inflammatory bowel disease, pregnancy, and pelvic inflammatory disease. Pyelonephritis, pancreatitis, and pneumonia may also present with an acute abdomen.

Management. The determination of the need for surgical intervention is the goal of the clinician in managing acute abdominal pain. Once the need for surgery is established, adequate volume status and electrolyte replacement is necessary. Nasogastric intubation may be needed for vomiting or abdominal distention. Antibiotics are required for suspicion of perforation. Frequent re-examination is recommended for acute changes (e.g., perforation, instability), until transfer of definitive care is made.

Pitfalls in Practice. The acute abdomen is a true surgical emergency. Transfer of care should be arranged early, and surgical intervention should be coordinated promptly.

Acute Appendicitis

Appendicitis is the most common surgical condition of children. Perforation occurs in up to 40% of patients, with infants and toddlers more often affected. Classical presentations are rare, and atypical features are exacerbated by the patient's inability to elaborate the history of the illness.

Low epigastric or periumbilical pain, with intermittent cramping is the typical initial history. Generally within 4–6 hours (range: 1–12), the pain localizes in the right lower quadrant. Anorexia is essentially invariable, and vomiting occurs in the majority of patients. The classic sequence of events is anorexia, pain, then vomiting. Examination reveals right lower quadrant tenderness (McBurney's point) with or without rebound and guarding. Rectal exam may elicit tenderness on the right lateral wall. Psoas and obturator signs, pain with extension of the right thigh while lying on the left side, and pain with passive rotation of the flexed thigh in the supine position respectively, may be present depending on the location of the appendix. In young children, examination may reveal an ill-appearing child, often in the fetal position, reluctant to change position. A diffusely tender abdomen is generally present with minimal or absent bowel sounds. Respiratory symptoms or distress may be present.

Diagnosis. No ancillary examination has been found to be statistically or clinically sensitive and specific for the diagnosis of appendicitis. Mild elevation in the WBC count with a left shift is suggestive, but significant elevation is not classically associated with the diagnosis. Abdominal radiographs are useful if a fecolith is noted, or other signs are seen suggestive of an alternative diagnosis. Computed tomography may be useful when special protocols are used (i.e., triple contrast).

Management. Definitive management is operative, after initial resuscitation if necessary. Intravenous access should be obtained, and fluids initiated if evidence of hemodynamic instability is present. If perforation is documented or suspected, parenteral antibiotic therapy should be initiated with coverage of gram-negative aerobic and anaerobic bacteria.

Pitfalls in Practice. Infants and toddlers may go undiagnosed or be misdiagnosed until perforation occurs. If considered within the differential diagnosis, appendicitis must be actively pursued, and transfer to an ED coordinated.

Intussusception

Intussusception is the most common cause of bowel obstruction in children between the ages of 3 months and 6 years. Intussusception is the telescoping of one segment of bowel into a more distal segment, most frequently ileocolic. If not recognized and treated early, edema of the bowel wall leads to ischemia and potential necrosis with its complications. The lead point of the intussusception is thought to be due to hypertrophied Peyer's patches (secondary to preceding viral infection), lymphoma, Meckel's diverticula, polyps, or redundant bowel.[12]

The clinical features vary, but classically the child has a preceding viral illness. The child then experiences recurrent brief episodes of marked irritability and apparent abdominal pain with the onset of symptoms. Episodes of spasm are marked by flexion of the thighs into the abdomen with crying; then the child returns to a relatively normal or lethargic state in the interim. Vomiting and diarrhea are common, and the classic currant jelly stool is passed as ischemia of the bowel occurs. A "sausage-shaped" mass may be palpated representing the intussuscepted bowel.

Diagnosis. A thorough history is generally the key to diagnosis of intussusception, including directed physical examination. Laboratory tests (CBC, electrolytes, type and crossmatch, and blood cultures) may be useful if sepsis is suspected in the ill-appearing child. Abdominal flat and upright films may display radiographic evidence of bowel obstruction with air-fluid levels, an intraabdominal mass, or free air if perforation has occurred. In highly suspicious cases, barium enema is the initial examination of choice as it is both diagnostic and therapeutic in the majority of cases. As barium is passed into the colon and up to the intussuscepted bowel, the hydrostatic pressure often reduces the segment. The same results may be obtained with an air-contrast enema. If perforation is clinically suspected, barium should not be used; a water-soluble contrast should be substituted.

Management. As discussed, the diagnosis and treatment typically occur with a barium enema. The rate of recurrence after barium enema ranges between 1 and 10%.[12] Reduction with a second enema may be attempted, but failure or a third recurrence generally necessitates operative management. Surgical consultation should be obtained early, particularly if the course has been protracted or if perforation is suspected.

Pitfalls in Practice. Symptoms may be present for a variable time period. If the diagnosis is delayed, the child may become extremely ill quite rapidly. Notification of the surgeon is necessary, and transfer to definitive care should be arranged early.

Volvulus

Intestinal volvulus is commonly associated with the congenital anomaly of malrotation of the midgut or an abnormal mesenteric attachment. As a result, this loosely adherent bowel has the potential to rotate about the free axis and create a volvulus. Malrotation with volvulus may occur in utero, or more commonly in the neonatal period. However, it may not occur until childhood, when the diagnosis is less suspect.

In the neonate, bilious vomiting, apparent constant abdominal pain, and the delayed passage of bloody stools suggests midgut volvulus. Examination reveals varying degrees of abdominal distention and tenderness, and two prominent loops of bowel may be appreciated on abdominal palpation. Gross blood on rectal examination is concerning for significant ischemia and possible necrosis of bowel.

Diagnosis. Laboratory testing is generally not useful in diagnosis, except in preparation for surgical management or in ill-appearing patients. Decreased small bowel gas, small bowel loops superimposed on the liver, and a "double-bubble sign" (distention of the stomach and first part of the duodenum) are radiographic evidence of midgut volvulus. A barium enema may display abnormal positioning of the cecum; an upper GI study may reveal a lack of the typical duodenal C-loop. Both findings are suggestive of malrotation.

Management. Once the diagnosis of midgut volvulus is seriously considered, surgical consultation should be obtained. Preparation for intervention should include basic laboratory studies including blood type and crossmatch, IV rehydration, and nasogastric intubation for decompression.

Pitfalls in Practice. In less than four hours a neonate may undergo irreversible ischemia and necrosis of the midgut. If surgical correction is not prompt, the entire small bowel and ascending colon may be lost.

Gastrointestinal Foreign Bodies

Children may present to the UC setting with a history of swallowing a foreign object. Food, coins, button batteries, and safety pins are common offenders. No history of foreign body (FB) ingestion can be elicited in many cases, and this finding complicates the diagnosis. Morbidity is associated with the specific characteristics of the object (i.e., size, shape, and "edges"). Elongated, rigid, or sharp objects are most frequently associated with perforation of the GI tract. It is essential for the clinician to differentiate between a swallowed foreign body and one that has been aspirated.

Symptoms vary based on the location of the object at presentation. Acute symptoms of swallowed objects include esophageal complaints, dysphagia, and increased salivation. The inability to handle secretions suggests complete esophageal obstruction, and may result in aspiration. Similarly, a large esophageal FB may compromise a patient's airway, necessitating emergent management. Subcutaneous emphysema and substernal or back pain suggest esophageal perforation.

The longstanding presence of an esophageal FB can present as failure to thrive, diminished oral intake, or wheezing due to tracheal compression. Foreign objects in the pharynx or that have been aspirated can present with hoarseness, stridor, cough, respiratory distress, or an asymmetric lung examination. Passage of the swallowed object through the GI tract does not ensure relief of symptoms, because the FB may have caused abrasions or lacerations of the esophagus. More importantly, relief of symptoms does not ensure passage of the object into the stomach. If the FB does pass into the stomach, the majority will be eliminated spontaneously and asymptomatically. Obstruction or perforation are possible complications, and are suggested by increased or significant abdominal pain, recurrent vomiting, or bleeding.

Diagnosis. In the unstable patient, with a presumed diagnosis of esophageal or pharyngeal FB, airway management and transfer for definitive care are emergent. In the stable patient, neck, chest, and/or abdominal films are appropriate for identification and location of the FB. Endoscopy is the ideal for diagnosis and management.

A posteroanterior (PA) chest x-ray may be helpful in locating the foreign object. For flat objects (e.g., coins), the presence of the object's lateral aspect (edge) on a PA film suggests tracheal placement. A flat surface suggests esophageal placement. Not all objects can be seen on x-ray, but other radiographic findings may be helpful. Mediastinal shift away from the side of the aspirated object, or a hyperinflated lung represent a one-way valve mechanism created by the object as it obstructs expiratory air flow.

Management. Diagnosis of pharyngeal or esophageal FB in the stable patient requires early endoscopic treatment, if no evidence of perforation is found. Perforation at any level of the GI tract requires urgent operative management. If the object has passed into the stomach or proximal duodenum, endoscopic evaluation is recommended. Attempts at treatment with emetics, cathartics, or otherwise is not recommended. Once the object is distal, observation with strict stool inspection is the treatment of choice. Close follow-up is required, particularly if symptoms develop or if passage does not occur within less than 5 days.

Pitfalls in Practice. Failure to recognize potential airway compromise or perforation can be devastating. The missed diagnosis of FB may result in late sequelae such as fistulas or abscesses. Diligence in diagnosis is essential. "Button" batteries offer a unique concern in management due to their potential for alkaline leaks, and patients with a suspected or documented button battery ingestion should be referred immediately.

Hypertrophic Pyloric Stenosis

Hypertrophic pyloric stenosis (HPS) affects male infants more often than females and should be considered in the differential diagnosis of infants with nonbilious vomiting, particularly if it is projectile. The course of the disease is usually protracted compared with infectious causes of vomiting. The cause is unknown, but a family history is often present. A typical presentation is a male infant less than 6 weeks old with persistent vomiting, visible peristalsis, dehydration and a palpable mass, or "olive," in the epigastrium.

Diagnosis. Laboratory tests reveal a hypochloremic, hypokalemic alkalosis. Abdominal ultrasound is generally thought to be the study of choice, with barium swallow following if the ultrasound is inconclusive or unavailable. Further testing should be in preparation for surgery.

Management. Rehydration and correction of acid-base and electrolyte abnormalities is appropriate. The patient should avoid oral ingestion, and surgical consultation should be obtained. Pylomyotomy is the classic corrective procedure.

Pitfalls in Practice. Dehydration and metabolic derangement can be severe if the diagnosis is not recognized. Prompt referral to an appropriate center is necessary.

Intestinal Colic

A common cause of crying in the neonate is intestinal colic (IC). Usually IC occurs in the healthy infant between the second week and third month of life. Infants typically flex at the hips, drawing the lower extremities up to the chest, crying, and pass flatus with relief of symptoms.

Diagnosis. Understandably, the diagnosis should be treated as one of exclusion. A detailed history and physical is warranted, with any indicated laboratory or radiographic examinations. CBC, electrolyte panel, and urinalysis may be helpful in excluding more serious diagnoses.

Management. Reassurance is frequently the treatment of choice. Suggestions to parents are supportive in nature. If the diagnosis is in doubt, admission may be warranted for monitoring and supervised feedings. Close follow-up with the primary pediatrician is necessary.

Pitfalls in Practice. It is essential to look for and exclude more serious illness before the diagnosis of intestinal colic is made.

Crying Infants

Parents who present infants for medical evaluation of excessive crying are rightly concerned about the possibility of serious illness in a child who cannot communicate the cause of distress. Parents are usually exhausted and fearful by the time they decide to bring their child to a health care provider. Parental anxiety and the infant's inability to assist in the history or physical make the assessment of the crying infant a challenge for physicians. A persistently crying infant should be assumed to be in pain; the challenge for the UC physician is to determine its cause.

History and Physical Examination. Pertinent aspects of the history include characterization of the current crying episode compared with the infant's prior behavior. The onset of the episode, circumstances surrounding the onset, its duration, the ability for the infant to be consoled, associated symptoms, and history of recent vaccinations, trauma, illness, or infectious exposure may provide some clues to the diagnosis. In infants, early sepsis, meningitis, an acute abdomen, metabolic abnormalities, and occult trauma are just a few serious pathologies that may present with no other history or symptoms besides crying.[14] The physical examination should be meticulously done, with careful attention to possible occult trauma or illness. Ancillary diagnostic testing should be directed by the findings on physical examination. Once serious illness or injury has been ruled out, attention should be directed at less serious causes of crying. Table 5 lists considerations in the differential diagnosis of the crying infant.

Management. The management of the crying infant depends on identified etiologies. The most difficult disposition decision is for the irritable, inconsolable infant for whom no cause for crying has been determined. Poole et al. determined that the majority of crying infants who cannot be consoled and for whom no cause can be found harbor serious pathology.[15] Such children are therefore at high risk and may require observation until the cause of crying becomes apparent.[14]

Pitfalls in Practice. It is easy and tempting to cut short the physical examination of a disruptive patient, and the crying infant certainly may fall into this category. It is also easy to minimize parental concern, especially for first-time parents. Failure to consider serious causes or arranging appropriate follow-up for the crying infant may result in substantial morbidity.

Child Abuse and Neglect

Child abuse and neglect present unique challenges to physicians and health care personnel. The diagnosis is complicated by the frequent desire of caretakers or parents to conceal or ignore the origin of an injury or other problems, and there is a natural discomfort on the part of caregivers to confront parents with their suspicions. Once a report of suspected abuse or neglect is made, formidable difficulties are inherent in the social management of the problem. Nevertheless, it is a caregiver's ethical obligation to protect children in cases of suspected abuse or neglect. This obligation has been legislated into the legal code of every state, requiring all cases of suspected or known physical abuse to be reported. In addition, some jurisdictions require that activities such as prostitution by a juvenile be reported under the child abuse laws. Reporting laws do not require the

Table 5. Differential Diagnosis of the Crying Infant

Emergent Diagnoses		Urgent
Infection	**Medical/Surgical**	**Infection**
Meningitis	Cardiovascular	Otitis media
Encephalitis	Supraventricular tachycardia	Herpes stomatitis
Sepsis syndrome	Congenital abnormality	Oral thrush
Pneumonia	Gastrointestinal	Gastroenteritis
Urinary tract infection	Dehydration secondary to	Cellulitis
Osteomyelitis	gastroenteritis	Insect bites
Septic arthritis	Intussusception	Herpangina
	Volvulus	
Trauma	Appendicitis	**Trauma**
Nonaccidental	Bowel perforation—traumatic	Hair tourniquet
Intracranial bleeds, skull fracture	Infectious, ischemic	Digit
Rib fracture, pneumothorax	Ophthalmologic	Penis
Long bone fracture	Congenital glaucoma	Clitoris
Intraabdominal blunt trauma	Genitourinary	Open diaper pin
Accidental (i.e., falls, motor	Incarcerated hernia	
vehicle accident)	Torsion of testis	**Medical**
Skull fracture	Urinary tract infection	Postvaccine pain: diphtheria-pertussis-tetanus
Extremity fracture	Heme	Gastroesophageal reflux
Birth trauma	Sickle cell anemia and crisis	Foreign body
	Neglect	Oral
Metabolic	Starvation/infestation	Nasal
Inborn errors of metabolism		Ear
Electrolyte abnormalities		Pharynx
Acid/base derangements		Eye
Hypoglycemia		Corneal abrasion
		Teething
Toxic		Colic
Salicylate toxicity		
Illicit drug exposure (child abuse)		**Behavioral/Miscellaneous**
Inadvertent overdosage:		Feeding
decongestants, anti-		Milk allergy
histamines, beta agonist		Parental anxiety
Inadvertent drug exposure		Environmental stress
Carbon monoxide problems		Idiopathic

Adapted from Troncinski DR, Pearigen DD: The crying infant. Emerg Med Clin North Am 16:895–910, 1998.

reporter to have proof of abuse but rather "suspicion," "reason to suspect," or some other similar concept. Hence physicians, nurses, hospital administrators, or their agents are required to report suspected abuse or neglect.

Differential Diagnosis. Unless abuse or neglect is part of the presenting history, this diagnosis is most often considered when inconsistencies exist between the history and the findings of the physical examination. This is especially true for physical abuse. Factors that should be considered include characteristics of the child (Table 6), characteristic of the parent or caretaker (Table 7), and the nature of the injury or other problem (Table 8).

The medical evaluation of suspected abuse and neglect is summarized in Table 9. It is best to perform a sexual abuse evaluation in a setting that has a well-established protocol and experience with this problem unless injuries that require immediate attention are

Table 6. Common Indications of Child Physical Abuse or Neglect

Presence of unexplained injuries	Unusual degree of concern for parents' emotional needs
Evidence of repeated or unexplained injuries in the past	Parents offer a history of being physically abused
Extremes of interpersonal behavior	Repeated vague physical complaints
• Very aggressive or very withdrawn	
• Very fearful or fearless	

Table 7. Common Characteristics of Abusive Caretakers

History given does not explain injury or condition or contradicts physical examination findings	Cause of injury projected onto another individual
	Unrealistic expectations of child
Undue delay in seeking care	Loss of control
Excessive or insufficient level of concern for child	Concern about own needs greater than concern for those of child
Emotional detachment from child	Hospital or physician "shopping"
Reluctance to provide information	Excessive stress or depression
History given of repeated injuries to child	Childhood history of abusive home

Table 8. Types of Child Abuse and Neglect

Abuse causing cutaneous injury	Neglect
• Ecchymoses (multiple, variable ages: patterns reflecting instrument used)	• Emotional
	• Nutritional
• Bites	• Medical
• Hair loss	• Safety
• Burns (hot water immersion, cigarette, iron, hair curlers)	• Educational
	• Physical (clothing, shelter, hygiene)
Abuse causing skeletal injuries	Sexual abuse
• Long bone fractures (shaft, transverse, or spiral; metaphyseal)	• Penile-vaginal penetration or contact
	• Oral-genital contact
• Rib fractures	• Penile-rectal penetration or contact
• Skull fractures	• Sexual touching, fondling
• Other (small bones of hands, feet; scapula, spine)	• Exposure
	• Exposure to pornography
• Dislocation (especially in infants)	• Other sexual activity
Abuse causing internal soft tissue injuries	Other types of abuse
• Central nervous system (direct trauma, shaken baby syndrome)	• Emotional abuse
	• Intentional poisoning (drugs, water, other)
• Abdomen (solid or hollow organs)	• Munchausen's syndrome by proxy

present. The UC physician should be aware that sexual abuse in children is usually associated with subtle or no physical findings. Thus the diagnosis should not be dismissed solely because there are no physical findings. Cultures for sexually transmitted diseases are indicated.

The interview should focus on events leading to the patient's visit and should include details of where the patient was, who else was present, who was responsible for supervision, and the precise mechanism of any injury. Inquiries are accepted more readily if they

Table 9. Medical Evaluation for Child Abuse

Physical abuse: thorough history and physical examination
- Identify all individuals present or responsible for child during abuse
- Describe all physical evidence of injury in detail
- Laboratory: coagulation panel, platelet count, and other studies as indicated (e.g., urinalysis, electrolytes, toxicology)
- Radiographic studies: long bone, chest, skull if abuse present in child < 3 years or if fracture present; bone scan if x-rays negative and fracture suspected

Neglect
- Thorough history and physical examination
- Growth parameters and nutrition assessment as indicated

Sexual abuse
- Examination < 72 hours since last abuse
- Full evidentiary examination
- Document appearance of external genitalia, hymen; results of wet prep and potassium hydroxide prep; results of gonococcal culture (throat, rectum, and vagina) and chlamydia (rectum and vagina) culture

are made in a sensitive, nonaccusatory fashion. The past history of injuries, hospitalizations, chronic medical problems, and behavior problems should also be sought.

Management. The initial social management of child abuse and neglect is suggested in Figure 3. The goals of management are to provide treatment for medical problems as needed, to report to the appropriate protective or law enforcement agency, and to provide a safe environment for the child. Hospitalization is not always necessary, although in many settings it may be the best option even in the absence of specific medical necessity.

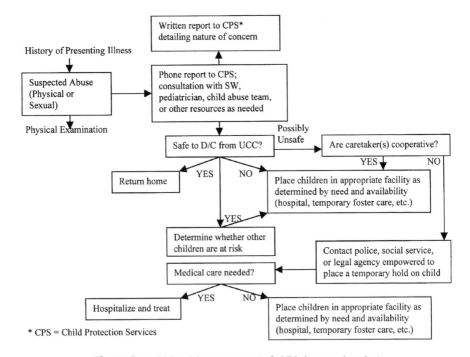

Figure 3. Initial social management of child abuse and neglect.

In almost all cases, it is preferable to discuss specific conclusions about abuse with the parents. Only in cases in which they are unavailable or present a real threat to health care givers should this not be done. Parents should be approached with a therapeutic and sympathetic attitude. The focus of the discussion should be everyone's concern for the health and safety of the child. It is also appropriate to convey the physician's legal responsibility to report a fact, which puts the focus on "the law."

Pitfalls in Practice. A willingness to accept the fact of child abuse and neglect is essential for health care providers. Recognition that, if suspected abuse goes unreported, the child is at a high risk for serious morbidity or even death should motivate UC physicians to report all suspected cases.

Intuition is often the first indication that something is wrong. These "gut feelings" should lead one to pursue the issue further. When addressing concerns, physicians should always have the welfare of the child as their primary concern; however, it is a mistake to assume that the parents do not share the same concern.

References

1. Slater M, Krug SW: Evaluation of the infant with fever without source: An evidence based approach. Emerg Med Clin North Am 17:97–126, 1999.
2. Graneto JW, Soglin DF: Maternal screening of childhood fever of by palpation. Pediatr Emerg Care 12:183–184, 1996.
3. Klassen TP, Rowe PC: Selecting diagnostic tests to identify febrile infants less than 3 months of age in being at low risk for SBI: A scientific overview. J Pediatr 121:671–676, 1992.
4. Jaffe DM, Fleisher GR: Temperature and and total WBC as indicators of bacteremia. Pediatrics 87:670–674, 1991.
5. Crain EF, Bulaz D, Bijur PE, et al: Is chest radiography necessary in febrile infants less than eight weeks of age? Pediatrics 88:821–824, 1991.
6. Baraff LJ, Bass JW, Fleisher GR, et al: Practice guideline for the management of infants and children 0 to 36 months of age with fever without source. Pediatrics 91:1–12, 1993.
7. Bosker G: Acute Otitis Media (AOM) Year 2000 Update. A rational and evidence based analysis of current controversies in antibiotic therapy and drug selection. Emerg Med Rep 21(7,8):75–94, 2000.
8. Rosenfield RM, Vertrees JE, Carr J, et al: Clinical efficacy of antimicrobial drugs for AOM: Meta-analysis of 5400 children from 33 randomized trials. J Pediatr 154:355–367, 1994.
9. Hoppe JE, Koster S, Bootz F, et al: Acute masoiditis: Relevant once again. Infection 22:178–182, 1994.
10. Wolf SM, Carr A, Davis DC, et al: The value of phenobarbital in the child who has had a single febrile seizure: A controlled prospective study. Pediatrics 59:378–385, 1977.
11. Glass RI, et al: Estimates of morbidity and mortality rate for diseases in American children. J Pediatr 118:S27, 1991.
12. Fleisher GR, Ludwig S: Textbook of Pediatric Emergency Medicine, 3rd ed. Baltimore, Williams & Wilkins, 1993, p 135.
13. Weber AL, Oh KS, Watts FB: Radiologic examination of the gastrointestinal tract in infants and children under 4 years of age. Radiol Clin North Am 9:5, 1971.
14. Trocinski DR, Pearigen PD: The crying infant. Emerg Med Clin North Am 16:895–910, 1998.
15. Poole SR: The infant with acute, unexplained, excessive crying. Pediatrics 88:450, 1991.

Appendix: Pediatric Triage

Marc Martel, MD
Cara Ellman Black, MD
Michelle H. Biros, MS, MD

Immediate intervention and transfer is required for the following:

Obstructed airway
- For a patient < 1 yr with an ineffective cough, alternate 4 back blows with 4 chest thrusts.
- For a patient > 1 yr with an ineffective cough, administer 4–6 abdominal thrusts until obstruction relieved.
- Do not perform finger sweep blindly.

Respiratory distress
- Supplemental oxygen, cardiac monitor, pulse oximeter.

Hemodynamic instability
- Supplemental oxygen, cardiac monitor, pulse oximeter, IV.

Multisystem trauma
- Evaluate airway, breathing, circulation; intervene as exam dictates.
- Immobilize (cervical collar, background).

Allergic reaction
- Epinephrine, 0.01 mg/kg (0.1 ml/kg) of 1:10,000 IV over 5 minutes (0.3 ml maximum), for wheezing, diffuse skin reaction and hemodynamic instability.
- Diphenhydramine for itching.

Seizure
- Supplemental oxygen, cardiac monitor, pulse oximeter.
- Benzodiazepines are first-line anticonvulsants: (1) diazepam (Valium), 0.3 mg/kg IV/IM, or 0.3–0.5 mg/kg PR; (2) lorazepam (Ativan), 0.1 mg/kg IV/IM/PR; (3) midazolam (Versed), 0.2 mg/kg IV/IM.

Prompt referral is recommended for the following:

Dermatologic conditions
- Purpura of uncertain origin (rule out meningococcemia)
- Maculopapular rash consistent with Kawasaki's disease, staphylococcal scalded skin syndrome, toxic shock syndrome.

Neonates (< 30 days old)
- Hyperbilirubinemia
- Temperature > 100.4°F
- Vesicular rash

Neurologic/neurosurgical conditions
- Altered mental status
- Traumatic closed head injury with neurological deficits, loss of consciousness, pupillary asymmetry
- Near drowning

Ophthalmologic conditions
- Perforated globe (cover with hard eye shield)
- Traumatic hyphema
- Lid margin laceration
- Acute decrease in visual acuity

Orthopedic conditions
- Fractures
- Hot or swollen joints
- Potential neurovascular compromise from any cause

Otolaryngologic conditions
- Periorbital cellulitis
- Posttonsillectomy bleeding

Surgical conditions
- Acute abdomen
- Acute scrotum
- Burns (>10% total body surface area; circumferential or across joints; involving face, hands, ears, feet, perineum; electrical; associated inhalation injury)

Chapter 19

Neurology in the Urgent Care Setting

William G. Heegaard, MD, MPH
Christopher L. Baker, MD

Headache

Headache is one of the most common disorders of humankind; in fact, it is the ninth most common reason for visiting a physician. In surveys, 64% of Americans report bothersome headaches at least occasionally and 10% see a doctor episodically for head pain.[1] Headache is generally a benign disorder, but it is the responsibility of the clinician to rule out serious causes in each patient. After serious disease has been excluded, benign causes can be identified and treated. Features of potentially life-threatening headaches are listed in Table 1.

Table 1. Features of Worrisome Headaches

First or worst headache of one's life	Headache associated with systemic symptoms
Change in established headache pattern	(fever, weight loss, polymyalgia, nausea, vomiting)
Abnormalities in the neurologic exam, papilledema,	Severe headache triggered by cough, coitus, or exertion
changes in mentation or consciousness	Headache associated with trauma
New headache onset in later adult life (> 65 years old)	Sudden onset, severe (thunderclap) headache
Pre- or postseizure headache	

Potentially Life-threatening Causes of Headache

Differential Diagnosis. Serious causes of headache can be life-threatening (Table 2). Headache is the main complaint in approximately one-half of patients with brain tumors, and the pain is usually resistant to relief by analgesics. It is rare, however, that headache is the sole finding in such patients.[2] The vast majority have seizure, weakness, cognitive changes, or abnormalities in the neurologic exam.

Posttraumatic headaches can result from a variety of causes, some of which are quite serious and require emergency referral. **Subdural hematoma** refers to a collection of blood in the space between the dura and the brain due to venous bleeding. Some patients can recall no traumatic event or a seemingly minor injury. The patient may present within a few hours after injury. A patient who presents with a headache 2–3 months after trauma may be harboring a chronic subdural hematoma. Chronic subdural hematomas typically present with more subtle findings, including unilateral weakness, alteration in consciousness, change in personality, and cognitive deficits.

Table 2. Potentially Life-threatening Causes of Headache

	Symptoms	Exam	Diagnosis	Treatment
Structural				
Tumor	Subacute and progressive pain, worse in the morning, N/V	Many will have focal deficits or papilledema	CT or MRI of the brain	Surgical Dexamethasone may be used to reduce edema
Subdural hematoma	Trauma recently or in past, common in elderly and alcoholics, cognitive and memory deficits	Many will have focal deficits, decrease in consciousness, trouble with cognition	Noncontrast CT	Surgical vs expectant management depending on the size and acuity Neurosurgical consultation mandatory
Epidural hematoma	Recent trauma with initial decrease in consciousness, recovery, and then subsequent decline	Most will have decreased level of consciousness and a focal exam	Noncontrast CT	Surgical
Infectious				
Meningitis	Fever, stiff neck, photophobia, altered mental status In children and elderly, symptoms more nonspecific Meningococcus can cause a characteristic rash	Nuchal rigidity, positive Brudzinski and Kernig signs, some may have focal signs	Lumbar puncture (LP)	Antibiotics (see text)
Encephalitis	Psychiatric changes, cognitive trouble, photophobia, fever	Memory difficulty, aphasia, confusion, depressed LOC	CT or MRI, LP, EEG	Supportive care Herpes encephalitis should be treated with acyclovir
Brain abscess	Nonspecific: headache, fever, neck stiffness, weakness, numbness, N/V; confusion may be present	Variable. Some will have fever, meningeal signs, papilledema, focal deficits, sinus tenderness, otitis, pneumonia	Contrast CT or MRI	Antibiotics, surgical drainage
Vascular				
Subarachnoid hemorrhage	Sudden, severe headache; may have neck pain as well	Focal signs, decreased LOC, although exam may be normal	Noncontrast CT followed by LP if CT is negative	Neurosurgical
Stroke	Acute onset of weakness, numbness, aphasia	Depends on location of stroke. Focal weakness or sensory changes, neglect, dysarthria, decreased LOC, dysmetria, and cranial nerve findings may be present	Largely clinical Noncontrast CT will differentiate ischemic from hemorrhagic	Hemorrhagic strokes require surgical consultation Anticoagulation and antiplatelet drugs are used to treat ischemic infarcts, and treatment is best initiated by a neurologist
Temporal arteritis	Severe throbbing frontotemporal headache, jaw claudication, symptoms of polymyalgia rheumatica Most patients > 50 years old	Tender temporal artery with decreased or absent pulse, sedimentation rate > 50 mm/hr	Temporal artery biopsy	Prednisone 40–60 mg/day must be started early to decrease risk of blindness
Hypertension	History of hypertension, medication noncompliance	Diastolic BP > 130	BP measurement	Lower BP
Carotid/ vertebral dissection	Headache with neck pain following exertion or trauma	TIA or stroke symptoms, cranial nerve palsies, Horner's syndrome, transient monocular blindness	Angiography	Neurosurgical

(Cont'd on next page)

Table 2. Potentially Life-threatening Causes of Headache *(Continued)*

	Symptoms	Exam	Diagnosis	Treatment
Referred Pain				
Sinusitis	Fever, purulent nasal discharge, maxillary toothache	Sinus tenderness, abnormal transillumination	Clinical, sinus CT	Antibiotics
Glaucoma	Blurry vision, eye pain, N/V	Increased intraocular pressure, cloudy cornea, midposition nonreactive pupil	Intraocular pressure measurement	Ophthalmology consultation
Temporo-mandibular disorder	TMJ noise and pain on movement, locking of the jaw, bruxism	Pain over TMJ worse with jaw movement	Clinical	Simple analgesics such as NSAIDs
Miscellaneous				
Pseudotumor cerebri	Young, obese patient with long-standing headache, N/V, oral contraceptive use, thyroid disorders	Normal LOC, nonfocal exam, papilledema	Increased pressure with LP in light of a normal head CT	Neurologic consultation
Trigeminal neuralgia	Paroxysms of severe unilateral pain in the trigeminal nerve distribution lasting seconds	Usually normal	Clinical	Carbamazepine
Post-lumbar puncture	Worse with sitting upright, LP within 24–48 hr	Normal	Clinical	Analgesics If severe, a blood patch may be required

N/V = nausea and vomiting, TMJ = temporomandibular joint, BP = blood pressure, LP = lumbar puncture.

Epidural hematomas are collections of blood between the inner table of the skull and the dura from rupture of the middle meningeal artery or a dural sinus. They typically require forceful trauma and are frequently associated with skull fractures. Symptoms appear within hours and include headache, dizziness, nausea, vomiting, and sleepiness. The classic presentation is head trauma producing a decreased level of consciousness followed by a lucid interval and then subsequent decompensation. This presentation occurs in only about one-third of all cases, however.

Postconcussive headaches may manifest in one-third to one-half of patients with significant head trauma. They may persist many months after the initial trauma and can present with any clinical picture, mimicking migraine, tension, or cluster headache.

Infectious causes of headache include meningitis, encephalitis, and brain abscess. Meningitis must be considered in every patient with headache and fever. Photophobia, malaise, altered sensorium, seizures, vomiting, and chills also may be present. A high level of suspicion must be maintained in the very old, very young, and immunocompromised patients, who commonly have an atypical presentation. Meningitis is commonly viral in origin and patients recover well with only symptomatic treatment. However, bacterial meningitis can be fatal within hours. Antibiotic therapy must be initiated as soon as possible, and it is appropriate to begin antibiotics even before lumbar puncture if meningitis is strongly suspected.

Patients with **encephalitis** typically present with fever, headache and a change in personality. Alteration in consciousness is universally present. Treatable causes include herpes simplex and varicella zoster viruses; prompt referral is mandatory.

Patients with **intracranial abscesses** present with subacute progression of symptoms over 2 or more weeks. Fever and headache are common, although the symptoms are often nonspecific. Meningeal signs, focal deficits, seizures, or signs of increased intracranial pressure (vomiting, papilledema) may be present. Patients may complain of symptoms pointing to potential sites of origin such as sinusitis, otitis media, dental infection, endocarditis, or pneumonia. Diagnosis is made with contrast computed tomography (CT) scanning or magnetic resonance imaging (MRI), and neurosurgical consultation is indicated.

A severe, unusual, acute-onset headache should prompt consideration of **subarachnoid hemorrhage** (SAH). It is classically described as "the worst headache of my life." Many patients have a normal neurologic examination. Others may have decreased level of consciousness or focal deficits. CT scan diagnoses more than 90% of all SAHs; lumbar puncture (LP) is mandatory when the CT scan is negative.[3] Emergent neurosurgical referral is necessary.

Temporal arteritis is an important cause of headache in patients older than 50 years. If left untreated, it can lead to irreversible blindness. The temporal artery is typically tender, swollen, and pulseless. Visual changes are common, as are systemic symptoms such as fever, myalgias, and weight loss. The diagnosis is strongly suggested by an erythrocyte sedimentation rate > 50 mm/hr and confirmed by temporal artery biopsy.

Headache can be associated with **stroke**, although only in approximately one-third of cases. **Hypertension** is a cause of headache, but generally only if the diastolic blood pressure is greater than 130 mmHg. Headache with neck pain after sustained exertion or trauma is characteristic of **vertebral or carotid dissection. Cerebral venous thrombosis** is a rare cause of headache, usually associated with infections, pregnancy, underlying malignancy, connective tissue disorders, or hypercoagulable states.

Pain from various **facial structures** may be referred to the head or directly cause headache. Sinusitis, tooth pain, and glaucoma are examples. Trigeminal neuralgia also may present as headache.

Pseudotumor cerebri is a condition in which intracranial pressure is elevated without mass lesion or hydrocephalus. This condition of unknown etiology can produce severe, nonspecific headaches, sometimes associated with transient visual loss and papilledema. Diagnosis is made with an increased opening pressure on lumbar puncture in the presence of a normal head CT. LP often is therapeutic as well.

After **lumbar puncture**, up to one-third of patients may experience headache. To minimize this complication, evidence supports using smaller needles (27-gauge), pencil-point needles, and minimizing the amount of fluid removed.[4] Treatment includes bedrest for mild cases and steroids or autologous blood patch for severe cases.

Management. The management of potentially life-threatening causes of headache generally requires resources not available in the urgent care setting. Therefore, prompt transfer to a center with adequate capabilities is necessary if any of the above disorders is diagnosed or suspected. Transfer should be made by ambulance with trained personnel because of the potentially life-threatening nature of such entities.

If meningitis is strongly suspected, antibiotics should be initiated before transfer if possible. For adults 18–50 years old, ceftriaxone, 2 gm IV every 12 hours, is the preferred initial antibiotic. Vancomycin may be added if concern exists about resistant streptococcal pneumoniae. If the patient is over age 50, ampicillin, 2 gm IV every 12 hours, should be added to cover *Listeria* spp. Patients with suspected temporal arteritis should receive steroids (prednisone, 1 mg/kg). Pain medication may be given while awaiting transfer.

Subdural and epidural hematomas require urgent diagnosis and potential surgical intervention and thus should be referred emergently to a facility with a CT scanner and neurosurgical expertise. The more recent the trauma, the more urgent the referral. Basilar skull fractures should be referred as well. For a patient with postconcussive headache, the character of the headache should dictate the treatment. Prognosis worsens the longer such headaches persist after the injury.

Pitfalls in Practice. Failure to distinguish serious from benign causes of headache can result in significant morbidity and mortality. Features that should elicit concern are summarized in Table 1. If any doubt exists concerning the benign nature of a particular headache, consultation with a specialist should be obtained. Trauma can lead to intracranial pathology, which potentially requires emergent surgical interventions. Such headaches should not be attributed to a benign process without full investigation.

Primary Headache Disorders

Migraine Headaches

Differential Diagnosis. Migraine headaches are extremely common, with a prevalence of 17.6% in women and 5.7% in men.[5] Recent evidence has implicated dysfunction in the serotonergic system as an important factor in the pathogenesis of migraines.[6] The migraine attack can be divided into five phases: prodrome, aura, headache, resolution, and postdrome.[7] Fifty percent to 80% of migraineurs experience a prodrome hours to several days before the onset of headache.[8] The prodrome may consist of aversion to light, noise, or smells; yawning; drowsiness; irritability; euphoria; increased thirst; polyuria; fluid retention; and food cravings. Approximately 10–20 minutes before the onset of the headache, 10–20% of migraineurs experience an aura.[9] The most common aura consists of visual changes such as scintillating scotoma, light sensitivity, uniform flashes of light, diplopia, and light sensitivity. Other manifestations include hemiparesis, paresthesias, ataxia, tinnitus, vertigo, and dysarthria. The headache is generally characterized as a unilateral, pulsatile pain, although up to 40% may have bilateral pain, and in some instances the pain may be constant. Other characteristics are listed in Table 3. Associated symptoms include nausea in as many as 90% of affected patients. The pain diminishes gradually in the resolution phase. Many have a postdrome of fatigue and limited food tolerance.

Migraines are commonly associated with triggers, which include certain medications (oral contraceptives, nitrites, reserpine, nifedipine, indomethacin, cimetidine, theophylline), menses, exertion, insufficient or excessive sleep, skipped meals, stress, emotional letdown, tobacco smoke, and strong odors.[10] Certain foods, such as alcohol, aged cheese, caffeine, chocolate, monosodium glutamate, meats with nitrites, and sulfites, can provoke an attack as well.

The most common type of migraines is migraines without aura (common migraine) and migraine with aura (classic migraine). Other less common subtypes are often grouped as complicated migraine and involve headaches in which the prodromal neurologic

Table 3. Characteristics of Benign Headaches

	Migraine without Aura	Migraine with Aura	Tension-type Headache	Cluster Headache
Prevalence	Common	Uncommon	Common	Rare
Gender	Females > males	Females > males	Females > males	Males > females
Age at onset	10–30 yr	10–30 yr	20–40 yr; rare after 50 yr	20–40 yr
Family history	Common	Common	Common	Rare
Prodrome	Common	Common	None	None
Aura	None	Present	None	None
Site of pain	Hemicranial/bilateral	Hemicranial/bilateral	Bilateral, occipital, frontal	Unilateral, periorbital
Character of pain	Pulsatile	Pulsatile	Aching, squeezing	Boring, severe
Onset	Gradual			
Onset to peak	Minutes to hours	Minutes to hours	Hours	Minutes
Duration	4–24 hours	4–24 hours	Hours to days	30–90 min
Frequency of attack	Variable	Variable	Variable	Daily during cluster
Associated symptoms	N/V, photophobia, phonophobia, osmophobia, blurred vision	N/V, photophobia, phonophobia, osmophobia	None	Nasal congestion, lacrimation, conjunctival injection, ptosis
Behavior during headache	Still and quiet	Still and quiet	No change	Pace
Nocturnal attacks	Can occur	Can occur	Rare	Frequent

N/V = nausea and vomiting.

manifestations last for the duration of the entire headache. In fact, neurologic deficits may occur in some cases without headache pain.[11]

Management. Nonpharmacologic treatment should begin with a wellness program with emphasis on regular exercise, regular sleeping patterns, and avoidance of alcohol, caffeine, and cigarette smoke. Avoidance of other recognized triggering factors also may prove beneficial. During an acute attack, placing an ice pack on the forehead or temples and finding a quiet environment may decrease the pain in some patients. Biofeedback and relaxation techniques may be useful as well.

Table 4 summarizes the pharmacological agents available for the treatment of acute migraine attacks and other acute primary headaches. Many drugs are effective in the prophylaxis of migraines. Beta blockers remain the treatment of choice, although calcium channel blockers, amitriptyline, valproic acid, methysergide, monoamine oxidase inhibitors, and others have been used with success. Prophylaxis, if successful, reduces the occurrence of migraines by 50%. Prophylaxis should be initiated in the urgent care setting only if reliable follow-up can be ensured, because the above medications have many potentially serious side effects.

Pitfalls in Practice. The most serious potential pitfall is failing to consider the many causes of life-threatening headache in all patients who present with head pain. The urgent care physician should be reluctant to give a patient a first-time diagnosis of benign headache until all other pathology has been excluded. Patients with chronic recurrent headaches (i.e., migraines) are often difficult to distinguish from drug-seekers, but with the new advances in nonaddictive migraine medications, such differentiation is easier. Drug overuse or rebound headaches may be common in this group of patients.

Cluster Headaches

Differential Diagnosis. The essential characteristics of cluster headache are described in Table 3. Attacks are grouped or clustered into periods of weeks or months during which headaches occur at extremely regular intervals, up to 10 times per day. These clusters are followed by remission for months or years. Most patients apply pressure or cold to the area of maximal pain but avoid lying down. Autonomic symptoms occur on the same side as the pain and commonly include lacrimation, conjunctival injection, rhinorrhea, or nasal stuffiness. A partial Horner's syndrome with ptosis and miosis occurs frequently on the side of attack. Cluster headaches are more common in men and commonly begin around age 30.[12]

Management. Treatment for cluster headache uses some of the same techniques that are effective for migraines (see Table 4). Patients should be advised to maintain a regular sleep schedule and to avoid alcohol and stress during a cluster period. Inhalation of 100% oxygen at 7–8 L/min for 15–20 minutes is effective in more than 70% of cases.[13] Ergotamines delivered by an inhaler (Medihaler, 1–3 puffs) or injection (DHE, 1 mg IM or IV) provide good relief for many patients. Sumatriptan may be effective if given near the beginning of an attack. Intranasal lidocaine also can be effective.[14]

Prophylactic therapy has been used to decrease the frequency, severity, and duration of attacks in a cluster period. Prednisone (40–80 mg/day) generally provides relief within 2 days and may be tapered after 1–2 weeks of therapy. Lithium (300 mg 2–4 times/day) can be helpful, although side effects are common and strict monitoring is critical to avoid hypothyroidism and renal dysfunction. Methysergide is now rarely used because of the potential to cause retroperitoneal fibrosis and cardiac valve damage. Other medications used for prophylaxis include calcium channel blockers, valproic acid, and indomethacin. Surgical procedures to ablate various components of the trigeminal nerve or autonomic pathways have been used for intractable cases with varying success.

Pitfalls in Practice. Because cluster headaches may resolve spontaneously, patients may not follow up as scheduled. Thus, prescriptions should not be refillable because many of the above medications can have dangerous side effects.

Tension-type Headache

Differential Diagnosis. Tension-type headaches (TTH) are mild-to-moderate headaches. Typical characteristics are listed in Table 3. Tension-type headaches are not aggravated by routine physical activity, and nausea, vomiting, photophobia, and phonophobia are generally absent. Jaw discomfort, neck pain, tender spots, and cervical or pericranial muscle spasm are present in some patients. Episodic tension-type headache occur less than 15 days per month, whereas chronic TTH averages 15 days or more per month. It was once postulated that TTHs result from muscle contraction; however, muscle contraction is now thought to be a secondary event triggered by abnormalities in central pain control.[15]

Management. Nonpharmacologic treatment modalities include stress management, relaxation techniques, and biofeedback, which can reduce the occurrence of TTHs as

Table 4. Drug Treatment for Acute Primary Headaches *(Columns continue opposite page)*

Drug	Headache	Route	Dose	Rebound
Aspirin	T, M	PO	1 gm every 6 hr	Yes
Acetaminophen	T, M	PO	1 gm every 6 hr	Yes
Ibuprofen	T, M	PO	800 mg every 6 hr	Unlikely
Naproxen	T, M	PO	825 mg, then 550 mg in 3–4 hr	Unlikely
Isometheptene, dichloralphenazone, acetaminophen (Midrin, Isocom)	M, T	PO	2 capsules at onset, can repeat 1 tablet each hr	Yes
Aspirin, butalbital, caffeine (Fiorinal)	M, T	PO	2 tablets at onset, can repeat 1 every 4–6 hr as needed	Yes
Metoclopramide	M, T	PO	10 mg 5–10 min before NSAID	No
Indomethacin	M, T	PR	50–100 mg at onset	Unlikely
Ergotamine tartrate	M, C	PR	1 suppository at onset, can repeat in 1 hr	Yes
Ketorolac	T, M	IM	30–60 mg initially, then 15–30 mg every 6 hr	Unlikely
Prochlorperazine	M	IV, IM	10 mg	No
Chlorpromazine	M	IV	12.5 mg, can repeat every 30 min to total dose of 37.5 mg	No
Dihydroergotamine	M, C	IV, IM	0.5–1 mg IV; can repeat every 8 hr, or 1 mg IM; can repeat every 1 hr	Unlikely
Sumatriptan	M, C	SC, PO, IM	6 mg SC; can repeat once at 1 hr, 100 mg PO; can repeat every 2hr	Likely
Meperidine	M, T, C	IM	Max initial dose 150 mg; can repeat 50–100 mg every 3–4 hr	Yes
Oxygen	C	Face mask	7–8 L/min for 15 min	No

T = tension-type, M = migraine, C = cluster, PO = oral, PR = rectal, IM = intramuscular, IV = intravenous, SC = subcutaneous, GI = gastrointestinal, PVD = peripheral vascular disease, MI = myocardial infarction.

well as the pain of a particular headache. Hot or cold packs, ultrasound, electrical stimulation, trigger point injections, and occipital nerve blocks can be useful in an acute attack.

Symptomatic treatment with acetaminophen, aspirin, or NSAIDs is generally effective (see Table 4). Only in rare cases are combination analgesics or narcotics necessary. Amitriptyline is the first-line medication for prophylaxis, although other tricyclic antidepressants also may be effective. If some features of migraine are present, addition of beta blockers or calcium-channel blockers may increase efficacy.

Pitfalls in Practice. Patients with frequent tension headaches often overuse both prescription and over-the-counter (OTC) medications, leading to analgesic overuse or rebound headache (see below).

Chronic Daily Headache/Drug-Rebound Headache

Differential Diagnosis. Chronic daily headache (CDH), a low-grade daily headache that may develop migrainous features, is associated with near-daily use of prescription or

Table 4. Drug Treatment for Acute Primary Headaches *(Continued)*

Side Effects	Contraindications	Remarks
GI upset	Active ulcer disease, third-trimester pregnancy	
	Liver toxicity with > 4 gm/24 hr	
GI upset	Active ulcer disease, third-trimester pregnancy	
GI upset	Active ulcer disease, third-trimester pregnancy	
Use > 2 day/wk has potential to cause rebound headache	Hypertension, PVD, recent MI	Max = 5/day, 20/month
Drowsiness, dizziness Use > 2 day/wk has potential to cause rebound headache	Active ulcer disease, porphyria	Max = 5/day, 15/month
Dystonic reaction, dizziness	Pheochromocytoma	
Nausea, vomiting, headache, rarely pancreatitis	Proctitis	
Nausea (may need antiemetic pretreatment), overdose can cause vascular occlusion or gangrene, heart valve disease if used for many years, physical dependence	Coronary artery disease, renal failure, hepatic failure, PVD, hypertension, pregnancy	Max = 2/day
GI distress, somnolence, dry mouth, dizziness, palpitations	Active ulcer disease, third-trimester pregnancy, liver disease	
Dystonic reactions (treat with diphenhydramine)		
Dystonic reactions, orthostasis Pretreat with 500 ml normal saline	Pregnancy	
Nausea, cramps, sedation, local reaction Pretreat with antiemetic if given IV	Coronary artery disease, renal failure, hepatic failure, PVD, hypertension, pregnancy	
Weakness, dizziness, flushing, rebound headache May cause chest pain or MI in patients with CAD	Don't use if ergot given within 24 hr, ischemic heart disease, Prinzmetal's angina, uncontrolled hypertension, PVD, hemiplegic or or basilar artery migraine, pregnancy	Max per day = 12 mg SC or 300 mg PO
Tremors, muscle twitches, can cause respiratory depression or seizures in high dose High addiction potential		

T = tension-type, M = migraine, C = cluster, PO = oral, PR = rectal, IM = intramuscular, IV = intravenous, GI = gastrointestinal, PVD = peripheral vascular disease, MI = myocardial infarction.

OTC analgesics. Drug-rebound headaches occur daily or near daily, usually in the morning, and may vary in type, severity, and location. The patient generally uses larger and larger doses of medication with the development of tolerance. Symptoms are perpetuated when the patient discontinues analgesic use. The most common offending agents are ergotamines, narcotics, combination analgesics, NSAIDs, aspirin and acetaminophen. The frequency of use may be more important than the dose.

Management. Withdrawal of the abused analgesic medication is critical. Patients generally have a worsening of headaches for 48–72 hours, followed by gradual improvement. An analgesic wash-out period of up to 8–12 weeks may be necessary. The addition of amitriptyline (10–25 mg) as prophylaxis and an NSAID for breakthrough pain is an effective regimen. Select patients who abuse high doses of narcotics or barbiturates should be referred to a headache specialist for analgesic withdrawal and additional headache management.

Pitfalls in Practice. Analgesic overuse is a common cause of headache, and the clinician can often make the problem worse by prescribing more analgesic medication.

Spells

Patients who present after experiencing "a spell" present a significant diagnostic challenge to the urgent care physician. A spell can be defined as events that involve a change in normal mental status, which can include loss of consciousness that has resolved by the time the patient presents for evaluation. Spells can be categorized as seizures, transient ischemic attacks, syncope, vertigo, and psychological problems.

The key to the diagnostic work-up of spells is a focused but thorough neurologic history and examination with appropriate adjunct tests. Of the six parts of the neurological exam (mental status, cranial nerves, motor response, sensory, coordination, and reflexes), a thorough mental status examination and coordination testing, including gait, are the most often neglected and most informative. Specific tests, such as pronator drift and walking on heels and toes, are often excellent indicators of focal weakness or focal neurologic causes of spells.

Seizure

Differential Diagnosis. Seizures are caused by an abnormal or aberrant electrical discharge of neurons, which result in abnormal neurologic functioning. Approximately 10% of the United States population has at least one seizure during their lifetime.[16]

Seizures are classified most easily into generalized and partial types. **Generalized seizures** can further be classified into absence (petit mal) and tonic-clonic (grand mal) seizures. **Partial seizures** are subclassified into partial simple seizures (without an alteration of consciousness) and partial complex types (with altered consciousness).

The clinical presentation of seizures can vary greatly. Seizure onset may be sudden or proceeded by actual sensations (e.g., nausea, epigastric pain, overwhelming fear). The classic presentation is the **generalized tonic-clonic seizure**, which results in repetitive motor activity involving all motor groups in a symmetrical fashion. Urinary incontinence and tongue biting are common. Duration is typically less than 5 minutes, and the seizure is followed by a postictal period of confusion and lethargy. Some patients display postseizure focal neurologic deficits (e.g., paresis, sensory, changes); however, most deficits resolve within 2 hours. Hemiparesis that persists for any substantial period after a seizure is referred to as Todd's paralysis and usually resolves within 24 hours. Prolonged postictal paresis may be caused by stroke, hemorrhage, or extra-axial hematoma; these clinical entities must be ruled out if suspicion exists. Seizures often cause short-term amnesia.

Patients who have a first-time seizure after the age of 50 years often have an identifiable structural lesion. Generalized tonic-clonic seizures also may be caused by axonal, toxic, or metabolic abnormalities. Nonstructural causes include hyponatremia, hypoglycemia, drug use (e.g., cocaine, stimulants), overdose of medications (e.g., tricyclic antidepressants, isoniazid), and withdrawal from alcohol and benzodiazepines.

Pseudoseizures are nonepileptic or behavioral seizures. They commonly occur in patients who also have epileptic seizures. At times they are impossible to distinguish from true seizures even by experienced neurologists who witness the event. Pelvic thrusting, alternating arm movement, leg kicking, and obvious volatile behavior are correlated with pseudoseizures.[17] In an urgent care setting, it is probably best to document the activity seen or described and to let the patient's primary care physician or neurologist decide the course of evaluation and treatment; if in doubt, the urgent care physician must assume the event to be a real seizure.

Management. Until recently first-time seizure patients were almost always admitted to the hospital. Depending on the patient's history, physical examination, and living situation, some patients can be discharged from the urgent care setting with close neurologic follow-up after an appropriate examination and work-up has been conducted—if they can be watched by a reliable observer. Work-ups include noncontrast CT to rule out possible hemorrhage or hematoma or an MRI if the seizure appears uncomplicated. Further studies that need to be conducted in the urgent care setting include anticonvulsant medication levels, electrolytes, glucose, calcium, magnesium, complete blood cell count, and, in selective cases, a toxicology screen. Lumbar puncture should be considered if an infectious etiology is a possibility. Electroencephalograms (EEGs) are very helpful, but are not generally available. EEGs should be set up within 24–48 hours and are especially helpful in determining whether anticonvulsant medications are needed. Approximately 30% of patients with first-time seizures have recurrent seizures.[18] Decisions about starting anticonvulsants usually should be left to a neurologist. Acute and chronic anticonvulsant therapy is described in Table 5.

TABLE 5. Acute and Chronic Anticonvulsant Therapy

Drug	Initial Dose	Maintenance	Therapeutic Range (µg ml)
Lorazepam	0.1 mg/kg	2 mg/min or less	
Diazepam	0.15 mg/kg	None	
Phenobarbital	15 mg/kg	2–3 mg/kg	20–30
Carbamazepine	None	600–1200 mg/day	8–12
Valproic acid	None	15–60 mg/kg/day	50–100
Phenytoin	18 mg/kg at 50 mg/min IV	5–6 mg/kg/day	10–20
Fosphenytoin	18 PE/kg at 150 mg/min IV	None	10–20

PE = phenytoin sodium equivalent units.

Patients with previous seizures who present to the urgent care setting with a changing seizure pattern should first be interviewed about possible changes in lifestyle, medication use, or any new or sustained alcohol or drug use. Almost all patients who have a therapeutic anticonvulsant level should undergo a thorough urgent neurologic evaluation by a neurologist, and hospital admission is highly recommended with either emergent CT scan or MRI.

If the seizure is due to medication noncompliance, oral loading is appropriate. For phenytoin, use 18 mg/kg orally, divided into two doses 30–60 minutes apart. Carbamazepine should be started at 100 mg orally 2 times/day for 1 week and gradually increased to the original dosage over the ensuing next 2 weeks.

A patient who experiences an alcohol withdrawal seizure may present to an urgent care center. If the examination and work-up are negative for other causes of seizures, diazepam is appropriate for withdrawal symptoms. However, no long-term anticonvulsant therapy is needed for true alcohol withdrawal seizures.[19,20]

On occasion, a patient who develops status epilepticus may be brought to an urgent care facility. Such patients need treatment in an emergency department. While arranging for advanced life support transport, the urgent care physician must stabilize the patient using the ABCs (airway, breathing, and circulation), establish an IV line, and draw blood for measurement of anticonvulsants, electrolytes, and complete blood count. Glucose (25 mg) should be given if the patient's finger-stick glucose reading is low. Thiamine (100 gm) should be considered also. If the patient's airway and breathing are stable, a benzodiazepine should be administered.

Lorazepam is the most effective anticonvulsant for aborting status epilepticus.[21] Phenytoin is an appropriate long-term anticonvulsant after lorazepam has been given. Phenytoin should be infused at a dosage of 18 mg/kg at 25–50 mg/minute with monitoring blood pressure during the infusion. Fosphenytoin (a new variant of phenytoin) can be infused at a faster rate with less hypotension, but its use should be reserved for ongoing status epilepticus unresponsive to conventional benzodiazepine administration. Fosphenytoin is an expensive drug with specific indications. It can be given intramuscularly; in status epilepticus, fosphenytoin should be given IV if prompt venous access is available.[22]

Since 1993, five new anticonvulsant medications have been introduced:[23] felbamate, gabapentin, lamotrigine, tiagabine, and topiramate. In general, immediate drug levels for these agents are not available in most hospitals. Each drug has specific indications, and felbamate has been associated with fatal idiosyncratic aplastic anemia and hepatitis. If patients taking these anticonvulsants arrive at the urgent care center after a seizure, management should be discussed with the on-call neurologist.

Pitfalls in Practice. Common errors in the management of seizures include administration of only phenytoin for status epilepticus without including benzodiazepines, specifically lorazepam, as the first-line medication. If significant sedation is necessary for management, a propofol or a lorazepam drip is appropriate. In this situation, most patients have to be intubated and transferred to an emergency department.

Using large amounts of benzodiazepines can cause intermittent hypoxia. Therefore, the patient's respiratory status needs to be monitored carefully and continuously; a long-term antiepileptic agent should be used after the administration of benzodiazepines; Phenytoin or phenobarbitol is the most appropriate choice. Current literature does not support the use of phenytoin with alcohol withdrawal seizures. It cannot be overemphasized that any structural or infectious cause of seizures must always be considered. The diagnosis of idiopathic epilepsy requires confirmation by an EEG.

Transient Ischemic Attacks

Differential Diagnosis. In sharp contrast to most seizures, transient ischemic attacks (TIAs) are relatively uncommon in younger people, rarely affect consciousness, and usually last 5–30 minutes. By definition, a TIA is a brief neurologic event that results in reversible deficits, which resolve within 24 hours. Approximately 20% of patients who experience a TIA later suffer a stroke.[24]

It is critical to determine the cause of TIAs. Causes include but are not limited to carotid, vertebrobasilar, and cardiac sources. Other causes of TIAs are listed in Table 6. Most TIAs are associated with cerebral atherosclerosis and thrombotic events and thus are usually associated with the distribution one of the carotid arteries. The carotid system includes the anterior, middle, and, in 25% of the population, a posterior cerebral artery. Carotid thrombotic TIAs often present with unilateral sensory and/or motor deficits of the contralateral upper and lower extremities.

Table 6. Common Causes of Transient Ischemic Attack and Stroke

Cardiac embolism	Trauma	Fibromuscular dysplasia
Septal defects	Dissection	Vasculitis
Valve disease	Irradiation with premature	Coagulopathy
Endocarditis	atherosclerosis	Sickle cell disease
		Drug-induced (especially cocaine)

The vertebrobasilar (posterior) circulation consists of the vertebral arteries, posterior cerebral arteries, and cerebellar artery as well as small brainstem arteries. TIAs involving this arterial distribution often result in coordination problems and vertigo. Other signs and symptoms of carotid and vertebrobasilar circulation TIAs are summarized in Table 7.

Table 7. Localization by Symptoms of Transient Ischemic Attack

Carotid Distribution	Vertebrobasilar Distribution
Hemiparesis	Vertigo
Hemisensory deficit	Nystagmus
Aphasia	Diplopia
Amaurosis	Perioral numbness
Cognitive deficits	Incoordination
	Dysphagia
	Persistent vomiting
	Lethargy, stupor, coma

Management. Two critical management decisions need to be made early in the treatment of TIAs. First, is the patient having a stroke? If focality has lasted longer than 30 minutes or significant neurologic deficits are present (e.g., loss of speech, cranial nerve deficits, contralateral extremity paralysis), the urgent care physician must assume a that stroke is in progress. This assumption is important because potentially life-saving therapeutic interventions with thrombolytics are now available. Patients who may be having a stroke must be expediently transported to a hospital with an available neurologist who is qualified to give thrombolytics. Patients should not wait for radiologic imaging at the urgent care center; neuroimaging should be performed at the receiving hospital's emergency department.

The second major decision is whether radiologic imaging should be performed while the patient is at the urgent care center. This decision is based on the character and duration of signs and symptoms, risk assessment for the individual patient, and capabilities of the urgent care center. Radiologic imaging of choice for TIAs still remains the noncontrast CT scan, because the first priority of the urgent care physician is to rule out a cerebral hemorrhage. Although MRI is better at detecting early ischemia, CT scan is more sensitive than MRI in detecting early acute intracranial hemorrhage (subarachnoid, extraaxial, or intracerebral) and therefore is the diagnostic choice in patients presenting with symptoms consistent with either acute TIA or stroke.[24]

Patients presenting to an urgent care setting with a new TIA probably should be admitted to the hospital to evaluate the source of the TIA. Anticoagulation therapy in the urgent care setting should be limited to the use of aspirin (325 mg/day) or ticlopidine (250 mg/orally 2 times/day). The addition of heparin should be discussed with the admitting neurologist; in most cases, heparin should not be started before a noncontrast CT scan is performed.[25]

Blood pressure control in stroke and TIAs is controversial. Most authors recommend treatment only with systolic blood pressure > 230 mmHg, diastolic pressure > 130 mmHg, obvious evidence of left ventricular failure, or evolving stroke pattern.[26–28] Acute reduction of blood pressure may precipitate further ischemic damage to the penumbra region surrounding the ischemic foci. If blood pressure control is initiated, a short-acting beta blocker or sodium nitroprusside should be considered in consultation with a neurologist.[27,28]

Pitfalls in Practice. Not recognizing and quickly referring a stroke patient for potential thrombolytic therapy is a major pitfall. In general, thrombolytic candidates must be treated within 3 hours of the onset of symptoms. Treating hypertension in the setting of focal ischemia can exacerbate a TIA or stroke. Heparinization before a CT scan is fraught with potential problems and should be avoided. Although TIAs are easy to diagnose, the urgent care physician must consider atypical presentations of subarachnoid hemorrhages in the differential diagnosis. Other obvious causes include toxic or metabolic, infectious, and peripheral neurologic disease. Failure to consider other causes of TIA in younger patients can result in missing a potentially reversible cause. Although still low in absolute numbers, the incidence of younger adults suffering TIAs or strokes may be increasing, especially with crack cocaine drug use.[29,30] The causes of stroke in young adults are summarized in Table 6.

Syncope

Differential Diagnosis. From a neurologic perspective, the causes of syncope are quite limited. The primary neurologic question is whether the syncopal event was a seizure. Seizure as a cause of syncope is suggested if an aura preceded the event, a prolonged postictal state exists, or physical signs of a seizure are present (e.g., tongue biting, urinary incontinence). Cardiac dysrhythmias, which can cause inadequate cerebral perfusion, can result in hypoxia-induced seizures, thus allowing syncope and seizures to coexist.

Management. An EEG can be diagnostic for determining that the spell was a seizure rather than a syncopal event. An EEG is indicated during the work-up of syncope if the diagnosis of seizure is seriously entertained. The main goal of a syncopal work-up should be to rule out life-threatening causes of syncope; therefore, a seizure work-up must be done in conjunction with a broad syncopal evaluation.

Pitfalls in Practice. Failure to appreciate a sudden cardiac dysfunction as a cause of syncope can be disastrous. In addition, attributing syncope to a vasovagal episode without considering more serious pathology can result in potential morbidity and mortality.

Vertigo

Differential Diagnosis. Vertigo is an abnormal sensation of movement that affects normal perception of balance. The great majority of patients with vertigo seen in the urgent care setting have peripheral nervous system lesions. After eliminating central nervous system (CNS) and systemic causes, the urgent care physician must decide whether the patient has **benign positional vertigo** (BPV), the most common cause of acute vertigo, or some other disorder. Patients with BPV experience acute attacks with rotational vertigo when they change head position. Diagnosis of BPV is made by the Dix-Hallpike maneuver.[31] The patient is brought rapidly from sitting position to a horizontal position with the head below the plane of the body and laterally positioned. This maneuver causes a reproduction of symptoms and torsional nystagmus toward the affected ear.

Management. Any suspicion of an acute CNS cause of vertigo should trigger a thorough neurologic work-up, which includes a CT scan (if acute hemorrhage is a concern) or MRI scan and a neurologic consultation. If the condition is chronic, consultation with the treating neurologist is indicated before further imaging is performed.

Treatment of systemic causes of vertigo is aimed at the underlying medical problem and should include consultation with the patient's primary physician. Symptomatic treatment of peripheral causes of vertigo often begins with an antiemetic; meclizine, 25 mg IV, is a commonly used medication. Otolith repositioning has been found to be extremely effective in resolving the symptoms of BPV.[32]

Pitfalls in Practice. Urgent care patients with vertigo must receive a thorough history and physical examination to differentiate central, peripheral, and systemic causes of vertigo. Failure to recognize CNS vertigo can lead to delayed diagnosis of potentially life-threatening pathology.

Psychological Spells

Differential Diagnosis. Psychological problems causing abnormal, stereotyped "spells" have certain features that suggest nonorganicity. No type of organic amnesia results in loss of orientation to self. When a patient complains of amnesia and cannot recall his or her name, psychological factors are invariably involved. Psychogenic stupor and coma often can be determined by observing how the patient avoids hitting his or her face when a raised arm is dropped over it. Another method is to wave money in the patient's field of vision and to watch his or her gaze follow it. If cold caloric testing is performed by instilling ice water in the ear, the presence of nystagmus indicates an awake patient; tonic eye deviation or no response is seen in coma. Fugue states and other dissociative states are generally easy to distinguish from neurologic disorders by the maintenance of neurologic function and alteration of the patient's identity as a primary feature. When in doubt, however, the physician must rule out possible serious causes of the event; psychological etiologies of spells are a diagnosis of exclusion.

Pitfalls in Practice. Determining that the cause of a spell is psychological without seriously considering other causes is fraught with problems. Psychological causes of syncope are always a diagnosis of exclusion. Simple diagnostic tests, such as cold calorics, help to differentiate life-threatening pathology from psychological presentations. Failure to refer patients who present with psychological causes of spells to a psychologist or psychiatrist is a disservice.

Neuropathies

Bell's Palsy

Differential Diagnosis. Bell's palsy is the acute onset of unilateral facial nerve weakness. Patients often complain of sudden facial weakness, difficulty with articulation, problems with eye closure, or difficulty with keeping food and water in the mouth. The term Bell's palsy implies an idiopathic etiology; however, facial paralysis can result from a myriad of causes, some of which are serious diseases (Table 8).

Table 8. Differential Diagnosis of Facial Nerve Palsy

Infectious	**Congenital**
Otitis media/mastoiditis	Mobius syndrome
Osteomyelitis of the skull base	Marginal mandibularis palsy
Syphilis	**Neoplastic**
Mucormycosis	Parotid tumor
Infectious mononucleosis	Temporal bone tumor
Tuberculosis	Cholesteatoma
HIV	Cerebellopontine angle tumor
Lyme disease	Leukemia
Inflammatory	Facial nerve schwannoma
Sarcoidosis	Histiocytosis X
Wegener's granulomatosis	**Traumatic**
Guillain-Barré syndrome	Temporal bone fracture
Vascular	Lightning injury
Stroke	**Idiopathic**
Vasculitis	Bell's palsy

A thorough history and physical exam help to rule out the more serious causes of facial paralysis. Dysarthria, aphasia, hoarseness, dysphagia, extremity weakness, visual changes, imbalance, hearing loss, or incoordination suggests a central lesion. Examination should include evaluation of the ear canal (for masses, vesicles, or signs of infection), palpation of the parotid gland for masses, and a complete neurologic evaluation. Any abnormalities on exam other than facial nerve weakness suggest that the condition is not idiopathic and requires further evaluation. Eye closure and the ability to cover the cornea must be evaluated. It is important for prognostic purposes to determine whether the paralysis is complete or partial.

Management. Recent evidence suggests that herpes simplex virus may be related to Bell's palsy.[33,34] Antivirals are recommended by many authorities, even though conclusive studies have yet to prove their effectiveness. Acyclovir, valacyclovir, and famcyclovir are reasonable choices, and the recommended duration of treatment is 7 days.

Corticosteroids have never been conclusively proved to benefit patients with Bell's palsy[33]; however, many experts recommend their use. One suggested course is prednisone, 1 mg/kg for 5 days; the dose is then halved every 2 days for a total treatment duration of 2 weeks.

One area of treatment, which is not controversial, is of eye care. Because of the paralysis, the eyelids do not close completely, and the cornea is therefore at risk of dessication. Artificial tears and eye lubricants provide a protective barrier during the day. At night, ointment can be placed and the eyelids carefully taped closed.

Prognosis is related to the degree of paralysis. Most patients with facial paresis can expect complete return to normal function. However, in cases of complete paralysis, the rate of recovery of complete function is only 60%.[33] Even for those who do not recover completely, most have at least some recovery of function. Typically, function begins to return by 3–4 months after onset.

Pitfalls in Practice. The diagnosis of Bell's palsy is a diagnosis of exclusion. The more serious causes of facial paralysis must be ruled out in every patient, and if worrisome signs or symptoms are present, urgent consultation with an otolaryngologist or neurologist must be obtained.

Guillain-Barré Syndrome

Differential Diagnosis. The only acutely life-threatening peripheral neuropathy is Guillain-Barré syndrome (acute demyelinating polyneuropathy). Symmetrical weakness develops over several days. The weakness typically first involves the legs and then spreads proximally. Deep tendon reflexes are lost. Cranial nerves may become involved, along with respiratory muscles. Autonomic manifestations, including tachycardia, facial flushing, fluctuating blood pressure, and disturbances of sweating, are common. Sensory loss is variable, and sensory exam is often normal. Frequently, patients report an antecedent viral illness, especially gastroenteritis. The cerebrospinal fluid shows an increase in protein with normal cellularity by the end of the first week of symptoms. The cause is unknown.

Management. Guillain-Barré disease requires immediate hospitalization to avoid respiratory collapse and consequences of autonomic instability. Intubation may be required for many patients. Plasmaphoresis may help to shorten the course, as may intravenous immunoglobulin.[35] Steroids have not been shown to be effective.

Pitfalls in Practice. Failure to recognize Guillain-Barré disease can result in rapid decompensation and death from respiratory failure or autonomic fluctuations.

Symmetric Peripheral Neuropathies

Differential Diagnosis. There are many causes of symmetric peripheral neuropathy, some of which are outlined in Table 9. Diabetes mellitus, one of the most common, typically manifests as a predominant sensory, distal, symmetric, small-fiber polyneuropathy, which primarily affects pain and temperature modalities. A large-fiber neuropathy can also occur, affecting vibration and position sense.

Table 9. Causes of Sensory Neuropathies

Metabolic	Drugs	Toxins	Miscellaneous
Diabetes	Pyridoxine	Arsenic	Parainfectious
Uremia	Cisplatin	Acrylamide	Paraneoplastic
Paraproteinemia	Thalidomide	Thallium	Rheumatoid arthritis
Amyloidosis	Isoniazid	Trichlorethylene	

Management. For management of painful sequelae, see Table 10. Aldose reductase inhibitors may be effective therapy for diabetic neuropathy.

Table 10. Treatment of Painful Neuropathies

Drug	Dosing
NSAIDS	Round the clock dosing
Amitriptyline	10–25 mg to start, max 100 mg/day
Carbamazepine	Begin at 100 mg twice daily; can increase
Clonazepam	Begin at 0.5 mg twice daily
TENS	Use as needed

Pitfalls in Practice. A multitude of other conditions can cause symmetric peripheral neuropathy. Some are potentially reversible (such as heavy metal overexposure). All patients require close follow-up after the urgent care evaluation.

Compression Neuropathies

Differential Diagnosis. Nerves can be damaged by repeated wear and tear against firm surfaces, resulting in motor and sensory loss. Common sites of compression include the median nerve at the wrist (carpal tunnel), the ulnar nerve at the elbow, the peroneal nerve at the fibular head, and the tibial nerve at the ankle (tarsal tunnel). Table 11 lists the clinical manifestations of these compression syndromes.

Table 11. Common Entrapment Neuropathies

Nerve	Features	Causes
Median	Numbness of first, second and third fingers; thenar weakness; positive Tinel's and Phalen's signs	Occupation, diabetes, pregnancy, hypothyroidism
Radial	Numbness on dorsum of hand, wrist drop	Lying on outstretched arm
Ulnar	Numbness in fourth and fifth fingers, claw hand, intraosseous atrophy	Pressure or trauma at elbow
Peroneal	Foot dorsum numbness, foot drop, weakness of eversion	Leg crossing
Posterior tibial	Pain and numbness of sole, weak toe flexors	Compression in tarsal tunnel

Management. Treatment of any underlying condition is important. Splinting often alleviates the condition, although in some cases surgical decompression is necessary. NSAIDs may provide symptomatic relief.

Pitfalls in Practice. All patients need close follow-up to ensure resolution of symptoms. Surgical treatment is necessary if conservative management fails.

Back Pain

Back pain is one of the most frequent complaints of patients presenting to urgent care centers. It is estimated that up to 80% of American experience some type of thoracic or low back pain during their lifetime.[36] Back pain is a leading cause of disability in the United States and frequently is due to a work-related injury. For most cases of back pain, management occurs on an outpatient basis unless intractable pain or loss of function occurs. Table 12 lists some causes of back pain.

Table 12. Causes of Back Pain

Visceral Causes (Referred Pain)	Disease of the Spine	Mass Lesions	Trauma
Abdominal aortic aneurysm	Herniated lumbar disc	Epidural or spinal abscess	Fracture
Pancreatitis	Ankylosing spondylitis	Hematoma	Muscular and ligamentous
Prostate disease	Scoliosis	Granuloma	
Renal disease	Degenerative arthritis	Tumor strain	
Bowel obstruction	Facet joint disease	(primary or metastatic)	
Visceral perforation	Spinal stenosis		
Spondylolisthesis			
Spondylosis			
Metastatic cancer			

Thoracic Back Pain

Differential Diagnosis. Although low lumbar back pain is much more common, thoracic back pain is also a frequent complaint. A thorough history and physical exam establish exactly where the thoracic back pain is originating. If the person has been involved in a motor vehicle accident or some other trauma, direct palpation of the spinous processes should be done. If the patient has midline spinous process pain, then thoracic x-rays (both anteroposterior and lateral) may help to rule out fractures. Thoracic spinal fractures commonly occur in the lower thoracic region, with either a direct fracture of the vertebrae or a vertebral compression fracture. Spinal compression fractures in women with known osteoporosis have been estimated to occur in approximately 10% of women over the age of 80 years.[37] Any patient who may have a thoracic fracture needs a thorough physical exam, which includes evaluation of reflexes, upper and lower extremity strength and bowel and bladder function. If any abnormalities are found, the patient should be transferred by ambulance to an emergency department for further evaluation and emergent radiographic imaging.

Most of thoracic back pain involves more localized paravertebral pain, which is often associated with acute musculoskeletal strain. The strain can be quite debilitating and may be associated with acute facet syndrome. Other possibilities include rheumatoid spondylitis, which typically affects young men. Herpes zoster may present as atypical acute thoracic pain with hyperesthesia and pain out of proportion to the physical exam. The pain is not consistent with muscular skeletal pain and is distributed along a dermatome.

Management. If findings are consistent with musculoskeletal pain, the best management is rest and short-term acute pain relief. Short-term narcotic use may be appropriate for acute thoracic muscle spasm and strain. Early follow-up with a primary physician and early initiation of physical therapy also should be arranged. NSAIDs are the mainstay for muscular strain and back pain and should be used if no contraindications exist.

Pitfalls in Practice. Back pain may be a sign of serious systemic illness (Table 13). Failure to consider these may result in delayed diagnosis. Any evidence of neurologic focality associated with thoracic back pain mandates immediate evaluation and often will necessitate transfer to an emergency department.

Table 13. Primary Back Pain Syndromes and Management

Syndrome	Presentation	Etiology	Management
Cord compression	Back pain, progressive limb weakness, bowel or bladder retention or incontinence, sensory deficits, upper motor neuron signs (brisk reflexes, Babinski's sign, spasticity)	Tumor, abscess hematoma	Immediate neurosurgical consultation and transfer for emergent surgery, dexamethasone (10 mg IV) while awaiting transfer
Herniated lumbar disc	Possible history of acute injury, back pain (lumbar, unilateral buttock, sciatic notch, referred to a sacroiliac joint, radiating down posterolateral leg); unilateral radiculopathy (less of foot dorsiflexion, toe extension); L4–S1 sensory losses; diminished or absent ankle reflex	Lifting or bending injury	Bed rest for 2–3 days, NSAIDs, heat, physical therapy
Vertebral fractures	Sudden onset of back pain, history of significant trauma, possible history of systemic disease	Trauma	Immobilize, transport for specialty consultation
Lumbar strain	Relapsing, remitting low back pain, worsened by activity; possible radicular pain; possible myofascial pain	Diagnosis of exclusion	Bed rest for 2–3 days, NSAIDs, heat, physical therapy

Low Back Pain

Differential Diagnosis. Most urgent care patients with low back pain have either mechanical low back strain or herniated disk syndrome. Mechanical low back strain is a diagnosis of exclusion. To differentiate mechanical back pain from back pain secondary to a herniated lumbar disk, a thorough physical exam is essential. The physical exam should include careful motor assessment in the dermatomes of all the lumbar nerves, especially the L5–S1 region, and a full sensory examination.

The straight-leg test can differentiate mechanical from herniated disk back pain. With the patient supine, the leg of the affected side is raised to 60°. If radicular pain is reproduced in a specific dermatome, a herniated disk is suggested. Often a partially positive straight-leg test occurs with the patient in the supine position; therefore, it is sometimes preferable to perform a straight-leg test with the patient seated. When the patient is sitting, the test is performed by extending the leg and knee; if this maneuver again causes pain in the dermatome distribution, a herniated disc is suspected.

In contrast, mechanical back pain is often worsened by activity, located throughout the lower portion of the back, and may or may not radiate into the buttock. There is usually no reported posterior thigh or calf pain, and rest will often resolve the patient's symptoms.

Management. The management of lumbar strain is described in Table 13. Chronic low back pain occurs in patients who have either undergone multiple laminectomies with microdiskectomies, and have degenerative disease (Table 14), or who have had numerous episodes of low back strain. These patients present with significant pain and often have been frustrated with the failure of medical management. The management of these patients includes NSAID administration and early physical therapy. Narcotics are very poor long-term pain relievers for patients with low back pain, and should be avoided. Low back exercises are effective. Individuals with acute or chronic syndromes may benefit from a short course of bedrest Other modalities that have been found to be somewhat effective are use of amitriptyline if no contraindications exist, transcutaneous electrical nerve stimulation and the referral to chronic pain syndrome clinics for long term pain management. If the patient has a primary care provider, that practitioner should be contacted to discuss the treatment plan.

Table 14. Degenerative Diseases of the Spine

Disease	Features	X-Ray Findings
Ankylosing spondylitis	Men affected more often than women; stiffness, limited motion; possible family history of early back pain; possible concurrent Reiter's disease, psoriasis, inflammatory bowel disease, cauda equina syndrome	Sacroiliac degeneration, bony bridging of vertebral bodies (bamboo spine), vertebral body destruction (late)
Facet syndrome	Low back pain: may radiate down legs but not below knees; radiated pain is bilateral, simultaneous	Degenerative; inflammatory lesions of facet joint
Spondylolysis	Common cause of low back pain in young athletic patients	Defect in pars interarticularis (usually bilateral), forward slipping of vertebra on next inferior vertebra (spondylolisthesis)
Spinal stenosis	Low back pain radiating down legs, aggravated by repeated activity	Osteoarthritic changes

Pitfalls in Practice. The responsibility of the urgent care physician is to evaluate carefully the cause of the back pain to ensure that no serious systemic illness is involved. Patients with low back pain often suffer exacerbations. It is easy for a practitioner to label such patients as drug seekers or to minimize their pain, thereby failing to recognize serious pathology.

Herniated Lumbar Disk

Differential Diagnosis. The usual location of a herniated disk involving the nucleus pulposus is the L4–L5 or the L5–S1 region. Usually the inciting event is an acute injury, which may involve lifting or bending. The patient often complains of something popping or snapping or immediate severe pain. From the pathologic standpoint, the nucleus pulposus has extruded from the annulus fibrosus of the intervertebral disk and impinges on the nerve root (Fig. 1). The herniation can be lateral or central. Any maneuver that stretches the dural sheath of the nerve root, such as straight-leg testing, exacerbates the pain and causes pain in the distribution of the impinged nerve root. A number of cases are atypical. However, if a careful physical exam is done with a full neurologic exam, including straight-leg testing, a great majority of even atypical herniated disk syndromes can be identified and referred to the appropriate physician (either an orthopedic surgeon or neurosurgeon). Radiographs are not needed if trauma or infection is not a concern. The diagnosis of herniated lumbar disks is based on physical findings.

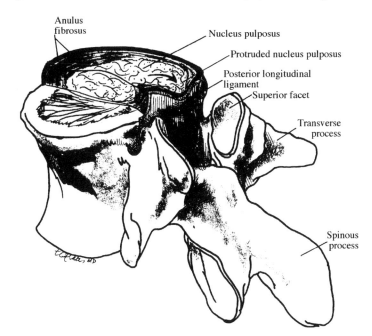

Figure 1. Disk protrusion at L4–L5. (From Cole AJ, Herring SH: The Low Back Pain Handbook. Philadelphia, Hanley & Belfus, 1997, with permission.)

Management. Suggested management is described in Table 13. Most herniated lumbar disks can be managed on an outpatient basis. If the patient does not have an acute foot drop (inability to dorsiflex the toe and foot), or rectal or bladder incontinence, and if the pain is manageable, the patient does not require admission. The patient should improve with bed rest for 2–3 days, narcotics, and NSAIDs. Follow-up should include an MRI and referral to a neurosurgeon or orthopedic surgeon. The surgical management of herniated depends on neurologic deficits, the progression of symptoms over time, and the failure of conservative management measures. Steroids have been found to be helpful in certain situations for acute herniated disk with nerve root inflammation. However, consultation with a neurosurgeon or orthopedic back surgeon should precede steroid administration.

Pitfalls in Practice. Emergent specialty consultation should be obtained if the patient presents with severe symptoms such as incontinence or acute foot drop. A thorough neurologic exam, including perirectal sensation and rectal tone, should be performed on all patients with complaints of back pain. Subtle presentations of herniated disk syndromes may be missed if a thorough exam is not performed. Patients with back pain are often undertreated for pain. Adequate pain medication is necessary.

Vertebral Fractures

Differential Diagnosis and Treatment. The history and physical exam often identify patients with vertebral fractures presenting to the urgent care center. Plain films of the thoracic or lumbar region are needed to identify the significance of the fracture. Any patient with neurologic deficit associated with an acute vertebral fracture should be immobilized and transferred immediately to the emergency department for further evaluation and management. Pathologic fractures due to metastatic, endocrine, or infectious causes need further evaluation in the hospital. Any patient who presents with acute neurologic deficit secondary to traumatic injury should receive high-dose steroids.[38]

Pitfalls in Practice. Failure to recognize the possibility of a fracture with resultant traumatic spinal cord injury can have devastating consequences. Failure to consider other traumatic injuries, either thoracoabdominal or other spinal injuries, in patients who have suffered a traumatic thoracic or lumbar back injury can result in mortality or further morbidity. Failure to immobilize a patient with vertebral fractures during transport can result in progressive neurologic deficit and paralysis.

Neck Pain

Differential Diagnosis. The first goal of the urgent care physician is to decide if the neck pain is a sign of a life-threatening disease such as meningitis or subarachnoid hemorrhage. Table 15 describes the signs, symptoms, diagnosis, and treatment of various neck pain complaints. In adults with meningitis, other meningeal signs should be present, such as meningismus (pain with flexion or extension of the neck), Brudzinski's sign (elicited by passively flexing the neck of the supine patient and watching for involuntary flexion of the knees), and Kernig's sign (pain in the posterior thigh when the knee is extended passively from a position of 90° flexion with the hip). Most adults with meningitis present with a severe headache, fever, and alteration in consciousness. The clinician should be aware of subgroups that present with atypical presentations of meningitis, including patients with AIDS, immunosuppressed patients, children less than 2 years of age, and elders.

Table 15. Signs, Symptoms, Diagnosis, and Treatment of Neck Pain

Syndrome	Symptoms and Signs	Diagnosis/Treatment
Meningitis	Fever, headache, photophobia, neck stiffness	CT scan, lumbar puncture, early antibiotics
Subarachnoid hemorrhage	Stiffness/tightness, worst headache of life, syncopal episode, confusion	CT scan, lumbar puncture if CT scan is unclear, transfer to emergency department with urgent neurosurgery evaluation
Cervical spondylosis	Nerve root impingement, patients often > 65, osteophyte formation	Symptomatic treatment with NSAIDs and follow-up with rheumatologist
Trauma	Post trauma with midline pain	Cervical spine series (anteroposterior, lateral, odontoid), transfer to emergency department if any cervical spine fractures
Neck spasm/ strain	Most common, tender paracervical muscles without midline pain, pain with range of motion	NSAIDs, possible short-term muscle relaxants and/or narcotics, early physical therapy

Other causes of serious underlying diseases manifesting as neck pain include tuberculosis or tumor invasion of the cervical spine. Although rare, they must be kept in the differential diagnosis. If these entities are suspected, a cervical spine x-ray should be performed. Rheumatoid arthritis can also involve the spine, and odontoid fractures and subluxations are quite common in this population.

The most frequent cause of presentation of neck pain to the urgent care center is traumatic or positional injury. Any traumatic injury that appears to have a mechanism possibly causing a cervical spine fracture should be treated with great care, prompt cervical immobilization, and early cervical spine x-rays. To determine whether a neck injury is potentially serious , the patient should be interviewed about the mechanism of injury and initial symptoms of extremity numbness or weakness. If there is any indication or concern, cervical spine films need to be performed immediately. A patient can present with neurologic findings despite a normal cervical spine—a condition termed spinal cord injury without radiologic abnormality (SCIWORA).[39] SCIWORA is particularly common in children but also occurs among the elders. The patient can present with central cord compression from an extension injury that buckles the ligament flavum into the spinal cord column. If this is a concern, a neurosurgical or neurologic consultation or transfer to an emergency department is needed

The great majority of patients with neck pain fall into the category of cervical strain. The pain is usually unilateral, and the muscle spasm can often be palpated along the sternocleidomastoid muscle, pericervical strap muscles, or trapezius muscle. Range of neck motion is often limited, and the syndromes can be quite debilitating if left untreated.

Management. As noted earlier, a cervical collar should be placed in any patient presenting with neck pain and history of acute trauma. The NEXUS cervical spine study identified certain patients who can be clinically cleared without x-rays.[40,41] This approach involves a careful history and physical exam, excluding any factors that may cloud the judgement of the patient (most notably alcohol intoxication), distracting injury, and pain on palpation along the midline of the cervical spine. If, after performing this assessment, the patient's neck is nontender and the mechanism of injury makes cervical spine injuries unlikely, the patient may be clinically cleared for a cervical spine fracture.

Patients with cervical strain often require intervention to stop the cycle of spasm and pain. A number of options can be used. First, the clinician should identify or eliminate any causes of neck pain such as occupational position and stress factors. If a trigger point is identified, injection of 1% lidocaine (2–3 ml) with a 22–25 gauge needle can relieve the painful spasm and provide immediate relief. The trigger point, if identified, should be immobilized between two fingers and an injection made into the center of the trigger zone. Flexion extension of the affected muscle should occur after the injection. Marcaine can be substituted for lidocaine; it has a longer duration of relief.

The most common treatment for neck spasm is NSAIDs on a scheduled basis for approximately 1 week. Muscle relaxants may provide additional benefit, primarily through sedation and relaxation. Ophenedrine is a central-acting muscle relaxant that is less sedating than others; the dose is 100 mg twice daily. If the patient is in severe pain, a dose of narcotic medication can be used to help break the spasm. While diazepam is effective at sedating and relieving some muscle spasm, it should be used with caution because of its addictive properties. Elavil should be considered for any chronic painful condition and started at 10–25 mg at night and increased weekly until it is effective or side effects occur. Such patients should be referred to a chronic pain clinic for further evaluation and treatment. Physical therapy should be started early and is extremely effective in relieving muscle spasm and strain neck pain.

Pitfalls in Practice. The clinician must consider serious causes of neck pain such as meningitis or subarachnoid hemorrhage, especially in patients with atypical presentations. Misinterpretation of cervical spine films resulting in a missed fracture or subluxation can result in significant morbidity. Failure to maintain patients in cervical immobilization until the cervical spine is cleared can result in spinal cord injury. Failure to initiate early physical therapy in neck spasm can result in unnecessary pain and discomfort.

References

1. Raskin NH: Headache. In Isselbacher KJ, et al (eds): Harrison's Principles of Internal Medicine, 13th ed. New York, McGraw-Hill, 1994.
2. Dodick D. Headache as a symptom of ominous disease. Postgrad Med 101:46–64,1997.
3. Morgenstern LB, et al: Worst headache and subarachnoid hemorrhage: Prospective, modern computed tomography and spinal fluid analysis. Ann Emerg Med 32(3 Pt 1):297–304, 1998.
4. Lambert DH, Hurley RJ, Hertwig L, Datta S: Role of needle gauge and tip configuration in the production of lumber puncture headache. Reg Anesth 22:66–72, 1997.
5. Saper JR: Diagnosis and symptomatic treatment of migraine. Headache 37 (Suppl 1):S1–S14, 1997.
6. Capiobianco DJ, Cheshire WP, Campbell JK: An overview of the diagnosis and pharmacological treatment of migraine. Mayo Clin Proc 71:1055–1066, 1996.
7. Blau JN: Migraine prodromes separated from the aura: Complete migraine. BMJ 281:658–660, 1980.
8. Silberstein SD, Lipton RB: Overview of diagnosis and treatment of migraine. Neurology. 44(Suppl 7):S6–S16, 1994.
9. Campbell JK: Manifestations of migraine. Neurol Clin 8:841–855, 1990.
10. Moore KL, Noble SL: Drug treatment of migraine. Am Fam Physician 56:2039–2048, 1997.
11. Kumar KL, Kooney TG: Headaches. Med Clin North Am 79:261–281, 1995.
12. Walling AD: Cluster headache. Am Fam Physician 47:1457–1463, 1993.
13. Ekbom K: Treatment of cluster headache: Clinical trials, designs and results. Cephalgia 15:33–36, 1995.
14. Mathew NT: Advances in cluster headaches. Neurol Clin 8:867–890, 1990.
15. Silberstein SD: Tension-type headaches. Headache 34:S2–S7, 1994.
16. Roth HL, Drislane FW: Seizures. Neurol Clin North Am 16:257–284, 1998.

17. Kuyk J, Leijlen F, Meinharl H: The diagnosis of psychogenic non-epileptic seizures: A review. Seizure 6:243–253, 1997.
18. Berg AT, Shinnar S: The risk of seizure recurrence following a first unprovoked seizure: A quantitative review. Neurology 41:965–972, 1991.
19. Jagoda A, Richardson L: The evaluation and treatment of seizures in the emergency department. Mt Sinai J Med 64(4&5):249–257, 1997.
20. Rathlev N, D'Onofrio G, Fish S, et al: The lack of efficacy of phenytoin in the prevention of recurrent alcohol related seizures. Ann Emerg Med 23:513–518, 1994.
21. Treiman DM, Meyer PD, Walton NY, et al: A comparison of four treatments for generalized convulsive status epilepticus. N Engl J Med 339:792–798, 1998.
22. Runge JW, Allen FA: Emergency treatment of status epilepticus. Neurology 46(Suppl): 520–521, 1996.
23. Marks WJ, Garcia PA: Management of seizures and epilepsy. Am Fam Physician 57:1589–1600, 1998.
24. Von Kommer R, Allen KL, Holle R, et al: Acute stroke: Usefulness of early CT findings before thrombolytic therapy. Radiology 205:327–333, 1997.
25. Feinberg WM, Albers SW, Barnett HM, et al: Guidelines for the management of transient ischemic attacks of the stroke council of the American Heart Association. Stroke 25:1329–1335, 1994.
26. Brown RD, Evans BA, et al: Transient ischemic attack and minor ischemic stroke; an algorithm for evaluation or treatment. Mayo Clin Proc 69:1027–1039, 1994.
27. Broderick J, Brott T, Barsan W, et al: Blood pressure during the first few minutes of focal ischemia. Ann Emer Med 22:1438–1443, 1993.
28. Phillips SJ: Pathophysiology and management of hypertension in acute ischemic stroke. Hypertension 23:131–135, 1994.
29. Levine SR, Welch KMA: Cocaine and Stroke. Stroke 19:779–783, 1987.
30. Klonoff DC, Andrews BT, Obana WG: Stroke associated with cocaine use. Arch Neurology 46:989–993, 1989.
31. Dix MR, Hallpike LS: The pathology, symptomology and diagnosis of certain common disorders of the vestibular system. Proc R Soc Med 45:341–354, 1952.
32. Epley JM: The canalith repositioning maneuver for treatment of benign paroxysmal positional vertigo. Otolaryngol Head Neck Surg 107:399–104, 1992.
33. Hashisaki GT: Medical management of Bell's palsy. Comp Ther 23:715–718, 1997.
34. Burgess RC, Bale JF, Michaels L, Smith RJH: Polymerase chain reaction amplification of herpes simplex viral DNA from the geniculate ganglion of a patient with Bell's palsy. Ann Oto/Rhinol Laryngol 103:775–779, 1994.
35. Van Der mèche FGA, Schmitz PIM, and the Dutch Guillain-Barre Study Group: A randomized trial comparing intravenous immune globulin and plasma exchange in Guillain-Barre syndrome. N Engl J Med 326:1123, 1992.
36. Anderson GB: Epidemiological features of chronic low back pain. Lancet 354:581–585, 1999.
37. Glasser DL, Kaplan FS: Osteoporosis: Definition and presentation. Spine 22:125–165, 1997.
38. Bracken MB, Shepard MJ, Collins WF, et al: A randomized controlled trial of methylprednisolone or naloxone in the treatment of acute spinal cord injury. N Engl J Med 322:1405, 1990.
39. Pang D, Pollack IF: Spinal cord injury without radiographic abnormality in children-the SCIWORA syndrome. J Trauma 29:654–664, 1989.
40. Meldon SW, Brant TA, Cydulka RK, et al: Out of hospital cervical spine clearance: Agreement between emergency medical technicians and emergency physicians. J Trauma 45:1058–1061, 1998.
41. Hoffman JR, Mower WR, Wolfson AB, et al: Validation of a set of clinical criteria to rule out injury to the cervical spine in patients with blunt trauma. N Engl J Med 343:94–99, 2000.

Chapter 20

Psychiatric Urgencies

James R. Miner, MD
James P. Winter, MD

General Approach to Psychiatric Urgencies

Patients with psychiatric conditions present to urgent care centers with a variety of symptoms, ranging from exacerbations of chronic disorders, problems with medications, or acute changes in behavior of psychiatric origin. Although often less obvious than patients with medical conditions, patients with psychiatric emergencies may have life-threatening medical and psychiatric disorders. Urgent care physicians need to develop a system for determining which patients suffering from psychiatric disorders need immediate and aggressive care and which can have psychiatric follow-up on an outpatient basis. Common causes of urgent need for medical care among patients with psychiatric disorders include worsening of an underlying mental disorder, suicidal behavior, assaultive behavior, extrapyramidal or other medication side effects, and medical complications of an underlying mental disorder.

The goals of treating patients with a psychiatric urgency include recognition and reversal of all life-threatening conditions, recognition of the potential for suicide or violent behavior, assessment of the patient's current neurologic and mental status, determination of whether the change in behavior is organic or functional in origin, prevention of progression or complications of the disorder, appropriate treatment of the patient, and appropriate disposition. Patients whose needs cannot be met in urgent care need to be transferred to an appropriate setting.

Psychiatric Exam

The psychiatric exam must take place in a calm environment and in a relaxed manner. A thorough history must be obtained, with emphasis on both medical and psychiatric causes of the current complaint. Patients with acute behavior changes should be specifically asked about suicidal ideation, hallucinations, mood, drug use, social situation, and a family history of psychiatric disorders. During the examination, patients should be evaluated for general behavior, affect, attention, level of consciousness, language skills, orientation, memory, thought content, perception, judgment, and conceptualization. A quick way to briefly assess a patient's mental status is the mini-mental status exam (Table 1). Although it is a nonspecific evaluation of a patient's mental status, it often clues the examiner to specific changes that need further assessment.

Table 1. Mini-Mental Status Exam and Scoring System

Maximum Score	
	Orientation
5	What is the (year)(date)(season)(month)?
5	Where are we (city)(state)(country)(hospital)?
	Registration
3	Name three objects, and ask the patient to repeat all three after you have said them.
	Attention and calculation
5	Count by sevens back from 100 (five digits back) or spell the word *world* backwards.
	Recall
3	Ask the patient to repeat the three objects noted above (one point each).
	Language and praxis
2	Show a pencil and a watch; ask the patient to name them.
1	Ask the patient to repeat the following: "No ifs, ands, or buts."
3	(Three-stage command): "Take this paper in your right hand, fold it in half, and put it on the floor."
1	Read and obey the following: "Close your eyes" (written on a piece of paper).
1	Write a sentence (must contain a noun, verb, and be sensible).
1	Copy this design (interlocking pentagons).

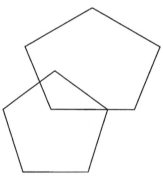

The copy must contain all angles, and the two must intersect

Adapted from Smith J: Organic brain syndrome. In Rosen B (ed): Emergency Medicine Concepts and Clinical Practice. St. Louis, Mosby, 1998, p 2139.

Medical Causes of Psychiatric Emergencies

A psychosis is defined as a dysfunction of thought processes from any cause and manifests as an impaired sense of reality. It is important and challenging to determine early in treatment whether the psychosis has a medical or functional etiology. Medical dysfunction has a known physiologic or biochemical basis. Functional etiologies probably have a neurobiochemical basis but are not currently definable on a physiologic basis and are therefore diagnosed by symptoms. Medical psychoses include delirium and dementia. Functional psychoses include schizophrenic disorders and affective disorders.

Patients who present with symptoms due to medical abnormalities often are delirious, with decreased rather than altered level of consciousness (Table 2). Several characteristics of medical vs. psychiatric disorders are listed in Table 3.

Table 2. Delirium vs. Psychosis

Characteristic	Delirium	Psychosis
Onset	Acute	Acute
Vital signs	Typically abnormal	Normal
Prior psychiatric history	Uncommon	Common
Course	Rapid, fluctuating	Stable
Psychomotor activity	Variable	Variable
Involuntary activity	Possible asterixis, tremor	Absent
Cognition function		
Orientation	Usually impaired	Occasionally impaired
Attention	Globally impaired	May be disorganized
Concentration	Globally impaired	Impaired
Hallucinations	Visual, visual and auditory	Primarily auditory
Delusions	Transient, poorly organized	Systematized
Speech	Pressured, slow, incoherent	Usually coherent
Course	Typically resolves	Responds to therapy, recurs

Adapted from Smith J: Organic brain syndrome. In Rosen B (ed): Emergency Medicine Concepts and Clinical Practice. St. Louis, Mosby, 1998, p 2139.

Table 3. Medical vs. Psychiatric Psychosis

Feature	Psychiatric		Medical	
	Schizophrenia	*Affective*	*Delirium*	*Dementia*
Onset	Variable	Variable	Acute	Gradual
Age (yr)	< 40	30–40	Any age	> 60
Course	Progressive	Fluctuating	Fluctuating	Progressive
Vital signs	Usually normal	Often abnormal	Often abnormal	Normal
Symptoms	Consistent	Fluctuating	Fluctuating	Consistent
Wakefulness	Normal	Increased	Fluctuating	Normal
Attentiveness	Fluctuating	Impaired	Fluctuating	Impaired
Disorientation	Rare	Intermittent	Intermittent	Constant
Hallucinations	Auditory	Auditory	Visual	None
Delusions	Complex-fixed	Grandiose	Simple-variable	Variable
Sleep-wake dysfunction	Rare	Frequent	Frequent	Frequent
Cognition	Intact (lack of insight)	Abnormal (cannot attend)	Abnormal (fluctuating)	Abnormal
Recent memory	Intact	Variable	Decreased	Decreased
Motor movements	Normal	Hyperactive	Variable	Normal or hypoactive
Neurologic signs	None	None	Occasional deficit	No acute changes
Most common cause for acute psychosis	Nonmedical compliance		Intoxicants withdrawal	Alzheimer's disease, alcohol dementia

It should be assumed that a patient's behavioral abnormality has a medical cause until all possibilities have been reasonably ruled out. Identified medical causes should be treated appropriately. Until the medical condition has resolved, patients sometimes require treatment of the psychiatric symptoms. Whether the behavioral abnormality has a medical or functional cause, the patient must be assessed for risk to self (suicide or self-neglect) and risk to others (violence).

Suicide

Differential Diagnosis. Suicide is one of the major causes of mortality in psychiatric patients, and all patients presenting with acute changes in behavior should be assessed for suicidal ideation. Questions about suicidal intent should be a routine part of every psychiatric exam. Any patient with suicidal ideation should be immediately assessed to determine risk. Suicidal patients may appear depressed or confused with chaotic mentation and disorganized thinking. Potentially suicidal patients must be observed and/or restrained until it can be adequately determined that they are not suicidal. The Hennepin County Medical Center Crisis Intervention Center uses a critical item assessment to determine suicide risk (Table 4). A tool such as this ensures a uniform and thorough evaluation of potentially seriously suicidal patients and assists consultants in their evaluation.

Management. Establishing a relationship with the patient is important. The interviewer must remain calm and attentive and demonstrate a level of concern. The interviewer should accept what is stated without challenge or criticism. Listening is the key in an open interview style.

If the patient establishes telephone contact with the urgent care center, it is essential that contact be maintained until specific crucial information is obtained. If the patient is reluctant to supply any information and appears to be at serious risk, the interviewer should ask for his or her phone number or have the call traced. Help (e.g., police, ambulance) can then be dispatched to the site of the call.

Suicidal planning is probably the most significant and alarming criterion of suicidal risk. Of concern are the lethality and availability of the method and specificity of detail. Shootings and hangings are worse threats than overdoses and wrist slashings. An available gun in the home is worse than a plan to buy one. Also, the more time and ingenuity spent in making a plan, the greater the risk. The interviewer must determine whether the patient has a definite, dangerous plan.

Stress must be evaluated from the patient's perspective. If increased stress results in increased symptoms, action is necessary to protect the patient. Personal or interpersonal stresses, physical health, loss of a job, and financial or social status play major roles in suicide risk. The interviewer also should search for symptoms related to depression, agitation, hopelessness, and psychosis. Most worrisome is a person with an agitated depression who voices an inability to cope with pressures at hand or who has evidence of tension and restlessness.

The suicidal threat must be assessed openly with the patient's family and friends. Generally, it is best to establish shared responsibility for the suicidal patient; this approach supplies a sense of concern about the patient that he or she lacks for himself or herself and indicates to the patient the concern of loved ones. An important issue is whether communication still exists between the suicidal patient and other people. This issue determines the limit of supportive resources or the possibility of rescuing activity. If

Table 4. Hennepin County Crisis Intervention Center Critical Item Suicide Risk Assessment

Primary suicide risk factors: Place the patient on a hold and obtain psychiatry consultation if any one factor is present:
Attempt
  1. Suicide attempt with lethal method (firearms, hanging/strangulation, jumping from high places)
  2. Suicide attempt resulting in moderate-to-severe lesions/toxicity
  3. Suicide attempt with low rescue ability (no known communication about the attempt, discovery unlikely because of chosen location and timing, no one nearby or in contact, active precaution to prevent discovery)
  4. Suicide attempt with subsequent expressed regret that it was not completed and continued expressed desire to commit suicide or unwillingness to accept treatment
Intent
  1. Suicidal intent to commit suicide imminently
  2. Suicidal intent with a lethal method selected and readily available
  3. Suicidal intent and preparations made for death (writing a testament or a suicide note, giving away possessions, making certain business or insurance arrangements)
  4. Suicidal intent with time and place planned and foreseeable opportunity to commit suicide
  5. Suicidal intent with ambivalence or ability to see alternatives to suicide
  6. Presence of acute command hallucinations to kill self whether or not there is expressed suicidal intent
  7. Suicidal intent with current active psychosis, especially major affective disorder or schizophrenia
  8. Suicidal intent or other objective indicators of elevated suicide risk but mental condition or lack of cooperation preclude adequate assessment

Secondary suicide risk factors: Obtain consultation from a psychiatrist if, in addition to some increased risk, 7 out of 13 factors are present:
  1. Recent separation or divorce
  2. Recent death of significant other
  3. Recent loss of job or financial setback
  4. Other significant loss, stress, life changes interpreted by patient as aggravating (e.g., victimization, threat of criminal prosecution, unwanted pregnancy, discovery of severe illness)
  5. Social isolation
  6. Current or past major mental illness
  7. Current or past chemical dependency/abuse
  8. History of suicide attempts
  9. History of family suicide (include recent suicide by close friend)
  10. Current or past difficulties with impulse control or antisocial behavior
  11. Significant depression (whether clinically diagnosable or not, especially if accompanied by guilt, worthlessness or hopelessness)
  12. Expressed hopelessness
  13. Rigidity (difficulty with adaptation to life changes)

Major demographic factors (not included in rating but may be included in assessment of overall risk)
  1. Male (especially older, white male)
  2. Living alone
  3. Single, divorced, separated, widowed
  4. Unemployed
  5. Chronic financial difficulties

Source: Adapted from the Hennepin County Crisis Intervention Center Policy and Procedures (unpublished), Hennepin County Crisis Intervention Center, Minneapolis, MN, with permission.

no supportive resources are available or if they are exhausted, the situation demands hospitalization of the suicidal patient.

If serious attempts at suicide have been made before, the risk is increased for further attempts. Chronic suicidal behavior is found typically in unstable patients, such as those with character disorders, borderline psychotics, or chronic maladaptors of employment and relationships.

The patient must be assessed medically. Chronic or debilitating illness diminishes the sense of self-worth and self-image. A fatal illness may cause a preoccupation with pain and fear; a physician whom the patient trusts can be helpful in such cases.[1] Intoxicated patients must become sober in a structured environment before an adequate evaluation can be made about their suicide risk.

When it has been determined that a patient is at risk for suicide or when there is any doubt concerning the evaluation of a suicide situation, the patient should be placed on a 72-hour hold and psychiatric consultation should be obtained emergently. Patients who are suicidal should be constantly supervised and/or placed in restraints for their own protection. Patients who attempted suicide but are currently denying suicidal intentions also should have emergent psychiatric consultation, and should be placed on medical hold and restrained and observed. In most circumstances, this requires transfer of the patient from the urgent care center to an ED or hospital capable of providing acute psychiatric consultation.

Pitfalls in Practice. Failure to identify a suicidal patient can lead to a missed opportunity to help the patient before suicide is attempted. Suicide is the most common form of avoidable mortality among psychiatric patients,[2] and the risk of completed suicide must be assessed constantly. When there is any doubt as to a patient's risk of completing suicide, the patient should be placed on medical hold and constantly observed or restrained until psychiatric consultation can be obtained.[2]

Violent Patients

Differential Diagnosis. Although violence is not always related to mental illness, certain mental disorders can be associated with violent behavior. Examples include acute psychotic states, alcohol and drug abuse, organic brain syndrome with medication, attention disorder with hyperactivity in adults, and paranoid schizophrenia with command-type hallucinations.[3]

The differential diagnosis must consider toxic and metabolic causes of agitation as well as drug-induced and psychotic causes. A urine toxicology screen may be of value but usually is not beneficial acutely. Laboratory studies of electrolytes and a complete blood count should be considered. The cause of the precipitating factors should be elicited in the history.

Management. Violent threats must be taken seriously. An urgent care center should have a plan for dealing with violent patients, including available security officers, holding areas, medicolegal hold forms, transfer holds, and medication available for immediate use. Patients with abnormal behavior should be assessed for risk of violence. Violent behavior can be a symptom of an underlying medical or psychiatric disorder, and once appropriate measures are taken to protect the patient and the medical staff, the cause must be investigated (Table 5).

Table 5. Nonpsychiatric Causes of Violent Behavior

Delirium	Anemia	Dementia	Vitamin deficiency
Trauma	Endocrine disorder	CNS infection	Drug reaction
Seizures	Alcohol	Neoplasm	Amphetamines
Cerebrovascular accident	Cocaine	Hypoglycemia	Phencyclidine
Vascular malformation	Lysergic acid	Hypoxia	Anticholinergics
AIDS	Aromatic hydrocarbons	Electrolyte abnormality	Steroids
Hypothermia	Sedative-hypnotics	Hyperthermia	

The critical item assessment for assessing violence potential that is used at the Crisis Intervention Center at Hennepin County Medical Center is presented in Table 6. An instrument such as this can be used to help determine overall violence rating and in assessment of violence potential.

Table 6. Hennepin County Medical Center, Critical Item Violence Potential Assessment

Primary risk factors: Obtain psychiatric consult if any one factor is present:
Assault
1. Assault with a lethal weapon
2. Assault resulting in serious injuries that require medical treatment
3. Assault with subsequent expressed regret that victim escaped, did not die, etc. *and* continued expressed intent to commit further violence or unwillingness to accept treatment
4. Destruction of property if it endangers other people (such as arson)

Threats
1. Threats of violence and fear of losing control and asking for help
2. Threats of violence and patient carries lethal weapon
3. Threats of violence and readily available and lethal method chosen
4. Threats of violence and there is a concrete plan with time and place set and a foreseeable opportunity to commit the planned act of violence
5. Threats of violence and currently active schizophrenia combined with anger and agitation
6. Threats of violence and history of violent behavior with weapons and without provocation
7. Threats of violence and current alcohol/drug intoxication, especially PCP or amphetamines
8. Command hallucinations to commit violence
9. Threat of violence or other objective indicators of elevated risk of violence but mental status or lack of cooperation preclude adequate assessment

Secondary risk factors: Obtain psychiatric consult if, in addition to some indication of increased risk, 9 out of 17 factors are present:
1. Male
2. < 35 years old
3. Referral by police or courts
4. History of violence or threats of violence
5. Previous domestic calls by police
6. History of mental illness, especially schizophrenia, organic brain syndrome, explosive disorder, or antisocial personality disorder
7. History of alcohol/drug use or dependency
8. Criminal record, especially involving felonies
9. History of parental brutality
10. Hypersensitivity to physical closeness (large "body buffer zone")
11. Hypersensitivity to challenges to one's masculinity (obviously for men only)
12. Fear of being closed in
13. Chronically low frustration tolerance, poor impulse control, accompanied by temper tantrums or rage reactions
14. Absence of empathy
15. Explosive appearance as subjectively judged
16. Presence of significant stressors (e.g., spouse threatening to leave, actual or suspected infidelity of spouse, job loss, or business failure, significant victim provocations)
17. Social isolation

Adapted from the Hennepin County Crisis Intervention Center Policy and Procedures (unpublished), Hennepin County Crisis Intervention Center, Minneapolis, MN, with permission.

Patients deemed at risk for violence to others should be placed on hold and in restraints until the evaluation is complete. Restraints require constant supervision and frequent reassessment of the patient, but their use is protective of both patient and staff. Generally, patients can be placed on their backs supine, with either two-point restraints on the opposite arm and leg or four-point restraints on all four extremities.

A patient who is acutely out of control should be managed first by restraints and medication such as droperidol, 5 mg IM.[4,5] Staff should be prepared when approaching a violent patient. Help should be immediately available, staff should stay between the patient and the door, and restraints should be kept in place until a patient is calm and has a normal mental status. Whether a patient will continue to be violent can be difficult to predict, and most patients should be transferred to an emergency department with facilities to care for violent patients and provide psychiatric consultation, if necessary.

Pitfalls in Practice. Failure to be prepared for a violent or potentially violent patient can be dangerous for the patient and medical staff.[6] Furthermore, such patients can be a threat to others if discharged without appreciation of their their violent potential.[7,8] Patients should be assessed for risk of committing acts of violence, and all patients who are potentially violent should be managed with in a careful and systematic manner.[9]

Thought Disorders

Differential Diagnosis. Schizophrenic disorders are defined as disturbances in content and expression of thought. There are 200,000 new cases of schizophrenia diagnosed in the U.S. each year. Cases tend to present in the third decade and are disproportionately high in lower socioeconomic classes, probably because of a gradual decline in level of function. Patients are genetically susceptible to schizophrenia, but the onset is probably affected greatly by biologic and environmental stressors. Clinical manifestations include active psychosis, self-inflicted injuries, personal neglect, and "soft" neurologic findings (Table 7).

Table 7. Characteristics of Schizophrenia

1. Two or more of the following present for most of one month
• Delusions
• Hallucinations
• Disorganized speech
• Grossly disorganized or catatonic behavior
• Flat affect
2. Social or occupational dysfunction below previous levels
3. Continuous signs of disturbance persist for 6 months including the one-month period for above criteria
4. No evidence of schizoaffective or mood disorder
5. Disturbance not related to the physiologic effects of a substance or general medical condition
6. No history of autistic disorder or pervasive developmental disorder

Adapted from American Psychiatric Association: Diagnostic and Statistical Manual of Mental Disorders, 4th ed. Washington, DC, American Psychiatric Association, 1994.

The differential diagnosis of thought disorders is broad, including toxic, metabolic, endocrinologic, and primary neurologic disorders (Table 8). A broad systematic approach must be undertaken to assess a patient with the new onset of schizophrenia. Patients with worsening of previously stable symptoms also must be assessed for new factors contributing to their disorder.

Management. Patients with active schizophrenia are at risk of injury to themselves through both self-injury and self-neglect. They also may present a risk of violent behavior toward others. Careful assessment of suicidal intent, intent to harm self, ability to

Table 8. Differential Diagnosis of Thought Disorders/Schizophrenia

Medical conditions that induce disorganized delusional thoughts	
Endocrine disorders	Hypoadrenalism
	Hypoparathyroid
	Hyperparathyroid
	Hypothyroidism
	Hyperthyroidism
Neurologic disorders	Cerebrovascular disease
	Encephalitis
	Neoplasms
	Epilepsy
Metabolic disorders	Hypoxia
	Hypercarbia
	Hypoglycemia
	Electrolyte abnormality
Other	Autoimmune disorders
	Hepatic failure
	Renal failure

Substance-induced thought disorder: benzodiazepenes, anticonvulsants (phenytoin, phenobarbital), tricyclic antidepressants, isoniazid, rifampin, antihistamines, corticosteroids, disulfiram, heavy metals, propranolol, digoxin, captopril, reserpine, and drugs of abuse (alcohol, amphetamines, cannabis, cocaine, hallucinogens, opioids, sedative-hypnotics)

Other mental disorders

care for self, and intent to harm others are important issues in the evaluation of schizophrenic patients. Complications from concurrent substance abuse syndromes also must be considered.

The area surrounding the acutely psychotic patient should be made safe, secure, and quiet. If the patient is agitated or at risk of injuring self or others, a legal hold and use of restraints may become necessary. Pharmacologic intervention can be done with droperidol, 5 mg IM,[5] which may be repeated after 30 minutes if necessary.[10] Once medical causes of acute psychosis have been ruled out, psychiatric evaluation for admission must be considered, especially if the patient continues to decompensate, is suicidal, or poses a risk to others. Admission is also advised for patients experiencing a first-time psychotic episode. Transportation to an emergency department with suitable staff and facilities should be considered early for acutely psychotic patients.

Patients with previously diagnosed schizophrenia or, on occasion, patients with a suspected new disorder who do not appear to be at risk of injuring themselves through suicidal behavior or self-neglect, do not appear to be a risk to others, have strong and available support systems at home, and do not have other medical conditions causing a change in psychiatric condition, can be referred for close follow-up with a psychiatrist.

Pitfalls in Practice. Medical causes of acute psychosis must be ruled out. Electrolyte and metabolic derangements as well as pharmacologic interaction should be considered. Noncompliance with a therapeutic regimen is a typical presentation. An intensive search for treatable causes and a thorough medical examination must be done. Without this depth, reversible causes of psychosis may be overlooked. Care must be taken to assess accurately whether a patient is at risk of violence, suicide, or inability to care for self. When in doubt, consultation should be obtained.

Affective Disorders

Affective disorders are disturbances in mood, such as depression, mania, and bipolar disorder.

Depression

Differential Diagnosis. Depression usually manifests with a loss of interest or pleasure in all or almost all usual activities and pastimes, coupled with a depressed mood. The signs and symptoms are presented in Table 9. There may be mood swings from sadness to anger to anxiety, but dysphoria is a consistent historical finding.

Table 9. Characteristics of Depression

Depressed mood most of the day
Diminished pleasure or interest in activities most of the day
Significant weight loss or loss of appetite
Insomnia or hypersomnia
Psychomotor retardation or agitation almost every day
Fatigue or loss of energy almost every day
Feelings of worthlessness, excessive/inappropriate guilt
Diminished ability to think or concentrate during the day
Recurrent thoughts of death, recurrent suicidal ideation
Symptoms are not accounted for by bereavement
Symptoms cause significant impairment in social, occupational, or other important areas of functioning
Symptoms are not due to the direct physiologic effects of a substance or general medical condition

Adapted from American Psychiatric Association: Diagnostic and Statistical Manual of Mental Disorders, 4th ed. Washington, DC, American Psychiatric Association, 1994.

The diagnosis of depression is made if four of eight specified symptoms are present almost daily for at least 2 weeks: (1) poor appetite or weight loss, (2) insomnia or hypersomnia, (3) psychomotor agitation or retardation, (4) loss of pleasure in usual activities or loss of sexual drive, (5) fatigue, (6) feelings of worthlessness or inappropriate guilt, (7) diminished concentration, and (8) death thoughts.[11]

The differential diagnosis of depression is broad (Table 10). Laboratory assessment in the urgent care setting should include an electrolyte screen; additional work-up should be done by the primary care physician.

Table 10. Differential Diagnosis of Depression

Medical disorders causing depressive symptoms
Neurologic : Alzheimer's disease, neoplasm, chronic subdural hematoma, seizure disorder, multiple sclerosis, Parkinson's disease, cerebrovascular accident, amyotrophic lateral sclerosis
Endocrine: Addison's disease, Cushing's disease, hypothyroidism
Medications: beta blockers, barbiturates, benzodiazepines, corticosteroids, H_2 blockers, methlydopa, carbidopa, other antihypertensives
Other: pancreatic tumor, HIV infection, mononucleosis, renal failure, post-viral infection syndrome, hypokalemia, environmental toxins

Substance-induced depression
Alcohol, amphetamines, anxiolytics, cocaine, hallucinogens, opioids, sedative-hypnotics

Other mental disorders
Manic-depressive episode (depressive phase), reactive depression, and chronic schizophrenia

There is a 5% lifetime prevalence for major depression, with over 10–14 million patients affected every year in the US. The onset is most likely to occur in early adulthood, but depression is observed in all age groups. There is a genetic susceptibility to major depression, although there are many cultural influences. Major depression is the primary cause of completed suicide. Table 11 presents characteristics differentiating depression from anxiety.

Table 11. Anxiety vs. Depression

Depression	Anxiety
Insomnia	Insomnia
Chronic fatigue	Palpitations
Weight loss	Increased or decreased appetite
Dyspnea with sighing	Dyspnea or hyperventilation
Constipation	Nausea or diarrhea
Changes in menses	Hyperhidrosis
Decreased libido	Increased or decreased libido
Guilt	Fear of dying
Excessive crying	
Social withdrawal	
Psychomotor retardation	

Management. When depression is suspected in a patient who has not been previously diagnosed with depression, the initial evaluation should rule out medical causes, including drug use or abuse. After medical causes have been ruled out, it must be determined whether the patient is at risk for suicide. Direct questioning of the patient is important. Patients who appear to have intact judgment and deny suicidal intent can be discharged with close follow-up to begin therapy for depression. If the patient has risk factors for suicide or does not have intact reasoning or judgment, emergency consultation is warranted.

Antidepressant therapy under psychiatric guidance is the definitive treatment. Antipsychotic agents have benefit in depressions with psychotic features or delusional components.[12] Depending on the agent used, treatment response is usually seen after 1–2 weeks of therapy. Underdosing is common. Antidepressant therapy probably should not be initiated in the urgent care setting. Rather, evaluation should be directed toward determining the patient's current level of functioning and presence of support systems. Patients at imminent risk of injury to themselves or greatly incapacitated in function should be hospitalized.

Pitfalls in Practice. Failure to appreciate a patient's risk of suicide can lead to preventable death. Depression can be difficult to recognize, especially in children and elders.[13] Care must be taken to recognize depressed patients, assess them for risk, and refer them as necessary. Appropriate and timely follow-up must be arranged for all patients discharged from the urgent care setting. Significantly depressed patients should be discharged only if a responsible adult is available to stay with the patient.

Medical conditions that mimic clinical depression must be considered and ruled out before a diagnosis of depression is made.

Mania

Differential Diagnosis. Mania presents as an elevated and expansive mood or irritability for at least 1 week. Symptoms also include decreased need for sleep, pressured speech, excesses, elevated self-esteem, grandiosity, distractibility, flight of ideas, agitation, and racing thoughts. The onset is generally in the third or fourth decade and is equally distributed between the sexes. Almost all patients with mania have a history of depression. The major concern in the evaluation of manic patients is to assess the patient's degree of impulsiveness and the risk of the behavior.

Mania can be caused by many of the same disorders that cause depression (see Tables 9 and 10). High-dose steroids, cocaine, amphetamine, phencyclidine, and other stimulants can also induce mania.

Management. Patients experiencing acute mania are often brought to the emergency department by police, emergency medical services, or their families. Because of the fluctuating nature of the disorder, it is important to observe patients closely and to consider a medical hold if the patient's or caregiver's safety is at risk. Once medical causes of manic behavior have been ruled out, patients with a first episode of mania should have psychiatric consultation and probably be admitted for the initiation of therapy. Patients with severe exacerbations of known disease also should have psychiatric consultation. Patients with chronic disease and mild symptoms controlled easily with neuroleptics or benzodiazepines in the urgent care center may be discharged home with close follow-up with their psychiatrist if a family member is available to assist them. Patients with a history of bipolar disorder who present to the urgent care center for problems with their chronic medications, especially lithium, should be referred to their primary psychiatrist, or emergent psychiatric consultation should be obtained.

Pitfalls in Practice. Because of their heightened level of mental and physical activity, manic patients can be difficult to manage. They must be assessed patiently so that the cause of the problem can be appreciated and the patient's risk of harm to self and others can be assessed. Agitated patients with mania must be approached like any violent patient, and measures should be taken to calm the patient so that thorough assessment is possible.

Anxiety Disorders

Differential Diagnosis. Anxiety represents an unpleasant and unjustified sense of apprehension and can be associated with physiologic symptoms. An anxiety disorder represents anxiety with dysfunction.

Anxiety and apprehension are normal responses to many conditions that prompt patients to seek medical care. When a patient presents with acute anxiety, a high level of suspicion that the cause is organic must be maintained.

Anxiety is the primary symptom of many medical as well as functional disorders (Table 12). Anxiety also can be a symptom of other psychiatric disorders such as mania, schizophrenia, somatization, depressive disorder, posttraumatic stress disorder, mimicry, social phobia, phobic disorder, panic disorder, and agoraphobia. The diagnosis of anxiety or should be made only when medical causes of the symptoms have been ruled out.

The signs and symptoms of anxiety are listed in Table 12. The urgent care physician must consider possible medical causes of anxiety before appropriate disposition can be arranged. A metabolic evaluation with measurement of electrolytes and arterial blood gases may be useful to rule out medical causes of anxiety; additional work-up is usually beyond the capacities of urgent care laboratory facilities.

Table 12. Differential Diagnosis of Anxiety Disorders

Normal anxiety	Hypoparathyroidism	Carbon monoxide
Hypoglycemia	Reactive hypoglycemia	Amphetamine/cocaine abuse
Agitated depression	Pheochromocytoma	Caffeine/methlyxanthine abuse
Acute psychosis	Hyperthyroidism	Yohimbine
Psychomotor epilepsy	Respiratory diseases	Cannabis
Hyperventilation syndrome	Asthma	Khat
Panic attack	Pulmonary embolism	Amyl nitrate
Phobias	Transient ischemic attack	Lysergic acid
Hypocalcemia	Huntington's chorea	Sedative withdrawal
Hypokalemia	Encephalitis	Alcohol withdrawal
Myocardial infarction	Subarachnoid hemorrhage	Seizure disorder
Hyperdynamic adrenergic state	Wilson's disease	Akathisia
Cardiac dysrhythmias	Combined systemic disease	Multiple sclerosis
Mitral valve prolapse syndrome	(Vitamin B12 deficiency)	Post concussive syndrome

Management. Patients should be placed in calm surroundings, and the situation should be discussed. Taking a complete history and expressing interest and empathy with the patient's concerns can be therapeutic. After organic, toxic, or other psychiatric causes of acute anxiety have been ruled out, the patient may be referred for outpatient psychiatric care. Patients who are unresponsive to calm surroundings may be treated pharmacologically. Morphine is helpful in anxiety caused by medical conditions such as pulmonary embolism and acute myocardial infarction. Lorazepam can be used in 0.5-mg IV increments for substance withdrawal and severe agitation. Droperidol, 2.5 mg IV or 5 mg IM, can be highly effective in anxious patients but may be associated with hypotension.[10] Great care must be taken in prescribing oral benzodiazepines for acute exogenous stress in the outpatient setting. Such patients can become quickly addicted to benzodiazepines, and the medications may mask underlying disorders, which can be treated more effectively if diagnosed accurately. Acute control of the current crisis is preferred, with close psychiatric follow-up if the patient is deemed safe. In any case, benzodiazepines should not be prescribed from the urgent care center for more than 1 week.

Pitfalls in Practice. Anxiety is the primary symptom in a vast array of disorders, and patients presenting with typical symptoms should not be quickly dismissed as having "anxiety" or a "panic attack." Careful assessment should be made to rule out life-threatening causes of the anxiety state.

Hyperventilation Syndrome

Differential Diagnosis. Hyperventilation is an abnormal respiratory pattern characterized by rapid, deep breathing. Prolonged hyperventilation results in a hypocarbic state that has several physiologic effects. Continued hypocarbia can lead to cerebral vasoconstriction, lightheadedness, and syncope. Continued hypocarbia and the resulting respiratory alkalosis also leads to a transient decrease in calcium, causing carpopedal spasm and paresthesias. These symptoms often contribute to the anxiety state that triggered the hyperventilation, causing the syndrome to progress.

Hyperventilation can represent the body's response to anxiety or stress but also may represent response to hypoxia, pain, metabolic acidosis, aspirin toxicity, and other life-threatening conditions. In one study, 87% of patients who were eventually diagnosed with hyperventilation syndrome had presented with cardiac or pulmonary complaints, including dyspnea (61%), chest pain (43%), palpitations (13%), and paresthesias (35%).[14] Medical causes of hyperventilation must be ruled out before it can be ascribed to anxiety. Common causes of hyperventilation are listed in Table 13.

Table 13. Differential Diagnosis of Hyperventilation Syndrome

Hypoglycemia	Tinnitus
Hyperthyroidism	Asthma
Pheochromocytoma (high blood pressure, headache)	Emphysema
Postconcussive syndrome	Mitral valve prolapse
Vertigo	Atrial tachydysrhythmias

The use of laboratory studies must be determined on the basis of clinical instinct and the results of the physical examination; however, arterial blood gases confirm hyperventilation syndrome with a resultant respiratory alkalosis.

Management. Patients can be placed on a nonrebreather oxygen mask, which often slows the respiratory rate and corrects the syndrome. Anxiolytics are often helpful, including oral benzodiazepines in less acutely ill patients. More severely distressed patients respond to parenteral benzodiazepines. Droperidol is also useful.

Pitfalls in Practice. The practice of breathing into a mask without oxygen or a paper bag is not recommended, because it can lead to hypoxia and relative worsening of the symptoms. Furthermore, if the hyperventilation has an underlying medical cause, it may be exacerbated by the induced hypoxia. The most important aspect of treating hyperventilation syndrome is to assess the patient for life-threatening causes of hyperventilatory states. Once it has been established that the cause is nonmedical and the patient has been treated and reassured, the patient may be safely discharged home.

Complications of Neuroleptic Drugs

Differential Diagnosis. **Dystonic reactions** are the most common side effects of the use of neuroleptic agents. They most likely result from an upset of the dopaminergic-cholinergic balance in the nigrostiatal pathways of the basal ganglia, leading to an overabundance of cholinergic stimulation.[15] Acute dystonic reactions involve a sustained involuntary skeletal muscle contraction, usually of sudden onset. The jaw is most frequently involved; torticollis, carpopedal spasm, oculogyric crisis, and opisthotonus are also produced. These symptoms have a varied course, with changes and fluctuations in severity. Such reactions occur within the first days of treatment in up to 10% of patients.[16] The diagnosis of acute dystonia is made by the combination of clinical impression and history of medication use. No laboratory studies are indicated.

Extrapyramidal symptoms, such as sedation, hypotension, and anticholinergic side effects, are common with antipsychotic drug therapy. Typically the butyrophenones, dibenzoxazepines, piperazines, and phenothiazines cause the most severe extrapyramidal symptoms. These reactions are common, worsen with stress, disappear with sleep, and wax and wane over time.

Another complication of neuroleptics is **akathisia**, which manifests as a restless feeling. The patient may appear agitated and move constantly. This reaction can occur any time in the first few months after the onset of therapy. It is easily mistaken for acute decompensation of the underlying psychosis.

Tardive dyskinesia usually appears several years after the initiation of therapy and presents as involuntary movements of the face and tongue.[17] Its onset is related directly to the total cumulative dose of the agent; once the symptoms have begun, there is no effective therapy. Lowering the dose or discontinuing the agent reverses the symptoms in some patients.

Neuroleptic malignant syndrome is a life-threatening complication of the use of neuroleptics. It usually occurs early in the course of treatment, after changes in dosing, or after recent high doses. High fever, muscle rigidity, altered mental status, autonomic instability, and high serum creatinine kinase levels are characteristic signs. It is thought to be due to depletion of dopamine stores in the brain.

Management. Severe dystonic reactions can be treated with diphenhydramine, 25 mg IV/IM. Less severe reactions can be treated with oral diphenhydramine (25–50 mg) or benztropine (1–2 mg). Patients should continue oral therapy for 48–72 hours to prevent recurrent symptoms.[18]

Akathisia can be treated with beta blockers or benzodiazepines. Generally, the medication causing this reaction can still be used if the dose is lowered. Akinesia or pseudoparkinsonism also can be seen in patients taking neuroleptics. Treatment with anti-parkinson agents or benztropine is generally effective.

Treatment of neuroleptic syndrome includes discontinuation of the causative agent, rehydration, and antipyresis. Dantrolene and bromocriptine also have been used with some success.[19,20]

Pitfalls in Practice. Failure to control muscle spasms secondary to a dystonic reaction can lead to acidosis and respiratory arrest.

Eating Disorders

Anorexia Nervosa

Differential Diagnosis. Anorexia nervosa involves a disturbed perception of body weight, often coupled with an intense fear of becoming obese. Patients are diagnosed after having lost at least 25% of their original body weight; they refuse to maintain a normal minimal body weight. Anorexia occurs primarily in young women, with prevalence rates among teenagers reported as high as 13% in the U.S.[21] Patients appear emaciated, often have abnormal vital signs, and may be cold-intolerant.

Management. Complications of anorexia include cardiovascular instability, medication side effects, malnourishment, chemical imbalances, anemia, leukopenia, and ECG abnormalities. Patients presenting with acute exacerbations of known disease must be evaluated for hydration status and metabolic abnormalities. Patients with a possible new diagnosis should be evaluated similarly, and if the patient is medically stable and seems likely to follow up, outpatient therapy can be arranged. If the patient is unstable or has a poor social situation, psychiatric consultation and admission should be considered.

Pitfalls in Diagnosis. Other medical causes of weight loss must be considered when the diagnosis is entertained, as well as the possibility that another mental disorder is the cause of weight loss.

Bulimia Nervosa

Differential Diagnosis. Bulimia nervosa is characterized by episodic rapid consumption of large amounts of food, usually accompanied by compensatory behavior. Patients are generally able to maintain their weight. Clinical manifestations include chronic constipation or diarrhea, cardiac and skeletal myopathies, gastric dilation or rupture, synthroid abuse, Mallory-Weiss tears, and substance abuse. Complications are similar to those of anorexia and include cardiovascular instability, medication side effects, malnourishment, chemical imbalances, anemia, leukocytopenia, ECG abnormalities, dental erosions, and dental caries.

Management. If a new diagnosis is considered in a medically stable patient, outpatient therapy can be arranged. If the patient is medically unstable, decompensating psychiatrically, or not a good candidate for outpatient therapy, psychiatric consultation should be arranged.

Pitfalls in Practice. As with anorexia, other causes of the patient's symptoms must be considered and ruled out.

Drug-Seeking Behavior

Differential Diagnosis. A problem frequently encountered in urgent care medicine is drug-seeking behavior. Because of the lack of long-term relationships with urgent care patients, this problem can be difficult to assess. Although patients with drug-seeking behavior tend to present with a wide variety of complaints that are generally nonpsychiatric, the root of the problem is addictive behavior (Table 14). Often summarization disorders and malingering present with drug seeking characteristics as well. When patients present with a given complaint, even when drug-seeking behavior is suspected, they must be given the benefit of the doubt and evaluated for the presenting complaint. Many painful conditions that require therapy have no objective findings, and the history is critical to determining the nature of a patient's pain.

Table 14: Common Signs of Drug-seeking Patients

Frequent visits for various nonspecific complaints
Visits after regular office hours for non-urgent complaints
"Just visiting from out of town and I'm out of my regular medications"
"My medications were stolen" or "I lost my medications"
Requests for specific pain medications for problems not generally requiring narcotics
Multiple drug allergies to non-narcotic pain medications
Failure to follow up with primary physician for chronic complaints
Agitation/hostility when specific requests for pain medications denied
Agitation/hostility when questioned about drug seeking behavior

Management. In dealing with a patient who is suspected of drug-seeking behavior, it is important to remember that the patient may be seeking treatment for a truly painful problem. Attempts should be made to assess the potential for drug-seeking, including directly addressing the issue, attempting to contact the patient's primary physician for more information, and discussing alternative pain management strategies with the patient. Other strategies include using pharmacies that keep a patient database of current medicine use, and prescribing only quantities of medicines sufficient for a short period until the patient can follow up with his or her primary care physician.

Pitfalls in Practice. Failure to take the time to assess a patient's request for addictive medicines can lead both to prescribing medications to patients who abuse them and to failure to prescribe medications to patients who truly need them. It is important to identify patients who have developed addictive behaviors with a prescription medication. Often they present only to the urgent care setting, and the continuing use of what is intended to be temporary care allows them to develop the problem. Once identified, such patients can be approached for treatment of both medication abuse and any underlying causes that may have contributed to the behavior.

Conclusions

The most important aspects of treating patients with psychiatric complaints in the urgent care setting is determining whether a life-threatening medical condition is the cause of the disturbance. Once life-threatening conditions or conditions that may deteriorate rapidly are ruled out, the patient must be assessed for potential danger to self and others. Maintaining a high degree of suspicion for medical causes of psychiatric symptoms, suicidal ideation, and potential violence helps to guarantee the patient's safety and protect long-term continuing health.

References

1. Stelmachers ZT: Basic Principles of Suicide Prevention. Minneapolis, MN, Hennepin County Crisis Intervention Center, 1987.
2. Butcher JN, Stelmachers ZT, Maudal CT: Crisis intervention and emergency psychotherapy. In Weinter IB (ed): Clinical Methods in Psychology, 3rd ed. New York, Wiley, 1985, pp 572–632.
3. Ringback Weitoft G, Gullberg A, Rosen M: Avoidable mortality among psychiatric patients. Soc Psychiatry Psychiatr Epidemiol 33:430–437, 1998.
4. Richards JR: Chemical restraints for the agitated patient in the emergency department. J Emerg Med 16:567–573, 1998.
5. Resnick M: Droperidol vs. haloperidol in the initial management of acutely agitated patients. J Clin Psychiatry 45:298–299, 1984.
6. Fernandes CM, et al: Violence in the emergency department: A survey of health care workers [see comments]. Cmaj 161:1245–1248, 1999.
7. Tardiff K, et al: A prospective study of violence by psychiatric patients after hospital discharge. Psychiatr Serv 48:678–681, 1997.
8. Simon RI: Psychiatrists' duties in discharging sicker and potentially violent inpatients in the managed care era. Psychiatr Serv 49:62–67, 1998.
9. McNiel DE, Binder RL, Fulton FM: Management of threats of violence under California's duty-to-protect statute [published erratum appears in Am J Psychiatry 155:1465, 1998]. Am J Psychiatry 155:1097–1101, 1998.
10. van Leeuwen AM, Parent M, et al: Droperidol in the acutely agitated patient: A double blind, placebo-controlled study. J Nerv Mental Disord 164:280–283, 1977.
11. American Psychiatric Association: Diagnostic and Statistical Manual of Mental Disorders, 3rd ed (revised). Washington, DC, American Psychiatric Association, 1987, pp 251–253.

12. Mason AS, Granacher RP: Clinical Handbook of Antipsychotic Drug Therapy. New York, Bruner/Mazel, 1980, p 152.
13. Alexopoulos GS, et al: Clinical determinants of suicidal ideation and behavior in geriatric depression. Arch Gen Psychiatry 56:1048–1053, 1999.
14. Saiach SG, Gardner WN: Patients with acute hyperventilation presenting to an inner-city emergency department. Chest 110:952–957, 1996.
15. Lee A: Treatment of drug-induced dystonic reactions. J Am Coll Emerg Physicians 8:453–457, 1979.
16. Mason AS, Granacher RP: Clinical Handbook of Antipsychotic Drug Therapy. New York, Bruner/Mazel, 1980, pp 197–198.
17. Fleischhacker WW, Kane JM: The pharmocological treatment of neuroleptic-induced akathesia. J Clin Psychopharmocol 10:12–21, 1990.
18. Corre KA, Bessen HA: Extended therapy for acute dystonic reactions. Ann Emerg Med 13:194, 1984.
19. Tsutsumi Y, et al: The treatment of neuroleptic malignant syndrome using dantrolene sodium. Psychiatry Clin Neurosci 52:433–438, 1998.
20. Kusumi I, Koyama T: Algorithms for the treatment of acute side effects induced by neuroleptics. Psychiatry Clin Neurosci 53(Suppl):S19–S22, 1999.
21. Battle EK, Brownell KD: Confronting a rising tide of eating disorders and obesity: treatment vs. prevention and policy. Addict Behav 21:755–765, 1996.
22. Folstein MF, Folstein SE, McHugh PR: "Mini-mental state": A practical method for grading the cognitive state of patients for the clinician. J Psychiatr Res 12:189–198, 1975.
23. Smith J: Organic brain syndrome. In Rosen B (ed): Emergency Medicine Concepts and Practice. St. Louis, Mosby, 1998, p 2139.
24. American Psychiatric Association: Diagnostic and Statistic Manual of Mental Disorders, 4th ed. Washington, DC, American Psychiatric Association, 1994, p 285.
25. Papp LA: Generalized anxiety disorders. In Sandock KA (ed): Comprehensive Textbook of Psychiatry, vol. VI. Baltimore, Williams & Wilkins, 1995, p 1244.

Chapter 21

Urgent Care Pharmacology

E. Corradin Vogel, MD

The medical disorders dealt with in urgent care centers often necessitate prescribing medications that alone have few deleterious effects. When given to patients with underlying medical disorders or complicated medical regimens, commonly prescribed medications have many potential adverse reactions of which the urgent care physician must be aware. Many interactions simply must be memorized to avoid their occurrence.

Certain patients in the urgent care population carry red flags that should warn the physician that they are at increased risk for drug interactions. Studies have shown that patients with congestive heart failure, hypertension, diabetes, and renal disease are at high risk for adverse drug reactions.[1] Other risk factors include female gender, extremes of age, previous drug reactions, liver and renal dysfunction, obesity, and dehydration.[2] The total number of medications that a patient is taking also indicates increased risk. According to Goldberg et al., "13% of patients taking two medications are at risk for adverse drug interactions, as compared to 38% of patients taking five medications, and 82% taking seven or more medications."[1] In addition, certain medications are notorious for their potential to interact with commonly prescribed medications. Table 1 (next page) provides a list of drugs that commonly interact with other medications. The physician should consider the potential for interactions before prescribing a new medication or multiple medications simultaneously.

Potential Drug Interactions with Commonly Prescribed Drug Classes

Many patients encountered in the urgent care setting take medications prescribed by their primary doctor that carry an increased potential for drug interactions. These "notorious" medications may cause toxicity when a patient's balanced medical regimen is altered by prescription of usually benign medications. It is important to become familiar with these medications and prescribe with caution when they appear on a patient's drug list. The list does not include all interactions possible, but it is meant to present medications that are commonly prescribed in the urgent care center and may interact significantly with common maintenance medications.

Antiarrhythmics

Digoxin. This cardiac glycoside is used to control arrhythmias (atrial fibrillation/flutter, supraventricular tachycardia) and for congestive heart failure treatment. Digoxin functions with a narrow therapeutic range in serum, and levels are altered by numerous

Table 1. Notorious Drug Interactions

Medication	Drugs That Increase Toxic Potential	Drugs That Decrease Effect	Effects on Other Medications	Comments
Antihistamines (astemizole, terfenadine)	Metronidazole, macrolide antibiotics, triazole antifungals, bepridil, cimetidine, nefazodone, CNS depressants			Cardiotoxicity, ↑ QT interval, torsades de pointes Increased sedation
Beta blockers	Other antihypertensives, ciprofloxacin, haloperidol, H₂ blockers, MAOIs, oral contraceptives	Aluminum/calcium salt antacids, barbiturates, cholestyramine, colestipol, NSAIDs, penicillins, rifampin, salicylates	Increased toxicity of antihypertensives, acetaminophen, benzodiazepines, haloperidol	
Calcium channel blockers	Other antihypertensives, H₂ blockers	Rifampin	Increased toxicity of antihypertensives, carbamazepine, digitalis, quinidine, theophylline	
Carbamazepine	Erythromycin, propoxyphene, verapamil, diltiazem, cimetidine			
Cisapride	Antibiotics (macrolides), antifungals (triazoles), cimetidine, ranitidine, diazepam, warfarin, CNS depressants			Cardiotoxicity, ↑ QT interval, torsades de pointes Increased sedation
Clonazepam	CNS depressants			Increased sedation
Corticosteroids		Anticholinesterase agents, barbiturates, diuretics, phenytoin, rifampin	Increased toxicity of NSAIDs (ulcers), diuretics (hypokalemia) Decreased effect of warfarin, salicylates, vaccines	
Digoxin	Calcium channel blockers, fluoroquinolones, macrolides, tetracycline			
Diuretics	Other antihypertensives		Increased toxicity of digitalis, lithium, aminoglycosides, tetracyclines Decreased effect of oral hypoglycemics	
H₂ blockers			Increased toxicity of diazepam, glipizide, glyburide, metoprolol, midazolam, lidocaine, metronidazole, pentoxifylline, phenytoin, propranolol, theophylline, triamterene, TCAs, warfarin Decreased effect of antifungals, cefpodoxime, cyanocobalamin, oxaprozin	

(Cont'd on next page)

Table 1. Notorious Drug Interactions *(Continued)*

Medication	Drugs That Increase Toxic Potential	Drugs That Decrease Effect	Effects on Other Medications	Comments
Lithium	ACE inhibitors, carbamazepine, diuretics (thiazides), fluoxetine, haloperidol, NSAIDs, phenothiazines		Increased toxicity of alfentanil, CNS depressants, Iodine Decreased effect of caffeine, theophylline	Increased hypothyroid effects
MAO inhibitors	Disulfiram, SSRIs, TCAs, meperidine, dextroamphetamines, dextromethorphan, phenothiazines, barbiturates, tyramine foods			Increased risk of serotonin syndrome Increased hypertension via tyramine effect
Oral contraception (ethinyl estradiol/ norgestrel)		Antibiotics (peni-cillins, rifampin, tetracyclines), antifungals, barbiturates, phenytoin	Increased toxicity of acetaminophen, anticoagulants, benzodiazepines, caffeine, corticosteroids, metoprolol, theophylline, TCAs	
Phenytoin	Chloramphenicol, disulfiram, doxycycline, fluconazole, itraconazole, oral contraceptives, quinidine, rifampin, steroids, theophylline	Folate, rifampin		
Proton pump inhibitors			Increased toxicity of digoxin, phenytoin, warfarin Decreased effect of antifungals, theophylline	
SSR inhibitors	MAOIs, TCAs		Increased toxicity of lithium, diazepam, trazodone	Fluvoxamine causes torsades de pointes with astemizole, terfenadine, triazole antifungals and decreased clearance; CNS depressants such as alcohol, antipsychotics, barbiturates, benzodiazepines
Sulfonylureas	Antifungals, beta blockers, chloramphenicol, H_2 blockers, other hypoglycemics, oral anticoagulants, MAOIs, NSAIDs, phenytoin, salicylates, sulfonamides, tricyclic antidepressants	Corticosteroids, rifampin, thiazide diuretics		Highly protein bound sulfonylureas interact with other protein bound drugs
Theophylline	Allopurinol, beta blockers, calcium channel blockers, cimetidine, ciprofloxacin, corticosteroids, disulfiram, ephedrine, erythromycin, influenza vaccine, macrolides, mexiletine, oral contraceptives, quinolones, thiabendazole, thyroid hormones	Barbiturates, charcoal ketoconazole, phenytoin, rifampin, sulfinpyrazone		

(Cont'd on next page)

Table 1. Notorious Drug Interactions *(Continued)*

Medication	Drugs That Increase Toxic Potential	Drugs That Decrease Effect	Effects on Other Medications	Comments
TCAs	Cimetidine		Increased toxicity of CNS depressants, anticholiner-gics, adrenergic agents	Cimetidine decreases theophylline metabolism
Valproic acid	CNS depressants		Increased bleeding risk with aspirin, warfarin	
Warfarin	Acetaminophen, some cepha-losporins, chloramphenicol, cimetidine, ciprofloxacin, co-trimoxazole, dipyridamole, erythromycin, fluconazole, indomethacin, ketaconazole, metronidazole, miconazole, nalidixic acid, penicillins, propoxyphene, quinine, ranitidine, salicylates, sulfonamides, sulfonylureas, sulindac, tetracycline	Aluminum hydroxide antacids, barbiturates, carbamazepine, cholestyramine, colestipol, dicloxa-cillin, griseofulvin, nafcillin, oral con-traceptives, phenytoin, rifampin, spironolactone, sucralfate		

The preceding text and table were adapted from information obtained from Lacy C, Armstrong LL, Ingrim NB, Lance LL: The Drug Information Handbook. Hudson, NY, Lexi-comp, 1996.

medications. Toxic potential is increased by fluoroquinolones, macrolides, tetracycline, and calcium channel blockers.

Anticoagulants

Warfarin is a common anticoagulant that produces anticoagulant effects by inhibition of the vitamin K-dependent coagulation factors II, VII, IX, and X. Interactions with warfarin are secondary to its highly protein-bound state in the serum, absorption rates, and induction or inhibition of cytochrome P-450 enzymes by other medications. Anticoagulant effects are increased by acetaminophen, some cephalosporins, chloramphenicol, cimetidine, ciprofloxacin, co-trimoxazole, dipyridamole, doxycycline, erythromycin, fluconazole, indomethacin, ketoconazole, metronidazole, miconazole, nalidixic acid, penicillins, propoxyphene, quinine, ranitidine, salicylates, sulfonamides, sulfonylureas, sulindac, and tetracycline. Anticoagulant effects decreased by aluminum hydroxide antacids, barbiturates, carbamazepine, cholestyramine, colestipol, dicloxacillin, griseofulvin, nafcillin, oral contraceptives, phenytoin, rifampin, spironolactone, and sucralfate.

Anticonvulsants

Carbamazepine. Toxic potential is increased by erythromycin, propoxyphene, verapamil, diltiazem, and cimetidine.

Clonazepam. Increased sedation with other central nervous system (CNS) depressants.

Phenytoin has a propensity to interact with other medications because it induces cytochrome P-450 enzymes. Medications that inhibit this enzyme system cause increased phenytoin levels. Toxic potential is increased by chloramphenicol, disulfiram, doxycycline, fluconazole, itraconazole, oral contraceptives, quinidine, rifampin, steroids, and theophylline. Phenytoin levels are decreased by folic acid and rifampin.

Valproic acid. Toxic potential is increased by CNS depressants and bleeding risk by warfarin and aspirin.

Antidepressants

Monoamine oxidase inhibitors (isocarboxazid, phenelzine sulfate, tranylcypromine sulfate). Use of this class of antidepressants has become less common since the introduction of the selective serotonin reuptake inhibitors (SSRIs), but they are mentioned because of their ability to produce the life-threatening serotonin syndrome and hypertensive emergencies when they interact with other commonly prescribed medications. Toxicity is increased by disulfiram, SSRIs, tricyclic antidepressants (TCAs), meperidine, amphetamines, dextromethorphan, phenothiazines, barbiturates, and tyramine-containing foods.

Selective serotonin reuptake inhibitors (fluoxetine, fluvoxamine, paroxetine, sertraline) are commonly prescribed for depression, anxiety disorders, and obsessive-compulsive disorder. Toxic potential is increased by TCAs and monoamine oxidase inhibitors (MAOIs). SSRIs increase toxic potential of lithium, diazepam, and trazodone .

Special attention is warranted for patients taking fluvoxamine (Luvox) as it inhibits cytochrome P-450, resulting in toxic levels of the antihistamines terfenadine (Seldane) and astemizole (Hismanal) and the antifungal ketoconazole, resulting in cardiotoxicity (including torsades de pointes). In addition, fluvoxamine decreases the clearance of other medications, including CNS depressants such as alcohol, barbiturates, and benzodiazepines.

Tricyclic antidepressants (e.g., amitriptyline, desipramine, doxepin, imipramine). Cardiotoxic effects are seen with overdoses and concomitant use of other antidepressants. TCAs also may increase effects of CNS depressants, anticholinergics, and adrenergic agents. TCA metabolism is decreased by cimetidine.

Antihypertensives

Beta blockers (e.g., atenolol, metoprolol, propranolol).Toxic potential is increased by other antihypertensives (e.g., calcium channel blockers, clonidine, hydralazine, diuretics), ciprofloxacin, haloperidol, H_2-blockers, MAOI antidepressants, oral contraceptives. Beta-blocker effect is decreased by aluminum/calcium salts, antacids, barbiturates, cholestyramine, colestipol, nonsteroidal anti-inflammatory drugs (NSAIDs), penicillins, rifampin, and salicylates. Beta blockers increase effects/toxic potential of other antihypertensives, acetaminophen, benzodiazepines, and haloperidol.

Calcium channel blockers (e.g., nifedipine, diltiazem, amlodipine). Toxic potential is increased by other antihypertensives (e.g., beta blockers, clonidine, hydralazine, diuretics), and H_2-blockers. Calcium channel blocker effect is decreased by rifampin. Calcium channel blockers increase effects/toxic potential of other antihypertensives, carbamazepine, digitalis, quinidine, and theophylline.

Diuretics (e.g., loop, thiazides). Toxic potential is increased by other antihypertensives and diuretics (e.g., beta blockers, calcium channel blockers, clonidine, and hydroxyzine). Diuretics may increase effects/toxic potential of digitalis, lithium, aminoglycosides, and tetracyclines. Diuretics may decrease effects of oral hypoglycemics.

H_2 blockers (cimetidine, famotidine, nizatidine, ranitidine) are commonly prescribed medications. They are also taken over the counter by patients who may not consider them to be a prescription medication. Be sure to ask patients specifically before prescribing a medication with potential interactions. Of the medications included in this class, cimetidine appears to have the greatest potential for drug interactions.[12] H_2 blockers may increase the toxic potential of diazepam, glipizide, glyburide, metoprolol (ranitidine), midazolam (ranitidine), lidocaine (cimetidine), metronidazole (cimetidine), pentoxifylline (ranitidine), phenytoin, propranolol (cimetidine), theophylline, triamterene, tricyclic antidepressants, and warfarin. H_2 blockers may decrease the effects of antifungal medications, cefpodoxime, cyanocobalamin, and oxaprozin.

Oral contraceptives (Ethinyl estradiol and norgestrel) are common forms of contraception, taken for convenience and reliability. They may be adversely affected by other medications. Oral contraceptive efficacy is decreased by antibiotics including penicillins, rifampin, tetracyclines; antifungals, including fluconazole, griseofulvin, itraconazole, and ketoconazole; barbiturates; and phenytoin. Oral contraceptives may increase the toxic potential of acetaminophen, anticoagulants, benzodiazepines, caffeine, corticosteroids, metoprolol, theophylline, and TCAs.

Sulfonylureas

The delicate serum glucose levels controlled by these oral hypoglycemics may be altered by prescription medications that are also highly protein-bound. Toxic potential is increased by antibiotics (chloramphenicol, sulfonamides), beta blockers, antifungals, H_2 blockers, other hypoglycemics, oral anticoagulants, MAO inhibitors, NSAIDs, phenytoin, salicylates, TCAs, and any highly protein-bound medication. Sulfonylurea effects are decreased by corticosteroids, rifampin, and thiazide diuretics.

Miscellaneous

Astemizole and terfenadine antihistamines. Antihistamines may have deadly cardiotoxic effects (prolonged QT interval leading to torsades de pointes) when prescribed with metronidazole, macrolide antibiotics, triazole antifungals, bepridil, cimetidine, or nefazodone. Increased sedation is seen with CNS depressants such as carbamazepine. The toxic potential of these antihistamines has led to their withdrawal from the market.

Cisapride induces gastric motility and is used in patients with gastroparesis, gastroesophageal reflux disease, and other gastrointestinal disorders. Be aware of its notorious electrocardiotoxic potential. Toxic potential (manifested as an increased QT interval with risk of torsades de pointes) is increased by antibiotics (macrolides), antifungals (e.g., ketoconazole, miconazole), cimetidine, ranitidine, diazepam, warfarin, and CNS depressants.

Corticosteroids are widely used for their anti-inflammatory effects and are used by patients with allergic, autoimmune, and inflammatory disorders, including Crohn's disease, COPD, rheumatoid arthritis, and others. Potential for drug interactions is based on the ability to induce cytochrome P-450 enzymes. Corticosteroid effect is decreased by anticholinesterase agents, barbiturates, diuretics, phenytoin, and rifampin. Corticosteroids increase the toxic potential of NSAIDs (ulcers) and diuretics (hypokalemia). Corticosteroids decrease the effects of warfarin, salicylates, and vaccines.

Lithium is used to treat patients with bipolar disorder. It has a significant potential for toxicity because of its narrow therapeutic range. Toxic potential is increased by angiotensin-converting enzyme (ACE) inhibitors, carbamazpine, diuretics (thiazides), fluoxetine, halperidol, NSAIDs, and phenothiazines. Lithium effect is decreased by caffeine and theophylline. Lithium increases the effect/toxic potential of alfentanil, CNS depressants, and hypothyroid effects of iodine.

Proton pump inhibitors (omeprazole/lansoprazole) are used to control gastrointestinal disorders involving elevated acid production. Drug interactions are due to induction/inhibition of cytochrome P-450 enzymes and decreased production of acid, on which many medications rely for absorption. Absorption is decreased by sucralfate. Omeprazole increases the concentration/toxic potential of digoxin, phenytoin, and warfarin. Omeprazole decreases the effect of antifungals and theophylline.

Theophylline is used in chronic obstructive airway disease for its bronchodilatory effects. Although it is not as commonly prescribed now as in previous years, it is known for its plethora of drug interactions involving cytochrome P-450 1A2 enzyme. Toxic potential is increased by allopurinol, beta blockers, calcium channel blockers, cimetidine, ciprofloxacin, corticosteroids, disulfiram, ephedrine, erythromycin, influenza virus vaccine, macrolides, mexiletine, oral contraceptives, quinolones, thiabendazole, and thyroid hormones. Theophylline levels are decreased with barbiturates, charcoal, ketoconazole, phenytoin, rifampin, and sulfinpyrazone.

Special Conditions

Interactions with Alcohol

Because of widespread use of alcohol within the general population, the urgent care physician must take the time to educate their patients about the risk of unwanted side effects when certain prescription medications are taken concomitantly with alcohol. Interactions range from disulfiram-like reactions (nausea, vomiting, vasodilation, hypotension, chest pain, flushing/diaphoresis of weakness) to treatment failures.

Increased Effect of Alcohol

Antihistamines: increased CNS depression through additive sedative effect.
Barbiturates: increased CNS depression through decreased metabolism, additive sedative effect.
Benzodiazepines: increased CNS depression through decreased metabolism, additive sedative effect.
Cisapride: increased effect by increasing gastric emptying, intestinal absorption.
Erythromycin: increased effect by increasing gastric emptying, intestinal absorption.
Narcotics: increased CNS depression through decreased metabolism, additive sedative effect.
TCAs: increased CNS depression through additive sedative effect.

Increased Drug Toxicity

Acetaminophen: increased hepatotoxicity.
Aspirin: increased gastrointestinal (GI) bleeding.
Hydralazine: increased hypotensive effect.
Isoniazid: increased hepatotoxicity.
Methyldopa: increased hypotensive effect.
Nitroglycerin: increased hypotensive effect.

NSAIDs: increased GI bleeding.
Oral hypoglycemics: hypoglycemia through impaired gluconeogenesis.
Phenylbutazone: increased hepatotoxicity.

Disulfiram-like Reactions

Antibiotics: cefamandole, cefoperazone, metronidazole, sulfonamides.
Antifungals: griseofulvin.
Oral hypoglycemics: tolbutamide.
Oncologic agents: procarbazine.

Drug and Food Interactions

Although the interactions of prescription medications with foods are well established in the literature, they are often overlooked. Drugs can interact with foods as well as each other to produce subtherapeutic or toxic effects. Most commonly, drug-food interactions occur through the alteration of absorption, metabolism, and elimination. It is important to become familiar with these interactions, many of which involve commonly prescribed medications, to maximize the therapeutic benefit your patients receive from the medications you prescribe. Table 2 lists some of the more common drug-food interactions.

Table 2. Drug-Food Interactions

Medication	Food	Mechanism	Solution
ACE inhibitors	High potassium foods	Hyperkalemic potential	Avoid K+-containing salt substitutes
Ampicillin	Most foods	Decreased absorption	Dose 1 hr before or 2 hr after meals
Azithromycin	Most foods	Decreased absorption	Dose 1 hr before or 2 hr after meals
Captopril	Most foods	Decreased absorption	Dose 1 hr before or 2 hr after meals
Cefuroxime Cefpodoxime	Most foods	Increased absorption	Dose with food
Ciprofloxacin	Dairy products	Decreased absorption	With enteral feedings, dose 1 hr before or 2 hr after meals
Digoxin	Most foods	Decreased absorption	Dose 1 hr before or 2 hr after meals
Diuretics (potassium-sparing)	Foods/salt substitutes with high potassium concentrations	Hyperkalemic potential	Avoid K+-containing salt substitutes
Erythromycin base	Fatty foods	Decreased absorption	Avoid dosing with fatty foods
Erythromycin stearate	Most foods	Decreased absorption	Dose 1 hr before or 2 hr after meals
Felodipine	Grapefruit juice	Inhibits metabolism	Avoid dosing with grapefruit juice
Griseofulvin	Fatty foods	Increased absorption	Dose with meals
Ofloxacin	Most foods	Decreased absorption	Dose 1 hr before or 2 hr after meals
Phenytoin	Enteral feedings	Decreased absorption	Dose 2 hr before or 2 hr after meals
Rifampin	Most foods	Decreased absorption	Dose 1 hr before or 2 hr after meals
Tetracycline	Most foods including dairy products	Decreased absorption	Dose 1 hr before or 2 hr after dairy products
Theophylline	Fatty foods	Increased absorption	Avoid dosing with fatty foods
Warfarin	Vitamin-K rich foods (e.g., leafy green vegetables, beans, cauliflower, fish)	Increased vitamin K for generation of clotting factors	Limit foods with high vitamin K levels

Adapted from Yamreudeewong W, Henann NE, Fazio A, et al: Drug-food interactions in clinical practice. J Fam Prac 40:376–384, 1995.

Over-the-Counter Medications

The increasing prevalence of self-medication with over-the-counter medications (OTCs) must not be ignored by the urgent care physician. It has been estimated that 40% of all drug purchases in the U.S. are OTCs.[3] In certain high-risk populations, such as the elderly and immunosuppressed, the simple interactions can have deleterious effects. It is important to identify and use caution in prescribing medications to high-risk patients who not only take other prescription medications with toxic potential but also take OTCs. One series demonstrated that an estimated 82% of an elderly U.S. population takes OTCs on a regular basis.[4] Common OTCs interact with many of the prescription medications provided in urgent care, altering the efficacy of medications and possibly producing toxicity. These common OTCs include antacids and H_2 blockers, anti-asthma medications, cold remedies, and NSAIDs.

Adrenergic Agonists

Also classified as sympathomimetics, decongestants, and bronchodilators, adrenergic agonists include ephedrine, pseudoephedrine, and phenylpropanolamine. These medications stimulate a sympathetic response, leading to cardiostimulation at toxic levels when taken in excess or combined with other sympathomimetics, including MAO inhibitors.

Antacids

Antibiotics: Aluminum and magnesium hydroxide antacids cause a decrease in the bioavailability of quinolones, some cephalosporins, such as cefpodoxime[5] and cefuroxime, and pencillins, such as ampicillin[6] and tetracycline.[7] Give the antibiotic 2 hours before or 6 hours after the antacid to avoid interactions.[8]

Antifungals: Similar interactions have been noted with antifungals as with antibiotics.

NSAIDs: Decreased bioavailability has been noted with several NSAIDs, including indomethacin[9] and naproxen.[10,11]

Antihistamines

Often found in common "cold" remedies and sleep aids, the antihistamines are known to induce sedation. Be aware that anticholinergic and CNS depression are common side effects of these medications. Providing patients with medications with similar pharmacologic profiles can lead to toxicity.

H_2 Blockers

Clinically interactions involving H_2 blockers have been noted to be most serious with the use of cimetidine; milder interactions are noted with ranitidine, famotidine, and nizatidine.

Antiseizure medications: Cimetidine has been shown to effect the metabolism of phenytoin,[12] necessitating the avoidance of this combination.

Beta blockers: Cimetidine has been reported to interact with several beta blockers; ranitidine, however, has not been demonstrated to have similar clinical effects.[13]

Theophylline: Both cimetidine[12] and ranitidine[14] have been demonstrated to increase theophylline levels and produce toxicity.

Warfarin: Increased prothrombin time has been demonstrated with ranitidine and especially cimetidine.[12,15]

NSAIDs

This popular class of pain relievers is commonly prescribed by physicians, and often self-administered by patients. The many adverse interactions with other prescription medications are related to potential effects on platelet aggregation and renal clearance. Any patient with a history of impaired renal clearance should be warned about the potential risks of using these medications.

Anticoagulants: The concomitant inhibition of platelet aggregation by NSAIDs and anticoagulants, such as warfarin, results in an increased risk of bleeding.

Anticonvulsants: There is an increased risk of bleeding when the anticonvulsant valproic acid is prescribed with aspirin.[16]

Antihypertensives: NSAIDs may decrease the antihypertensive effects of beta blockers, thiazides, and vasodilators.[17]

Lithium: The risk of lithium toxicity is increased when lithium is combined with NSAIDs.

Methotrexate: Renal impairment secondary to NSAIDs contributes to methotrexate toxicity. This combination should be avoided.[18]

Drug-Herb Interactions

Trends suggest greater acceptance of alternative medicine, and many patients explore self-medication with herbal remedies. Unfortunately, these "natural" remedies lack regulation and often are not appreciated by patients or physicians for their potential interactions and side effects. It is prudent to question patients about herbal medicine use when they present to the urgent care center with poorly controlled chronic conditions such as cardiovascular disease, diabetes, and seizure disorders, among others. Many herbs have potential toxic effects when used alone; when combined with prescription medications, they may alter a medication's clinical effect.[22,23] Because of the lack of regulation, many herbal remedies have varying quantities and qualities of the active ingredient that they are marketed to contain. The literature to date lacks adequately controlled studies of many potential herb-drug interactions. The list in Table 3 is derived from a limited number of case reports and observations of some of the more commonly used herbal medicines in the United States. The herb-drug interactions are collected from the limited literature available and represent only previously reported interactions. Much of the available information comes from numerous popular websites, and the source of this information is not always clear. Limited, if any, controlled studies support claimed indications or verify the safety profiles of these herbs.

Toxicology

The average American household contains numerous medical, household, and industrial products with the potential to be accidentally or intentionally ingested. The urgent care physician should be aware of some of the common ingestions and able to initiate medical treatment until more definitive care can be implemented.

According to the American Association of Poison Control Centers (AAPCC), there were an estimated 4.6 million poisonings in 1998, 52.7% of which occurred in children < 6 years old. In all age groups, most poisonings were determined to be accidental (86.7%)

Table 3. Drug-Herb Interactions in Common Herbal Preparations

Herb	Common Uses	Interactions
Betel nut (*Arecu catechu*)	Prepared as a chew and utilized as a stimulant. Also regarded as a panacea for treatment of headaches, arthritis, fever, diarrhea, gonorrhea, malaria, and tapeworm infestation.	Bronchodilators (limits bronchodilating effect); fluphenazine, procyclidine (akasthisia, bradykinesia, rigidity, tremor).
Cayenne, chili pepper (*Capsicum* spp.)	"Treatment" of peripheral vascular disease, viral illnesses (including colds, chicken pox), and "kidney and prostate ailments."	Angiotensin-converting enzyme inhibitors (potentiates cough); theophylline (increased absorption).
Danshen (*Salvia miltiorrhiza*)	Marketed as a cholesterol-lowering agent and believed to increase coronary perfusion.	Warfarin (increases PT/INR).
Don quai tang-kuei (*Angelica sinensis*)	Allergies, premenstrual syndrome.	Warfarin (increases PT/INR).
Echinacea (*Echinacea* spp.)	Immune stabilizer for "treatment" of common cold, promotion of wound healing.	No significant drug interaction reported, but may cause immunosuppression with prolonged use.
Garlic (*Allium sativum*)	Marketed as a cholesterol-lowering agent, antioxidant, and for vascular protective effects. May also be used for asthma exacerbations, cold symptoms, toothaches, and snake, scorpion and bee stings.	Warfarin (increased PT/INR).
Gingko biloba	Marketed as an agent to improve cerebral and peripheral circulation and believed to improve memory, and relieve tinnitus and vertigo.	Aspirin (increased bleeding time), warfarin (increases PT/INR).
Ginseng (*Panax* spp, *Eleutherococcus* spp.)	Used as an anxiolytic, believed to provide general "strengthening" properties. Reported side effects include hypertension, insomnia, and even anxiety in large doses.	Alcohol (increased clearance), phenelzine (headache, mania, tremor), warfarin (decreased PT/INR).
Goldenseal (*Hydrastis canadensis*)	"Treatment" of acne, rashes, diarrhea, rhinitis, and pharyngitis.	Doxycycline, tetracycline (decreased absorption).
Guar gum (*Cyamopsis tetragonoloba*)	Used as a dietary suppressant and "treatment" of diarrhea.	Prolongs gastric retention and may delay or limit absorption of bumetanide, digoxin, and metformin.
Licorice (*Glycyrrhiza glabra*)	Steroid-like anti-inflammatory effect used to remedy rashes, and for "treatment" of cancer, Addison's disease.	Prednisolone (decreased clearance), oral contraceptives (hypertension, edema, hypokalemia.
Milk thistle (*Silybum marianum*)	Hepatitis, cancer, and used as an antioxidant.	No harmful drug interactions are reported. Milk thistle may actually be protective against the hepatotoxic effects of several medications including acetaminophen, clofibrate, haloperidol, lovastatin, pravastatin, metronidazole, and tacrine.
Papaya (*Carica papaya*)	Believed to be a panacea for "treatment" of arthritis, asthma, cancer, constipation, febrile illnesses, hypertension, peptic ulcer disease, skin infections, toothaches	Warfarin (increased PT/INR).
Psyllium (*Plantago ovata*)	Glucose control in diabetes, bowel irregularities including constipation and diarrhea.	Lithium (decreased serum levels).

(Cont'd on next page)

Table 3. Drug-Herb Interactions in Common Herbal Preparations *(Continued)*

Herb	Common Uses	Interactions
St. John's wort (*Hypericum perforatum*)	The active ingredient hypericin is commonly prescribed for depression in Europe and gaining popularity in the U.S. as "Nature's Prozac."	Cyclosporin, digoxin, theophylline (decreased serum levels); nefazodone, trazodone, sertraline (mild serotonin syndrome); oral contraceptives containing ethinyloestradiol, desogestrel (breakthrough bleeding); paroxetine (lethargy).
Saw palmetto (*Serenoa repens*)	Used as an aphrodisiac and for treatment of benign prostatic hypertrophy.	No significant drug interactions are reported, although mild gastrointestinal distress and headches have been noted.
Valerian (*Valeriana officinalis*)	Anxiolytic, sleeping agent, and relief of muscle spasms.	No significant drug interactions are reported, although headaches and palpitations are reported.
Yohimbine (*Pausinystalia yohimbe*)	Used as an aphrodisiac to increase libido, treatment of erectile dysfunction, and marketed as a "fat burner" secondary to thermogenic properties.	Tricyclic antidepressants (hypertension, which yohimbine alone in large quantities can produce).

PT = prothrombin time, INR = international normalized ratio.

vs. intentional (10.5%). Among poisoning fatalities, however, most (76.5%) were determined to be intentional. The most commonly overdosed substances included analgesics, street drugs, anxiolytics/antipsychotics, cardiovascular medications, and alcohol.[22] Because of the increased morbidity and mortality of many of these substances, definitive management at a referral center is mandatory.

Evaluation

Initial management of any overdose should involve measures to stabilize the patient by ensuring intact airway, breathing, and circulation (ABCs). Because many ingestions cause CNS depression along with the possibility of cardiotoxicity, initial assessment and repeat evaluations are essential with monitoring of vital signs, cardiac rhythm and oxygen saturation. It is important to obtain an adequate history from the patient and available relations to identify specific toxins. Be aware that the suicidal patient may offer misleading information. Important questions to ask include possible type of ingestion (patient's medication list, empty medication bottles, household products within reach), amount of ingestion, time of ingestion, evidence of trauma, and medical history/prior overdoses.

After a toxin has been identified, the clinician should assess the potential for the signs and symptoms of the toxidrome related to that medication/ingestion. This process helps determine the probable clinical course of the patient. Local and national poison centers provide excellent and immediate information to guide the initial patient management and determine need for referral to an emergency department. Table 4 provides specific antidotes for various toxic ingestions. Be aware that time may be the rate-limiting factor in the morbidity and mortality suffered by an overdose patient. Either memorize the phone number for local or national poison control, or have it posted in a readily available location. One toll-free number used by many states is 1-800-222-1222.

Table 4. Selected Toxins, Antidotes, and Administration Methods

Toxin	Antidote	Administration
Acetaminophen	N-Acetylcysteine	Loading dose of 140 mg/kg followed by 17 doses of 70 mg/kg every 4 hours. IV formula but currently not FDA-approved.
Benzodiazepines	Flumazenil	Initial dose of 0.2 mg IV over 30 sec, followed by 0.3–0.5 mg IV until response to a total of 3–5 mg.
Cyanide	Amyl nitrite, sodium nitrite, sodium thiosulfate	Inhale amyl nitrite ampule for 30 sec of every minute with 100% oxygen. Continue until IV sodium nitrite can be given at 300 mg IV at a rate of 2.5–5 ml/min. Then administer 12.5 gm sodium thiosulfate IV.
Digitalis glycosides	Digoxin-specific antibody, phenytoin	If unknown ingestion in presence of dysrhythmias, give 20 vials. If known amount of ingestion, number of vials equals dose in mg divided by 0.6.
Iron	Deferoxamine	Give 15 mg/kg/hr IV or 90 mg/kg IM every 8 hours to a total of 6 g in 24 hours.
Methanol, ethylene glycol	Ethanol *or* Fomepizole	Loading dose is 10 ml/kg of 10% ethanol in D5W IV over 30 min. Begin maintenance dose of 0.66–1.33 ml/kg/hr IV of 10% solution. Maintain blood ethanol concentrations at 100–150 mg/dl. Follow serum sodium and glucose levels. Give 15 mg/kg IV over 30 min, then 10 mg/kg every 12 hr × 4 doses.
Opiates	Naloxone	Give 0.01 mg/kg (0.4–2 mg) IV/IM/SC/ET to response.
Organophosphates	Atropine, 2-PAM	Test dose = 2 mg, then give 2–4 mg IV every 10–15 min as needed until secretions stop. Then administer 2-PAM chloride (pralidoxime) at 1–2 gm IV q 6 hr.

Adapted from Mengert TJ, Eisenberg MS, Copass MK: Emergency Medical Therapy. Philadelphia, W.B. Saunders, 1996, pp 875.

Management

In most circumstances, the management of the overdosed patient is beyond the scope of care possible in the urgent care setting. Because is it impossible to predict the magnitude or time course of toxicity in most overdoses, transfer by ambulance of overdosed UC patients to an emergency department is advisable. Table 4 lists selected toxins and their emergency management.

Early intervention to limit the body's exposure to a toxin is vital. This goal can be achieved through immediate gastric emptying (emesis, lavage), decreased absorption (charcoal), or whole-body irrigation. Other methods of limiting exposure include urine alkalinization and dialysis. Others are beyond the scope of this book and require referral to a tertiary care center. These decontamination procedures are performed *only* after initial stabilization of the patient's ABCs. Immediate activation of the local emergency medical services (dial 911) is necessary if this goal cannot be ensured.

Emesis. Although once widely accepted as the initial step in decontamination of poisonous ingestions, emesis is not a universal measure and many contraindications limit its use. Limited indications include awake and alert patients with a suspected ingestion without contraindications (listed below). Traditionally emesis is induced through the ingestion of syrup of ipecac. Common doses include 30 ml for adults and children over 5 years old, 15 ml for children aged 1–5 years, and 10 ml for children 6–12 months old. **Contraindications** include age less than 6 months, nontoxic ingestions, comatose patients, seizure activity, CNS depression, potential for deterioration in < 2 hours, decreased gag reflex, bleeding risk (esophageal varices, Mallory-Weiss tear), ingestion of sharp objects, remote (> 1–2 hours) ingestions, and ingestion of pure hydrocarbon or strong acids and bases.[23]

Gastric Lavage. A controversial issue with many questioning its exact indications, gastric lavage is typically indicated in the overdose patient who presents immediately after ingestion (< 1–2 hours) of a toxic substance and who has either failed a trial of emesis or for whom emesis is contraindicated. Again, the airway must be secured before any attempts to perform gastric lavage to avoid aspiration. This procedure is usually performed by insertion of a large-bore orogastric tube (36–40 French for adults, 16–28 French for children) to proper length. The patient is then placed in the left lateral decubitus position, and saline aliquots of 200 ml for adults and 50–100 ml for children is inserted until a total of several liters for adults or 500 ml to 1 L for children is lavaged. The tube is then left intact for the insertion of charcoal. **Contraindications** include ingestion of strong acid or base, bleeding risk, nontoxic ingestion, ingestion of sharp objects, or ingestion of drug packets.[23]

Activated Charcoal. A widely accepted method of decontamination by limiting absorption of toxin, activated charcoal should be provided to any patient without contraindications who has possibly ingested a toxic substance. Activated charcoal has a tremendous surface area for absorption of most organic and inorganic substances, with the exception of small ions. Initial dose includes 1gm/kg, with typical adult dose being 50–70 gm in liquid form. The initial dose only may be delivered with a cathartic, such as sorbitol, to aid in passage through the GI tract. Repeated doses of activated charcoal are indicated if vomiting prevents ingestion of first dose and for toxins with known small volume of distribution, low plasma protein binding, or enterohepatic circulation. **Contraindications** include ingestion of caustic acids or bases, ileus, or an unprotected airway. Contrary to previous reports, acetaminophen ingestion is not a contraindication to providing charcoal. According to Goldfrank, the amount of the acetaminophen antidote N-acetylcysteine absorbed by charcoal is not clinically significant.[23]

Whole-bowel Irrigation. This less frequently used method of GI decontamination involves the oral delivery of potent osmotic agents to speed passage of specific toxins from the GI tract. Indications for use include patients who are suspected "body packers" (i.e., they ingest packets of drugs such as cocaine to aid in concealment from authorities), massive ingestions, and ingestion of toxins that are not absorbed by charcoal (see above). Polyethylene glycol (GoLytely, Colyte) is delivered orally or down a nasogastric tube at a dose of 4 L over 4 hours until rectal output is clear. **Contraindications** include ileus, obstruction, or perforation.

Referral

The information provided above is meant for use in the initial evaluation and management of patients at risk for toxic ingestions. Any patient exhibiting signs or symptoms of systemic compromise warrants a primary survey for initial assessment and necessary interventions with immediate referral to an emergency department or hospital for definitive management. Never overlook the basic approach to any acutely ill or injured patient: assessment of airway, breathing, circulation, and disabilities (neurologic survey). Remember to reassess continually any patient with suspicion of a toxic ingestion because systemic effects may have a delayed presentation.

Never assume that a patient with suspicion of intentional overdose is completely truthful. Be suspicious of other etiologies for a patient with altered mental status, including coingestions, infection, trauma, and cardiopulmonary and CNS pathology. Administration of thiamine, glucose, and naloxone is indicated for any patient who presents with a decreased level of consciousness of unknown etiology.

Initial management, as described above, should serve as a general guideline for stable patients with protected airways who will be referred to an emergency department or primary care provider. In addition, it is important for both patient protection and legal reasons to secure a medical hold on all patients believed to have an intentional ingestion because they may be exhibiting suicidal ideations.

References

1. Goldberg RM, Mabee J, Chan L, Wong S: Drug-drug and drug-disease interactions in the ED: Analysis of a high risk population. Am J Emerg Med 14:447–450, 1996.
2. Anastasio GD, Cornell KO, Menscer D: Drug interactions: Keeping it straight. Am Fam Physician 56:883–888, 891–894, 1997.
3. Gebhart F: Rx-to-OTC switches to be mixed bag for pharmacists in future. Drug Top 134:58, 1990.
4. Ostrom JR, Hammarlund ER, Christenson DB, et al: Medication usage in an elderly population. Med Care 23:157–164, 1985.
5. Hughes GS, Heald DL, Barker KB, et al: The effects of gastric pH and food on the pharmocokinetics of a new oral cephalosporin, cefpodoxime proxetil. Clin Pharmacol Ther 46: 674–685, 1990.
6. Sommers DK, Van Wyk M, Moncrieff J, et al: Influence of food and reduced gastric acidity on the bioavailability of bacampicillin and cefuroxime axetil. Br J Clin Pharmacol Ther 18:535–539, 1984.
7. Garty M, Hurwitz A: Effect of cimetidine and antacids on gastrointestinal absorption of tetracycline. Clin Pharmacol Ther 28:203–207, 1980.
8. Nix DE, Watson, WA, Lener ME, et al: Effects of aluminum and magnesium and ranitidine on the absorption of ciprofloxin. Clin Pharm Ther 46:700–705, 1989.
9. Galeazzi RL: The effect of an antacid on the bioavailability of indomethacin. Eur J Clin Pharmacol 12:65–68, 1977.
10. Segre EJ: Effects of antacids on naproxen absorption. N Engl J Med 291:582–583, 1974.
11. Weber SS, Bankhurst AD, Mroszczak E, Ding TL: Effect of Mylanta on naproxen availability. Ther Drug Monit 375–383, 1981.
12. Somogyi A, Muirhead M: Pharmacokinetic interactions of cimetidine 1987. Clin Pharmacokinet 12:321–366, 1987.
13. Kelly SG, Salem SA, Kinney CD, et al: Effects of ranitidine on the disposition of metoprolol. Br J Clin Pharmacol 19:219–224, 1985.
14. Fernandez E. Ranitidine and theophylline. Ann Intern Med 100:459, 1984.
15. Baciewicz AM, Morgan PJ: Ranitidine-warfarin interaction. Ann Intern Med 112:76–77, 1990.
16. Lacy C, Armstrong LL, Ingrim N, Lance LL: Drug Information Handbook. Hudson, NY, Lexi-Comp, 1996, p 1221.
17. Lacy C, Armstrong LL, Ingrim N, Lance LL: Drug Information Handbook. Hudson, NY, Lexi-Comp, 1996, p 765.
18. Honig PK, Gillespie BK: Drug interactions between prescribed and over-the-counter medications. Drug Safety 13:296–303, 1995.
19. Mengert TJ, Eisenberg MS, Copass MK: Emergency Medical Therapy, 4th ed. Philadelphia, W.B. Saunders, 1996, pp 860–861.
20. Fugh-Berman A: Herb-drug interactions. Lancet 355:134–138, 2000.
21. Plontnikoff, GA, George J: Herbalism in Minnesota: What should physicians know? Minnesota Medicine 82:13–26, 1999.
22. Litovitz TL, Klein-Schultz W, et al: 1998 Annual Report of the American Association of Poison Control Centers Toxic Exposure Surveillance System. Am J Emer Med 117:435-487, 1999.
23. Goldfrank LR, Flomenbaum NE, Lwein NA, et al: Goldfrank's Toxicology Emergencies, 5th ed. Norwalk, CT, Appleton & Lange, 1994, pp 25–41.

Chapter 22

Medicolegal and Risk Management Issues in Urgent Care

Erich Zeitz, MD, JD

Despite the proliferation and success of urgent care clinics, few or no state or federal laws specifically regulate these health care facilities.[1] State and federal statutory regulation of outpatient clinics covers most urgent care clinics.[2] Many medicolegal and risk management concerns are universal to all health care providers, but the practice setting of urgent care lends itself to certain unique issues.

Malpractice

The elements of a medical malpractice claim are established by state common law, a body of law based on prior written judicial opinions on appellate cases. Although there are nuances from state to state and procedural requirements created by each state legislature, the main elements of a malpractice case are uniform across the jurisdictions of the United States. Each of the four elements of duty, breach of duty, causation, and damages must be met by the injured plaintiff; in the case of medical malpractice, the plaintiff is the patient.

A duty typically is proven with the establishment of the physician-patient relationship during patient examination. The patient expects to be treated with reasonable care, and a breach of duty by a physician or other health care practitioner occurs when treatment falls below the standard of care. Increasingly state courts define this standard by a national standard of care of similarly situated physicians. The plaintiff must then show causation, which in legal terms is proximate cause. Proximate cause is the legal requirement of connection between the negligent action and the injury that the patient ultimately sustains. The plaintiff must show that it was foreseeable that the physician's conduct might create a risk of harm to the victim and that the results of that conduct and intervening causes were foreseeable. Finally, the plaintiff must demonstrate economic damages to him- or herself or family members, measured both in special damages, such as lost wages, and in general damages, such as pain and suffering.

Consent

Consent to treatment has traditionally been necessary for the successful defense against a civil battery claim by a patient for unlawful touching of person. Express written consent is routinely provided in forms authorizing treatment and payment prior to a patient's evaluation. In addition, consent is often implied by patients by participating in a history or physical exam. Express consent also occurs when physicians ask permission from patients to perform a test, such as a blood draw, and patients agree.

A special form of consent is necessary involving minors because the law normally considers children under the age of eighteen incapable of making legally binding decisions. Statutory exceptions have been created to allow minors to consent when public policy dictates that children should be able to receive treatment without parental knowledge. These statutory exceptions vary from state to state, and local statutes should be reviewed. Below are common examples of a minor's right to consent.

In states such as Minnesota, "emancipated minors" may consent. Emancipated minors must maintain an address apart from their parents and maintain their own financial affairs.[3] Similarly, minors who have married or borne a child are competent to consent by statute.[4] Public policy dictates that minors can effectively consent to treatment for pregnancy, sexually transmitted diseases, and alcohol or drug abuse.[5] Finally, either by statute or case law, most states allow immediate treatment for any life- or limb-threatening illness without formal consent.[6] If there is any doubt whether a complaint constitutes an emergency, decisions should be made in favor of treatment. An attempt should be made to contact parents for telephone or written consent both before treating any nonemergent condition and after treatment within the emergency exception described above.

Documentation

Careful documentation of the patient encounter is important for several reasons. First, it provides a written record of what occurred during the visit and may be reviewed and relied upon by subsequent care providers. Preferably it should be transcribed to type. In many urgent care clinics, transcription is available, and typed records should be routinely reviewed for accuracy. If typed transcriptions are not available, every effort should be made to produce a thorough, *legible* written record. It often is said that if it was not recorded, it was not done. This generalization holds true both for billing requirements and possible future legal requirements. Federal regulations require documentation of procedures to allow proper Medicare and Medicaid billing. Third-party insurance claims often require the same documentation. In the rare case of subsequent legal action, it is difficult to recall accurately what transpired 2–10 years earlier during a single patient encounter. The medical record is the best opportunity to create lasting documentation.

In discussing documentation, it is appropriate to mention discharge instructions, which often are the only written documentation that the patient receives. In addition to outlining prescribed treatment, discharge instructions should clearly describe when to follow-up with a primary care physician, if indicated, and when to seek urgent or emergency care if the condition worsens. This information effectively provides a safety net for poor patient outcomes.

Many patients with minor work-related injuries may present to urgent care. Coverage for their care is often provided by workers' compensation insurance; insurance coverage may require additional paperwork completion. Standard forms are available that clearly delineate work restrictions and time off from work when medically indicated.

Transfer

Every urgent care clinic should have written protocols for the treatment of life-threatening emergencies when critically ill patients mistakenly present to an urgent care clinic or a patient's condition deteriorates while at the urgent care clinic. Typically the emergency medical system should be activated, and the patient should be transported by advanced life support ambulance to a nearby hospital. Receiving physicians should be given information about transfers to facilitate the best possible patient care.

The Emergency Medical Treatment and Labor Act (EMTALA) of 1986 provides protection for patients and hospitals against improper transfer of ill patients, termed "patient dumping." The act requires evaluation and stabilization of any presenting patient before transfer to another hospital. Specific requirements apply to the transferring and receiving hospital. Civil penalties and loss of Medicare reimbursement are possible consequences of violation. The act and its subsequent interpretation were intended to apply to hospitals and in most cases do not apply to urgent care except in a clearly defined exception. Any urgent care facility owned by a hospital is probably subject to the extensive requirements of EMTALA.[7] Questions regarding applicability of and conformance with EMTALA should be addressed to urgent care management or hospital counsel.

Even in the vast majority of urgent care cases, in which EMTALA does not apply, sound referral patterns should be followed to maximize good care. Although EMTALA liability may not be present, common law malpractice risk remains. Effective physician-to-physician communication lessens this risk by improving patient care. Receiving physicians at emergency departments should be notified about anticipated transfer, and patient data, such as a copy of medical records, laboratory tests, and x-rays, should be forwarded to the receiving physician. Appropriate transportation should be based on the patient's condition.

Often because of geographic restraints or patient preferences, there are only a few hospitals to which patients are referred. In such situations urgent care and emergency department management may wish to establish formal guidelines or written protocols for transfer of patients who require further diagnostic work-up but are not necessarily critically ill.

Confidentiality

In general, the patient-physician relationship is considered confidential, and no information gathered during the course of a patient encounter should be released to any third party without the patient's express consent. Exceptions to this general rule occur when the state has an overriding interest in the information. This information should be released only to state agencies under direction of state law or court order. Release of information occurs only on a limited basis and does not allow general disclosure.

Common reportable diseases include certain infectious diseases such as human immunodeficiency virus, hepatitis B, tuberculosis, or sexually transmitted diseases not previously reported. State health agencies determine which diseases are reported and how reports should be made. Physicians are also under statutory duty to report suspicion of child abuse or neglect[8] and suspicion of vulnerable adult abuse or neglect.[9] Other statutes may require reporting data about patients presenting with burns or gunshot wounds.[10] The urgent care practitioner should be familiar with the nuances of each state's reporting requirements.

In rare cases, there may be common law duty to report to a third party any knowledge of an impending danger. When a patient is assessed to be mentally ill and states that he or she intends to harm a third party, courts have determined that a duty is owed to the intended victim to ensure safety.[11]

Risk Management

Urgent care centers are designed for and predominantly cater to minor illnesses. It is therefore easy to become complacent and misdiagnose a minor illness when the patient may actually be suffering from a potentially life-threatening condition. Although no independent data are available for urgent care centers, it is likely that the most high-risk presentations mirror those of emergency departments. A review of published appellate decisions supports this view.[12] Therefore, it is worth reviewing the eight high-risk diagnostic areas for emergency physicians, including missed diagnoses of chest pain, abdominal pain, fractures, wounds, pediatric fever/meningitis, subarachnoid hemorrhage, aortic aneurysm, and epiglottitis. Additional liability was associated with lack of a radiograph follow-up system.[13] Effective risk reduction for poor patient outcomes should focus on understanding the proper work-up and treatment of these high-risk diagnostic areas, although they may often require diagnostic capabilities beyond that of an urgent care. Keeping a broad differential diagnosis prevents the patient with severe occult illness from leaving the urgent care center with a misdiagnosis.

Finally, studies have demonstrated that effective patient communications can reduce malpractice risk. The importance of good communication between physician and patient cannot be overestimated. Levison et al. found that physicians who explained more about the visit to patients (including anticipated wait time), used humor more often and attempted to understand patients more clearly are less likely to have malpractice claims against them.[14]

References

1. Katzman K: Freestanding Emergency Centers: Regulation and Reimbursement. Am J Law Med 11:105–123, 1985.
2. See, for example, Rhode Island Gen. Laws § 23-17-2 (1999) or California Welfare & Institution Code § 16946 (1999).
3. Minn. Stat. 144.341 (1999).
4. Minn. Stat. 144.342 (1999).
5. Minn. Stat. 144.343 (1999).
6. Minn. Stat. 144.344 (1999).
7. Frew D: Patient Transfers: How to Comply with the Law, 2nd ed. Dallas, American College of Physicians, 1995.
8. See, for example, Minn. Stat. § 626.556 (1999).
9. See, for example, Minn. Stat. § 626.557 (1999).
10. See, for example, Minn. Stat. § 626.52 (1999).
11. Waller T: Estates of Morgan v. Fairfield Family Counseling Center: Application of Traditional Tort Law Post-Tarasoff Akron L. Rev. 31:321, 1997.
12. See, for example, Murray v. United States, 36 F. Supp. 2d 713 (1999).
13. Karcz A, Holbrook J, et al: Massachusetts Emergency Medicine Closed Malpractice Claims: 1988–990, Ann Emerg Med 22:55–61, 1993.
14. Levison W, Roter DL, et al: Physician-patient communication: The relationship with malpractice claims among primary care physicians and surgeons. JAMA 277:553–559, 1997.

Index

Page numbers in **boldface type** indicate complete chapters.